THE BRONCHIAL CIRCULATION

LUNG BIOLOGY IN HEALTH AND DISEASE

Executive Editor

Claude Lenfant
Director, National Heart, Lung, and Blood Institute
National Institutes of Health
Bethesda, Maryland

1. *Immunologic and Infectious Reactions in the Lung,* edited by Charles H. Kirkpatrick and Herbert Y. Reynolds
2. *The Biochemical Basis of Pulmonary Function,* edited by Ronald G. Crystal
3. *Bioengineering Aspects of the Lung,* edited by John B. West
4. *Metabolic Functions of the Lung,* edited by Y. S. Bakhle and John R. Vane
5. *Respiratory Defense Mechanisms* (in two parts), edited by Joseph D. Brain, Donald F. Proctor, and Lynne M. Reid
6. *Development of the Lung,* edited by W. Alan Hodson
7. *Lung Water and Solute Exchange,* edited by Norman C. Staub
8. *Extrapulmonary Manifestations of Respiratory Disease,* edited by Eugene Debs Robin
9. *Chronic Obstructive Pulmonary Disease,* edited by Thomas L. Petty
10. *Pathogenesis and Therapy of Lung Cancer,* edited by Curtis C. Harris
11. *Genetic Determinants of Pulmonary Disease,* edited by Stephen D. Litwin
12. *The Lung in the Transition Between Health and Disease,* edited by Peter T. Macklem and Solbert Permutt
13. *Evolution of Respiratory Processes: A Comparative Approach,* edited by Stephen C. Wood and Claude Lenfant
14. *Pulmonary Vascular Diseases,* edited by Kenneth M. Moser
15. *Physiology and Pharmacology of the Airways,* edited by Jay A. Nadel
16. *Diagnostic Techniques in Pulmonary Disease* (in two parts), edited by Marvin A. Sackner
17. *Regulation of Breathing* (in two parts), edited by Thomas F. Hornbein
18. *Occupational Lung Diseases: Research Approaches and Methods,* edited by Hans Weill and Margaret Turner-Warwick

19. *Immunopharmacology of the Lung,* edited by Harold H. Newball
20. *Sarcoidosis and other Granulomatous Diseases of the Lung,* edited by Barry L. Fanburg
21. *Sleep and Breathing,* edited by Nicholas A. Saunders and Colin E. Sullivan
22. Pneumocystis carinii *Pneumonia: Pathogenesis, Diagnosis, and Treatment,* edited by Lowell S. Young
23. *Pulmonary Nuclear Medicine: Techniques in Diagnosis of Lung Disease,* edited by Harold L. Atkins
24. *Acute Respiratory Failure,* edited by Warren M. Zapol and Konrad J. Falke
25. *Gas Mixing and Distribution in the Lung,* edited by Ludwig A. Engel and Manuel Paiva
26. *High-Frequency Ventilation in Intensive Care and During Surgery,* edited by Graziano Carlon and William S. Howland
27. *Pulmonary Development: Transition from Intrauterine to Extrauterine Life,* edited by George H. Nelson
28. *Chronic Obstructive Pulmonary Disease: Second Edition, Revised and Expanded,* edited by Thomas L. Petty
29. *The Thorax* (in two parts), edited by Charis Roussos and Peter T. Macklem
30. *The Pleura in Health and Disease,* edited by Jacques Chrétien, Jean Bignon, and Albert Hirsch
31. *Drug Therapy for Asthma: Research and Clinical Practice,* edited by John W. Jenne and Shirley Murphy
32. *Pulmonary Endothelium in Health and Disease,* edited by Una S. Ryan
33. *The Airways: Neural Control in Health and Disease,* edited by Michael A. Kaliner and Peter J. Barnes
34. *Pathophysiology and Treatment of Inhalation Injuries,* edited by Jacob Loke
35. *Respiratory Function of the Upper Airway,* edited by Oommen P. Mathew and Giuseppe Sant'Ambrogio
36. *Chronic Obstructive Pulmonary Disease: A Behavioral Perspective,* edited by A. John McSweeny and Igor Grant
37. *Biology of Lung Cancer: Diagnosis and Treatment,* edited by Steven T. Rosen, James L. Mulshine, Frank Cuttitta, and Paul G. Abrams
38. *Pulmonary Vascular Physiology and Pathophysiology,* edited by E. Kenneth Weir and John T. Reeves
39. *Comparative Pulmonary Physiology: Current Concepts,* edited by Stephen C. Wood
40. *Respiratory Physiology: An Analytical Approach,* edited by H. K. Chang and Manuel Paiva

41. *Lung Cell Biology,* edited by Donald Massaro
42. *Heart-Lung Interactions in Health and Disease,* edited by Steven M. Scharf and Sharon S. Cassidy
43. *Clinical Epidemiology of Chronic Obstructive Pulmonary Disease,* edited by Michael J. Hensley and Nicholas A. Saunders
44. *Surgical Pathology of Lung Neoplasms,* edited by Alberto M. Marchevsky
45. *The Lung in Rheumatic Diseases,* edited by Grant W. Cannon and Guy A. Zimmerman
46. *Diagnostic Imaging of the Lung,* edited by Charles E. Putman
47. *Models of Lung Disease: Microscopy and Structural Methods,* edited by Joan Gil
48. *Electron Microscopy of the Lung,* edited by Dean E. Schraufnagel
49. *Asthma: Its Pathology and Treatment,* edited by Michael A. Kaliner, Peter J. Barnes, and Carl G. A. Persson
50. *Acute Respiratory Failure: Second Edition,* edited by Warren M. Zapol and Francois Lemaire
51. *Lung Disease in the Tropics,* edited by Om P. Sharma
52. *Exercise: Pulmonary Physiology and Pathophysiology,* edited by Brian J. Whipp and Karlman Wasserman
53. *Developmental Neurobiology of Breathing,* edited by Gabriel G. Haddad and Jay P. Farber
54. *Mediators of Pulmonary Inflammation,* edited by Michael A. Bray and Wayne H. Anderson
55. *The Airway Epithelium,* edited by Stephen G. Farmer and Douglas Hay
56. *Physiological Adaptations in Vertebrates: Respiration, Circulation, and Metabolism,* edited by Stephen C. Wood, Roy E. Weber, Alan R. Hargens, and Ronald W. Millard
57. *The Bronchial Circulation,* edited by John Butler

Additional Volumes in Preparation

Lung Cancer Differentiation, edited by Samuel D. Bernal and Paul J. Hesketh

Cytokines of the Lung, edited by Jason Kelley

Pulmonary Complications of Systemic Disease, edited by John F. Murray

Lung Vascular Injury: Molecular and Cellular Response, edited by Arnold Johnson and Thomas J. Ferro

THE BRONCHIAL CIRCULATION

Edited by

John Butler

University of Washington School of Medicine
Seattle, Washington

MARCEL DEKKER, INC. New York • Basel • Hong Kong

Library of Congress Cataloging-in-Publication Data

The Bronchial circulation / edited by John Butler.
p. cm. -- (Lung biology in health and disease ; v. 57)
Includes bibliographical references and index.
ISBN 0-8247-8443-X (alk. paper)
1. Bronchi--Blood-vessels. I. Butler, John.
II. Series.
QP121.B84 1992
612.2--dc20 91-45968
CIP

This book is printed on acid-free paper.

Marcel Dekker, Inc.
270 Madison Avenue, New York, New York 10016

Current printing (last digit)
10 9 8 7 6 5 4 3 2 1

Printed in the United States of America

INTRODUCTION

> Organs of extreme perfection and complications . . .
>
> In looking for the gradations by which an organ in any species has been perfected, we ought to look exclusively to its linear ancestors . . .
>
> Organs of little apparent importance . . .
>
> In the first place, we are much too ignorant in regard to the whole economy of any organic being, to say what slight modification would be of importance or not. . . . They [some naturalists] believe that very many structures have been created for beauty in the eyes of man, or for mere variety.
>
> Charles Darwin, 1859
> *On the Origin of Species*

One could make such statements about the bronchial circulation and, at the risk of being misunderstood, also about this volume!

In Volume 14 of the series Lung Biology in Health and Disease *(Pulmonary Vascular Diseases,* edited by Kenneth M. Moser), Leon Cudkowicz, also a contributor to this volume, vividly and comprehensively described the "Bronchial Arterial Circulation in Man." That chapter was a remarkable complement to his treatise *The Human Bronchial Circulation in Health and Disease,* published in 1968. His comments on the history of knowledge about the bronchial circulation clearly establish that over the years, opinions have wavered concerning its physiological importance.

But years of observations and investigations have demonstrated that the bronchial circulation is truly an organ "of extreme perfection and complications" that plays a major role in the homeostasis of the pulmonary circulation and its regulation. The road to this realization is paved with landmark studies by the most imaginative and creative investigators in this area of research.

Indeed, the bronchial circulation has not been "created for beauty in the eyes of man"—at least, not as man would relish the drawings of Leonardo da Vinci.

This new monograph of the series Lung Biology in Health and Disease, titled *The Bronchial Circulation*, is a culmination of much effort. Some, on my part, to convince John Butler—my mentor, my former boss, and my friend—to edit it. I knew he was the only possible choice because of his deep interest in this "pesky circulation." I knew that if he would accept this responsibility, the book would be the best! One needs only to peruse the Table of Contents and the List of Contributors to realize that John Butler's efforts have been limitless. As he and his fellow authors look at what they have accomplished, they should be proud.

This volume is not for "mere variety"; it is not for "beauty" either. It is for elegance, completeness, and importance. Much more needs to be learned about the bronchial circulation. There is no question that this monograph and the ideas it contains will be an inspiration to those who seek to discover the "riches from this pesky circulation." I have no doubt that John Butler found me a bit excessive when I repeatedly asked him to edit this volume, but I knew that if I succeeded, science and all of us would be well served.

Claude Lenfant, M.D.
Bethesda, Maryland

PREFACE

It is usual for an editor of a multiauthor treatise to introduce the work with a modest, but confidence-inspiring account of how this responsibility evolved from a single-minded, lifelong dedication to the subject. Yet I must confess that my interest in the bronchial circulation occurred quite by chance and is reprehensibly recent. A colleague and I were convinced that Clements (1961) and Pattle et al. (1962) were correct that the reduction of surface tension by surfactant protected against pulmonary edema. We had shown the edemagenic effect of removing surfactant by measuring the gain in weight of excised lungs. But who would believe the relevance of data from excised lungs? Could we possibly use the continuous weighing method in living lungs? Surprisingly, we found we could weigh one lung continuously in open-chested preparations (Agostoni et al., 1987). To fix pressures and flows, we had to isolate the pulmonary vasculature, perfusing the artery and collecting the effluent from the pulmonary vein in a closed circuit. Unfortunately, there was a continuous weight gain in the lungs, unrelated to any effort of ours to cause edema. After considerable cogitation, it finally dawned on us that this was caused by the input from the intact bronchial circulation in this living animal. Recording the excess of pulmonary venous return over the arterial input gave us a moment-to-moment measurement of all the anastomotic bronchial flow to the lung: a lung, moreover, in which we could easily alter both circulatory and airway pressures and flows. So we had blundered upon another opportunity, this one promising to provide new insights about the bronchial circulation.

I had no prolonged period of agonizing reappraisal, as would have been fitting before embracing a new focus for my thoughts and energies. Thus my confession that the modest amount of knowledge about the bronchial circulation that I have been able to apply to this book hardly reflects a life steeped in contemplation of the subject.

There has not been a book on the bronchial circulation since Leon Cudkowicz wrote *The Human Bronchial Circulation in Health and Disease* almost 25 years ago (Cudkowicz, 1968). That book is now a classic—a source of information for which all the contributors to this book, at one time or another, have felt grateful. Its scholarly style, thought-provoking glimpses of previous investigators, and unexpected observations of what still remains to be explained make its reading a pleasure. Its most unusual attribute (since it is a medical book) is its limited size. This new book is much bigger and will never be so famous. Nevertheless, there has been a need for a review of our present state of knowledge about the bronchial circulation for some time. Although the scope of the work remains unusually limited, the larger size of this book partly reflects the great increase in information on the subject.

The other reason for writing a follow-up book about the bronchial circulation came from frustrations in publication. (I suspect this is more frequently the reason for a book than the prior publication of a succession of relevant scientific papers.) Members of the Da Vinci Society, a group of biological scientists particularly interested in the bronchial circulation (the reason for the name becomes obvious after reading Cudkowicz's historical introduction), were understandably frustrated some years ago when they had anticipated rapid publication of manuscripts from a symposium that launched the new society. We had submitted about 200 manuscript pages. The journal concerned, I believe because he had inadvertently encouraged us to submit the proceedings of our symposium, had fired its editor and changed its format. There was little doubt about the new editor's decision:

> My letter of March 10th seems terribly clear. The entire symposium report must be limited to the 40 typewritten page limit. Obviously this format was not followed and therefore the communication is unacceptable.
>
> The second problem with this particular communication is that it arrives almost a year too late and well past the absolute final deadline for symposium reports to be published before the change in policy passed four months ago.

However, the frustrated seed of this group of papers remained alive. It can now be considered to have been successfully revived and even to have blossomed into the present form.

Having discussed the genesis of this book, I shall do something that has probably never been done before by an editor: give the reader reasons why he should not bother to read on. It has been said by some physiologists on more than one occasion that the bronchial circulation is an unimportant nonentity. It must be admitted that the normal bronchial circulation is trivial. Its anatomy is incompletely defined. Its flow is less than 1% of the cardiac output and not indispensable. In most species, no evident derangements can be shown when it is completely cut off. The clinician points out that the bronchial circulation does more harm than good. It causes hemoptysis and problems in lung transplantation. Only the radiologist who practices bronchial vascular angiography and embolic obstruction of bleeding bronchial vessels can be found to derive any riches from this pesky circulation.

However, I believe that those who read on will find that these are not valid arguments. The bronchial vasculature is capable of most important functional responses that are necessary to make the very act of breathing safe, to prevent pulmonary infarctions, and to aid in repair after lung injuries and infection. The bronchial circulation has been likened to Mother or the Red Cross, little praised in times of well-being, but coming in to provide essential sustenance when help is needed.

The literary successes within that do not come from the pens or word processors of the contributors are due to the dedicated work and inspired suggestions of Mel Figley, to whom I am profoundly grateful.

I give particular thanks to Cathy Greenbaum, whose help has been an important factor in coordinating this book, and to Rebecca Manring for her rapid, efficient transcription, careful editing, and meticulous reference reviews. Finally, my thanks go to Tina Walters and all the staff of the Respiratory Division of the University of Washington, who have coped with scheduling problems and all the other difficulties that seem to be inherent in the production of such a work.

John Butler

References

Agostoni, P. G., Deffebach, M. E., Kirk, W., Lakshminarayan, S., and Butler, J. (1987). Upstream pressure for systemic to pulmonary flow from bronchial circulation in dogs. *J. Appl. Physiol. 63*:485–491.

Clements, J. A. (1961). Pulmonary edema and permeability of alveolar membranes. *Arch. Environ. Health 2*:280–283.

Cudkowicz, L. (1968). *The Human Bronchial Circulation in Health and Disease.* William and Wilkins, Baltimore, pp. 1–424.

Pattle, R. E., Claireaux, A. E., Davies, P. A., and Cameron, A. H. (1962). Inability to form a lung lining film as a cause of the respiratory distress syndrome in the newborn. *Lancet 2*:468.

CONTRIBUTORS

Piergiuseppe Agostoni, M.D. Technical Director, Cardiology Institute, University of Milan, Milan, Italy

Jeffrey L. Ardell, Ph.D. Department of Physiology, University of South Alabama College of Medicine, Mobile, Alabama

Elisabeth M. Baile, M.Sc. Pulmonary Research Laboratory, University of British Columbia, St. Paul's Hospital, Vancouver, British Columbia, Canada

Scott A. Barman, Ph.D. Assistant Professor, Department of Pharmacology and Toxicology, Medical College of Georgia, Augusta, Georgia

John Butler, M.D. Professor of Medicine, Division of Pulmonary and Critical Care Medicine, Department of Medicine, University of Washington School of Medicine, Seattle, Washington

Paula G. Carvalho, M.D. Staff Physician, Pulmonary Section, Veterans Administration Medical Center, Boise, Idaho, and Department of Medicine, University of Washington School of Medicine, Seattle, Washington

Nirmal B. Charan, M.D. Chief, Pulmonary Section, Veterans Administration Medical Center, Boise, Idaho, and Associate Professor, Department of Medicine, University of Washington School of Medicine, Seattle, Washington

Joel D. Cooper, M.D. Chief, Lung Transplant Program, and Professor of Surgery, Washington University School of Medicine, St. Louis, Missouri

Leon Cudkowicz, M.D. Professor of Clinical Medicine, Department of Internal Medicine, University of Cincinnati School of Medicine, Cincinnati, Ohio

Mark E. Deffebach, M.D. Division of Pulmonary and Critical Care Medicine, Department of Medicine, University of Washington School of Medicine, Seattle, Washington

Kent Ellis, M.D. Professor, Department of Radiology, Columbia Presbyterian Medical Center, New York, New York

David John Godden, M.D. (Edinburgh) Department of Medicine and Therapeutics, University of Aberdeen, Aberdeen, Scotland

Michael P. Hlastala, Ph.D. Professor of Medicine, Physiology, and Biophysics, University of Washington School of Medicine, Seattle, Washington

Richard W. Hyde, M.D. Professor of Medicine and Toxicology, Pulmonary and Critical Care Unit, University of Rochester Medical Center, Rochester, New York

Annika Laitinen, M.D. Department of Anatomy, University of Helsinki, Helsinki, Finland, and Department of Medical and Physiological Chemistry, University of Lund, Lund, Sweden

Lauri A. Laitinen, M.D. Department of Pulmonary Medicine, University of Lund, and Astra Draco, Lund, Sweden

S. Lakshminarayan, M.D., F.R.C.P. Division of Pulmonary and Critical Care Medicine, Veterans Administration Medical Center, and Professor of Medicine, University of Washington School of Medicine, Seattle, Washington

William M. Long, M.D. Department of Physiology, North Dakota Medical School, Grand Forks, North Dakota

Michael A. Matthay, M.D. Associate Professor, Departments of Medicine and Anesthesia, University of California, San Francisco, San Francisco, California

Peter D. Paré, M.D. Professor of Medicine, Pulmonary Research Laboratory, University of British Columbia, St. Paul's Hospital, Vancouver, British Columbia, Canada

Carl G. A. Persson, M.D. Professor, Department of Clinical Pharmacology, University Hospital of Lund, Lund, Sweden

Jacques Rémy, M.D. Chief, Department of Diagnostic Radiology, Hôpital Albert Calmette, Lille, France

Martine Rémy-Jardin, M.D. Department of Diagnostic Radiology, Hôpital Albert Calmette, Lille, France

Hans Schreinemakers, M.D. Division of Cardiothoracic Surgery, Washington University School of Medicine, St. Louis, Missouri

Deborah Shure, M.D. Associate Professor, Department of Medicine, University of California, San Diego, and Division of Pulmonary and Critical Care, Veterans Administration Medical Center, San Diego, California

Julian Solway, M.D. Associate Professor, Department of Medicine, University of Chicago, Chicago, Illinois

Erik R. Swenson, M.D. Division of Pulmonary and Critical Care Medicine, University of Washington School of Medicine, Seattle, Washington

Aubrey E. Taylor, Ph.D. Department of Physiology, University of South Alabama College of Medicine, Mobile, Alabama

Cyr Voisin, M.D. Department of Diagnostic Radiology, Hôpital Albert Calmette, Lille, France

Elizabeth M. Wagner, Ph.D. Assistant Professor of Medicine, Division of Pulmonary and Critical Care Medicine, Asthma and Allergy Center, Johns Hopkins Medical Center, Baltimore, Maryland

Adam Wanner, M.D. Professor of Medicine and Director, Pulmonary Division, University of Miami and Mt. Sinai Medical Center, Miami Beach, Florida

Stephen E. Webber, Ph.D. Department of Physiology, St. George's Hospital Medical School, London, England

John G. Widdicombe, D.M. Professor, Department of Physiology, St. George's Hospital Medical School, London, England

CONTENTS

Part IV: REGULATION

Part VII: THERAPY

Part I

BACKGROUND

1

The Bronchial Circulation in the Human
A Historical Introduction

LEON CUDKOWICZ

University of Cincinnati School of Medicine
Cincinnati, Ohio

I. Introduction

The Museum of Alexandria in the Third Century BCE provided, through the practice of dissection of cadavers, a rich soil for anatomic observation. Erasistratus is credited with the concept of unidirectional movement of blood to the lungs and that of air to the left ventricle (Erasistratus, 270 BCE; Galen, 1562). The discovery of aortic branches entering the human lung is attributed to him (approximately 270 BCE) because of a reference made to him by Galen (Galen, 180), who visited Alexandria, participated in dissection, and transferred this skill to Rome. Galen became physician and friend of the Emperor Marcus Aurelius. Miller (1947), in his admirable review of the history of the bronchial circulation, points out that Galen (130–201) observed systemic blood vessels to the lungs but failed to name them. In the *Tractat de Arteria et Vena Dissectione* he wrote: "Arteries from the second thoracic vertebra emerge and are distributed to the adjacent lungs and break up into small branches which are then hard to see." With the end of the Middle Ages, the adherence to Galen's system of anatomy faded, and in the middle of the thirteenth century the Arab physician Ibn-An-Nafis, born in Damascus in

1210, rejected Galen's assumption of interventricular pores altogether and clearly stated (Meyerhof, 1935):

> . . . blood passes via the vena arterialis (pulmonary artery) to the lung for circulation and mixes with air in the pulmonary parenchyma. The aerated blood gets refined and passes through the arterio-venalis (pulmonary veins) to reach the left cavity of the two cavities of the heart. . . . The residuum of less rarified blood is used up by the lung for its own nourishment.

How exactly the lung derives this "nourishment" and by which conduits is not clear from Ibn-An-Nafis' *Commentary on Avicenna's Canon* (Bittar, 1956).

With the demise of the Roman Empire, Western Europe became deprived of much of Greek science, which was diverted to the Byzantine Empire. There it emerged in Arabic translations of Galen and Hippocrates by way of reconquered Spain, in conjunction with significant contributions of Arabic medicine.

In the Western European world Galen's scheme was first challenged in the early sixteenth century by Michael Servetus, the true martyr among the pulmonary circulation's discoverers. In his book, *Christianismi Restitutio* (Chapter V, pp. 159–171), published in 1533 and devoted to the search for true religion, he describes the passage of the blood through the lungs (Servetus, 1533):

> The notable size of the pulmonary artery confirms this: That is, it was not made of such size, nor does it emit so great a force of pure blood from the heart itself into the lungs merely for their nourishment, nor would the heart be of much service to the lungs merely for their nourishment, nor would the heart be of much service to the lungs, since at an early stage, in the embryo, the lungs, as Galen teaches, are nourished from elsewhere, because those little valvules of the heart are not opened until the time of birth.

Unfortunately, Michael Servetus failed to identify here the aortic branches to the lungs. This remarkable genius communicated his ideas to Calvin, who rejected them. He was arrested, judged, and burned at the stake at Champel, outside Geneva on October 27, 1553, with a copy of his book attached to his arm. Alas, only two authentic copies of the book remain.

The sixteenth century is replete with the rediscovery of Greek and Arabic texts of the pulmonary circulation, culminating in the work and sacrifice of Michael Servetus, but no references are known at that time to have been made concerning the extraordinary efforts and description of the pulmonary and bronchial circulations by Leonardo da Vinci (1911).

Born an illegitimate child in the small hill town of Vinci in 1452, Leonardo da Vinci received a very poor education and appeared to be able to read but not write Latin. He was extremely attached to his mother in early childhood but completely lacked paternal guidance. In fact, he had no guidance from anyone. Soon after the age of 16, in Verocchio's studio, he left his mark as a painter of unique individuality and brilliance. The angel he painted on a canvas by Verocchio almost extinguished the art of the teacher. He was alone, and he had the unique ability of knowing this. "One has risen before dawn and my companions are still asleep." Elsewhere: "Whoever refers to authorities in disputing ideas, works with his memory rather than with his reason." So vast were the interests of this genius that we must pause for a moment. A universe existed, and he set out without guide or compass to make it comprehensible to himself, relying entirely on his own observations and judgment.

Leonardo da Vinci questioned all he had read and disregarded most established forms of knowledge, except geometry. His contributions in the arts of painting and sculpture are well known and cannot be considered here, except perhaps that he did so many things at the same time that even his greatest paintings, such as the *Mona Lisa* and the *Last Supper*, remained incomplete. His observations in the sciences are also renowned. What is by no means fully established concerns our scholarship of Leonardo's knowledge of anatomy and physiology. Detailed, and conflicting, accounts of the fate of Leonardo's anatomic notebooks exist, probably the most beautiful of their kind ever compiled.

Before I venture to summarize da Vinci's observations, I must mention that, almost alone, he dissected over 30 human cadavers in Italy, in an age that knew neither formalin nor refrigeration. Not until the Quincentenary Exhibition held in 1952 at the Royal Academy, London and devoted to the drawings of Leonardo da Vinci was it possible to place his remarkable anatomic observations in their appropriate historical perspective. Much was written before the nineteenth century concerning bronchial arteries, but no references appear in those texts to the fundamental observations made 500 years earlier by Leonardo da Vinci regarding the bronchial circulation.

II. Leonardo da Vinci (Fig. 1)

In the Quincentenary Exhibition held in 1952 at the Royal Academy, London, and devoted to the drawings of Leonardo da Vinci, exhibit 301 showed a drawing from the *Quaderni d'Anatomia* II.I.V. (Fig. 2; Royal Windsor

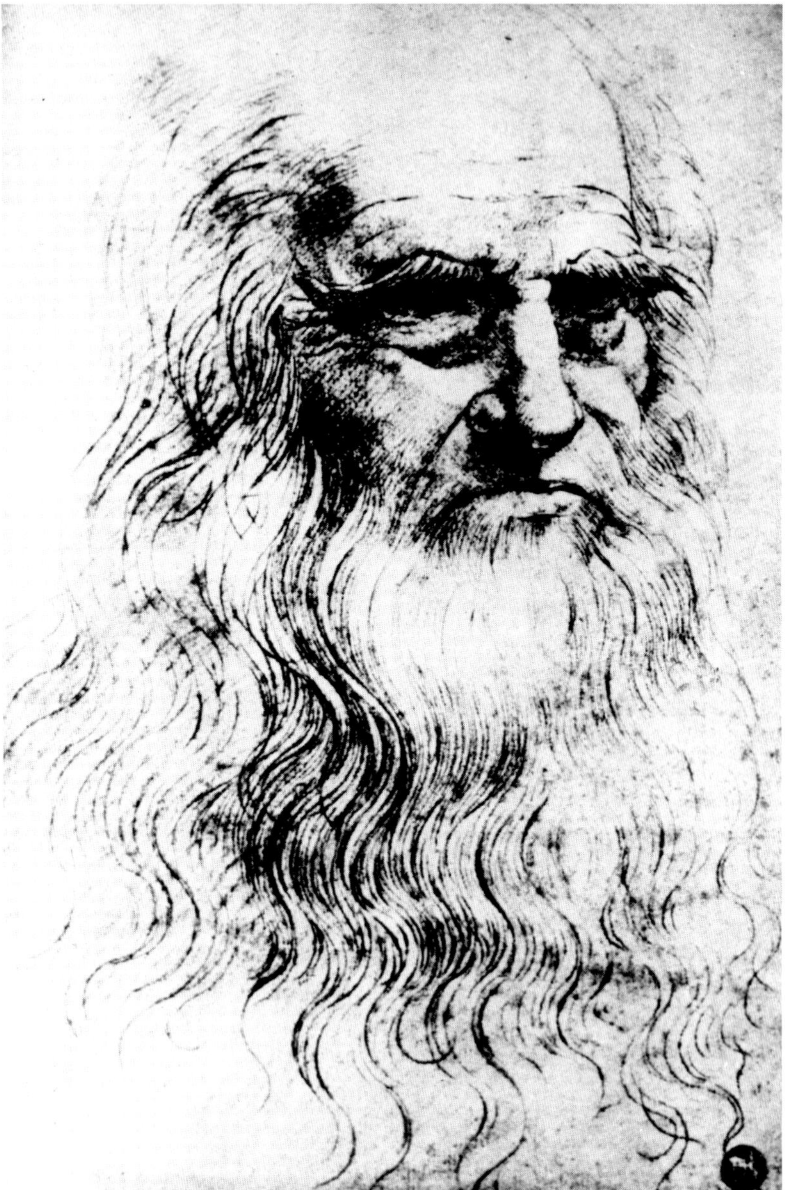

Figure 1 Leonardo da Vinci, self-portrait as an old man. (Royal Library, Turin.)

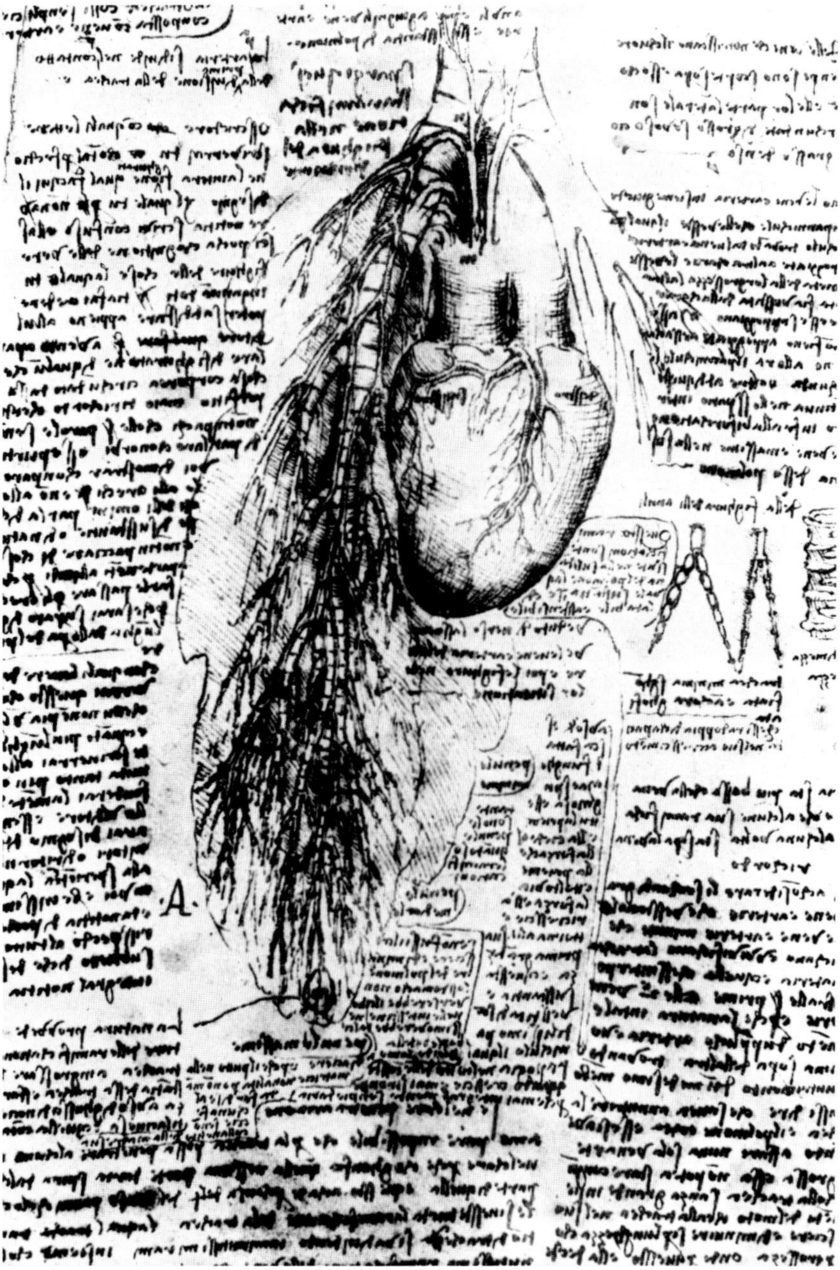

Figure 2 The bronchial arteries. Drawing by Leonardo da Vinci from the *Quaderni d'Anatomia*, II. I.r. (reproduced by gracious permission of Her Majesty Queen Elizabeth II.)

Library) in which Leonardo depicts the heart, the coronary arteries, the trachea, and the bronchial tree of a left lung with its accompanying bronchial arteries. It is thought that this drawing stems from 1513, when Leonardo worked in the hospitals of Rome, where he had gone after the return in 1512 of Maximillian Sforza, son of Duke Ludovico, to Milan. Leonardo, because he was previously in the service of the French invaders of Milan, was not a welcome person, and he departed with Francesco di Melzi for Rome. The subsequent years were restless, and with his patron, Giuliano de Medici dead and the Pope hostile to him, Leonardo found nothing to keep him in Rome. His former French patron had not forgotten him, and in 1517, he crossed the Alps with Francesco di Melzi to end his many years of wandering at the Chateau de Cloux near Amboise on the Loire.

Here he was visited by the Cardinal Luis of Aragon, whose secretary noted the event:

> On the tenth of October 1517, Monsignor and the rest of us went to see, in one of the outlying parts of Amboise, Messer Leonardo da Vinci the Florentine, an old man of more than seventy years, the most excellent painter of our time, who showed His Excellency three pictures: one of a certain Florentine lady, done from the life at the instance of the late Magnificent Giuliano de Medici, another of St. John the Baptist as a youth, and one of the Madonna and Child in the lap of St. Anne: all most perfect, and from one whom, since he was then subject to a certain paralysis of the right hand, none could expect any more good work. He has given good instruction to a Milanese pupil who works very well. And although the aforesaid Messer Leonardo cannot color with the same sweetness as he used to, he is still able to make drawings and to teach the others. This gentleman has written of anatomy with much detail showing, by illustration, the limbs, muscles, nerves, veins, ligaments, intestines, and whatsoever else there is to discuss in the bodies of men and women, in a way that has never yet been done by anyone else. All of this we have seen with our own eyes; and he said that he had dissected more than thirty bodies both of men and women of all ages. He has also written of the nature of water, of diverse machines, and of other matters, which he has set down in an infinite number of volumes all in the vulgar tongue, which if they should be published, will be profitable and enjoyable.

One cannot help feeling, as did the Cardinal's secretary, how profitable would have been the publication of that "infinite number of volumes." But this was never done (Keele, 1952).

After enjoying 2 years of tranquility at the Chateau de Cloux near Amboise, Leonardo da Vinci died there on May 2, 1519. At the time of his death, Francesco Melzi was only 20 years old. He left France and returned to his villa at Vaprio, near Milan, carrying with him all of Leonardo's priceless manuscripts. For 50 years, until 1570, Melzi kept those manuscripts untouched, worshipping the memory of Leonardo without offering a single one of the plates for publication.

Upon Francesco Melzi's death in 1570 they passed to his nephew, the lawyer Urazio Melzi, who was uninterested and careless. Toward the end of the century he sold them to the sculptor Pompeo Leoni. While in his possession, they were shown between 1601 and 1606 to Rubens when he visited Italy. Rubens described and appreciated their great beauty. Pompeo Leoni carried all the Leonardo drawings in his possession to Spain, with the thought of presenting them to King Philip. Philip died, however, before he could see them. Pompeo Leoni brought some of the drawings back to Italy but sold the major bulk of the manuscripts to someone in Spain. In 1638 they were purchased from a Spanish owner by Thomas Howard, Earl of Arundel, who brought them to England. The mode of transfer from Arundel to the Crown is not known. It is understood, however, that King Charles I himself placed the da Vinci drawings in a large and strong chest. Queen Mary II of England apparently showed them in 1690 to Huygens. The key to the chest was lost thereafter until the reign of King George III, when Dr. William Hunter saw them in 1760.

Thereafter, and until the exhibition at the Royal Academy in 1952, 600 of the original drawings were kept at Windsor Castle, including that of the bronchial circulation (No. 301; Fig. 2).

In December 1950, I completed my thesis for the degree of Doctor of Medicine, University of London, with "A Study of the Bronchial Arteries in Normal and Diseased Lungs," having been totally unaware of the drawings and descriptions provided by Leonardo da Vinci. In June 1952, I visited the Quincentenary Exhibition at the Royal Academy in London and saw for the first time the drawing from the *Quaderni d'Anatomia* II.I.V (Royal Windsor Library). The bronchial arteries were here shown to arise from the aorta and to follow the individual bronchi to their termination. It was, unfortunately, too late to include a copy of this magnificent drawing in my M.D. thesis. However, permission was obtained from the Royal Windsor Library and from H.M. Queen Elizabeth II to publish a paper entitled "Leonardo da Vinci and the Bronchial Circulation" and thus establish da Vinci as an illustrious reference (Cudkowicz, 1953).

In the same drawing a circle is seen at the inferior margin of the lung, which surrounds a terminal basal bronchus. A line runs from this circle to the adjacent script, which, translated on page 85 of the *Catalogue*, reads as follows: "Nature prevents the rupture of the ramifications of the trachea by thickening the substance of this trachea and making thereof a crust, like a nutshell, and it is cartilaginous and in the interior remains dust and watery humour." This, the catalogue emphasizes, is one of the "earlier descriptions of a tuberculous cavity" (Fig. 3) (Cudkowicz, 1952).

Closer scrutiny of this cavity reveals the additional and remarkable feature of small bronchial arteries within its periphery. Microscopy of the vasculature in the vicinity of tuberculous cavities has shown that the pulmonary arteries in the surrounding lung have usually undergone occlusive changes and that the only true, patent arteries in the walls of tuberculous cavities are dilated bronchial arteries (Fig. 4). It is impossible to say if Leonardo deliberately intended to show these systemic arteries reaching the walls of the cavity or if the vessels depicted were merely branches destined to follow the bronchus containing the peripheral cavity. The latter explanation is probably the more likely.

The circle indicating tuberculous cavitation in this drawing is therefore of some interest in that it indicates, either by chance or deliberately, Leonardo's awareness of the existence of cavities, their relationship to the bronchial tree, and possibly also their correct blood supply (Fig. 5).

Keele (1952) in his monograph on Leonardo's study of the heart and blood reproduces this same drawing and quotes from Leonardo's notebooks relevant passages appertaining to the bronchial circulation:

> Why nature duplicated artery and vein in such an instrument, one above the other, finding themselves for the nourishment of one and the same member (the lung).
>
> You may say that the trachea [whole bronchial tree] and the lung have to be nourished, but if you had to do it with a single large venarteria, this could not accompany the trachea without great interference with the movement which the trachea makes in dilatation and contraction as well as in length and thickness. Wherefore, for this, nature gave a vein and artery to the trachea which would be sufficient for its life and nourishment, and somewhat removed the other large branches from the trachea to nourish the substance of the lung with greater convenience.

This teleological view of the function of the bronchial circulation, expressed about 300 years before Reisseisen and von Sömmering's definition of the bronchial arteries as the "vasa nutritiva of the lungs" (1808), is so modern in conception that very little can really be added. It bears testimony to his grasp of the function of organs as much as the accuracy of his drawing emphasizes his exceptional skill as an academic anatomist. Those who have tried to dissect the bronchial arteries, even under most modern conditions, are well aware of the hazards involved in tracing these delicate structures. Without the use of contrast media to outline the intrapulmonary course of these vessels radiographically and careful microscopy to show up the relationship of the bron-

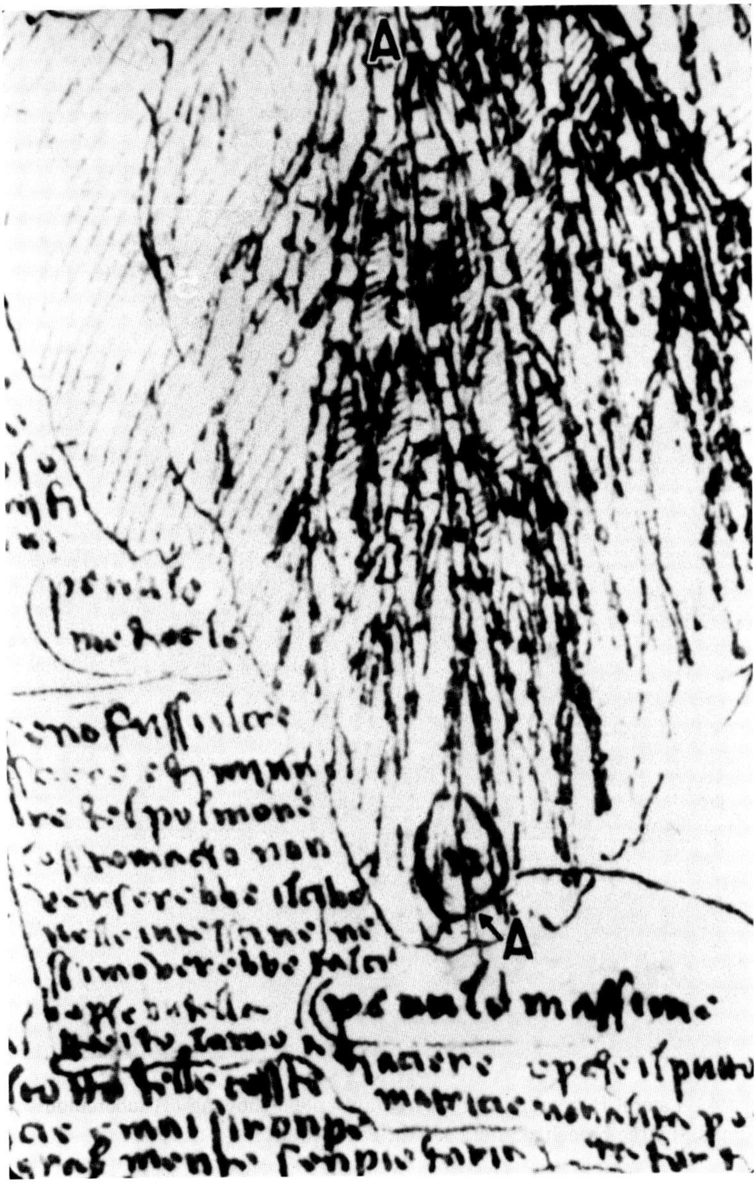

Figure 3 Detail of drawing by Leonardo da Vinci of the bronchial arteries following the left basal bronchi. A tuberculous cavity is depicted in the center of a basal segment. (A) Bronchial arteries are shown in the vicinity of the cavity. (Reproduced by gracious permission of Her Majesty Queen Elizabeth II.)

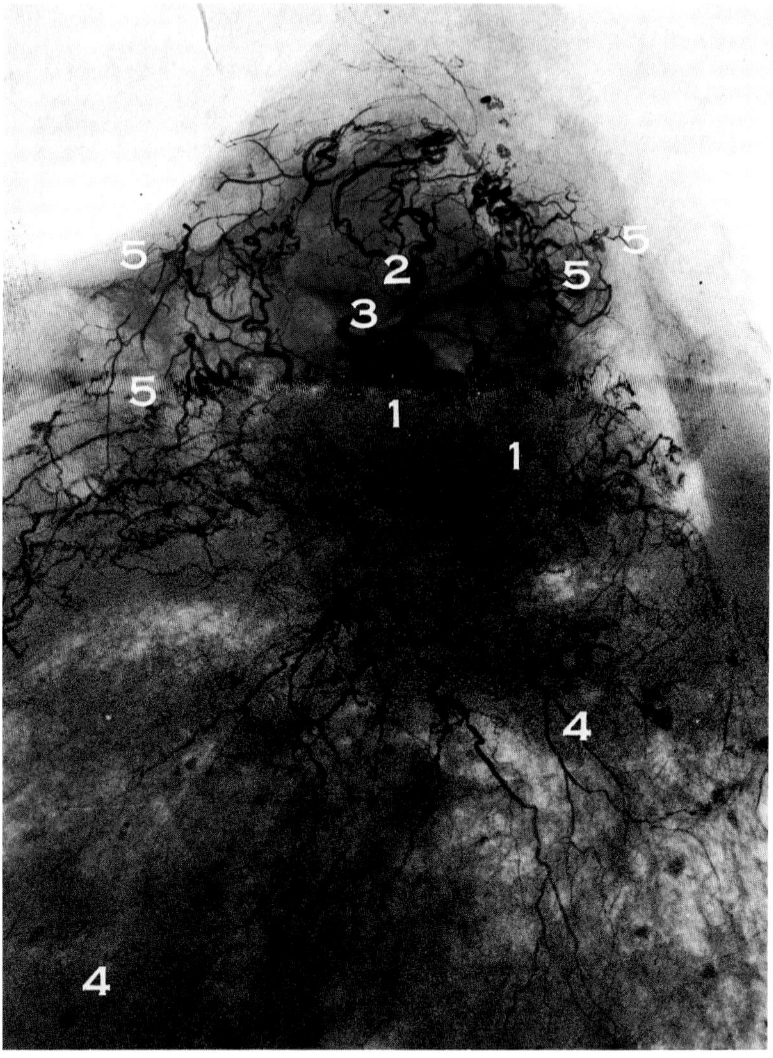

Figure 4 Lateral radiograph from a left upper lobe showing (1) tuberculous cavity; and (2 and 3) large bronchial arteries in the cavity wall.

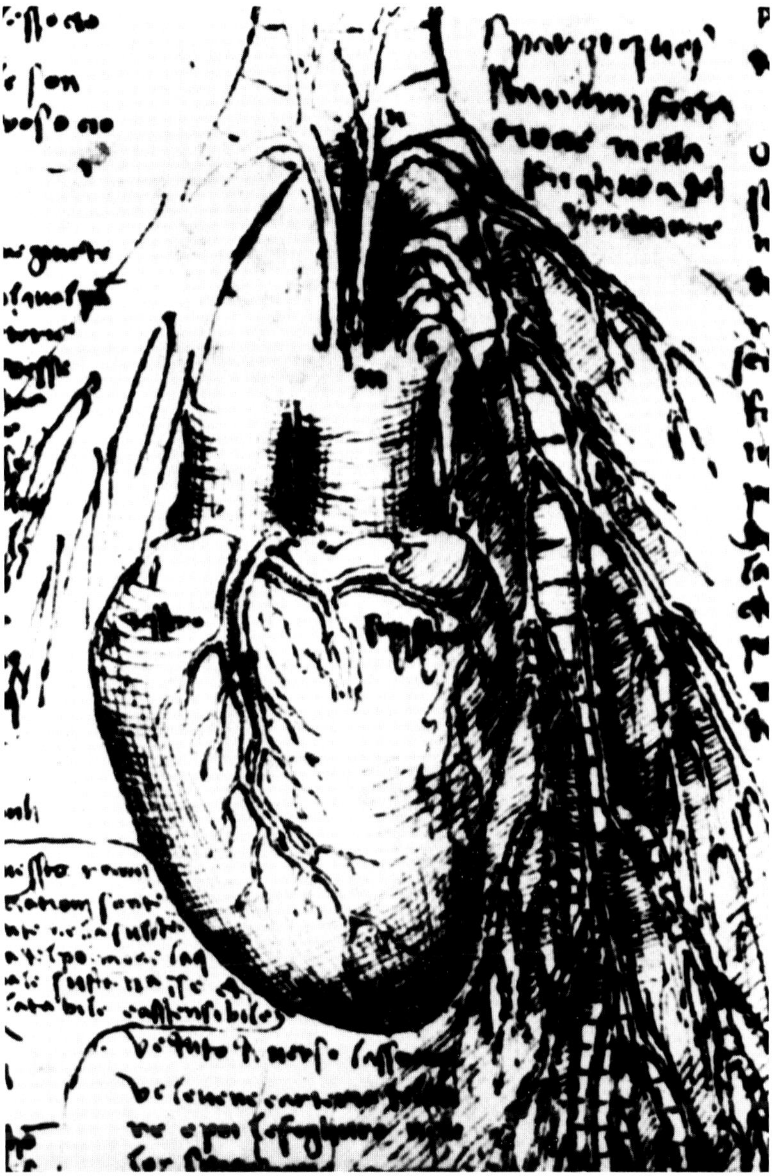

Figure 5 Detail of drawing by Leonardo da Vinci of the heart, aorta, and left bronchial arteries. The aortic origin of the left bronchial arteries is depicted, as is their course along the bronchial tree. The coronary arteries are also shown. (Reproduced by gracious permission of Her Majesty Queen Elizabeth II.)

chial arteries to the bronchial tree and other lung structures, modern studies of this circulation would be almost inconceivable (Fig. 6) (Wearn et al., 1934; Cudkowicz and Armstrong, 1951).

The drawing of the bronchial circulation by Leonardo, made at the time when such methods were unknown, is therefore an example of his great genius and ought to have pointed the way to an earlier recognition of vascular components in relation to lung pathology. Yet Leonardo depicted the coronary arteries and emphasized their nutritive function in respect to the myocardium, but myocardial ischemia as a concept in heart disease did not gain clinical relevancy until the present century (Fig. 5).

Leonardo da Vinci's mirror writing, his use of the "vulgar tongue," the intellectual indifference of his contemporaries, and the long incarceration in past centuries of his notebooks in private hands may perhaps have been responsible for medicine's disregard of those remarkable observations. There are, of course, many astounding facets to the life and work of Leonardo da Vinci that must overshadow his purely anatomic achievements. Those who are concerned with diseases of the lung, however, derive from this drawing of nearly 500 years ago much inspiration and encouragement to elucidate further the vascular factors in lung disease (Fig. 2).

III. Additional Historical Milestones

Claudius Galen, born in 130 in Pergamum, Asia Minor, found his way to Rome in the year 164. He became the friend and physician of Marcus Aurelius, who like him was a stoic philosopher and ardent Hellenist. Galen's knowledge of anatomy from personal dissection of animals was vast. The human was the animal of which he had the least direct knowledge. He reports vivisection of pigs, goats, sheep, horses, mules, asses, cows, stags, bears, mice, birds, and at least one elephant. His physiology was based on the principle of ablation. He cut, tied, and severed. The exposure of the beating heart and lungs in living animals he found too difficult because of deaths from pneumothorax. By removing the sternum, Galen observed the beating heart of pigs, but he could no more analyze this in the quickly moving heart than could Harvey 1500 years later. "It is impossible to ligate the pulmonary vein," he lamented, "it can be done around the base of the heart, but the animal dies at once." He was balked. He reached the limit of his technical skill, and so he failed to discredit Erasistratus' idea of active cardiac diastole. He did, however, establish that arteries contain blood in life.

In about 180 he provided the first observation of systemic blood vessels to the lung. In the *Tractat de Arteria et Vena Dissecitone* he wrote, "Arteries near the second dorsal vertebra descend and first distribute themselves to the

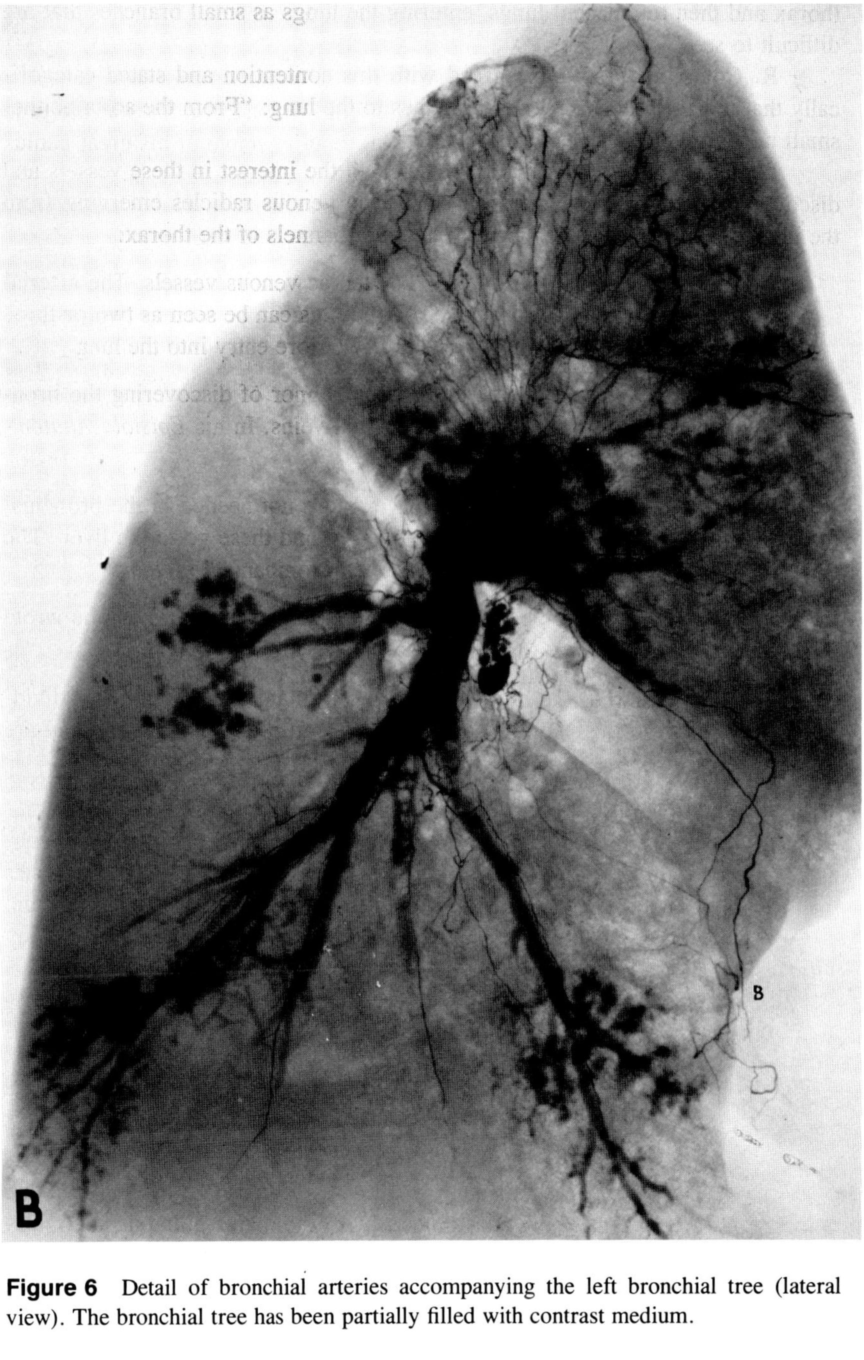

Figure 6 Detail of bronchial arteries accompanying the left bronchial tree (lateral view). The bronchial tree has been partially filled with contrast medium.

thorax and then to adjacent lungs, entering the lungs as small branches that are difficult to see."

R. Columbus (1559) disagreed with this contention and stated categorically that the aorta does not send branches to the lung: "From the aorta neither small nor large branches enter the lung."

Dominico de Marchettis (1654) renewed the interest in these vessels and discovered not only arterial branches but also venous radicles emerging from the lung and fusing with the systemic venous channels of the thorax:

> Arterial vessels exist in the lungs as well as venous vessels. The arterial vessels that supply the substance of the lungs can be seen as two or three arteries, or fused as a single large artery before entry into the lung.

Ruyisch (1732), who claims the primary honor of discovering the bronchial arteries, denied the existence of bronchial veins. In his *Epistola Anatomica* (1792, Amsterdam) he stated:

> In regard to the bronchial arteries, veins are not needed in the bronchial tree, because there are veins in the pleura, and these go to the liver. The liver has hepatic arteries, but they are unaccompanied by veins.

Of anastomoses between the pulmonary artery and bronchial arteries, he wrote as early as 1721 in *Epistola sexta, Opera omina*, Tom I:

> The distribution of the bronchial arteries in man: if traced along individual bronchi to their very end, having broken up into capillaries, they are lost to view.

He illustrated this distribution with drawings of the injected vessels.

In 1808 and 1822 Reisseissen and von Sömmering published a monograph *Concerning the Structure of the Lungs* in which the bronchial arteries are well described. They gave the following definition of the bronchial arteries: "The bronchial arteries are the nutritive vessels of the lungs." They summarized their distribution:

> Their branches insinuate themselves into the dividing bronchi, surround them in a plexiform manner, and follow them to their end, where these vessels become so extremely small, that it becomes nearly impossible to force colouring matter as far as their terminals.

With the anatomic recognition of the bronchial arteries, attention began to be focused on their function and purpose. In particular, evidence in the human was sought concerning anastomoses with the major pulmonary circulation. The first to attack this interesting problem was Guillot, who in 1838 and 1845 published his method of study and his conclusions.

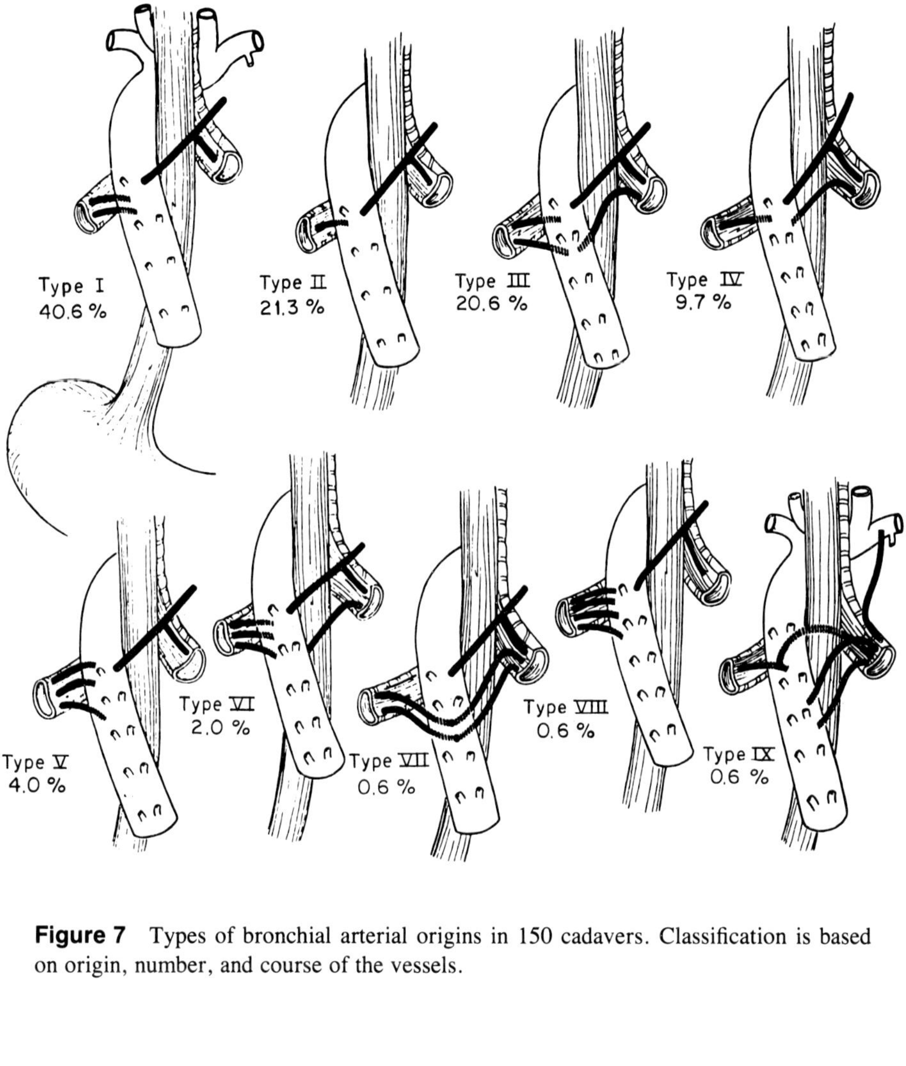

Figure 7 Types of bronchial arterial origins in 150 cadavers. Classification is based on origin, number, and course of the vessels.

Guillot injected gelatin, colored yellow by the addition of lead chromate, into the pulmonary artery of human cadavers and gelatin, colored red with vermilion, into the bronchial artery. He examined the specimen carefully for the anastomotic channels and admixture of the two dyes. No precapillary arterial communication between the two systems could be demonstrated, but a venous communication between the bronchial arteries and the pulmonary veins was found.

Le Fort, in 1859, followed the distribution of the bronchial arteries by dissection and microscopy and established evidence that the capillaries of the bronchial arteries cease near the respiratory bronchioli and that the capillary bed beyond is derived entirely from the pulmonary artery.

von Luschka (1863), in Vol. I of his *Anatomie des Menschen*, believed that an anastomosis between the two circulations exists at the level of their capillary beds. He was the first to draw attention to the capillary distribution of the bronchial artery to the bronchial mucosa:

> . . . that numerous branches enter the walls of the finer bronchi to disappear and emerge as the capillary bed of the bronchi . . . during the course of the bronchial artery, twigs penetrate the adventitia, and furnish a capillary bed for the mucosa which, without interruption, joins the capillaries of the pulmonary arteries.

R. Virchow, in 1847, occluded a major branch of the pulmonary artery in rabbits and dogs that was destined to supply a whole lung lobe and found that this occlusion did not result in necrosis of the dependent lobe. He concluded that the bronchial arteries must have maintained the nutrition of the lobe:

> . . . the bronchial arteries are sufficient, so that the functional vessel, i.e. pulmonary artery, can be interrupted in animals without untoward interference with the nutrition of the lung.

He also stated that the nutrition of the lung structures derive from intercostal arteries. Virchow reiterated these conclusions in 1856, and stress was also laid on the progressive enlargement of bronchial arteries resulting from the ligation of a main pulmonary artery branch to a lobe.

Rindfleisch (1878) considered the bronchial arteries as end arteries.

Cohnheim and Litten, in 1875, agreed with Rindfleisch and thought that, as end arteries, the bronchial arteries are unlikely to sustain the nutrition of the lung as a pulmonary blood supply. After the classic work of Kuettner (1878), however, this contention was abandoned and these authors accepted Virchow's view.

Kuettner (1878), of Heidelberg, injected silver nitrate, followed by a dye that would not penetrate capillaries, into the bronchial arteries of a rabbit and thus showed once more that the bronchial arteries extended as far as the respiratory bronchioli. In a second experiment, he tied the left branch of the pulmonary artery and proceeded to inject a saline solution of aniline blue proximal to the ligature. The right lung became blue at once, whereas the left lung showed a bluish tinge only in the bronchial mucosa. This observation led to the conclusion that a capillary anastomosis existed between the two systems. In a third experiment, paraffin emboli were injected into the jugular vein of a dog and were followed by an infusion of "chromic lead oxide" into the same structure. Subsequent microscopy showed that the lead particles were never found beyond the paraffin obstruction in the affected pulmonary artery branches. He concluded from this that "...the arterial divisions of the pulmonary artery anastomose nowhere with one another. They are end-arteries." This led him to believe that the terminal branches of the pulmonary artery do not communicate with vessels of similar caliber derived from the bronchial arteries and that if any anastomoses exist, they must be capillary only.

Zuckerkandl of Vienna reviewed the problem as he saw it in 1881 and 1883 and stated that the bronchial arteries are primarily nutritive to the lung, that they ramify in the bronchi, supplying the mucosae, and in addition, in the human, are the main blood supply to the pleurae. He also agreed with the distribution along the bronchi as outlined by Le Fort (1858): "the vessels end near bronchioli respiratorii, and from thence the bronchial capillaries fuse with the alveolar capillaries." He divided the venous drainage of the bronchial arteries into (1) an upper, that is, from larger bronchi, and (2) a lower. "The upper venous drainage occurs via venae azygos, and the lower, via the pulmonary veins." Zuckerkandl quoted Eppinger (1883), who suggested that damage to the bronchial arteries might lead to ischaemia, that is, emphysema with chronic bronchitis and compensatory right ventricular hypertrophy. Zuckerkandl states in addition that a venous anastomosis exists between pulmonary and systemic veins via the mediastinal veins. With the dual anastomoses in mind, he argues on teleological grounds that this is as it should be. Since the bronchi do not participate directly in the oxygenation of venous blood, they derive their oxygenated blood from the bronchial arteries, and the capillary bed of the pulmonary artery therefore needs only to extend as high as the ductus alveolaris. The venous blood in the alveolar bed is oxygenated there and becomes nutritive to the alveolar structures at the same time.

With the turn of the century, the problem of the role played by the bronchial arteries received a new impetus with the work of Miller (1947), who outlined in 1906 further methods of study of the two vascular beds and gave a good description of the anatomic arrangement and distribution of the bronchial arteries. In Chapter 5 of his monograph, *The Lung*, he summarizes the anatomy of the blood supply of the lung:

> Two sets of blood vessels to the lung exist. The first, the pulmonary arteries and veins, which constitute the functional respiratory circulation, and secondly, the bronchial arteries, which furnish the nutritive vessels to lungs. One right bronchial artery arises directly from the thoracic

aorta or from the first or the third intercostal artery. On the left side, two vessels often arise from the anterior wall of the thoracic aorta at the level of T.5. Both bronchial arteries may have a variable origin; i.e. they may arise from internal mammary arteries, or even the R. subclavian artery. (Fig. 7.)

Miller followed by dissection the course of the bronchial arteries along the posterior walls of the main bronchi from the hila, where they divide and follow the bronchi to their termination. Each bronchial division is accompanied by a corresponding subdivision of the bronchial artery, which often anastomose with each other and embed themselves in the connective tissue layer surrounding the bronchi. The general course of the vessels is at right angles to the muscular coat as far as the bronchioli, where they disappear with the emergence of the alveoli. From an arterial plexus within the fibrous coat, small branches penetrate the muscle layer to reach the tunica propria of the bronchus and continue to run in the long axis of the bronchus. Miller also provided a clear description of the venous component of the bronchial circulation. He demonstrated that bronchial veins found at the hila drain the first and second divisions of the bronchial tree. These veins drain into the venae azygos or intercostal veins.

He found that venous radicles form a plexus on the inner side of the muscle coat, penetrate the muscle, and constitute a second plexus between the muscle and fibrous layers from which a source of the pulmonary veins is produced. The capillary bed of the pulmonary artery breaks up into as many plexus as there are ductus alveolares, atria, sacculi, and alveoli, and from this capillary distribution the pulmonary veins receive their main blood supply.

Additional veins draining into the pulmonary veins arise as follows:

1. Within the walls and on the peripheral side of alveolar septa
2. Within the pleurae, which in the human derive their arterial blood via bronchial arteries
3. Within the ductus alveolares, forming there two venous radicles on either side of the ductulus
4. Within the bronchial walls, causing the formation of the two venous radicles, which leave the bronchioli and, as has been shown, are derived from the bronchial arterial capillary bed

Thus it follows that the pulmonary veins convey a certain proportion of systemic venous blood via the left heart into the systemic arterial circulation.

Miller's observation that some bronchial arterial capillaries fuse with the capillary bed of the pulmonary artery recapitulates the observations of Le Fort

(1858) and Kuettner (1878). In his studies of tuberculous lungs, Miller frequently found tubercles situated in the transition zone of the two circulations and suggested that this favored site may often stem from a retardation of flow of the two circulations.

Miller (1947) quotes Yates, whose experience in World War I suggested that injuries to the pulmonary artery were less fatal and severe than corresponding chest injuries also involving the bronchial arteries. He conjectured that the higher blood pressures in the latter and their proximity to the pleurae favored infarction, sometimes even gangrene of the lung. Also, with infarcts extending to the pleura, empyemata were an almost constant sequel.

The question of anastomosis between the two circulations, Miller thought, was not adequately dealt with by Reisseissen (1808), Kuettner (1878), or Zuckerkandl (1881). He believed that the use of a fluid injecting medium caused erroneous results in that such fluids would certainly traverse capillary beds. Postulating venous communication only, he associated himself with the findings of Guillot (1845) and Le Fort (1858).

Miller concluded that bronchial arteries are chiefly connected with pulmonary veins and that injection of the bronchial vessels via the pulmonary artery is only possible if the pulmonary veins are occluded as a result of back pressure along the venous radicles that participate in the formation of the pulmonary veins.

Miller's studies were later often confirmed, in particular by Ghoreyeb and Karsner (1913), Karsner and Ash (1912), Berry and Daly (1931), and Daly (1958).

Additional anatomic observations by Miller concern the distribution of the bronchial arteries to all the pulmonary nerves and lymphatic structures of the lung and the formation of vasa vasorum to the pulmonary artery. The latter, derived as they are from the bronchial arteries, proceed to the media of that vessel without actually communicating with its lumen.

Ghoreyeb and Karsner (1913), in studying the relation of the bronchial arteries to the nutrition of the lung (quoting Koenigstein, 1903, *H*, 1903, *Anat. Hefte*, 22, 309), used carmine and soluble Berlin blue as a viscid gelatin injection medium in the dog. Both solutions were warmed to 40°C before use. The carmine solution was injected at 40 mmHg into the pulmonary artery, and the Berlin blue simultaneously into the aorta at 140 mmHg. This experiment showed that, as long as physiological pressure was maintained in the pulmonary and the bronchial circuits, very little if any admixture of the injecting media occurred. As soon as the pressure in one bed was reduced to zero, however, the opposite system penetrated the bed of the other. This seems to agree with Virchow's (1856) contention that a lung lobe that has its main pulmonary arterial branch occluded may remain viable through the compensatory effects of a collateral bronchial circulation.

Karsner and Ash (1903) approached the problem of anastomoses between the two systems from the aspect of pulmonary embolization. Citing Kuettner (1878), who had demonstrated capillary anastomoses, Rindfleisch (1878), who originally denied such communication, and Miller (1947), who depicted partial communication in the capillary bed alone, they decided in view of Virchow's, Luschka's, and Miller's (1947, 1925) experiments to verify the true site of anastomoses by embolic occlusion of branches of the pulmonary artery. Rokitansky's (Karsner and Ghoreyeb, 1913) and Pannum's (1862) skepticism that emboli produced irreversible changes in the lung added an additional spur to their subsequent work. The live dog was used once more. The aorta was clamped below the origin of the left subclavian artery. Turnip seeds were introduced into the jugular vein. The branches of the pulmonary veins, emerging from lobes, were tied after injection of the seeds or the thorax was filled with oil. The finding after these proceedings was stated as follows:

> ...emboli will cause infarction after stopping flow in the bronchial arteries if the pulmonary veins are tied, or if the lungs are compressed from without.

These manipulations produce the requisite amount of vascular stasis favorable for the development of experimental infarction.

In 1931, Berry et al. first studied the relationship of the two pulmonary vascular systems by means of radiography in dogs. By this method they showed that there was no radioscopic or microscopic evidence of anastomoses, except the partial venous anastomosis demonstrated by Miller (1925). Microscopy outlined the bronchial arterial supply to the bronchial walls and mucosa, the vasa vasorum to the pulmonary artery, and the vasa nervosa to all the pulmonary nerves.

Referring to Reisseissen's "vasa nutritiva," the synonym for the bronchial arteries, Mathes et al. (1932) wondered if a characteristic pattern of these vessels could be obtained from radiography in the dog. They employed a radioscopic method of studying the pulmonary and bronchial circulations and provided the first radiological visualization of the bronchial arteries.

In 1931, Berry and Daly used the double-perfusion pump of Dale and Schuster (1928) in experiments in which the pulmonary artery and the bronchial arteries were (either directly or indirectly via the aorta) simultaneously perfused while blood collections were carried out from the left auricle or the azygos vein.

The pressure relationship of the two beds was found to behave in a consistent manner. Blood flow measurements showed that twice as much bronchial venous blood entered the pulmonary veins compared with the volume drained via the azygos veins. Another observation showed that the elevation of aortic pressure not only raised the pressure in the pulmonary circulation but also augmented the venous flow from the isolated lung.

Mathes et al. in 1932 published a second study concerning the pulmonary, bronchial, and lymphatic circulations of the lung under pathological conditions. The conditions were produced experimentally in the dog. They set out to examine the role of the two circulations by postmortem angiography in diseases affecting the parenchyma of the lung following pulmonary embolic effects.

The results of their normal studies showed that the pulmonary artery conveys venous blood to alveoli and nourishes the alveolar epithelium. The nutrition of the bronchial walls, lymphatics, fibrous stroma, and the walls of the pulmonary artery is solely effected by the bronchial arteries. Each pulmonary artery is an end artery, in the sense that no anastomosis exists proximal to the capillary bed. The position of emboli in the branches of the pulmonary artery demonstrated this point rather well. When there was occlusion of a branch of the pulmonary artery, the embolus lodged at the apex of a pyramidal area, which remained consistently free of injection material introduced into the main pulmonary artery. Provided the embolus was sterile, this pyramidal lung area remained viable and relatively normal in appearance. The bronchial arteries appeared as a tracery of small vessels coursing along the bronchi to their visible termination. Nowhere was an anastomosis with the pulmonary artery shadows in evidence. However, filling of the pulmonary artery and veins occurred via the bronchial arteries, as demonstrated by Karsner and Ash (1912), as long as the pulmonary artery pressure was reduced to zero.

Injection methods were used for studies of the bronchial arteries in a dog suffering from pneumonia as a result of distemper, and Mathes et al. (1932) observed considerable dilatation of the bronchial arteries coursing to the consolidated areas. The lymphatics showed the same dilatation. The generalized compensatory dilation of the bronchial capillary bed was thought to maintain the nutrition of the consolidated areas and accorded with the studies by Karsner and Ash (1912).

Mathes et al. (1932) also found that with infected emboli a transient pneumonitis ensued, with local consolidation and occasional abscess formation. In a few instances hemorrhagic infarcts resulted. The bronchial arteries became dilated in every case, even tortuous, and where abscesses had formed, the bronchial arterial branches traversed the abscess walls.

Mathes and others (1932) concluded from these experiments that bronchial arteries behave in the manner observed by Karsner and Ash (1912) (i.e., embolization leads to a pressure fall to zero in the pulmonary arterial branches, with dilatation and compensatory filling of affected areas by the bronchial vessels). The mechanism of this dilatation was not explained.

The work by these authors confirms the importance of the bronchial arteries after pulmonary embolization because of their ability to sustain the nutrition of the affected lobe by compensatory dilatation. Room for speculation is offered in that the healing of lung abscess cavities, including tuberculous cavities, also seems to depend on the systemic arterial blood supply to the lung (1925).

Horine and Warner (1932) initiated studies of the bronchial circulation in living animals. They confirmed the distribution of bronchial arteries along the entire length of the bronchi, giving origin to capillary plexus in the bronchial submucosa and the bronchi as far as the respiratory bronchioli. These plexus also disseminate through the lymphatic glands, interlobular septae, and pleurae. At regular intervals, the bronchial capillaries join venous plexus that follow the long axis of the bronchi. From these plexus venous radicles emerge, which contribute branches to the pulmonary veins. They reiterated Miller's (1947) findings regarding the separate venous drainage from the upper bronchial divisions via the bronchial veins.

Berry in 1935 published his review of the relationship of the two circulations to the lungs and added his own radiographic investigations in autopsied human lungs. He dwells on the opinions of Reisseissen and von Sömmering (1808), Kuettner (1878), and Zuckerkandl (1881) and the contrary experiences of Guillot (1845) and Miller (1947). Misconceptions about anastomoses between the two systems arose as a consequence of the use of fluid injection materials that were too thin to resemble the behavior of blood in the two systems. The radiopaque materials used by Berry et al. (1931) in the dog and by Mathes et al. (1932) (bisoxychloride, barium sulfate, and gelatin, respectively) did not traverse capillaries and reached arterioles with diameters in excess of 75 μm only. Berry and Daly (1931) used this same material in a study of the hemodynamic relationship between the two circulations in the dog.

Berry and Brenner (Berry, 1934), who tried the same method with human lung specimens, had to abandon the attempt because rapid autolysis allowed the perfusate to escape via the tracheal cannula. Berry thereafter studied the human bronchial vasculature by using histology and angiography after barium sulfate injections in stillborn infants, thus hoping to obviate the autolytic factor.

Berry (1934) refers to Hudson and colleagues, who in 1932, using a similar radiopaque technique, demonstrated small anastomotic channels between the bronchial arteries and branches of the extracardiac coronary arteries in the region of the ostia of the pulmonary veins and that the bronchial arteries could sometimes be injected via the cannulized coronary arteries. Twigs from the esophageal, pericardial, and vasa vasorum of the descending thoracic aorta ramify in the ligamentum pulmonale and communicate there with twigs from the bronchial arteries at the hilum. From the hilum the posterior bronchial artery sends a branch to the visceral pleura.

Berry's radiographic findings revealed that in the human lung there was no anastomosis between the pulmonary and bronchial circulations in vessels larger than 14 μm in diameter. This was subsequently confirmed by histology.

By microscopy of the peribronchial connective tissue, arterial twigs penetrate cartilaginous gaps, pierce smooth muscle, and become distributed in the submucosa. The cartilaginous plates have a small vessel deep in the perichondrium, which is also a twig of the bronchial artery.

These important observations confirm Reisseissen and von Sömmering's (1808) definition of "vasa nutritiva" for the bronchial arteries, as far as the human bronchi are concerned, and complete the anatomic approach to the human bronchial circulation.

IV. Pulmonary Nerves and the Bronchial Circulation

Berry (1934) also demonstrated that all intrapulmonary nerves in the human receive their blood supply from the bronchial arteries. At the lung roots, twigs from these systemic vessels penetrate the epineural sheath and become distributed in the subdivisions of the connective tissue, reaching the nerve fibers as tiny, discrete arterioles. In this connection, Berry quotes Daly and Von Euler (1931), who were able to maintain the excitability and conductivity of these nerves continuously for 3 h by perfusing the bronchial vasculature in the dog. Berry's (1934) conclusions supported the previous observations of Miller (1947). This special study by Berry, utilizing a radiographic injection techniques, was the first of its kind in human specimens and confirmed the experimental data of previous investigators who worked so diligently in the rabbit and the dog.

The normal anatomy of the bronchial vasculature, particularly its relationship to the pulmonary nerves and pleura, therefore seems well established. A very good account of the physiology of this system was presented by Daly (1936) in his *Harvey Lectures*, published in May 1936.

Daly reviewed existing knowledge of the bronchial circulation in broad outline. He accepted Miller's (1947) anatomic description as the most reliable and favored Zuckerkandl's teleological explanation of their function (1881). He went on to show that sympathetic twigs to the bronchial arteries come from the sympathetic ganglia at T3 and T4. In perfusion experiments of the isolated lung (perfusion via the bronchial arteries), excitation of the vagosympathetic nerve raised the pressure in the bronchial arteries, and the exhibition of ergotamine annulled this effect. His perfusion experiments in dogs (simultaneously perfusing bronchial and pulmonary arterial circulations in the isolated lung) yielded vasomotor responses that differed from those seen in dogs in which the pulmonary artery alone was perfused. The reason for this difference was attributed to the possibility that the pulmonary nerves could only be kept in a viable state provided their blood supply via the bronchial arteries was maintained throughout the experiment. Excitation of the cervical vagosympathetic, the cervical vagi, the stellate ganglion, or the thoracic vagosympathetic trunk resulted in vasoconstriction of the pulmonary vessels in every case. This effect was not altered by atropine but could be reversed by ergotamine. Vasodilatation occurred very infrequently, and when it did, it could be enhanced by physostigmine.

Daly stipulated that under resting conditions certain communicating channels, hitherto unrecognized, exist between the pulmonary artery and pulmonary veins, shunting blood away from alveolar capillaries. Only during exercise, he thought, do sympathetic stimuli, acting via the pulmonary nerves, close these channels (by active constriction) and divert the blood flow into the capillary bed, thereby augmenting the total capillary area available for oxygenation. This also explained the "paradoxical" diminution in the pulmonary artery pressure sometimes observed in exercise (1958).

Daly cited Olkon and Johanides (1930), who observed through a window in the thoracic cage of a dog lung capillaries directly below the visceral pleura and noticed that an increase in airway pressure diminished the number of visible open alveolar capillaries but that the velocity of blood corpuscles in larger capillaries increased. These studies are thought to support the possible existence of such shunts at precapillary sites in dogs.

It is interesting that Wearn et al. (1934) used a similar method and were able to report on the action of epinephrine on these superficial shunt capillaries. They witnessed a widening of and an intermittence of flow in the already visible loops.

Daly thought it conceivable that a deficiency in the bronchial blood supply due to bronchial arterial spasm or general systemic arterial disease, or even a lowered systemic blood pressure, might lead to modification in the function of the bronchial muscles, ganglia, and nerves. All tissues concerned in controlling intrinsic pulmonary mechanisms, Daly conjectured, depend on the bronchial arteries for their arterial blood supply.

It is, of course, conjecture to postulate a possible explanation of bronchial asthma (a disorder that may well be intrinsic to the muscle, its nerve supply, or even the neuromuscular junction itself) to the effects of an inadequate bronchial blood supply.

Daly refers to Virchow's observations (1847, 1856) that occlusion of a pulmonary artery branch to a whole lobe leads to extensive compensatory enlargement of the bronchial arteries; obstruction of small branches of the pulmonary artery appears to have no effect on the bronchial arteries. The bronchial arteries dilate (Mathes and others, 1932) and form new vessels to infected region and abscesses. It therefore seems that the bronchial vasculature is responsible for the defense and repair of the damaged organ.

In conclusion Daly stated: "The true understanding of the role of the bronchial arteries in modifying the intrinsic pulmonary mechanism will only be possible with new knowledge gained from the results of clinical studies that are correlated with histological examination of the lung." Subsequent to these experimental studies, efforts evolved slowly to quantify bronchial arterial blood arterial blood flows, and, with the advent of cardiac catheterization, to elucidate these in the human.

V. Development of Bronchial Arterial Blood Flow Measurement

Measurement of bronchial arterial blood flow in the human became possible with the advent of cardiac catheterization using an application of the indirect Fick's principle. Bing et al. used this method in 1947 for the measurement of bilateral bronchial arterial flows in children with Fallot's tetralogy. Bloomer et al., in 1949, used the direct Fick in dogs for the calculation of effective unilateral bronchial arterial anastomotic flow. Bronchospirometry is used to measure the uptake of 100% oxygen by the lung without pulmonary blood flow (bronchial flow only) while the contralateral normal side respires air. About 4 months after unilateral pulmonary artery ligation, the effective blood flow to the lungs usually exceeded 1.0 L/min/m^2 and increased the left ventricular minute volume by about one-third over that of the right.

Adapting this technique to patients, Madoff et al. (1952) found in a girl with a congenitally absent right pulmonary artery an effective right bronchial arterial flow of 950 ml/min. Fishman et al. (1958) also used the direct Fick method for the measurement of bilateral bronchial arterial flow in four patients with atresia of the pulmonary arteries in whom the precapillary flow constituted the entire circulation through the alveoli. The oxygen content of the precapillary bronchial arterial flow was assumed to be the same as in a systemic artery.

An alternative approach to the measurement of the bronchial arterial flow is offered by the simultaneous determination of right and left ventricular outputs utilizing an indirect dye dilution technique. Dye dilution curves obtained from the pulmonary artery after injection of an indicator close to the right atrium have been found to give accurate estimates of the right ventricular output (1957).

Although bronchopulmonary anastomoses may not be the only communication between the pulmonary and bronchial circulations, for the purpose of this technique it is assumed that in the steady state and in the absence of other known shunts, an excess in left over right ventricular output is a measure of the anastomotic bronchopulmonary flow. Figure 8 is a diagrammatic represen-

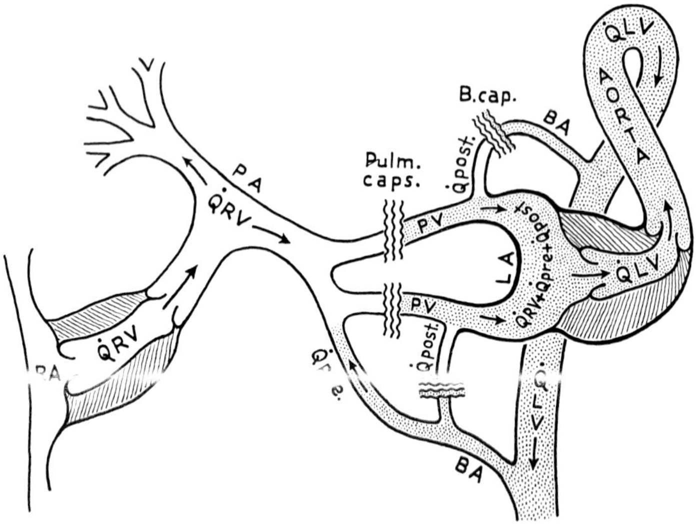

Figure 8 Components of left ventricular minute flow ($\dot{Q}\mathrm{LV}$), right ventricular minute flow ($\dot{Q}\mathrm{RV}$), precapillary bronchopulmonary minute flow ($\dot{Q}\mathrm{BP}_{\mathrm{pre}}$), and postcapillary bronchopulmonary minute flow ($\dot{Q}\mathrm{BP}_{\mathrm{post}}$)

tation of the components of the left ventricular minute flow. The small amount of bronchial venous blood returning to the right atrium through the azygous system is not specifically included.

It is assumed that the bronchial artery minute flows ($\dot{Q}\mathrm{B}$), derived indirectly from estimates of the difference between simultaneously recorded flows of the right ($\dot{Q}\mathrm{RV}$) and left ($\dot{Q}\mathrm{LV}$) ventricles, measure both postcapillary ($\dot{Q}\mathrm{B}_{\mathrm{postcap}}$) and precapillary ($\dot{Q}\mathrm{B}_{\mathrm{precap}}$) anastomostic flow between the bronchial and pulmonary vasculature, which returns to the left side of the heart through the pulmonary veins.

$$\dot{Q}\mathrm{LV} - \dot{Q}\mathrm{RV} = \dot{Q}\mathrm{B}_{\mathrm{precap}} + \dot{Q}\mathrm{B}_{\mathrm{postcap}}$$
$$\dot{Q}\mathrm{B}_{\mathrm{precap}} + \dot{Q}\mathrm{B}_{\mathrm{postcap}} = \dot{Q}\mathrm{BF}$$

Additional flows from other systemic arteries to the lungs, such as the intercostal and pericardiophrenic arteries, are included in this measurement but not the component entering the azygous system of veins, estimated by Bruner and Schmidt in 1947 as one-third of the total in dogs.

Fritts et al. in 1957 and Fox and Wood in 1957 established that $\dot{Q}\mathrm{RV}$/min could be calculated from dye curves in blood withdrawn from the pulmonary artery after the injection of an indicator fairly close to the right atrium. With

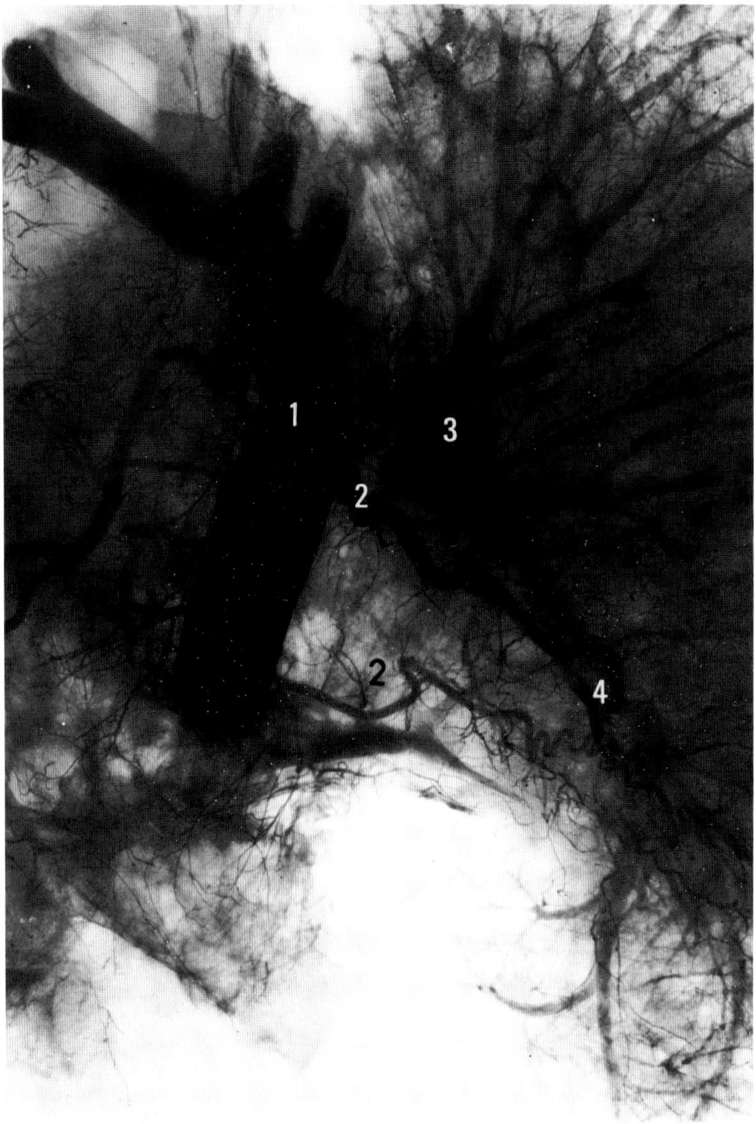

Figure 9 Precapillary bronchopulmonary anastomoses of the left lower lobe, the common denominator in clubbing of the fingers and certain lung diseases (see text for details): (1) aorta; (2) bronchial artery; (3) pulmonary artery; and (4) site of anastomoses.

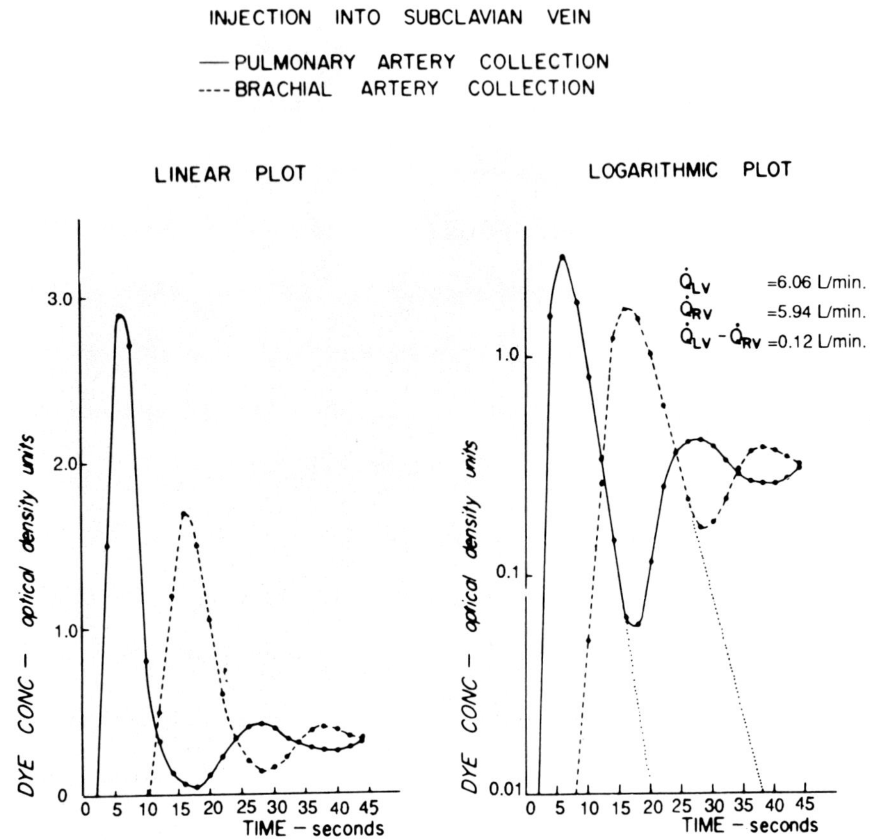

T.C. 46 M NORMAL

Figure 10 Normal bronchial arterial blood flow (indirect technique). Representative normal examples of simultaneously measured right and left ventricular outputs from dye dilution curves and their semilogarithmic plots (Evans blue).

the same indicator bolus, $\dot{Q}_{LV}$/min can be simultaneously obtained from a peripheral arterial dye curve.

In this technique, a small amount of dye is withdrawn during the inscription of the pulmonary artery curve before the blood carrying the indicator to the left heart is further diluted to form the peak of the systemic arterial curve. Apart from this effect on the $\dot{Q}_{LV}$/min curve peak, unsuspected early recirculation is also likely to distort the downslope of the systemic curve. Such small

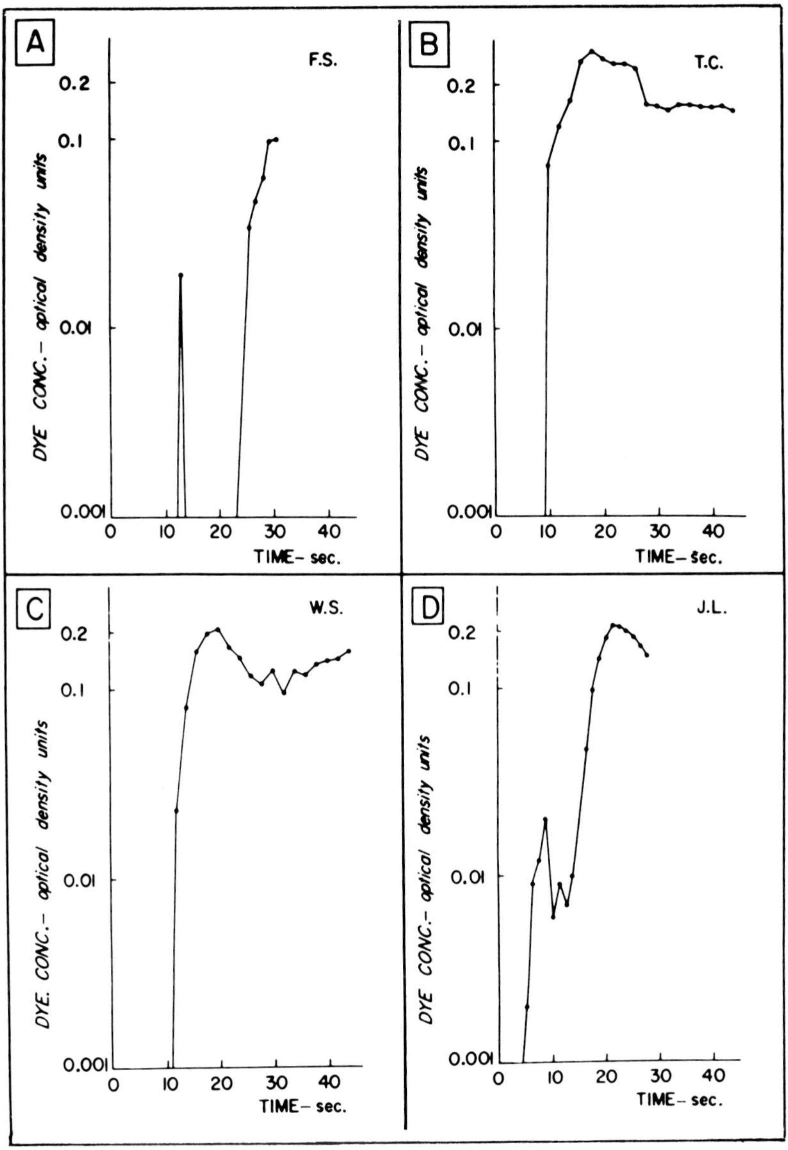

Figure 11 Left atrial dye dilution curves obtained after injection into the ascending aorta in four normal patients. (B and C) No dye appears before the curve of recirculation. (A) A small amount of dye appears before recirculation. (D) An early curve. (Reproduced from Cudkowicz et al. by permission of *Clinical Science*.)

aberrations affect the very small $\dot{Q}_{B}$/min derived in this manner. In the study by Fritts et al. (1957), the average difference between $\dot{Q}_{LV}$/min and $\dot{Q}_{RV}$/min in nine normal subjects was 0.9%, but there was a considerable variation among the individual patients. In another study (1959), three of the five patients without lung disease showed a mean increase in left over right ventricle outputs of 1.5%. In one subject no difference could be demonstrated, and in another the $\dot{Q}_{RV}$/min exceeded the $\dot{Q}_{LV}$/min. Nevertheless, the densitometric recordings of Evans blue by Fritts et al. (1957) in 13 studies of nine patients with normal cardiorespiratory systems showed no difference (±1.5% variation) between the dye dilution right ventricular flow and the cardiac output obtained by the direct Fick method (oxygen uptake) (Figs. 9–11).

Differences well in excess of 10.3% have been established between the left and right ventricular output in patients with bronchiectasis, pulmonary neoplasms, and occluded pulmonary arteries, however, suggesting that this method may be useful in the presence of a large bronchial arterial minute flow.

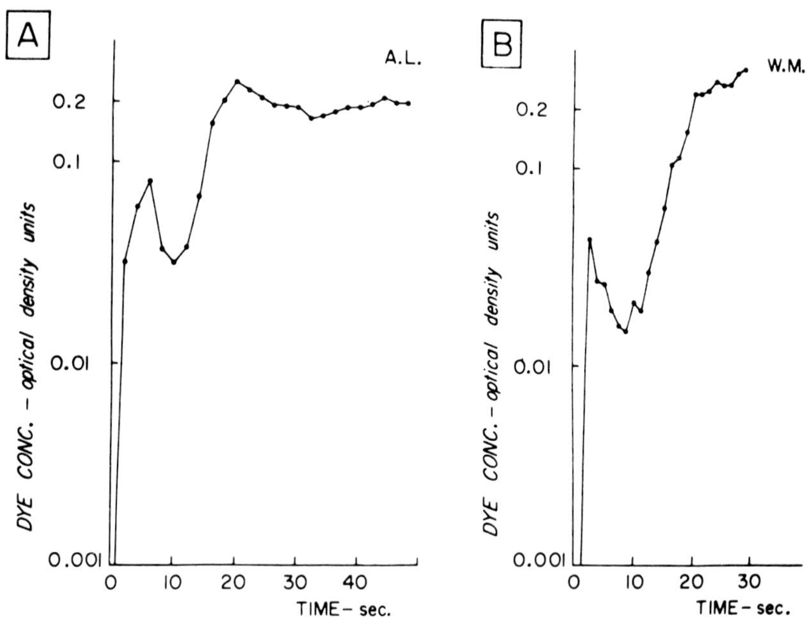

Figure 12 Left atrial dye dilution curves obtained in two patients with finger clubbing (A, patient A. L.; B, Patient W. M.). An early curve precedes the curve of recirculation. (Reproduced from Cudkowicz et al. by permission of *Clinical Science*.)

In disorders suspected of being associated with particularly poor systemic blood flow to the lungs, such as pulmonary emphysema (1961), this indirect method clearly would not be sufficiently sensitive (1968), so that a more precise and direct method of measurement is needed (Figs. 13–17).

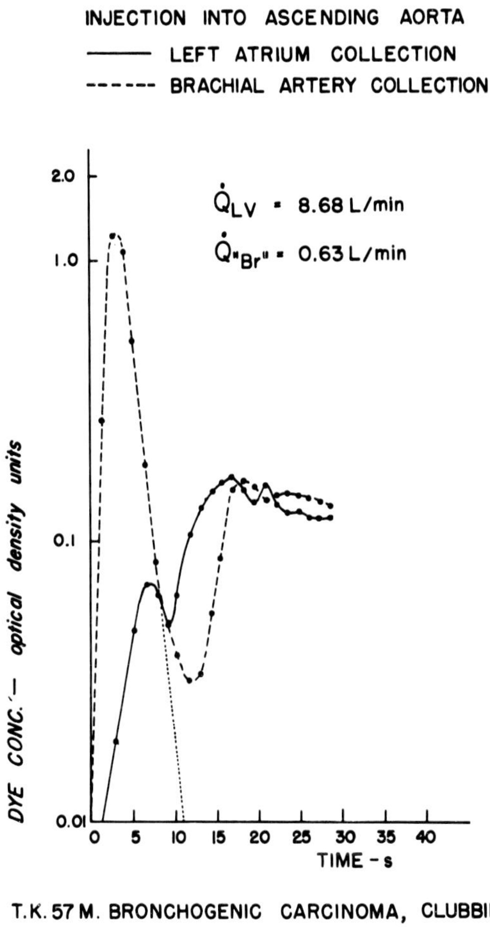

Figure 13 Simultaneously inscribed brachial arterial and left atrial dye dilution curves after injection into the ascending aorta in patient 10 with bronchogenic carcinoma. (Reproduced by Cudkowicz et al. by permission of *Clinical Science*.)

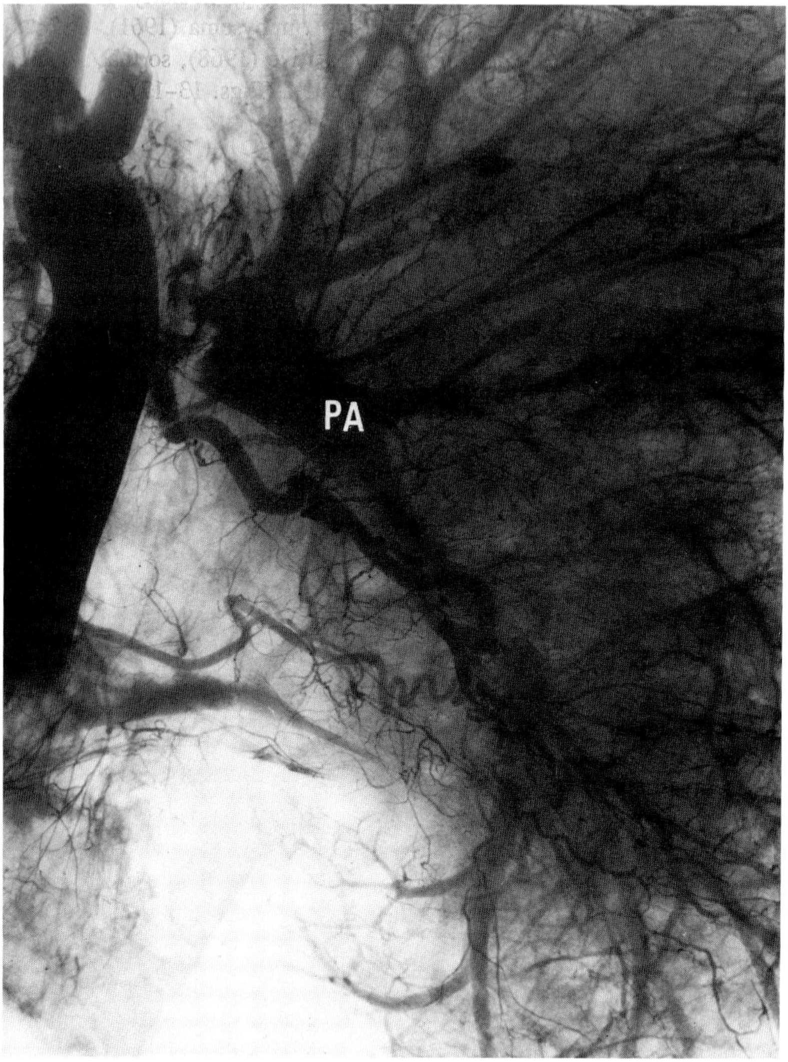

Figure 14 Left lower lobe bronchiectasis. PA view of left lung showing large bronchial arteries conveying injection medium into left lower lobe pulmonary arteries. The left main pulmonary artery is filled retrogradely and is occluded distal to the origin of the lingular branch.

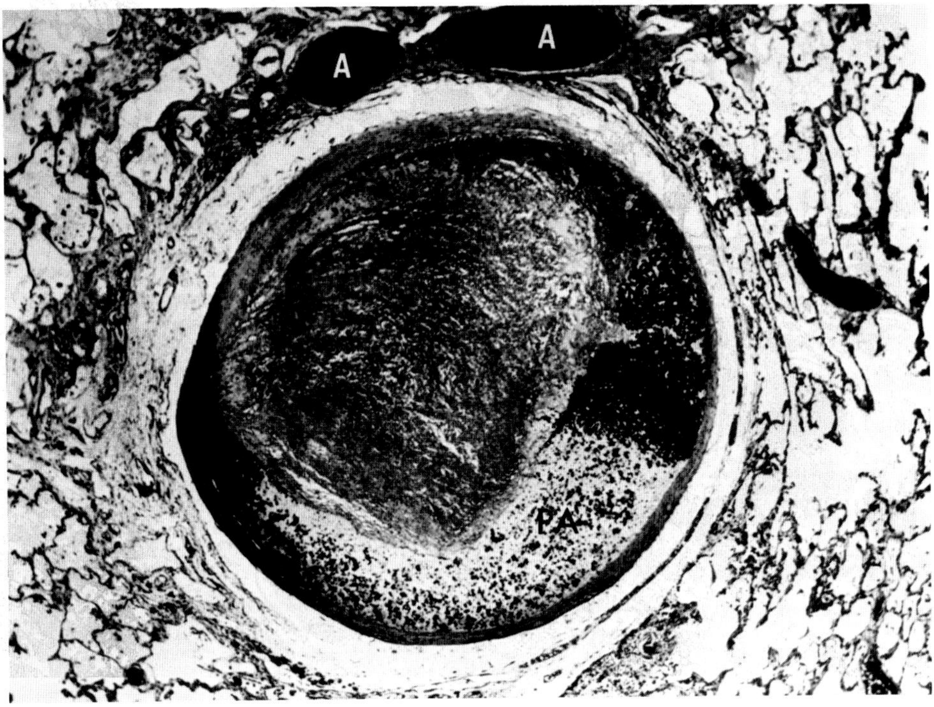

Figure 15 Bronchiectasis. Atheroma and intimal proliferation affect the proximal pulmonary arteries. (A) Grossly dilated vasa vasorum in the adventitial coat of the pulmonary artery not communicating as yet with the pulmonary artery lumen. (Reproduced from Cudkowicz and Armstrong (1953) by permission of *Thorax*.)

VI. Conclusion

As an idea, the bronchial circulation never seems to have existed before Leonardo da Vinci. It seems that he alone brought it from its platonic remoteness to human conception with his incisive intellectual chisel. Subsequently, Harvey nearly uncovered the total secret of the circulation but remained in ignorance of the terminal branches, the capillaries, in both the lungs and the periphery. This discovery of course required the microscope, and with its invention, Marcello Malpighi appeared to have finally closed the circle. How-

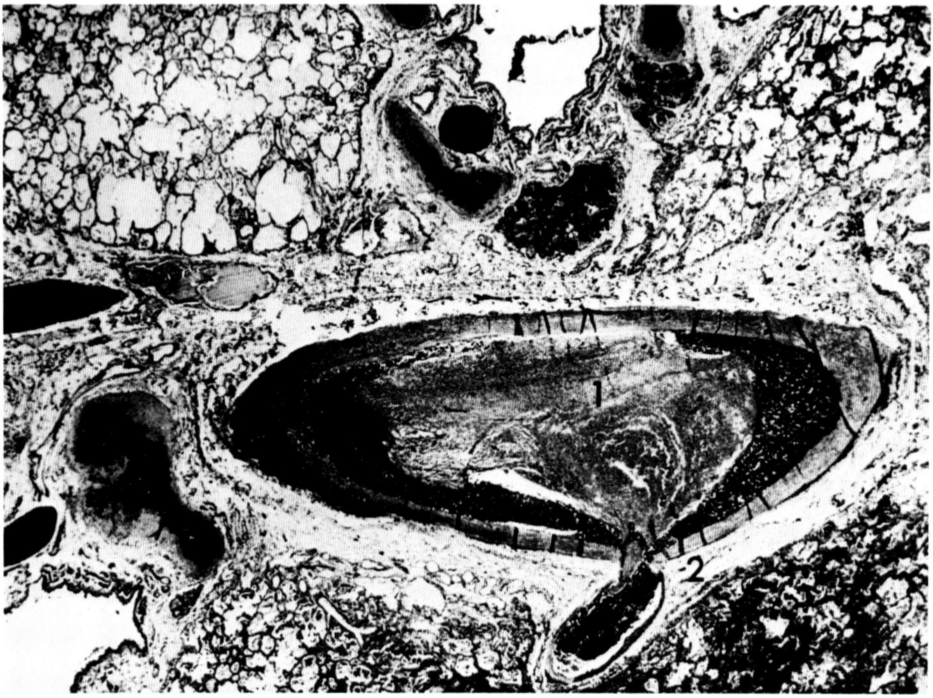

Figure 16 Bronchiectasis. (1) Thrombosed pulmonary artery lumen; (2) communicating vas vasorum conveys bismuth granules into patent part of pulmonary artery lumen (×100). (Reproduced from Cudkowicz (1952) by permission of the *British Journal of Tuberculosis and Diseases of the Chest*.)

ever, the precise capillary relationship between the bronchial and pulmonary circulations remains shrouded in controversy. The mystery has been addressed by many investigators, but a challenge still slumbers in our uncertainty. It is appropriate to close with Harvey: "from hence, the way being thus pervious, others, trusting to more pregnant wits, may take occasion to do better and search further."

References

Aramendia, P., Martinez, J., Deletona, L., and Aviado, D. M. (1962). Exchange of blood between the pulmonary and systemic circulation via bronchopulmonary anastomoses. *Circ. Res.* **11**:870.

Aviado, D. M., Daly, M., Lee, C. Y., and Schmidt, C. F. (1961). The contri-

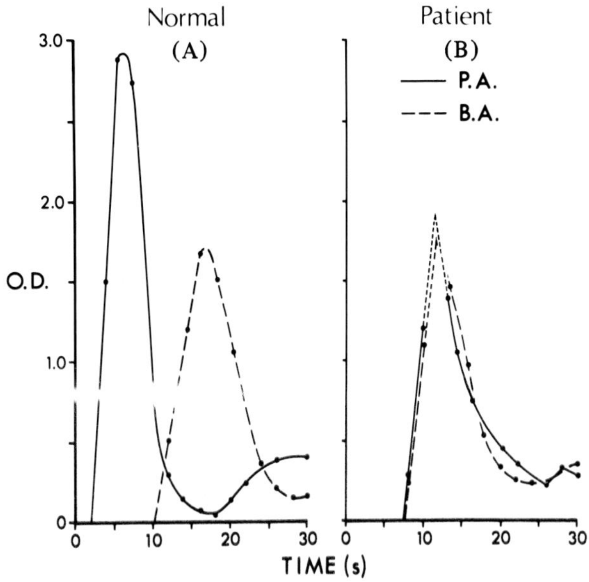

Figure 17 Dye dilution curves from pulmonary artery and brachial artery in (A) a normal patient and (B) a patient with severe left bronchiectasis. The appearance time and height (B) of the curves are identical, indicating that the catheter in the pulmonary artery sampled arterial blood.

bution of the bronchial circulation to the venous admixture in pulmonary venous blood. *J. Physiol. (Lond.)* **155**:602.

Berry, J. L. (1934). The relation between the bronchial and pulmonary circulations in the human lungs. *Q. J. Exp. Physiol.* **24**:305.

Berry, J. L., and Daly, I. de B. (1931). The relation between the pulmonary and bronchial vascular systems. *Proc. R. Soc. Lond. [Biol.]* **109**:319.

Berry, J. L., Brailsford, J. F., and Daly, I. de B. (1931). The bronchial vascular system in the dog. *Proc. R. Soc. Lond. [Biol.]* **109**:214.

Bing, R. J., Vandam, L. D., and Gray, F. D. Jr. (1947). Physiological studies in congenital heart disease II. Results of preoperative studies in patients with Fallot's tetralogy. *Bull. Hopkins Hosp.* **80**:12.

Bittar, E. E. (1956). The influence of Ibn Nafis; a linkage in medical history. *Univ. Michigan Med. Bull.* **22**:274.

Bloomer, W. E., Harrison, W., Lindskog, G. E., and Liebow, A. A. (1949). Respiratory function and blood flow in the bronchial artery after ligation of the pulmonary artery. *Am. J. Physiol.* **157**:317.

Bruner, H. D., and Schmidt, C. T. (1947). Blood flow in the bronchial artery of the anesthetized dog. *Am. J. Physiol.* **148**:648.

Cauldwell, E. W., Siekert, R. G., Lininger, R. E., and Anson, B. J. (1948). An anatomic study of 150 human cadavers. *Surg. Gynecol. Obstet.* **86**:395.

Cohnheim, J., and Litten, M. (1875). Uber die Folgen der Embolie der Lungenarterien. *Virchows Arch. Pathol. Anat.* **65**:99–115.

Columbus, R. (1559). *De re anatomica*. Lib. 15.2, cap. 2.

Cournand, A., and Richards, W. D. (1941). Pulmonary insufficiency. *Am. Rev. Tuberc.* **44**:123.

Cudkowicz, L. (1952). Some observations of the bronchial arteries in lobar pneumonia and pulmonary infarction. *Br. J. Dis. Chest* **46**:99.

Cudkowicz, L. (1953). Leonardo da Vinci and the bronchial circulation. *Br. J. Dis. Chest* **47**:23.

Cudkowicz, L. (1958). Pressure and oxygen content measurements distal to temporary and permanent unilateral occlusion of a pulmonary artery in dogs. *Circ. Res.* **6**:728.

Cudkowicz, L. (1967). Cardio-respiratory studies in patients with lung tumors. *Dis. Chest* **51**:427.

Cudkowicz, L. (1968). *The Human Bronchial Circulation in Health and Disease*. Baltimore, Williams and Wilkins Co., Chapter 13, p. 314.

Cudkowicz, L. (1974). The localization and management of pulmonary hemorrhage. *Critical Care Medicine*. Edited by W. Oaks. New York, Grune and Stratton, Chapter 23, pp. 263–299.

Cudkowicz, L. (1979). *Bronchial Arterial Circulation in Man in Pulmonary Vascular Disease*. Edited by K. M. Moeser, New York, Marcel Dekker, pp. 111–232.

Cudkowicz, L., and Armstrong, J. B. (1951). Observations on the normal anatomy of the bronchial arteries. *Thorax* **6**:343.

Cudkowicz, L., and Armstrong, J. B. (1953). The blood supply of malignant pulmonary neoplasms. *Thorax* **8**:152.

Cudkowicz, L., Abelmann, W. H., Levinson, G. E., Katznelson, G., and Jreissaty, R. M. Bronchial arterial blood flow in man. *Clin. Sci.* **19**:1–21.

Cudkowicz, L., Calabresi, M., Nims, R. G., and Gray, F. Jr. (1959). The simultaneous estimation of right and left ventricular outputs applied to a study of bronchial circulation. *Am. Heart J.* **58**:743.

Dale, H. H., and Schuster, E. H. J. (1928). *J. Physiol. (Lond.)* **64**:356.

Daly, I. de B. (1958). Intrinsic mechanisms of the lung. *Q. J. Exp. Physiol.* **43**:2–26.

Daly, I. de B., and Hebb, C. (1966). *Pulmonary and Bronchial Vascular Systems*. London, Edward Arnold.

Daly, T. de B. (1936). The physiology of the bronchial vascular system. *Harvey Lect.* 235–255.

Daly, T. de B., and von Euler, U. S. (1931). The functional activity of the vasomotor nerves to the lungs in the dog. *Proc. R. Soc. Med.* **110**(92):111.

da Vinci, Leonardo (1911). *Quaderni d'Anatomia* II.I.V. C. L. Vangensteen, A. Fonahn, and H. Hosplock, Vols. I–VI. Christiania, Denmark.

de Marchettis, D. (1654). *Anatomia Patavii*. Edited by I. Padovia.

Erisistratus (ca. 270 BCE), cited by Claudius Galen, *De Affectorum Locorum Notita*, Lib. V, cap II.

Ferguson, F. C., Kodilak, R. E., and Dietrick, J. E. (1944). Varices of the bronchial veins as a source of hemoptysis in mitral stenosis. *Am. Heart J.* **28**:445.

Finley, T., Lenfant, C., Haab, P., Piper, J., and Rahn, H. (1960). Venous admixture in the pulmonary circulation of anesthetized dogs. *J. Appl. Physiol.* **15**:48.

Fishman, A. P., Turino, G. M., Brandfonbrenner, M., and Himmelstein, A. (1958). The "effective pulmonary" collateral blood flow in man. *J. Clin. Invest.* **37**:1071.

Fox, I. J., and Wood, E. H. (1957). Application of dye dilution curves recorded from the right side of the heart or venous circulation with the aid of a new indicator dye. *Proc. Staff. Meet. Mayo Clin.* **32**:541.

Fritts, H. E., Jr., Harris, P., Chidsey, C. A., III, Clauss, R. H., and Cournand, A. (1957). Validation of a method for measuring the output of the right ventricle in man by inscription of dye dilution curves from the pulmonary artery. *J. Appl. Physiol.* **11**:362.

Galen, C. (1562). *Tractat*. Basel, Frobeniane edit. Lib. 6 cap. 3.

Galen, C. (ca. 180). *De venarum arterioramque dissectione*, 9. K. II.819.

Ghoreyeb, A. A., and Karsner, H. T. (1913). A study of the relation of pulmonary and bronchial circulation. *J. Exp. Med.* **18**:500.

Gray, F. D. Jr., Jurie, P. R., and Whittemore, R. (1951). Circulatory changes in chronic pulmonary disease. *Yale J. Biol. Med.* **23**:380.

Gross, L. (1919). Preliminary report on reconstruction of circulation of liver, placenta and lung in health and disease. *J. Can. Med. Assoc.* **3**:632.

Guillot, N. (1845). *Arch. Gen. Med.* Series 4. **7**(1):151–258.

Harvey, W. (1628). *De Motu Cordis*. Holland, J. M. Fleischman.

Horine, C. F., and Warner, C. G. (1932). Distribution of the pulmonary and bronchial circulation. An experimental study. *J. Thorac. Surg.* **2**:80.

Hudson, C. L., Moritz, A. R., and Wearn, J. T. (1932). The extra cardiac anastomoses of the coronary arteries. *J. Exp. Med.* **56**:919.

Karsner, H. T., and Ash, J. E. (1912). Studies in infarction. II. Experimental bland infarction of the lung. *J. Med. Res.* **27**:205–224.

Karsner, H. T., and Ghoreyeb, A. A. (1913). Studies in infarction. III. The circulation in experimental pulmonary embolism. *J. Exp. Med.* **18**:507.

Keele, K. D. (1952). *Leonardo da Vinci: Movement of the Heart and Blood.* London, Harvey and Blythe.

Koenigstein, H. (1903). *Anat. Hefte.* **22**:309.

Kuettner, C. (1878). Beitrag zur Kenntniss der Kreislaufsverhältnisse der Saugethierlunge. *Virchows Arch.* **73**:476–523.

Le Fort, L. (1858). *Recherches sur l'anatomie du poumon chez l'homme.* These, Paris.

Levinson, G. E., Cudkowicz, L., and Abelmann, W. H. (1959). Measurement of regional blood flow by indicator dilution. *Science* **129**:640.

Liebow, A. A. (1953). The bronchopulmonary venous collateral circulation with special reference to emphysema. *Am J. Pathol.* **29**:251.

Liebow, A. A. (1959). Discussion of structural alterations of pulmonary vessels in response to pulmonary hypertension. *Pulmonary Circulation.* Edited by W. Adams and I. Veith. New York, Grune and Stratton, p. 124.

Liebow, A. A., Hales, M. R., and Lindskog, G. E. (1949). Enlargement of the bronchial arteries and their anastomoses with the pulmonary arteries in bronchiectasis. *Am. J. Pathol.* **25**:211.

Madoff, I. M., Gaensler, E. A., and Strieder, S. W. (1952). Congenital absence of the right pulmonary artery. *N. Engl. J. Med.* **247**:149.

Mathes, M. E., Holman, E., and Reichert, F. L. (1932). A study of the bronchial pulmonary and lymphatic circulation of the lung. *J. Thorac. Surg.* **1**:339.

Meyerhof, M. (1935). Ibn an Nafis (13th century) and his theory of the lesser circulation (1515). **23**:100.

Miller, W. S. (1925). The vascular supply of the bronchial tree. *Am. Rev. Tuberc.* **12**:87.

Miller, W. S. (1947). *The Lung*, 2nd ed. Springfield, Illinois.

Nakamura, N. (1924). Zur Anatomie der Bronchialarterien. *anat. Anz.* **58**:508.

Nakamura, T., Katori, R., Miyazawa, K., et al. (1961). Bronchial blood flow in patients with chronic pulmonary disease. *Dis. Chest* **39**:192.

Olkon, D. M., and Johanides, M. (1930). *Arch. Intern. Med.* **45**:201.

Panum, P. L. (1862). Experimentale Beitrage zur Lehre der Embolie. *Virchows Arch. [A]* **25**:308.

Reisseissen, F. D., and von Sömmering, S. T. (1808). *Über den Bau der Lungen*. Berlin.

Rindfleisch, E. (1878). *Handbuch der Gewebelehre*, 5th ed. Leipzig.

Rossignol, H. (1848). *Recherches sur la structure intime du poumon de l'homme*. Bruxelles.

Royal Academy of Arts, London (1952). *Catalogue*. Quincentenary Exhibition of Drawings by Leonardo da Vinci, p. 85.

Ruyisch, F. (1732). *Epistola anatomica.* Amsterdam, Probl. Sexto.

Ryan, T. J., and Abelmann, W. H. (1961). Response of bronchial blood flow to tissue proliferation in the human lung. *J. Clin. Invest.* **40**:1077.

Schlaepfer, K. (1926). The effect of the ligation of the pulmonary artery of one lung with and without resection of the phrenic nerve. *Arch. Surg.* **13**:623–629.

Servetus, M. (1533). *Christianismi restitutio*. Translated by C. D. O'Malley. American Philosophical Society, 1953.

Stewart, G. N. (1921). The pulmonary circulation time, the quantity of blood in the lungs and the output of the heart. *Am. J. Physiol.* **58**:20.

Suslow, K. I. (1895). *Some Investigations on the Anatomy of the Bronchial Arteries in Man*. Translated from Russian. Thesis, University of St. Petersburg.

Töndury, G., and Weibel, E. (1956). Über das Vorkommen von Blutgefässanastomosen in der menschlichen Lunge. *Schweiz. Med. Wochenschr.* **86**:265.

Virchow, R. (1847). Über die Standpunkte in der Wissenschaftlichen Medizin. *Virchows Arch. [A]* **1**:1–19.

Virchow, R. (1856). *Gesammelte Abhandlungen zur Wissenschaftlichen Medizin*. Frankfurta. M. Vol. 20, p. 385.

von Luschka, H. (1863). *Die Anatomie des Menschen*, Vol. I. Tubingen.

Wagner, H. N., Jr., Sagiston, M., Jr., Iio, J. C., McAfee, J. K., Meyer, K., and Langan J. K. (1964). Regional pulmonary blood flow in man by radioisotope scanning. *JAMA* **187**:601.

Wearn, J. T., Ernstene, A. C., Bromer, A. W., Barr, J. S., German, W. J., and Zschiesche, L. J. (1934). The normal behavior of pulmonary blood vessels with observations on the intermittence of the flow of blood. *Am. J. Physiol.* **109**:236–256.

Weibel, E. (1958). Die Entstehung der Längsmuskulature in den Ästen der Arteria Bronchialis. *Z. Zellforsch.* **47**:440.

Weibel, E. (1963). *Morphometry of the Human Lung*. New York, Academic Press.

Zuckerkandl, E. (1881). Über die Anastomosen der Venaepulmonales mit den Venae bronchiales. *Sitzungsberichte Akad. Wiss. Wien.* **3**:84–110.

Zuckerkandl, E. (1883). Verbindungen der arteriellen Gefässe der menschlichen Lunge. *Math.-Nat. Kl. Sitzungsberichte Akad. Wiss. Wien.* **2**:87–171.

Part II

STRUCTURE

2

Anatomy of the Normal Bronchial Circulatory System in Humans and Animals

NIRMAL B. CHARAN and PAULA G. CARVALHO

Veterans Administration Medical Center
Boise, Idaho
and University of Washington School of Medicine
Seattle, Washington

I. Introduction

The lung has two distinct circulatory systems. The pulmonary circulation is a low-pressure vascular system that has predominantly a gas-exchange function. In contrast, the bronchial circulation is a high-pressure system that provides nutrition to the walls of the bronchial tree, the large pulmonary blood vessels, some hilar structures, including lymph nodes, the lung parenchyma, and the visceral pleura. Since these two circulatory systems have different functions, their development and consequently their structure are also different. The anatomy of the pulmonary circulation has been studied extensively; however, the anatomic details of the bronchial circulation have received attention only in recent years.

The importance of the bronchial circulation has been known for centuries. For example, Virchow (1847) demonstrated that ligation of a pulmonary artery did not result in lung infarction. He also showed that the bronchial arteries supplying the occluded lung increased in size and postulated that they must be responsible for providing nutrition to the lung. Despite this finding over 100 years ago, the functional importance of the bronchial circulatory system was largely ignored until recent years. The role of the bronchial circulation in providing nutrition to the airways became evident following lung transplantation, when ischemia and infarction of the bronchus developed in the transplanted lung (Veith et al., 1983; Mills et al., 1970). In addition, it was found that life-threatening hemoptysis was most often from the bronchial circulation, and techniques have been developed to cannulate and embolize the bronchial artery (Viamonte et al., 1965; Roberts, 1990; Cohen et al., 1990). The bronchial circulation has also been shown to play an important role in the conditioning of inspired air (Baile et al., 1985) and may be involved in exercise-induced asthma (Cabanes et al., 1989). The anatomy, physiology, and clinical relevance of the bronchial circulation continue to be under active investigation.

Because we have only begun to understand the physiological and clinical importance of the bronchial circulation, it is pertinent to have an understanding of the anatomy of this system. Therefore, the purpose of this chapter is to review the anatomy of the bronchial circulatory system in humans as well as in some commonly used laboratory animal species.

II. Embryology

The embryology of the bronchial circulatory system has not been studied in detail. A few reports have described the embryology in humans; however, similar information is not yet available for other animals.

The pulmonary and bronchial circulatory systems in the human embryo develop from the primitive aortic arches, which appear during the first month. Tobin (1952) systematically studied the embryology of the bronchial blood vessels in serially sectioned human embryos varying in age from 4 to 7 weeks. He also studied sections of lungs from fetuses 2–9 months of age. These studies were performed in uninjected fetuses or fetuses injected with solutions of India ink, liquid latex, vinyl acetate, or colored gelatin. Other studies were made of vascular casts obtained by injecting the pulmonary vessels with vinyl acetate or liquid latex. He found that during the fourth week of gestation branches from the paired dorsal aortas form a capillary plexus around the developing lungs, trachea, and esophagus. Thus, the initial blood supply to the developing lungs is associated with the systemic circulation. Additional arterial branches are also derived from the developing fourth aortic arch and the aortic sac.

The pulmonary arteries develop from the sixth aortic arch and fuse with the pulmonary plexus around the developing lungs. With this fusion, the blood supply of the pulmonary plexus reverts to the pulmonary arteries and the ventral branches of the aorta regress. There is a stage, however, when the pulmonary plexus is supplied by both sources, implying that during early development anastomoses exist between the aortic branches and the pulmonary arteries. Tobin (1952) suggested that these aortic branches do not regress completely and later form the bronchial arteries. On the other hand, Boyden (1970a) described development of the bronchial artery from the aorta. By examining stained sections, he found that by the sixth to seventh week (25 mm embryo), the bifurcation of the trachea descends to a level below the ductus arteriosus. At this time there is an outgrowth of a capillary sprout from the aorta, which becomes the future tracheobronchial artery. The bronchial arteries assume their definitive form by approximately eight weeks. Thus it is not until the ninth week that growth alters these relations and the maturing of tissue favors induction of the lower bronchial arteries.

Boyden (1970a) described the presence of a bronchial artery to the trachea and left main bronchus in a 9 week (41 mm) fetus and suggested that it was the first to appear. On the other hand, in a 12 week fetus, there are three bronchial arteries to the left lung and one to the right lung (Boyden, 1970b). Hence, in humans, the bronchial arteries tend to appear between the eighth and the ninth weeks of gestation. Subsequently, these bronchial arteries grow out into the lungs along the segmental bronchi, keeping pace with cartilage formation. Figure 1 shows the relationship of the esophagus, aorta, pulmonary trunk, aortic trunk, and bronchial arteries in a 12 week fetus.

Boyden (1970b) suggests that the development of the bronchial arterial system is complete by 26 weeks, which incidentally corresponds with the time that the fetus becomes viable.

The presence of anastomoses between the bronchial and pulmonary circulations have been demonstrated in human fetuses. Wangenvoort and Wangenvoort (1967), using sectioned material, found extensive bronchial arterial and bronchopulmonary anastomoses (20–110 μm in diameter) in 10 fetuses 26–37 weeks of age.

III. Anatomy

The origin and distribution of the bronchial arteries vary greatly from species to species (McLaughlin 1983). The anatomy of the bronchial circulatory system has been studied in detail in humans and sheep and, to a lesser degree, in other mammals and some avian species.

A. Humans

In humans the bronchial arteries usually arise from the aorta or intercostal arteries. The number of bronchial arteries for each lung has been studied by several investigators with somewhat different findings (Cauldwell et al., 1948; Liebow, 1965; Kasai and Chiba, 1979; Meckel (1831–1832); Hovelacque et

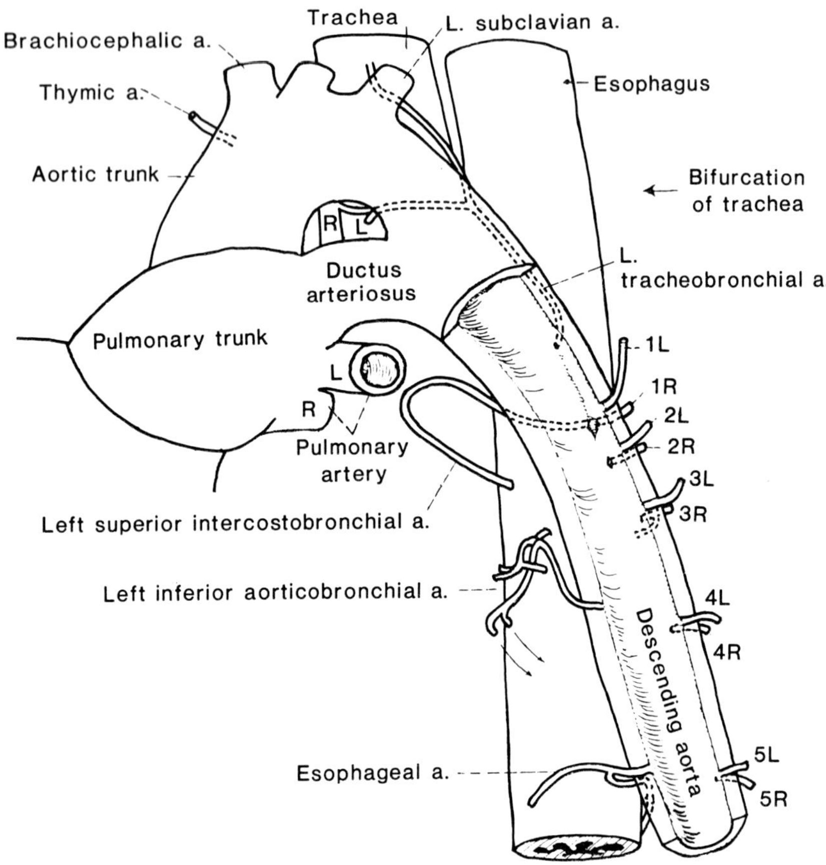

Figure 1 Bronchial arteries of a 83 gestational day human fetus (85 mm length). The numbering indicates order of paired intercostal arteries (L, left; R, right). (From Boyden, 1970b, with permission.)

al., 1936). Cauldwell et al. (1948) dissected the origin of the bronchial arteries in 150 human cadavers and concluded that the majority of the vessels originated directly from the aorta. They found that the most common presentation was two arteries to the left lung and one to the right lung (41%), as shown in Fig. 2. The next most common presentation was one artery to each lung (21%), followed by two arteries to each lung (21%). This study has been criticized because the anatomic relationships of the bronchial artery with other structures were not adequately described and cardiac malformations in these subjects were not excluded.

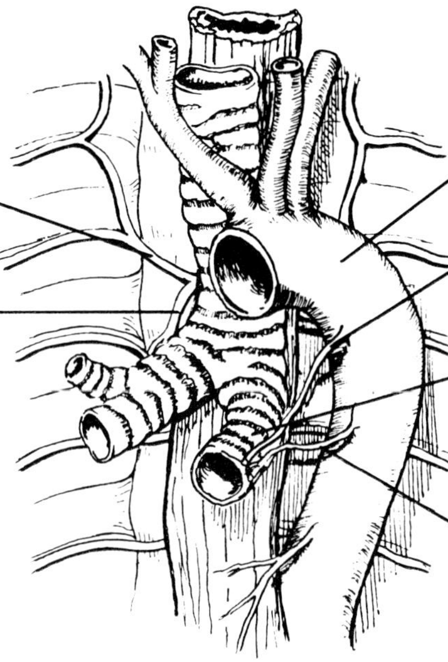

Figure 2 Origin of the bronchial arteries.

Liebow (1965) studied 50 normal human lungs by injecting vinyl plastic into the aorta. He found that the main bronchial arterial supply came either directly from the aorta or by mediation of an intercostobronchial artery. He referred to these vessels as posterior bronchial arteries. On the other hand, he used the term "accessory bronchial arteries" for blood vessels reaching the bronchi from branches of the aorta other than the aortic intercostal arteries. He found that the most common arrangement, accounting for 30% of all specimens, consisted of two posterior bronchial arteries to each lung. This pattern was confirmed by a more recent study by Kasai and Chiba in 1979 and is also consistent with an earlier observation by Meckel in 1831–1832. These four arteries may be identified as right superior, right inferior, left superior, and left inferior bronchial arteries. The second most common arrangement (20%) was that of two left and one right bronchial artery, a pattern thought to be "classic" by Cauldwell et al. (1948). Liebow (1965) found that the inverse arrangement, two right and one left bronchial artery, was almost as common as the classic pattern, although it was only one-fourth as frequent in the Cauldwell series. On the other hand, Schreinemakers et al (1990) studied 30 autopsy cases and found that the most common pattern, accounting for 26.6% of cases, was one right and two left bronchial arteries, followed by two right and two left bronchial arteries. Fourth in frequency was a single main trunk to each bronchus. These four groups accounted for 76% of the specimens in the Liebow (1965) series and for 92% of those in the Cauldwell et al. (1948) series.

The origin of the bronchial arteries is also quite variable. The posterior bronchial artery may originate either directly from the aorta or from a branch that also yields an intercostal artery (intercostobronchial trunk). In Liebow's study (1965), 66% of the specimens exhibited bronchial arteries of both modes of origin; in 26% there was an aortic origin only, and in 8% all bronchial arteries came from an intercostobronchial trunk. The respective percentage in an older series was 80, 18, and 2% (Nakamura, 1924). At least one intercostobronchial trunk was present in 37 of the 50 specimens (74%). In Cauldwell et al.'s series (1948), the intercostobronchial trunk was present in 89% of specimens, and in Nakamura's series (1924) it was present in 81%. This vessel also yields the first aortic intercostal artery. In the majority of cases, there is only a single intercostobronchial trunk. All intercostobronchial trunks originate from the right side of the aorta, even those that supply a bronchial artery to the left bronchial tree (Liebow, 1965). Of all right bronchial arteries 43% are of intercostobronchial origin, whereas 84% of left bronchial arteries arise directly from the aorta.

A fairly recent Japanese study found two right and two left bronchial arteries to be the most common pattern (Kasai and Chiba, 1979). They found that the right superior artery usually arose from the right first aortic intercostal artery. A small branch sometimes arose from the right subclavian artery and connected to the right superior bronchial artery. The right inferior artery had the most variable course. It frequently arose directly from the aorta and crossed ventral to the left bronchus. In more than 50% of cases it formed a common trunk with the left inferior artery. The left superior artery arose from the aortic arch or from the descending aorta close to the left recurrent laryngeal nerve. Small branches sometimes arose from the left subclavian artery and joined the left superior bronchial artery. The left inferior artery usually arose from the descending aorta behind the left bronchus. In about half of the cases it formed a common trunk with the right inferior artery.

A single bronchial vessel may supply both lungs and is called the common trunk. In 85% of cases there is at least one common trunk that supplies both lungs.

In 75% of cases, all major bronchial arteries arise at the level of the first or second aortic intercostal arteries, that is, at the level of the fifth or sixth thoracic vertebrae (Liebow, 1965). In approximately 50% of cases, some smaller bronchial arteries may arise above the first aortic intercostal artery on the anterior or the right lateral surface of the aorta. Infrequently, the accessory bronchial arteries may arise from the innominate artery, the subclavian artery, and the internal mammary, pericardiophrenic, and esophageal arteries (Viamonte et al., 1965).

At their site of origin within the mediastinum, a bronchomediastinal plexus is formed that supplies most of the mediastinal structures, including the esophagus, hilar lymph nodes, vasa vasorum of the thoracic aorta, pericardium, mediastinal pleura, and vagus nerves (Viamonte et al., 1989). Upon reaching the main bronchus on each side, the vessels form an annulus surrounding the bronchus (Cudkowicz, 1979). They enter the lungs through the hilum and divide upon reaching the mainstem bronchus on each side in the peribronchial connective tissue sheath and then follow the branches of the bronchial tree (Nakamura, 1924; Cudkowicz and Armstrong, 1951). Generally, two or three branches of the bronchial artery wind around and supply the wall of the bronchus. They follow the airways as far as the terminal bronchioles. The branches anastomose freely with each other, forming a plexus in the peribronchial space. They also give rise to small branches that penetrate the muscular layer to reach the bronchial mucosa, where they form the submucosal plexus. Thus, there is a submucosal as well as a peribronchial vascular plexus along the entire length of the bronchial tree to the terminal bronchioles. The bronchial arteries also supply the walls of the pulmonary artery and the pulmonary vein. Figure 3 shows the submucosal bronchial microvascular plexus just underneath the bronchial epithelium.

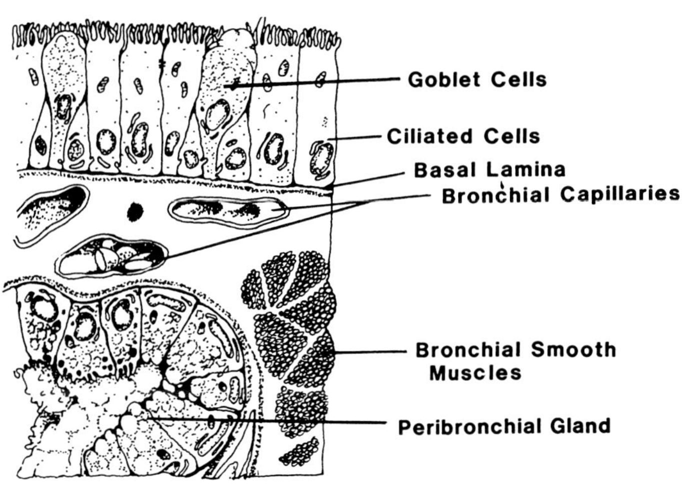

Figure 3 Cross section of a main bronchus showing the relationship of the bronchial microvasculature with bronchial epithelium, bronchial smooth muscles, and submucosal glands.

Cudkowicz (1979) injected 10 pairs of human lungs with contrast material and found that branches of the bronchial arteries also supplied the visceral pleura. The medial surface of the visceral pleura receives vessels from the annulus formed by the branches of the bronchial arteries at the hilum. The anterior, lateral, and interlobar visceral pleurae receive their blood supply from the distal branches of bronchial arteries that supply the airways and penetrate the lung parenchyma to reach the pleura (Cudkowicz and Armstrong, 1951; Cudkowicz, 1979).

At the hilum the bronchial arteries have a diameter of approximately 1.5 mm, which decreases to approximately 0.75–0.5 mm at the point of entry into a bronchopulmonary segment (Pump, 1972). There appears to be no relationship between the lumina of the bronchi and the size of the bronchial arteries (Liebow, 1965).

The dense arteriolar network around the bronchi terminates in the bronchial capillaries and bronchial venous plexus, which have an irregular shape and course (Murata et al., 1986). The vessels in the bronchial venous plexus have thin walls and are irregular compared to the bronchial arteries. They are present along the entire length of the bronchial tree as far distally as the terminal bronchioles (Fig. 4). The number of vessels decreases in proportion to the reducing caliber of the bronchi and bronchioles.

Bronchopulmonary Connections

The bronchial microvascular plexus anastomoses with the pulmonary microvasculature along the airway and beyond the terminal bronchioles (Fig. 5). Wagenvoort and Wagenvoort (1967) found, in perinatal lungs, branches arising from medium-sized bronchial arteries that did not supply the bronchi but ended in the pulmonary alveolar microvessels. They termed these vessels "bronchopulmonary arteries." These arteries are evident but are seen less frequently in older children and adults (Wagenvoort and Wagenvoort, 1967; Wagenvoort et al., 1964). Tobin (1952) described two types of large anastomoses: one relatively short (1–2 mm) and narrow (50–100 μm in diameter) found within lobular subdivisions of the lung, and the other longer (10–40 mm) and wider (300–400 μm), found between branches of the bronchial artery at segmental bronchi and connecting to more distally placed branches of the pulmonary artery. The anastomotic vessels appeared to be coiled, possibly because of the spiral musculature in their walls. He suggested that the coiled structure may help to regulate the pressure gradient from bronchial to pulmonary vessels. Cudkowicz (1979), using radiopaque injections of the lung, was unable to find precapillary anastomoses between the bronchial artery and the pulmonary artery.

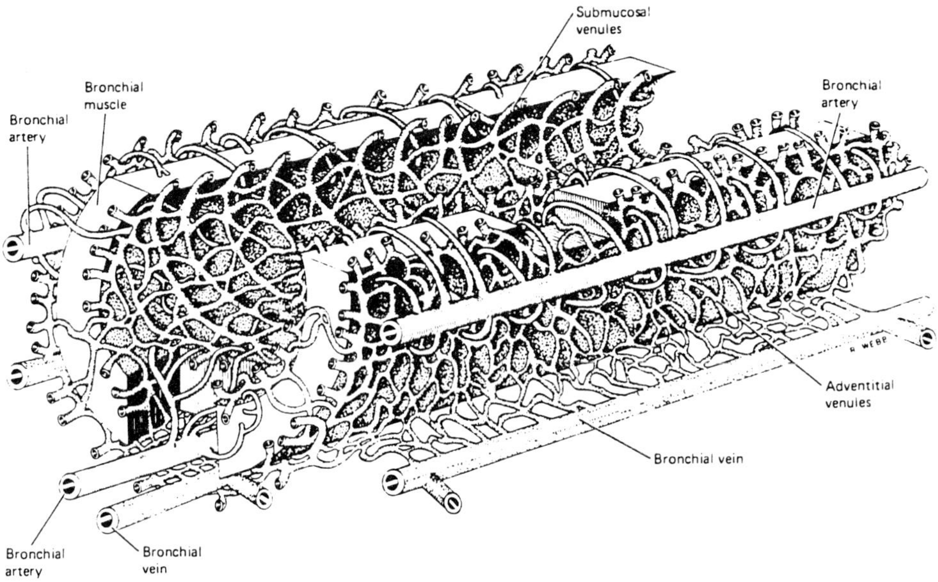

Figure 4 The bronchial venous network in a segment of the tracheobronchial tree illustrating the submucosal location of the plexus and interconnections with a venous plexus on the adventitial side of the muscle. (From Fishman, A. P., *Pulmonary Diseases and Disorders*. © 1980 McGraw-Hill, New York, p. 400.)

Murata et al. (1986) studied 10 normal adult lungs obtained at autopsy using radiopaque injection techniques. They described communications between bronchial vessels and small branches of the pulmonary veins. These communications were better visualized when the pulmonary veins were infused with radiocontrast material. Histological studies revealed that the vascular network communicating with the pulmonary vein consisted of a bronchial venous plexus that had a characteristic thin wall and irregular shape. These communications were found even in the 1 mm bronchioles. The bronchial vessels around the pulmonary vein also communicated with small branches of the pulmonary vein. Thus, the entire bronchial venous system around the airways and blood vessels was connected with the pulmonary vein through small branches.

Murata et al. (1986) also found direct communications of the bronchial venous plexus with the surrounding alveolar capillaries through small venules present in both bronchi and bronchioles. The bronchial venous plexus in the

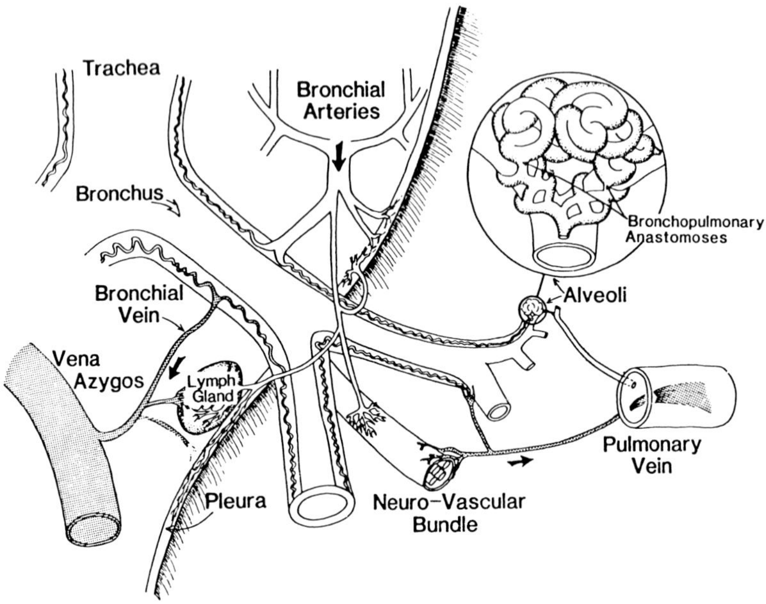

Figure 5 The systemic blood supply to the lung. The blood flow from the extrapulmonary airways and supporting structures returns to the right heart, whereas blood from the intrapulmonary airways becomes anastomotic with the pulmonary circulation and returns to the left atrium. (From Deffebach et al., 1987, with permission from the *American Review of Respiratory Disease.)*

pleura also appeared to have communications with the branches of the pulmonary vein.

Bronchopulmonary anastomoses may have functional implications. Because of the dense vascular communications that exist between the pulmonary veins and the bronchial venous plexus, it is possible that a rise in pulmonary venous pressure is reflected into the bronchial venous plexus. Furthermore, because the peribronchial interstitial pressure is more negative than that in the alveolar wall, it is possible that increases in the hydrostatic pressure in the pulmonary vein could result in fluid transudation from the bronchial venous plexus. This may explain the presence of peribronchial interstitial cuffs of edema fluid in early interstitial pulmonary edema.

It has been shown that when the pulmonary artery becomes occluded, the bronchial circulation hypertrophies and bronchial blood flow increases. Because the bronchial circulation anastomoses with the pulmonary circulation at the precapillary level, it is possible that the bronchial blood perfuses the pulmonary capillaries after pulmonary artery occlusion and thus may have a role in gas exchange. A few studies have indicated that oxygen uptake and significant CO_2 elimination can occur from the bronchial circulation in the absence of pulmonary blood flow (Charan and Carvalho, 1989; Lilker and Nagy, 1975). Bronchopulmonary anastomoses have been shown to increase in number and size in many other cardiopulmonary diseases (Turner-Warwick, 1963).

Other Bronchial Arterial Anastomoses

The bronchial arteries also have anastomoses with other vascular beds. There is normally an extensive extrapulmonary anastomosis between the bronchial arteries and those vessels supplying adjacent structures in the mediastinum, including the coronary, esophageal, thymic, inferior thyroid, intercostal, internal mammary, left subclavian, innominate, right vertebral, pericardiophrenic, and thyrocervical arteries (Daly and Hebb, 1966; Rees, 1981).

The anastomosis between the bronchial and the coronary circulation may become important in certain clinical conditions. Normally anastomoses between the coronary circulation and the bronchial circulation are small and nonfunctional. However, these anastomoses may become functional when a gradient develops between the coronary and the bronchial vascular beds. In certain conditions shunting of blood from coronary to bronchial arteries may develop, and this has been termed "bronchial artery steal syndrome" (Steffas et al., 1990). This may occur in aortic stenosis (Villar do Valle et al., 1969), Takayasu's arteritis (Halon et al., 1987), and the tetralogy of Fallot (Bjork, 1966; Zureikat, 1980). In patients with normal coronary arteries and a chest pain syndrome, coronary to bronchial artery anastomosis with the bronchial steal syndrome has been incriminated for causing myocardial ischemia (Steffas et al., 1990).

Bronchial Veins

The venous blood from the proximal tracheobronchial tree (first two or three subdivisions, mainly extrapulmonary) drains into the bronchial veins, which become continuous with mediastinal vessels (Fig. 5). These proceed to the azygous system and drain through the superior vena cava to the right heart (Gilroy, 1952; Liebow, 1959). These veins may have valves, and if so, the venous drainage is unidirectional toward the right heart (Liebow, 1953). The major portion of the intrapulmonary bronchial venous flow drains into the pulmonary circulation and subsequently into the left atrium (Fig. 5). Marchand et al. (1950) injected vinylite through the left atrial appendage and described "deep or true bronchial veins." These veins terminated either directly into the left atrium or into the main pulmonary vein close to the left atrium. They found one such vein for each lung. The presence of these veins has not been confirmed in subsequent human studies.

Chiba et al. (1990) studied extrapulmonary bronchial veins in one patient with an azygos lobe. They found one or two small bronchial veins that took almost the same course as the bronchial arteries but diverged from them near their junctions with the major veins and around the thoracic aorta. The bronchial veins from each side communicated with each other. There were about nine bronchial veins on each side that drained into the brachiocephalic veins, left atrium, inferior thyroid vein, left pericardiophrenic, and the upper intercostal veins. In this case, they could not find bronchial venous drainage into the azygos vein.

B. Sheep

The anatomy of the bronchial circulation in sheep has been studied by several investigators (Magno and Fishman, 1982; Charan et al., 1984; Charan et al., 1987) using corrosion casting techniques. More recently, single-photon emission computed tomography (SPECT) has been utilized as a noninvasive means of studying the bronchial circulation (Chiles et al., 1990). Sheep have several distinct arterial branches that supply the tracheobronchial tree, and different investigators called them different names. Therefore, in 1987, the da Vinci Society for Study of the Bronchial Circulation adopted a uniform nomenclature for description of the bronchial circulation in sheep (Magno et al., 1987).

The bronchoesophageal artery usually originates from the ventral surface of the aorta and gives off a cranial branch called the thoracic tracheal artery (Figs. 6, 7 and 8). The caudal branch of the bronchoesophageal artery bifurcates into the esophageal and common bronchial arteries. The esophageal artery supplies the caudal mediastinal node, esophagus, and pleura. From its origin, the common bronchial branch travels cranially and to the right to reach the bifurcation of the trachea (Figs 7 and 8). Here, it divides into a right bronchial branch (ramus bronchialis dexter) and a left branch (ramus bronchialis sinister). These branches further divide into smaller branches and follow the bronchial tree to the terminal bronchioles. The common bronchial branch is the main source of blood supply to the bronchial tree, with the exception of the right cranial lobe (Fig. 9).

The tracheal bronchial branch (ramus bronchialis trachealis) measures <1 mm in diameter and originates from the brachiocephalic trunk (truncus brachiocephalicus) near the thoracic inlet (Figs. 6 and 8). It may also occasionally arise from the left subclavian or the bicarotid trunk. After its origin, the artery travels caudally and to the right to reach the tracheal bronchus (bronchus trachealis). It then divides, forms a plexus around the bronchus, and supplies the bronchial tree of the right cranial lobe (lobus cranialis dexter).

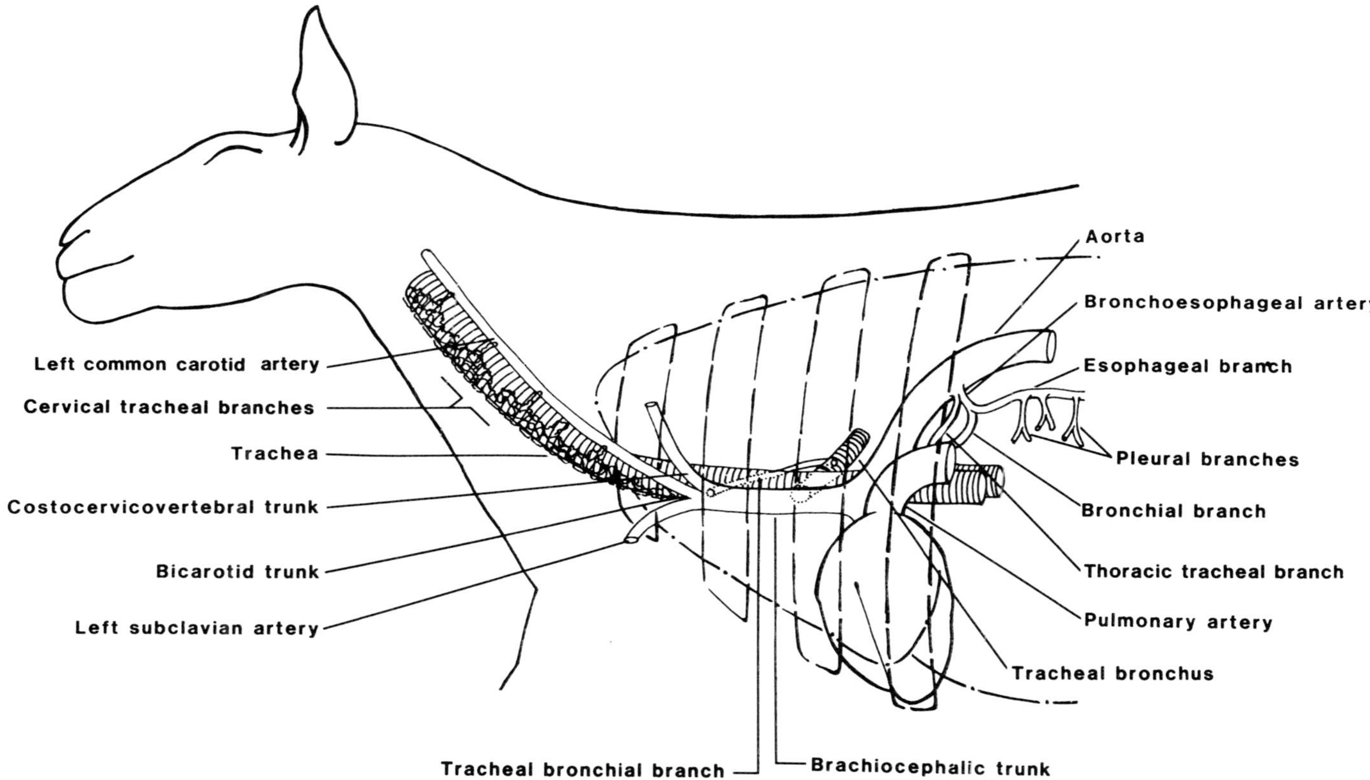

Figure 6 The systemic arterial blood supply to the tracheobronchial tree in sheep. (From Charan et al., 1987, with permission from the *Journal of Applied Physiology.*)

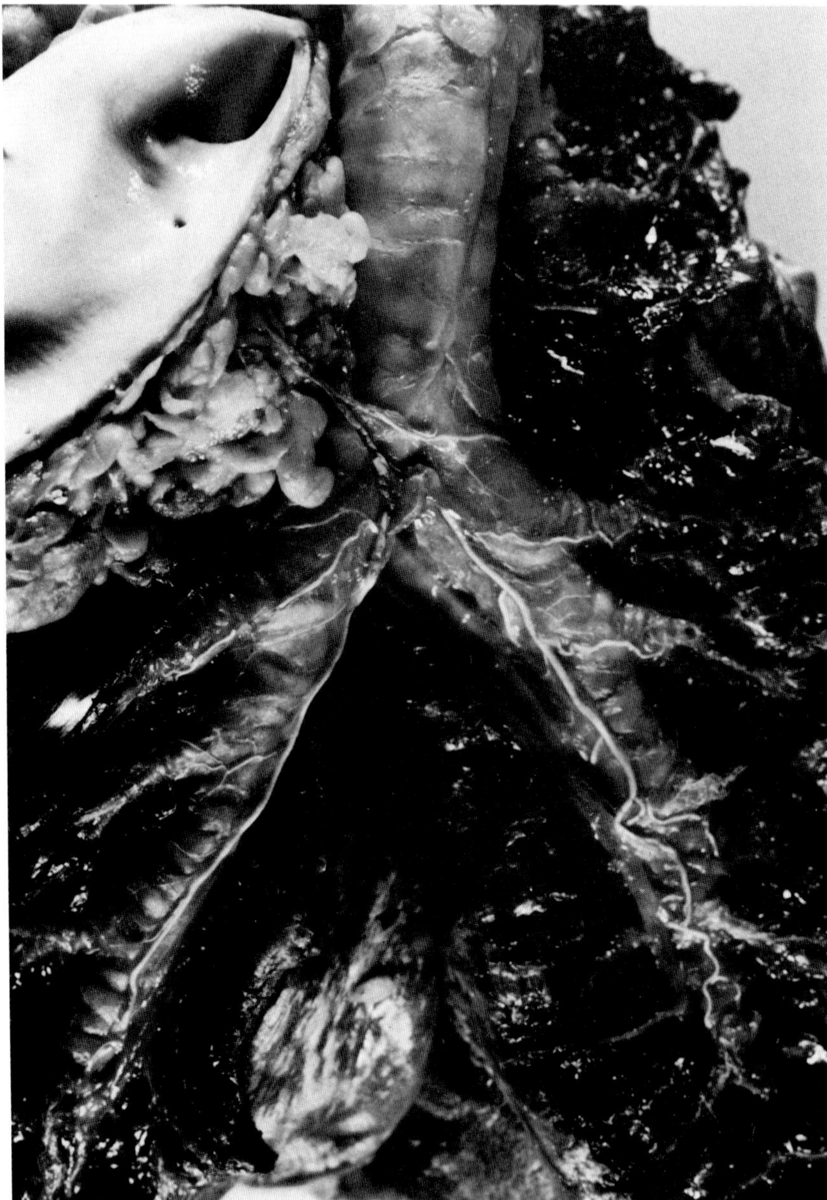

Figure 7 Dorsal view of the tracheobronchial tree of sheep. Batson's solution was injected into the bronchoesophageal artery. The specimen shows filling of the common bronchial artery and its division into the left and the right bronchial arteries.

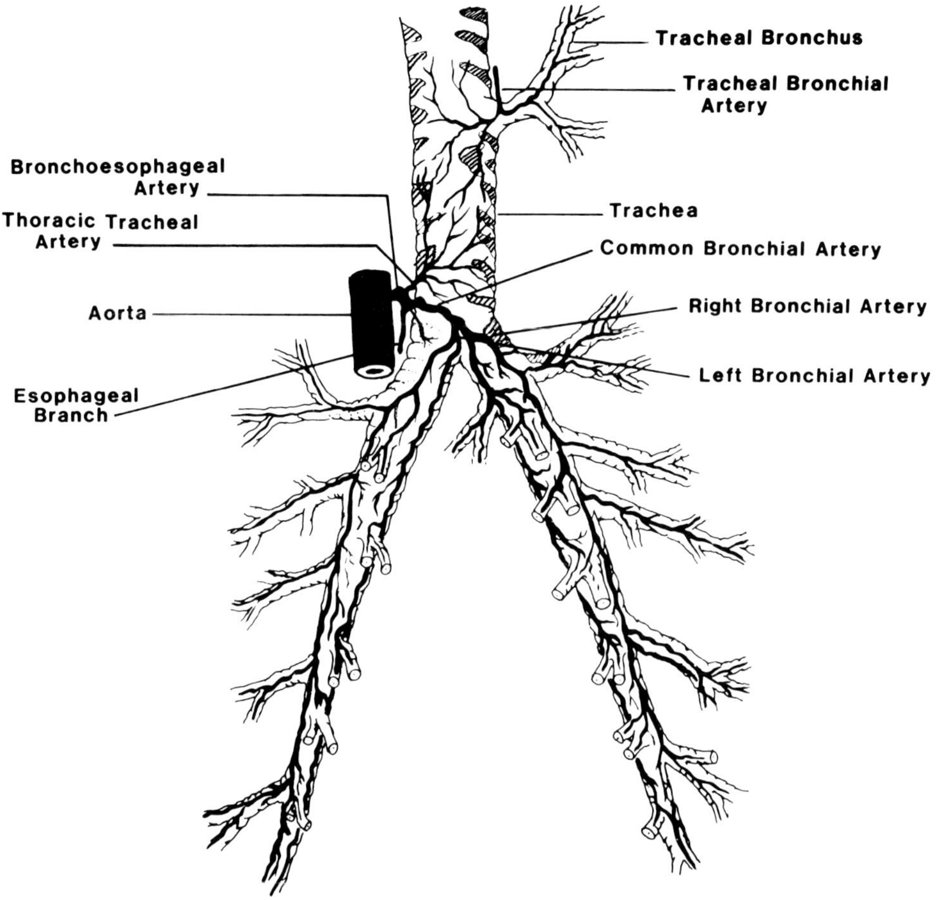

Figure 8 Detailed dorsal view showing the systemic arterial blood supply to the tracheobronchial tree in sheep.

Branches are also given off to the submucosa of the bronchus, to the pleura of the right cranial lobe, and to the portion of the thoracic trachea between the origin of the tracheal bronchus and the thoracic inlet (Fig. 9). This artery anastomoses with the common bronchial artery, the thoracic tracheal artery, and the cervical tracheal arteries. The venous blood from the intrapulmonary bronchial tree returns via bronchopulmonary anastomoses into the pulmonary circulation. The venous blood from the extrapulmonary bronchi drains into the cranial vena cava via small tributaries that join veins from other mediastinal

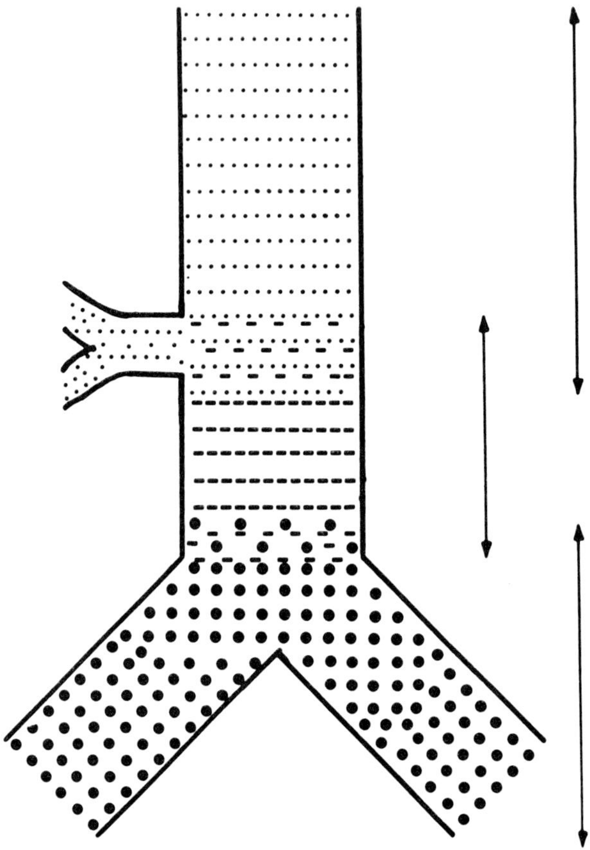

Figure 9 The relative distribution of arterial blood supply by three intrathoracic arteries to the tracheobronchial tree. (From Charan et al., 1987, with permission from the *Journal of Applied Physiology.)*

structures and form a medastinal vein. This vein terminates in the cranial vena cava 3–4 cm above the right atrium.

There is a small branch that supplies a portion of the thoracic trachea and is called the thoracic tracheal branch (ramus trachealis thoracica; (Figs. 6 and 8). This branch originates from the bronchoesophageal artery in about 50% of animals and from the thoracic aorta in 43% of animals ~3–5 cm craniad to the origin of the bronchoesophageal artery. It is not present in ~7% of the animals. The thoracic tracheal branch is <1 mm in diameter. From its origin, this branch travels cranially and to the right to reach the bifurcation of the trachea. The thoracic tracheal branch divides into several small branches and forms a rather sparse plexus around the trachea as well as a submucosal plexus. This branch supplies blood to the trachea from the origin of the tracheal bronchus to the tracheal carina (Fig. 10). A portion of the venous blood from the tracheal branch returns to the right heart via a bronchial vein, which in turn empties into the left azygos vein. In approximately half the animals, the thoracic tracheal branch also supplies the pleura of the left cranial

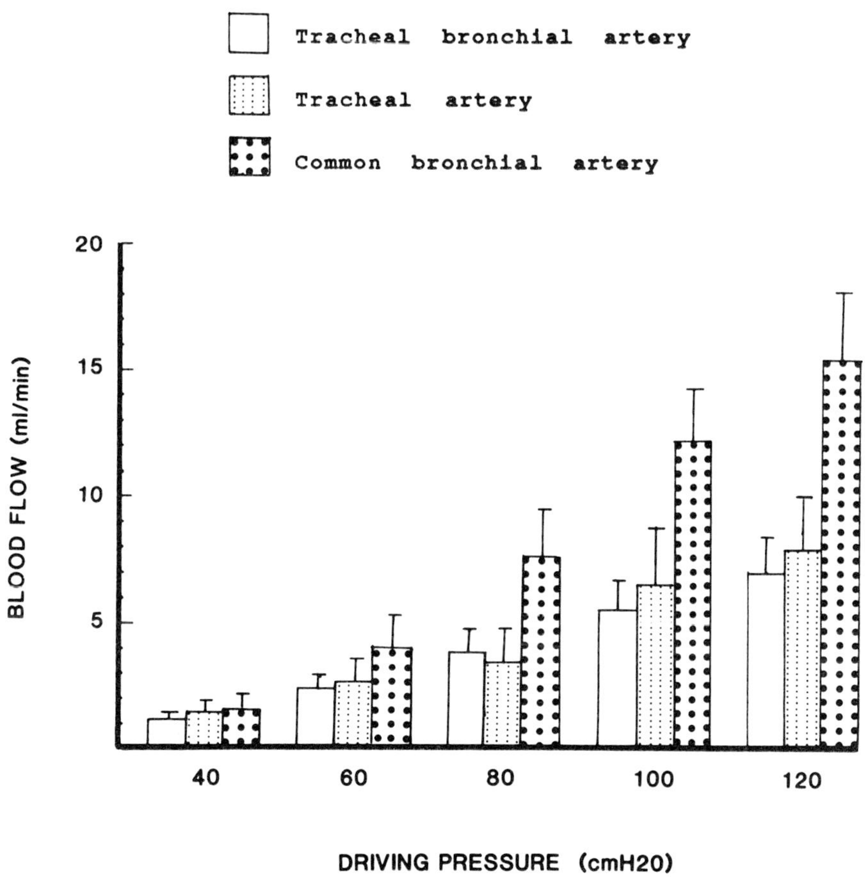

Figure 10 Relative blood flow of three systemic arteries supplying the intrathoracic tracheobronchial tree of the sheep. As the driving pressure (hydrostatic level above the left atrium) rises, the flow in the common bronchial artery increases relatively more than in the other arteries. (From Charan et al., 1987, with permission from the *Journal of Applied Physiology.*)

lobe (lobus cranialis sinistra). Anastomoses are present between the thoracic tracheal branch, the tracheal bronchial branch, and the common bronchial branch of the bronchoesophageal artery.

It has been estimated that the common bronchial branch contributes ~50% and the thoracic tracheal and the tracheobronchial artery ~25% each to the total tracheobronchial blood flow (Fig. 10) (Charan et al., 1987).

Vessels originating from either intercostal or coronary arteries have not been found to supply the tracheobronchial tree in sheep as they have in humans and dogs.

The intrapulmonary course of the bronchial artery in sheep is similar to that described in humans. The bronchial arteries descend the bronchi and give branches that form a microvascular plexus around the bronchi (Fig. 11). In sheep there is a peribronchial as well as a submucosal plexus (Fig. 12). These two plexus are connected with each other by small vessels. Figure 13 shows the arrangement of vessels in the wall of the bronchus. Beyond the terminal bronchioles the bronchial circulation merges with the pulmonary circulation. Figure 14 shows pulmonary capillary filling following the infusion of Batson's solution into the bronchial artery, suggesting that the bronchial circulation joins the pulmonary circulation at the precapillary level. It appears that bronchopulmonary anastomoses in sheep are more numerous on the pulmonary arterial side than on the pulmonary venous side (Charan et al., 1985). Blood from the extrapulmonary bronchi drains into the left azygos vein by a single small bronchial vein at a point close to the pericardium (Fig. 15). The intrapulmonary bronchial blood flow drains into the pulmonary circulation (Magno and Fishman, 1982).

Hill et al. (1989) studied the vascular network in the large airways of sheep by light, transmission, and scanning electron microscopy. They found an extensive plexus of large submucosal sinuses, up to 500 μm in diameter, deep in the mucosa close to the airway cartilage of the trachea and main bronchi (Fig. 16). They speculated that these sinuses could have a role in the conditioning of inspired air, helping to warm and humidify it. These sinuses were not described by other investigators (Magno and Fishman, 1982; Charan et al., 1984).

The anatomy of the bronchial circulation in the goat is quite similar to that described in the sheep.

C. Dogs

In dogs, the bronchial arteries usually arise from the first to the fifth right aortic intercostal arteries, but occasionally they arise from the sixth or the seventh intercostal arteries (Notkovich, 1957; Collier, 1979). Collier (1979) found that the bronchial artery arose from the fifth right intercostal artery in 74% of

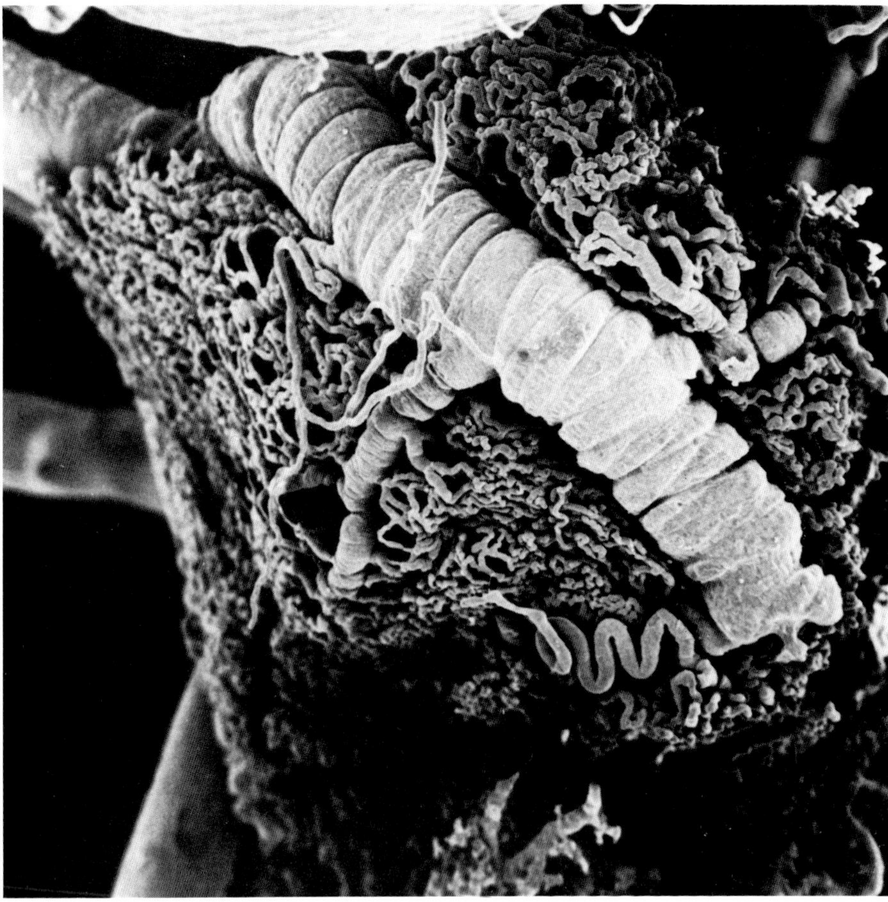

Figure 11 Scanning electron micrograph showing the bronchial microvascular plexus originating from the bronchial artery in a sheep bronchus. The bronchoesophageal artery was filled with Batson's solution, and the tissue was digested with potassium hydroxide solution. The cast was then examined with a scanning electron microscope.

dogs. An origin from the left intercostal arteries or directly from the aorta is uncommon. In about 66% of animals there is one right and one left bronchial artery.

Laitinen et al. (1989) studied the tracheobronchial circulation in dogs using light, transmission, and scanning electron microscopy. They described a

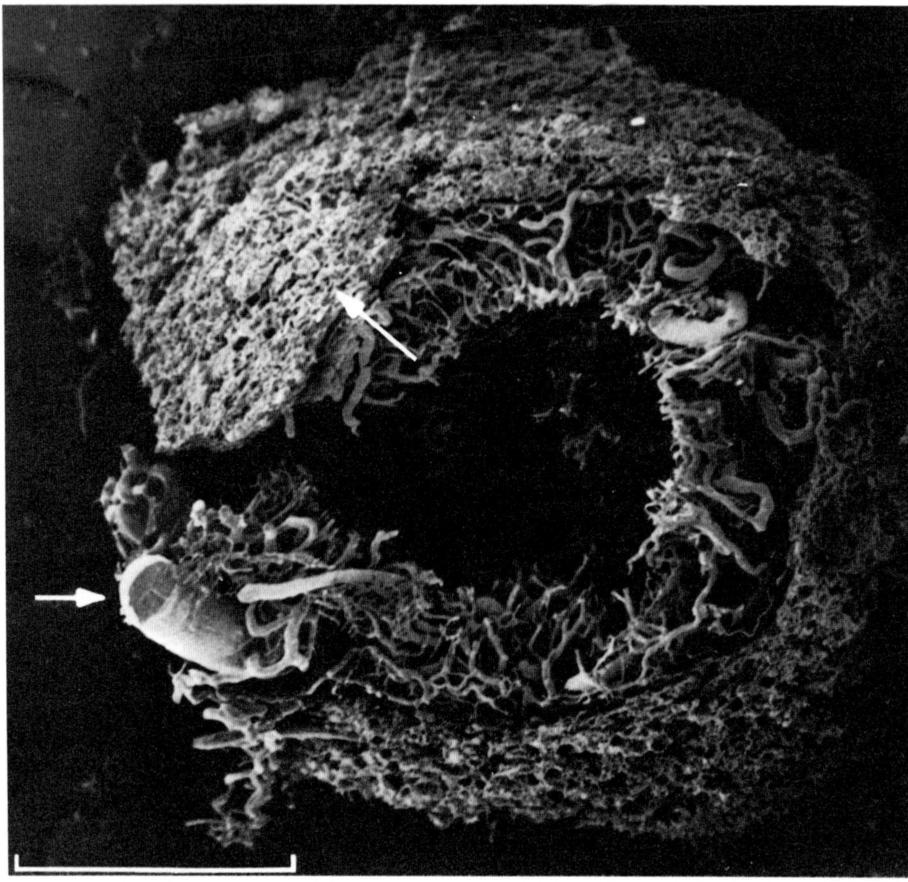

Figure 12 Scanning electron microscopy of a cross section of a small (1.5 mm) airway (bar = 500 μm) after filling the bronchial microvasculature with Batson's solution. Lower arrow points to the bronchial artery, which is approximately 300 μm in diameter. Bronchial capillaries are seen as a dense plexus of relatively thin vessels. Upper arrow points to the blanket of alveolar capillaries surrounding this plexus. (From Charan et al., 1984 with permission from the *Journal of Applied Physiology*.)

dense network of small vessels that ran in the trachea and bronchi close to the tracheobronchial lumen around and along the airway wall. This vascular network was just under the epithelial basement membrane. This capillary bed converged to form venules that extended to a deeper mucosal plexus formed by large venules and arterioles. The diameter of most vessels in the airway

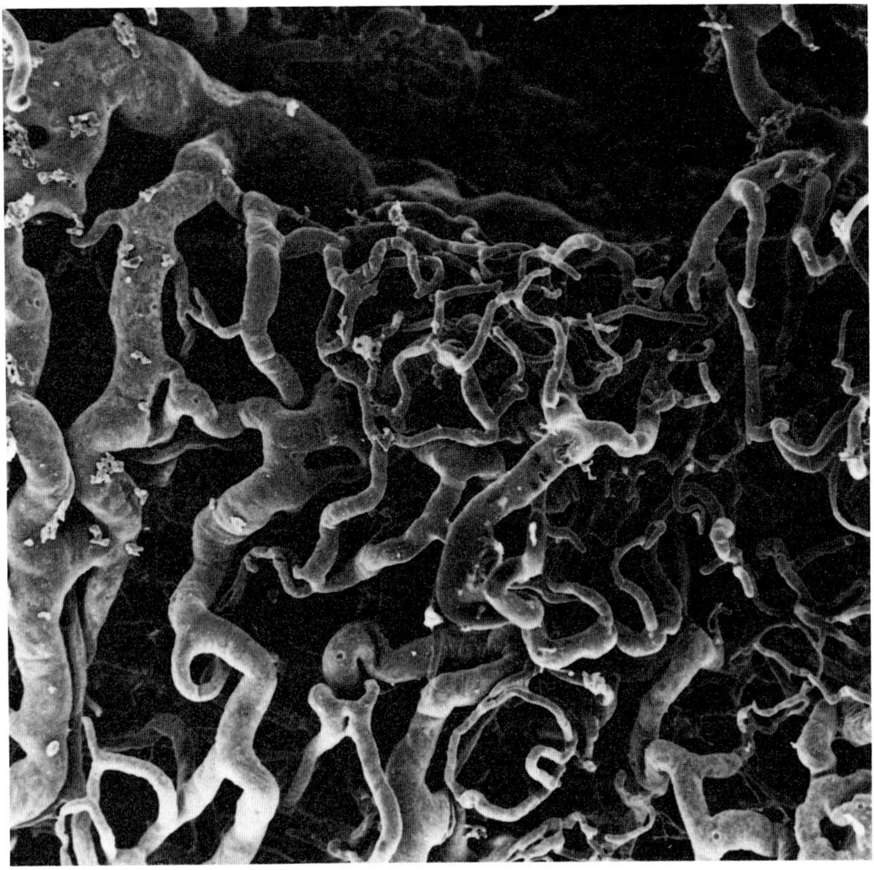

Figure 13 Relationship between bronchial and pulmonary microvasculature. Alveolar spaces are clearly seen in the capillary nctwork at the top. Capillaries can be seen to be somewhat flattened as a result of the geometry of the alveoli. Pulmonary capillaries are approximately the same diameter as the length between branches. Bronchial capillaries are seen in the lower half. The arrows point to distinct bronchopulmonary communications clearly visible along the interface of the two circulations. (From Charan et al., 1984, with permission from the *Journal of Applied Physiology*.)

mucosa was less than 30 μm. They did not find arteriovenous anastomoses. The trachea and the bronchi had similar vascular patterns, except that in the bronchi the capillaries had a more conspicuous longitudinal orientation.

Bronchial veins are formed near the hilum of the lung and collect venous blood from the extrapulmonary airways (Mathes et al., 1932). These veins

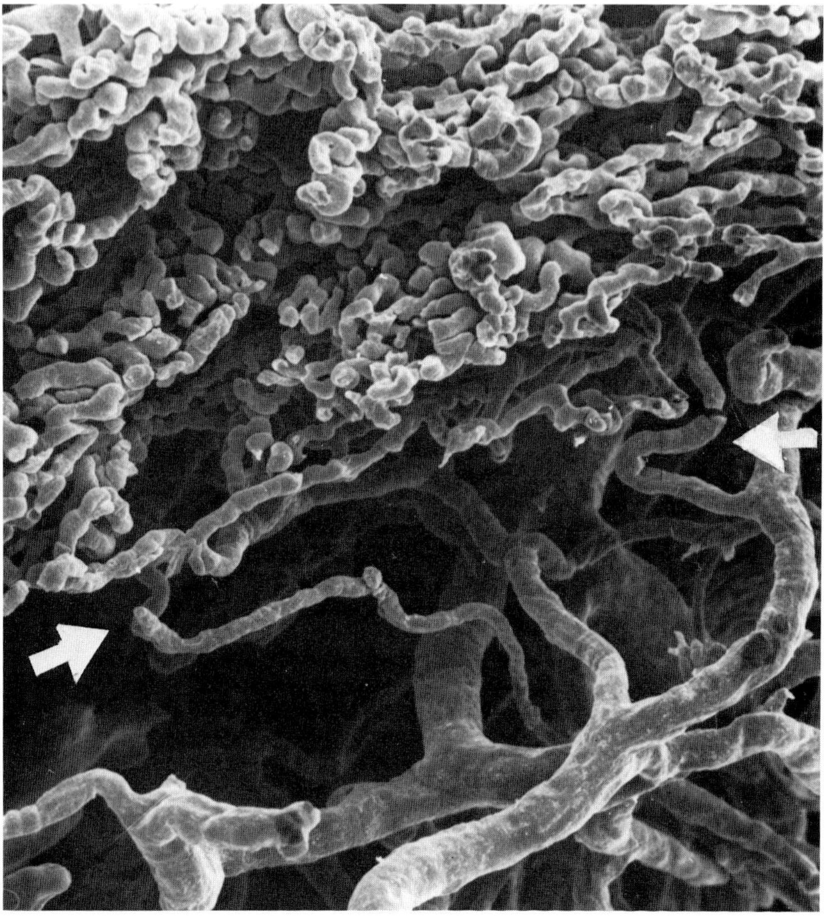

Figure 14 Higher magnification of bronchial microvascular plexus in the wall of a small bronchus.

drain into the azygos, the hemiazygos, and intercostal veins and may have valves. The intrapulmonary bronchial blood flow is drained into the pulmonary circulation. In a few physiological studies, it has been demonstrated that approximately 75% of bronchial-to-pulmonary anastomoses are on the pulmonary venous side (Charan et al., 1986; Modell et al., 1981).

The pulmonary and bronchial circulatory contributions to the tracheobronchial tree have been examined in a recent study utilizing radiolabeled microsphere techniques (Barman et al., 1988). This study indicates that the

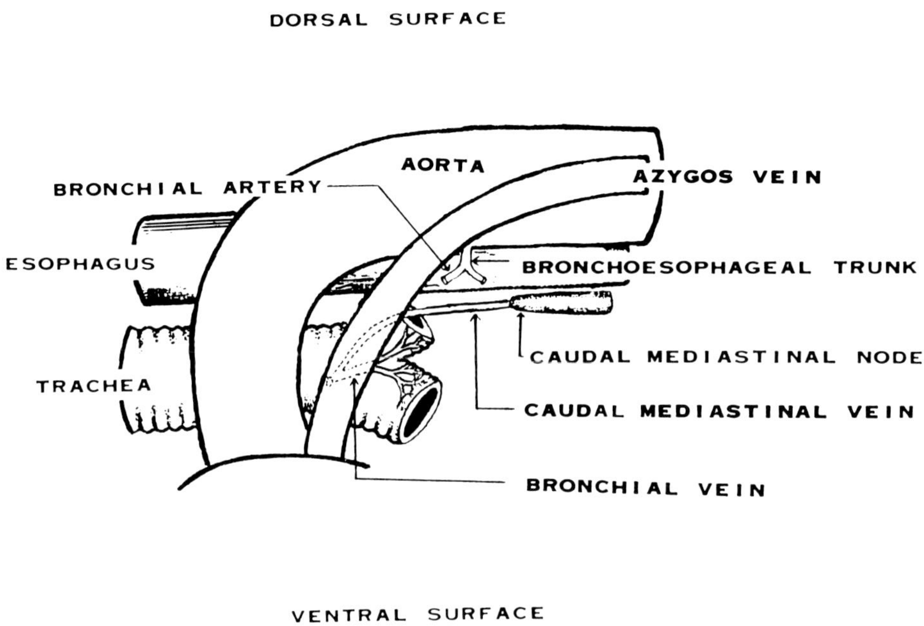

Figure 15 Bronchial venous drainage. (From Charan et al., 1984, with permission from the *Journal of Applied Physiology*.)

systemic (bronchial) circulation is the primary source of tracheal blood flow and that both the pulmonary and systemic circulations may contribute about 50% of the blood flow to the main bronchi in dog lungs.

D. Rabbits

The anatomy of the bronchial circulation has not been studied in detail in rabbits. Rabbits appear to have one bronchial artery for each lung, and the origin of these vessels is quite variable (Balding et al., 1964; Verloop, 1949). The right bronchial artery originates from the highest right intercostal artery, whereas the left bronchial artery may originate from the same artery, the aorta, or the left common carotid artery.

We recently studied the anatomy of the bronchial circulation in 18 adult New Zealand white rabbits (Charan and Carvalho, 1990). The animals were anesthetized and sacrificed. The upper abdominal wall was opened, and the chest cavity was entered through the diaphragm. By this technique we were able to prevent structural damage to the thoracic vascular bed. The pericardium was opened, and the ascending aorta was cannulated through the left

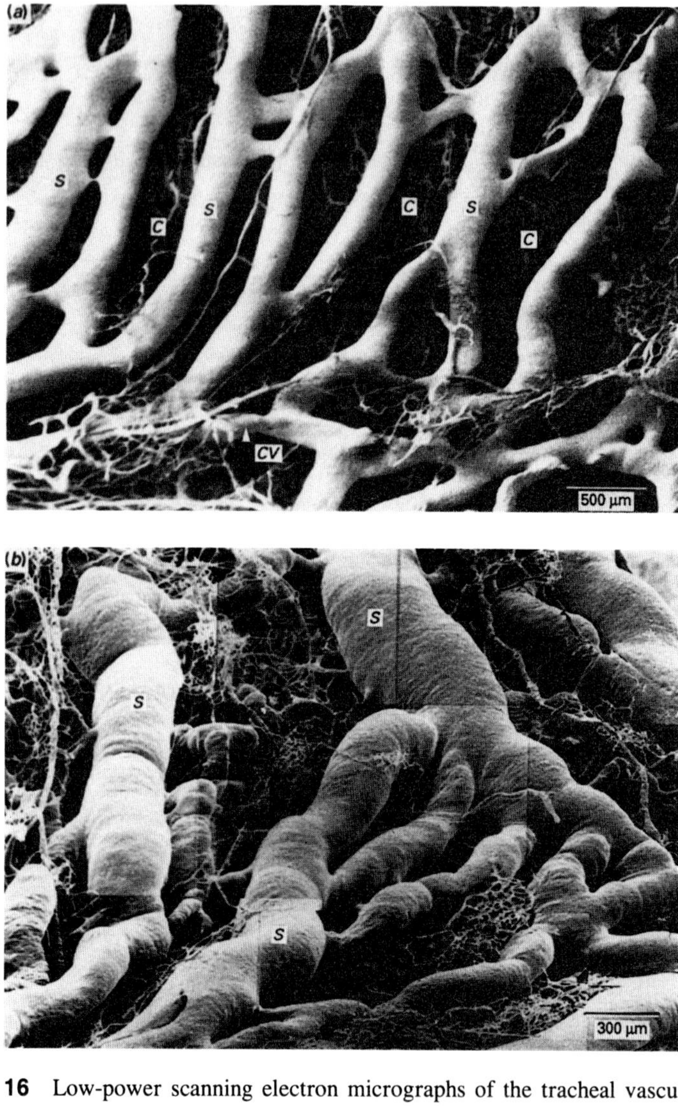

Figure 16 Low-power scanning electron micrographs of the tracheal vasculature of the sheep. (a) View from the submucosal surface showing network of sinuses (*S*), with subepithelial capillaries (*C*) lying deeper. The transverse diameter of the trachea is across the figure, the sinuses running mainly longitudinally. The intercartilaginous space is transverse at the bottom of the picture, showing connecting vessels (*CV*) joining the sinuses. (b) Scanning electron micrograph of the tracheal sinuses (*S*) showing their network connections. (From Hill et al. Blood sinuses in the submucosa of the large airways of the sheep. *J. Anat.* **162**:235–247, 1989, with permission of Cambridge University Press and the authors.)

ventricle. The pulmonary artery and the trachea were also cannulated. The lungs were inflated with air, and Batson's #17 anatomic corrosion compound was simultaneously infused into the aorta and pulmonary artery. After the vascular cast had hardened, the airways were filled with clear Batson's solution. The entire thoracic contents, including the rib cage, were then removed and submerged in potassium hydroxide. After the tissue had digested, the casts were dissected and the anatomy was studied. The blood supply to the cervical trachea came from small arteries originating from the innominate artery on the right side and from the left subclavian artery on the left side. On the right side, one or two bronchial arteries originated from the right highest intercostal artery at the level of about the first rib (Fig. 17). The origin of the left bronchial artery was variable. In approximately 60% of the animals it originated from the right highest intercostal artery, traversed caudally and to the left, and supplied the left bronchial tree. In the other 40% of the animals it originated from the left highest intercostal artery (Fig. 18). The microvascular plexus around the airways was remarkably sparse. The casting material that filled the bronchial arteries did not appear in the pulmonary artery or the pulmonary vein, suggesting that bronchopulmonary anastomoses are not pronounced in the rabbit lung. The visceral pleura was not supplied by the bronchial arteries.

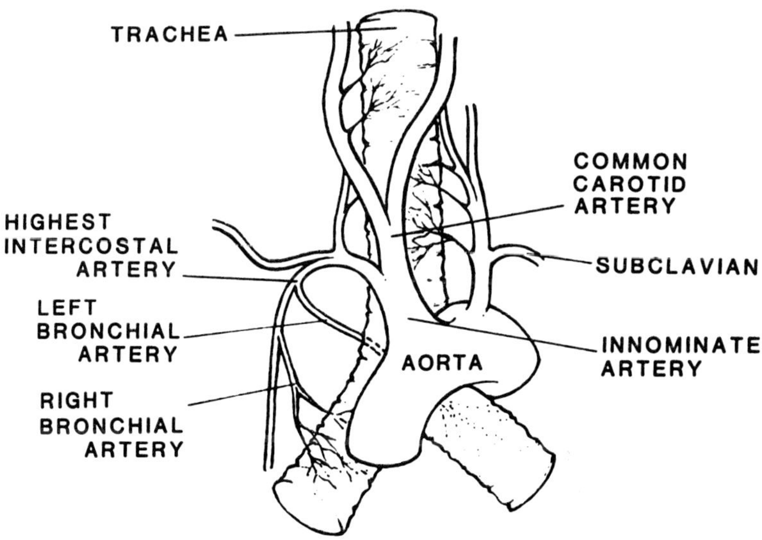

Figure 17 The tracheobronchial blood supply in rabbits. The right bronchial arteries originate from the right highest intercostal artery. In approximately 60% of the animals the left bronchial arteries also originate from the right highest intercostal artery.

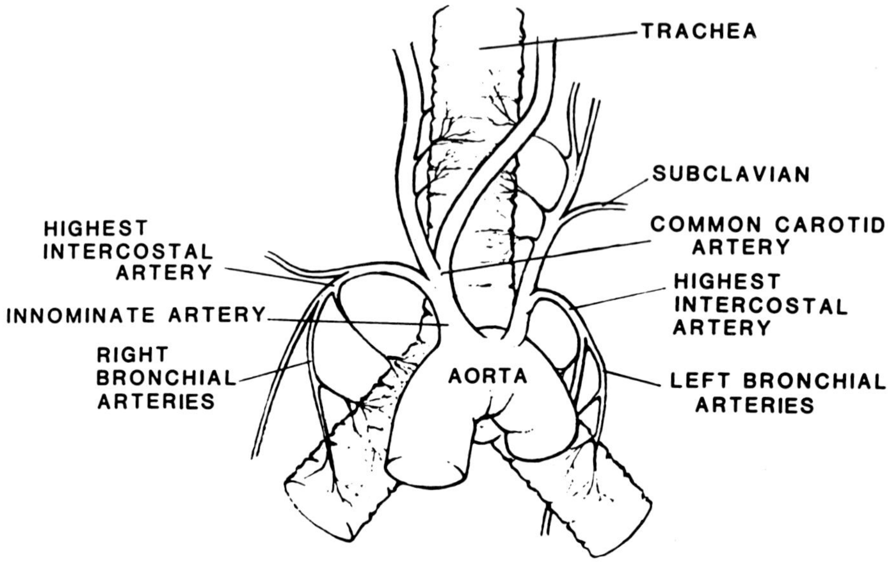

Figure 18 Origin of the left bronchial artery from the left highest intercostal artery in the rabbit lung. This arrangement was observed in 40% of the animals.

A pathway for the bronchial venous drainage could not be identified in this study.

Hughes (1965) described a network of blood sinuses, similar to that found in sheep, in the trachea of the rabbit. These are fed by venules draining radially outward from the superficial capillary network of the mucosa. The sinuses drain into collecting veins that run circumferentially with the arteries in the intercartilaginous spaces to pierce the tracheal wall on its lateral aspect.

E. Rats

Recently, rats have been used as an animal model in pharmacokinetic studies involving the tracheobronchial circulation. However, the anatomy of the bronchial circulation in rats has not been studied in detail. From a few preliminary studies, it appears that rats have multiple bronchial arteries and that numerous bronchopulmonary anastomoses exist (Schraufnagel, 1989; Munoz et al., 1989).

F. Avian Species

General studies of the avian arterial system have indicated that the bronchial arteries arise from the esophagotracheobronchial branch (ductus shawi) of each common carotid artery in many species (Bahaduri et al., 1957; Abdalla and King 1975, 1976, 1977). In most species, three or four branches from the esophagotracheobronchial artery supply the trachea, the syrinx, and the esophagus. However, in domestic pigeons and domestic fowl there is a single bronchial artery on each side; that is, a true left and right bronchial artery. This pair of bronchial arteries arise, via a common trunk, either from the right esophagotracheobronchial artery, as in fowl, or from the left, as in the pigeon. They also give rise to small bronchial arteries that supply the extrapulmonary part of the primary bronchus. The bronchial artery gives brances to the wall of the extra- and intrapulmonary parts of the primary bronchus. Minor anastomoses are present between the bronchial arteries and the pulmonary artery in the goose, muscovy duck, and turkey (group I) but not in the guinea fowl, quail (group II), or pigeon (group III) (Abdalla and King, 1977). In group I, the bronchial arteries supply the entire length of the extra- and intrapulmonary bronchi, but in groups II and III and domestic fowl they are confined to the extrapulmonary bronchi only, whereas the intrapulmonary part is supplied by the pulmonary artery. The small bronchial veins drain the extrapulmonary part of the primary bronchus into the esophageal vein of the same side, which empties into the cranial vena cava near its junction with the jugular vein. The intrapulmonary part of the primary bronchus is drained by the pulmonary vein.

G. Other Mammals

Significant anatomic differences exist in the distribution of the bronchial artery among various mammalian species. In general, its distribution appears to depend upon the amount of supportive or non–gas-exchanging pulmonary structures present in a given species. McLaughlin et al. (1961) studied thin-slice latex injection preparations of lung in 10 individual species and humans. They were able to classify them into three distinct subgross lung types by considering several morphological characteristics, including bronchial artery distribution.

In a subsequent study, McLaughlin (1983) examined sections of latex-injected lungs from 10 mammalian species, including humans, and determined the subgross distribution of the bronchial artery in each. The bronchial artery was variable in its distribution to the pleura, interlobular septa, distal airways, and alveoli and also in the presence or absence of bronchopulmonary anastomoses (Table 1).

In lung types I and III, the pleura and interlobular septum are both thick and are supplied by the bronchial artery. In lung type II, the pleura is thin and derives its vascular supply from the pulmonary artery. Interlobular septa and interlobular bronchial arteries do not appear to be present.

The bronchi were found to be supplied by the bronchial artery to the level of the distal terminal bronchioles in all lung types. However, in rabbit

Table 1 Subgross Distribution of Bronchial Artery[a]

	Cow	Lamb	Pig	Dog	Cat	Rhesus monkey	Rabbit	Rat	Guinea pig	Horse	Human
Pleura	+	+	+	−	−	−	−	−	−	+	+
Septa	+	+	+	−	−	−	−	−	−	+	+
Bronchi	+	+	+	+	+	+	+	+	+	+	+
Terminal bronchioles	+	+	+	+	+	+	−	+	+	+	+
Alveoli	−	−	−	−	−	−	−	−	−	+	+
Hilar nodes	+	+	+	+	+	+	+	+	+	+	+
Vasa vasorum	+	+	+	+	+	+	+	+	+	+	+
BA-PA anastomoses	+	+	−	−	−	−	+	+	+	+	+

[a] Abbreviations: + = distributed to structure; − = not distributed to structures; BA-PA anastomoses = bronchial artery-pulmonary artery anastomoses.
Source: From McLaughlin (1961).

lungs, a variant type II, the bronchial artery could not be traced beyond the second or third division of the mainstem bronchus.

In all lung types, the vasa vasorum to the pulmonary artery and vein and branches to the hilar lymph nodes were derived from the bronchial artery.

Venous drainage of all structures in all lung types was accomplished by the pulmonary vein; however, the first few divisions of the trachea and the hilar lymph nodes were drained by the azygous system.

In summary, the distribution of the bronchial artery varies greatly from species to species and appears to depend on the presence of tissues that are more likely to require a systemic blood supply. These differences in the distribution of the bronchial circulation between species necessitates caution in selecting laboratory animals, particularly if the findings obtained are to be extrapolated to humans.

References

Abdalla, M. A., and King, A. S. (1975). The functional anatomy of the pulmonary circulation of the domestic fowl. *Respir. Physiol.* **23**:267–290.

Abdalla, M. A., and King, A. S. (1976). The functional anatomy of the bronchial circulation of the domestic fowl. *J. Anat.* **121**:537–550.

Abdalla, M. A., and King, A. S. (1977). The avian bronchial arteries: Species variations. *J. Anat.* **123**:697–704.

Bahaduri, J. L., Biswas, B., and Das, S. K. (1957). The arterial system of the domestic pigeon (*Columbia livia* Gmelin). *Anat. Anz.* **104**:1–14.

Baile, E. M., Dahlby, R. W., Wiggs, B. R., and Pare, P. D. (1985). Role of tracheal and bronchial circulation in respiratory heat exchange. *J. Appl. Physiol.* **58**:217–222.

Balding, J. D., Jr., Oglivc, R. W., Hoffman, C. L., and Knisely, W. M. (1964). The gross morphology of the arterial supply to the trachea, primary bronchi and esophagus of the rabbit. *Anat. Rec.* **148**:611–614.

Barman, S. A., Ardell, J. L., Parker, J. C., Perry, M. L., and Taylor, A. E. (1988). Pulmonary and systemic blood flow contributions to upper airways in canine lung. *Am. J. Physiol.* **255**(Heart Circ. Physiol. 24):H1130–1135.

Bjork, L. (1966). Anastomoses between the coronary and bronchial arteries. *Acta Radiol. (Diagn.) (Stockh.)* **4**:93–96.

Boyden, E. A. (1970a). The developing bronchial arteries in a fetus of the twelfth week. *Am. J. Anat.* **129**:357–368.

Boyden, E. A. (1970b). The time lag in the development of bronchial arteries. *Anat. Rec.* **166**:611–614.

Cabanes, L. R., Weber, S. N., Matran, R., Regnard, J., Richard, M. O., Degeorges, M. E., and Lockhart, A. (1989). Bronchial hyperresponsiveness to methacholine in patients with impaired left ventricular function. *N. Engl. J. Med.* **320**:1317–1322.

Cauldwell, W. E., Siekert, R. G., Lininger, R. E., and Anson, B. J. (1948). The bronchial arteries. *Surg. Gynecol. Obstet.* **86**:395–412.

Charan, N. B., and Carvalho, P. (1989). Gas exchange with the bronchial circulation. *Am. Rev. Respir. Dis.* **139**:A445.

Charan, N. B., and Carvalho, P. (1990). Anatomy of the tracheal-bronchial circulation in rabbits. *FASEB J.* **4**:A1182.

Charan, N. B., Turk, G. M., and Dhand, R. (1984). Gross and subgross anatomy of the bronchial circulation in sheep. *J. Appl. Physiol.* **57**:658–664.

Charan, N. B., Turk, G. M., and Ripley, R. (1985). Measurement of bronchial arterial blood flow and bronchovascular resistance in sheep. *J. Appl. Physiol.* **59**:305–308.

Charan, N. B., Albert, R. K., Lakshminarayan, S., Kirk, W., and Butler, J. (1986). Factors affecting bronchial blood flow through bronchopulmonary anastomoses. *Am. Rev. Respir. Dis.* **134**:85–88.

Charan, N. B., Turk, G. M., Czartolomny, J., and Andreazuk, T. (1987). Systemic arterial blood supply to the trachea and lung in sheep. *J. Appl. Physiol.* **62**:2283–2287.

Chiba, S., Suzuki, T., Takahasi, D., and Kasai, T. (1990). An autopsy case of azygous lobe and the extra-pulmonary course of the bronchial veins in man. *Okajimas Folia Anat. Jpn.* **66**:313–338.

Chiles, C., Newman, G. E., and Blinder, R. A. (1990). A method for evaluating the bronchial circulation. *Invest. Radiol.* **25**:52–57.

Cohen, A. C., Doershuk, C. F., and Stern, R. C. (1990). Bronchial artery embolization to control hemoptysis in cystic fibrosis. *Radiology* **175**:401–405.

Collier, P. S. (1979). Bronchial arteries of the dog. A pharmacoanatomical study. *J. Anat.* **128**:887–888.

Cudkowicz, L. (1979). Human bronchial arterial circulation. In *Pulmonary Vascular Diseases*. Edited by K. M. Moser. *Lung Biology in Health and Disease*, Executive Editor Claude Lenfant. New York, Marcel Dekker.

Cudkowicz, L., and Armstrong, J. B. (1951). Observations on the normal anatomy of the bronchial arteries. *Thorax* **6**:343–358.

Daly, I. de B., and Hebb, C. (1966). *Pulmonary and Bronchial Vascular Systems*. London, Edward Arnold.

Gilroy, J. C., Marchand, P., and Wilson, V. H. (1952). The role of bronchial veins in mitral stenosis. *Lancet* **2**:957–959.

Halon, D. A., Turgeman, Y., Merdler, A., Hardoff, R., and Sharif, T. (1987). Coronary artery to bronchial artery anastomosis in Takyasu's arteritis. *Cardiology* **74**:387–391.

Hill, P., Goulding, D., Webber, S. E., and Widdicombe, J. G. (1989). Blood sinuses in the submucosa of the large airways of the sheep. *J. Anat.* **162**:235–247.

Hovelacque, P., Monod, O., and Evrard, H. (1936). Note au sujet des arteres bronchiques. *Ann. Anat. Pathol.* **13**:129–141.

Hughes, T. (1965). Microcirculation of the tracheo-bronchial tree. *Nature (Lond.)* **206**:425–426.

Kasai, T., and Chiba, S. (1979). Macroscopic anatomy of the bronchial arteries. *Anat. Anz.* **145**:166–181.

Laitinen, A., Laitinen, L. A., Moss, R., and Widdicombe, J. G. (1989). Organization and structure of the tracheal and bronchial blood vessels in the dog. *J. Anat.* **166**:133–140.

Liebow, A. A. (1953). The bronchopulmonary venous collateral circulation with special reference to emphysema. *Am. J. Pathol.* **29**:251–289.

Liebow, A. A. (1965). Patterns of origin and distribution of the major bronchial arteries in man. *Am. J. Anat.* **117**:19–32.

Liebow, A. A., Hales, M. R., and Bloomer, W. E. (1959). Relation of bronchial to pulmonary vascular tree In *Pulmonary Circulation: An International Symposium, 1958.* Edited by W. R. Adams and I. Veith. New York, Grune and Stratton, pp. 79–98.

Lilker, E. S., and Nagy, E. J. (1975). Gas exchange in the pulmonary collateral circulation of dogs. *Am. Rev. Respir. Dis.* **112**:615–620.

Magno, M. G., and Fishman, A. P. (1982). Origin, distribution, and blood flow of bronchial circulation in anesthetized sheep. *J. Appl. Physiol.* **53**:272–279.

Magno, M., Charan, N., Parsons, G. H., Baile, L., Albertine, K. H., and Butler, J. (1987). Nomenclature for the bronchial circulation (letter). *J. Appl. Physiol.* **62**:2512.

Marchand, P., Gilroy, J. C., and Wilson, N. H. (1950). Anatomical study of the bronchial vascular system and its variations in disease. *Thorax* **5**:207–221.

Mathes, M. E., Holman, E., and Reichert, F. L. (1932). A study of the bronchial, pulmonary and lymphatic circulations of the lung under various pathologic conditions experimentally produced. *J. Thorac. Surg.* **1**:339–362.

McLaughlin, R. F. (1983). Bronchial artery distribution in various mammals and in humans. *Am. Rev. Respir. Dis.* **128**:S57–S58.

McLaughlin, R. F., Tyler, W. S., and Canada, D. O. (1961). Subgross pulmonary anatomy in various mammals and man. *JAMA* **175**:694–697.

Meckel, J. F. (1831–1832). *Manual of General Descriptive and Pathological Anatomy*. Translated from German into French, with additions and notes by A. J. L. Jordan and G. Breschet, and from the French by A. S. Doane, Vol. 2. New York, Collins, Hannoy and H. C. Sleight, pp. 287–288.

Mills, N. L., Boyd, A. D., and Geranpong, C. (1970). The significance of bronchial circulation in lung transplantation. *J. Thorac. Cardiovasc. Surg.* **60**:866–874.

Modell, H. I., Beck, K., and Butler, J. (1981). Functional aspects of canine bronchial pulmonary vascular communications. *J. Appl. Physiol.* **50**:1045–1051.

Munoz, N. M., Chang, S., Murphy, T. M., Stimler-Gerard, N. P., Blake, J., Mack, M., Irvin, C., Voelkel, N. F., and Leff, A. R. (1989). Distribution of bronchoconstrictor responses in isolated-perfused rat lung. *J. Appl. Physiol.* **66**:202–209.

Murata, K., Itoh, H., Todo, G., Itoh, T., Kanaoka, M., Furata, M., and Torizuka, K. (1986). Bronchial venous plexus and its communication with pulmonary circulation. *Invest. Radiol.* **21**:24–27.

Nakamura, N. (1924). Zur Anatomie der bronchialarterien. *Anat. Anz.* **58**:508–517.

Notkovich, H. (1957). The anatomy of the bronchial arteries of the dog. *J. Thorac. Surg.* **33**:242–253.

Pump, K. K. (1972). Distribution of bronchial arteries in the human lung. *Chest* **62**:447–451.

Rees, S. (1981). Arterial connections of the lung: The inaugural Keith Jefferson lecture. *Clin. Radiol.* **32**:1–15.

Roberts, A. C. (1990). Bronchial artery embolization therapy. *J. Thorac. Imaging* **5**:60–72.

Schraufnagel, D. E. (1989). Microvascular casting of the lung: Bronchial versus pulmonary artery filling. *Scanning Microsc.* **3**:575–578.

Schreinemakers, H. H. J., Weder, W., Miyoshi, S., Harper, B. D., Shimokawa, S., Egan, T. M., McKnight, R., and Cooper, J. D. (1990). Direct revascularization of bronchial arteries for lung transplantation: An anatomical study. *Ann. Thorac. Surg.* **49**:44–54.

Steffas, L., Assayag, P., Brochet, A. E., Faraggi, B. M., Gamerman, G., and Valere, P. E. (1990). Coronary to bronchial artery anastomosis with bronchial steal syndrome demonstrated by thallium-201 myocardial tomoscintigraphy. *Eur. Heart J.* **11**:275–279.

Tobin, C. E. (1952). The bronchial arteries and their connections with other vessels in the human lung. *Surg. Gynecol. Obstet.* **95**:741–750.

Turner-Warwick, M. (1963). Precapillary systemic-pulmonary anastomoses. *Thorax* **18**:225–237.

Veith, F. J., Kamholz, S. L., Mollenkopf, F. P., and Montefusco, C. M. (1983). Lung transplantation 1983. *Transplantation* **35**:271–278.

Verloop, M. C. (1949). On the arteriae bronchalis and their anastomoses, with the arteriae pulmonales in some rodents; a micro-anatomical study. *Acta Anat. (Basel)* **7**:1–32.

Viamonte, M., Parks, R. E., and Smoak, W. M. (1965). Guided catheterization of the bronchial arteries. *Radiology* **56**:205–229.

Viamonte, M., Jr., Viamonte, M., Camacho, M., and Liebow, A. A. (1989). Corrosion cast studies of the bronchial arteries. *Surg. Radiol. Anat.* **11**:215–219.

Villar Do Valle, P., Barcia, A., Bargeron, L. M. Jr., Karp, R. B., and Kirklin, J. W. (1969). Angiographic study of supravalvular aortic stenosis and associated lesions. Report of five cases and review of literature. *Ann. Radiol.* **12**:779–786.

Virchow, R. (1847). Uber die Stadpunkte in den wissenschaftlichen Medizin. *Virchows Arch [A]* **1**:1.

Wagenwoort, C. A., and Wagenwoort, N. (1967). Arterial anastomoses, bronchopulmonary arteries and pulmobronchial arteries in perinatal lungs. *Lab. Invest.* **16**:13–24.

Wagenwoort, C. A., Heath, D., and Edwards, J. E. (1964). *The Pathology of the Pulmonary Vasculature*. Springfield, Illinois, Charles C Thomas.

Zureikat, H. Y. (1980). Collateral vessels between the coronary and bronchial arteries in patents with cyanotic congenital heart disease. *Am. J. Cardiol.* **45**:599–603.

3

The Bronchial Circulation
Histology and Electron Microscopy

LAURI A. LAITINEN

University of Lund and Astra Draco
Lund, Sweden

ANNIKA LAITINEN

University of Helsinki
Helsinki, Finland
and University of Lund
Lund, Sweden

I. Introduction

Information on the number and structure of the microvessels in the airways contributes to a better understanding of the function of the airway mucosa. During recent years the importance of the bronchial circulation has been emphasized as a possible contributing factor in the development of various airway diseases. Thus, morphological studies in this field have expanded. Such studies can reveal the differences between species in the structure of the microcirculation. This is essential knowledge when interpreting physiological results and extrapolating circulatory mechanisms from different animal species to the human.

Although the gross anatomy of the tracheobronchial circulation has been described frequently (Marchand et al., 1950; Cudkowicz and Armstrong, 1951; Hughes, 1965; Daly and Hebb, 1966, Charan et al., 1984; Baier et al., 1985), there are only a few descriptions of the detailed organization and structure of the mucosal microvasculature. In several species bronchial arteries from the peribronchial connective tissue give rise to smaller branches that reach the airway mucosa and form a capillovenular plexus (Pietra et al., 1971; Magno and Fishman, 1982; Charan et al., 1984; Laitinen et al., 1989). However, very little information is available about the organization and structure of the human airway microcirculation (Cudkowicz, 1979; McLaughlin, 1983; Deffebach et al., 1987).

In general, the vessels seen with the naked eye (vessels larger than 100 μm) are considered within the macrovasculature. Vessels that can only be visualized with the light microscope (with diameters less than 100 μm) and form a dense network are called the microvasculature.

As the microvascular bed is approached, the caliber of the arteriole gradually diminishes. The network of the microvessels lying between the smallest recognizable arteries and veins is formed by ramifications of arterioles, capillaries, and postcapillary venules. The capillary bed is drained by vessels having increasing diameters, the venules (Zweifach, 1957). This microvascular network represents the terminal portion of the bronchial vascular system and plays a role in the transfer of gases, nutrients, and metabolic waste products.

In several species, including the human, light microscopy confirms the pattern of vessels in the mucosa that is suggested by the more detailed scanning electron microscopy (SEM) findings. Using light and electron microscopy in cross sections of airway mucosa from different species, capillaries lie just under the epithelial basement membrane, usually at a distance less than 10 μm from the epithelium. Small postcapillary venules are located deeper in the mucosa (Fig. 1). The number of arterioles in the mucosa is much less than that of the capillovenular structures.

II. Gross Structure and Morphology of the Bronchial Vasculature

There are great differences between species in the size and type of the vessels, as well as in the location of the microvascular network.

A. Scanning Electron Microscopy

Without three-dimensional casts of the airway microcirculation, it has been difficult to evaluate the richness of the microcirculation as well as its continuity along the trachea and bronchi using only light microscopic plane sections.

Developments in scanning electron microscopy and related techniques have been essential to allow visualization of the airway microcirculation in a three-dimensional way. Since the first attempts of Murakami (1971) to use polymerizing media in connection with the corrosion cast/technique, scanning electron microscopy has become a very important tool for examining the vascular organization of different organs.

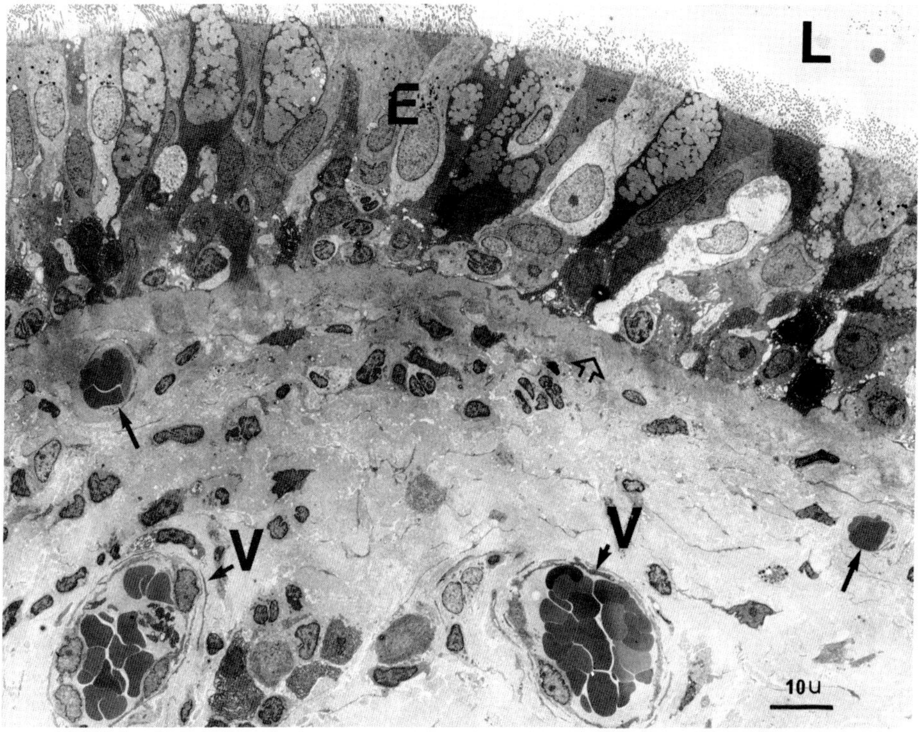

Figure 1 Transmission electron micrograph. Biopsy specimen from human airway, right upper lobe bronchus. The epithelium (E) consists of ciliated and goblet cells. Underneath the airway epithelial basement membrane (open arrow) are located small capillaries (black arrows). Deeper in the mucosa are postcapillary venules (V). L = airway lumen. Magnification × 1300. Bar = 10 μm.

To study the airway microcirculation, vascular corrosion casts are made by exposing the bronchial artery and injecting it with a polymerizing compound, such as Batson's compound #17 (Polysciences, Inc.). This compound, in contrast to some used previously, allows the filling of capillaries that are less than 10 μm in diameter. After the resin has hardened in the vasculature, the other tissues are digested away and the cast is prepared for scanning electron microscopy by routine methods using critical point drying. As a result of this process, the airway microcirculation is seen as a tube made up of a vascular network that is presumably similar to that around the bronchus in vivo. The relationships of the resin-filled vessels to the other airway structures can be followed by studying them during the dissolving process (Laitinen et al., 1989).

The vascular casts can be evaluated by comparing the dimensions of the vessels, their patterns of ramification, and their surface features. Usually an arteriole is smaller than the corresponding venule. When arterioles are traced from the capillary level the origins are constricted. This constriction is not seen on the venular side. Arterioles often appear to be in a state of constriction, which causes the surface of the cast to reveal a coarse pattern of longitudinal foldings and ruffles caused by the corresponding profile of the endothelium. The venules remain smooth. Tracing capillaries from the feeding arterioles to the draining venules helps to identify the vessels (Castenholtz, 1983, 1989).

B. Species Differences

In the greyhound, scanning electron microscopy has demonstrated that arteries approximately 100 μm in diameter run on each lateral wall of the trachea in a circular manner between adjacent cartilaginous half-rings. These vessels branch to form the mucosal microvascular network. Close to the airway lumen runs a dense superficial network consisting of capillaries and their loops (Fig. 2). In the deeper half of the mucosa a less dense network is formed by venules draining the superficial capillary network. Small arteriolar branches that supply the capillaries are also located at the level of this venular network.

At least two arteries (0.5–1.0 mm in diameter) accompany each bronchus (0.5–5.0 mm in diameter), running in the peribronchial connective tissue. When the bronchi divide, the arteries also divide into equally sized branches. During their course the arteries give off relatively small branches that penetrate the bronchial wall to supply the mucosal vascular layer. As in the trachea, a dense network of vessels is located in the mucosa close to the airway lumen (Fig 3). The network is obvious even in the smallest (0.5 mm diameter) bronchi examined (Laitinen et al., 1989).

The sizes of the vessels vary between species. In contrast to those of the greyhound, rat tracheal vessels are smaller; pairs of arterioles approximately 100 μm in diameter extending the length of the trachea give rise to branches approximately 30 μm in diameter. These arterioles run between adjacent cartilaginous rings. Terminal arterioles arising from these arterioles and providing the blood supply to the airway mucosa measure about 12 $\pm 8 \mu m$ (McDonald, 1988).

Some similar features are present in many species. In rats, guinea pigs, cats, dogs, rhesus monkeys, and humans, the tracheobronchial microcirculation is characterized by the rich subepithelial network (Sobin et al., 1963; Hughes, 1965; McDonald, 1988; Laitinen et al., 1989). In the most peripheral

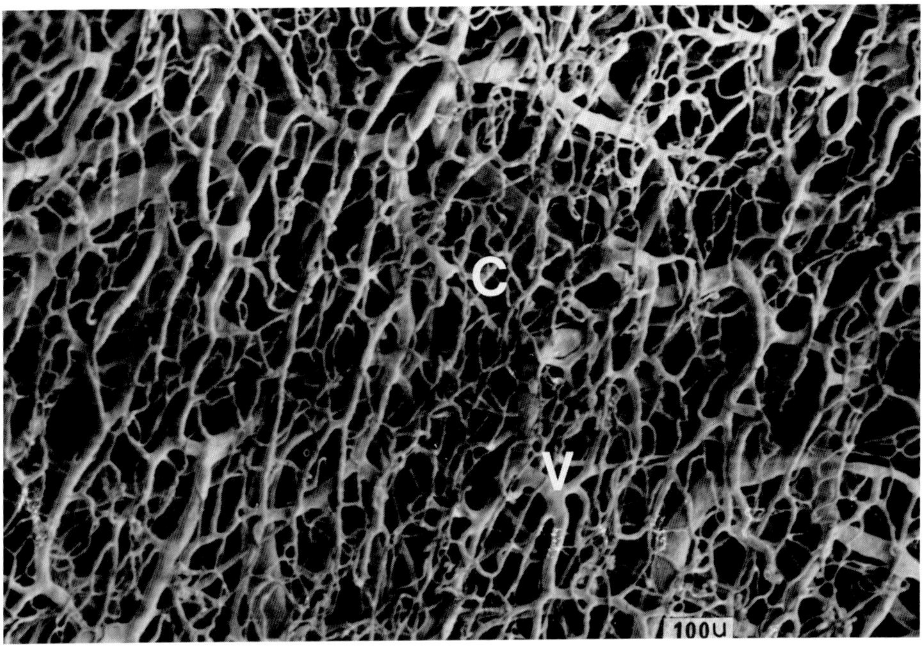

Figure 2 Scanning electron micrograph taken from the luminal side of a vascular cast from the lateral wall of the trachea over the fifth cartilage half-ring. A dense vascular network is shown in the tracheal mucosa. Small superficial capillaries (C) are draining into deeper veins (V). Bar = 100 μm. (From Laitinen et al., 1989.)

bronchioles the longitudinally arranged capillary bed anastomoses with the alveolar capillaries (Pump, 1972).

In sheep and rabbits the venules of the large airways drain to sinuses located deeper in the airway wall (Sobin et al., 1963; Hill et al., 1989). In sheep the sinuses are described as having a diameter of up to 0.5 mm with a preferred location between the cartilaginous rings (Hill et al., 1989). In rabbits the bronchial arterial supply ends at the level of relatively large airways and the capillary bed is less extensive.

C. Comparison with the Human

At present we lack information from microvascular casting techniques in the human, especially knowledge of the smallest vessels (Laitinen and Laitinen, 1990). Although the bronchial artery can be exposed and injected immediately after lobectomy in lung cancer patients (Fig. 4), a "cul-de-sac" phenomenon

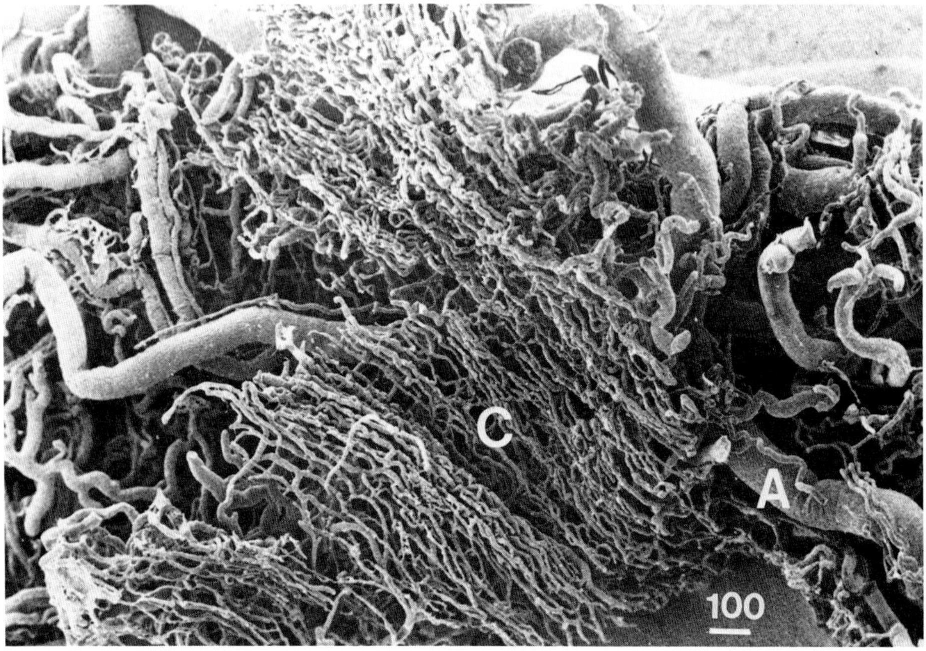

Figure 3 Scanning electron micrograph of a cast of the microvascular network in the mucosa of a 3 mm diameter bronchus in the dog. The capillaries run longitudinally along the course of the bronchus. A = arteriole, C = capillaries. Magnification × 110. Bar = 100 μm. (From Laitinen et al., 1989.)

appears. Part of the microvessels are not filled with the resin because of blood clots (Fig 5). Animals can be heparinized before injection of the plastic, and this diminishes the obliteration of small blood vessels with blood clots.

Another problem in obtaining information about the human airway microcirculation is in acquiring normal material to be studied. Surgically excised lungs are usually not healthy and often show pathological changes caused by the underlying disease. The changes in the airway microcirculation caused by the disease are impossible to predict.

However, the basic structure of the bronchial vasculature in the human is similar to that in the dog. A dense network of capillaries runs close to the epithelium at all levels of the lower airways. The capillaries converge to form venules extending to a deeper plexus of larger venules and arterioles (Fig. 4). The networks are continuous around and along the airways.

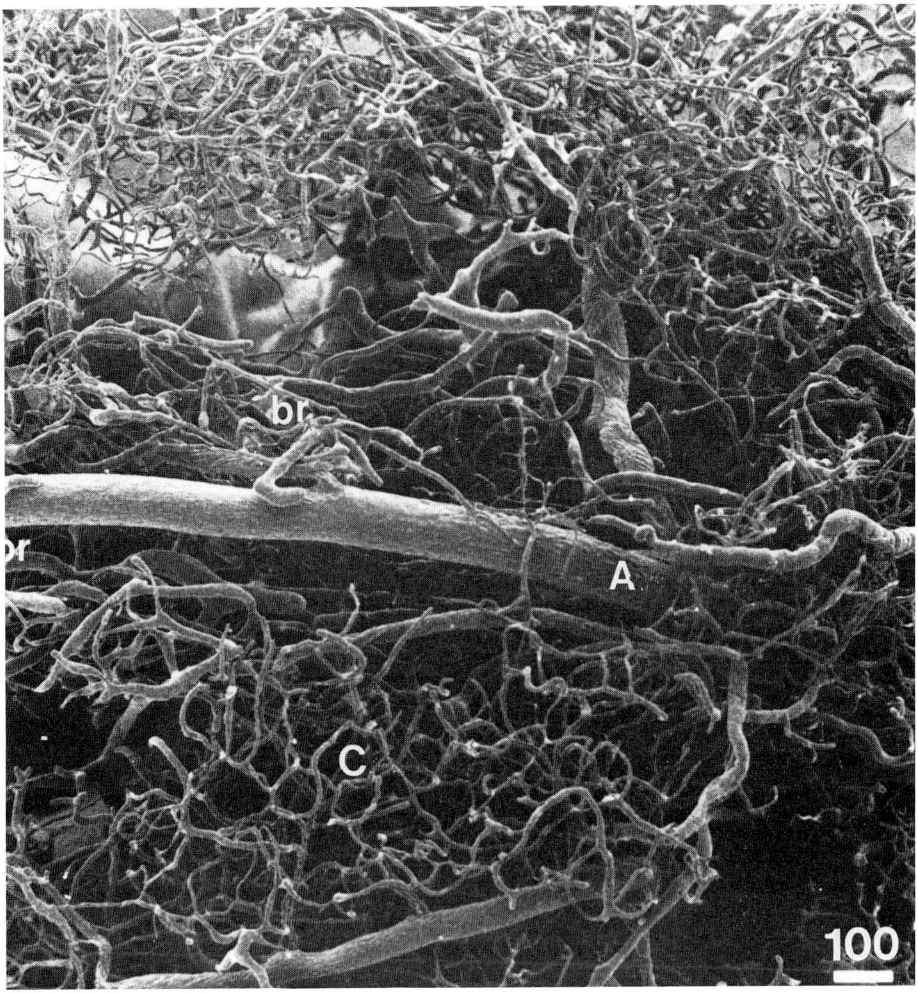

Figure 4 Scanning electron micrograph of a cast of the human airway microcirculation prepared in the same way as the cast in Fig. 3. The bronchial artery was catheterized and injected after lobectomy for lung cancer. The network of capillaries (C) runs close to the airway surface and drains to venules deeper in the mucosa. The arteriole (A) gives off small branches (BR) to supply the capillary network. Magnification × 125. Bar = 100 μm.

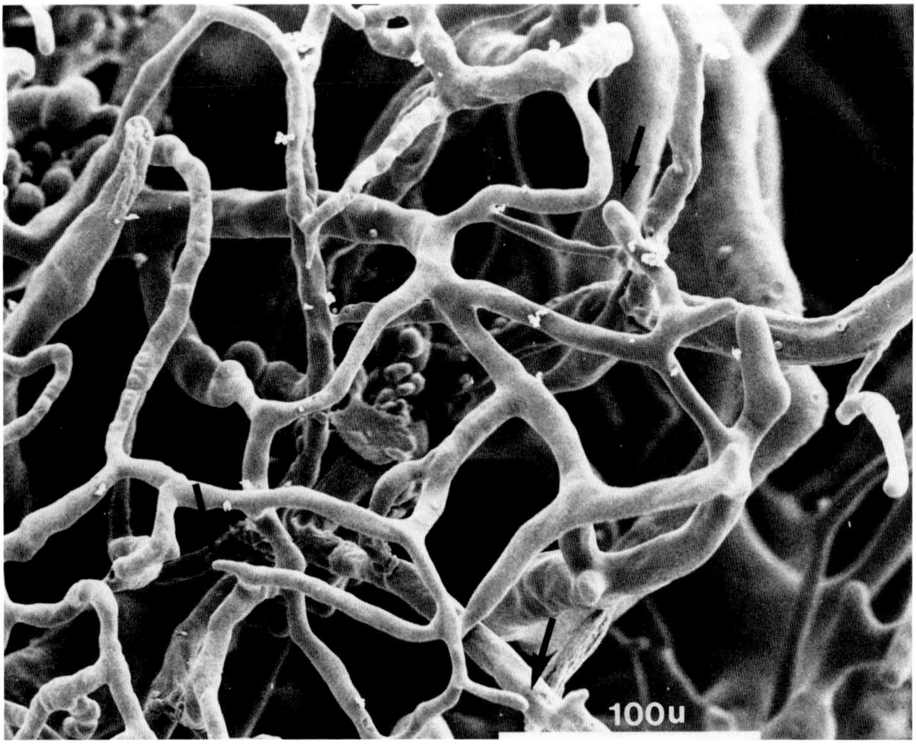

Figure 5 Enlargement of part of Fig. 4. Many capillaries end as culs-de-sac (arrows) indicative of unfilled vessels. The difference between the dog and the human cast was caused by the delay in injecting the bronchial artery in the human and because the dog could be heparinized to prevent blood clots in the vessels. Bar = 100 μm.

D. Anastomoses Between the Bronchial and Pulmonary Vessels

Branches of the bronchial circulation have been found to anastomose with the pulmonary artery in several species (Charan et al., 1987; McLaughlin et al., 1983). In the human the bronchial capillary bed has been described as anastomosing with the alveolar capillaries in the most peripheral bronchioles (Pump, 1972). Thus, in the distal branches of the airways the blood may flow from the bronchial arteries via the bronchial capillaries to the pulmonary capillaries and veins.

III. Histology and Ultrastructure

A. Arteries and Arterioles

During the course of the bronchial artery there is repeated branching along with the bronchial tree, giving a vast increase in the total cross-sectional area of the arterial bed. The arteries give rise to arterioles with progressively diminishing caliber in the mucosa. In arterioles of 100 μm there is usually a tunica media of two or more layers of smooth muscle cells. As the arteriole becomes progressively smaller in diameter, there is a corresponding decrease in the thickness of its three tunicae: intima, media, and adventitia. In the terminal arteriole the tunica media contains only a single layer of smooth muscle cells. Thus, the distal portion of the arteriolar stem is gradually thinned into extremely fine terminal arterioles of capillary dimensions (see Leak, 1980).

The smooth muscle cells in the media are surrounded by a basal lamina except for junctions formed with adjoining smooth muscle and endothelial cells. The endothelial cells lining the arteriole are flat on the luminal side and held together by tight junctions. They rest on the basal lamina and are separated from the smooth muscle cells by elastic and collagenous fibers. In the terminal arterioles the endothelial cells are separated from the single layer of smooth muscle cells by a basal lamina. Membrane-to-membrane contacts exist between the smooth muscle cells and endothelial cells (Fig. 6). The outermost layer of the arterioles, the adventitia, contains occasional fibroblasts and collagenous fibers. The adventitia contains nonmyelinated nerves, which may regulate the contractile properties of the smooth muscle in the arteriolar wall and thus the blood flow to the mucosa.

In rat airways the terminal arterioles are densely innervated (Fig. 7). Electron microscopy shows that two-thirds of the nerves to these vessels are located within 1 μm of the arterial wall smooth muscle. The nerves contain 50 nm diameter, clear core vesicles or a mixture of these and larger (80–100 nm) dense core vesicles typical of cholinergic and peptidergic nerves. Nerves morphologically resembling adrenergic nerves are also seen (McDonald et al., 1988).

Data from histochemical studies support the finding that bronchial vessels are innervated by cholinergic and adrenergic nerves, as well as peptidergic nerves (Hebb, 1969; Mann, 1971; Partanen et al., 1982; Dey et al., 1981; Laitinen et al., 1985). Neuropeptides like substance P and calcitonin gene-related peptide that have been associated with an afferent, sensory type of innervation have also been found close to airway vessels (Lundberg et al., 1984; Springal et al., 1988).

In the human, nerves containing different kinds of vesicles have been

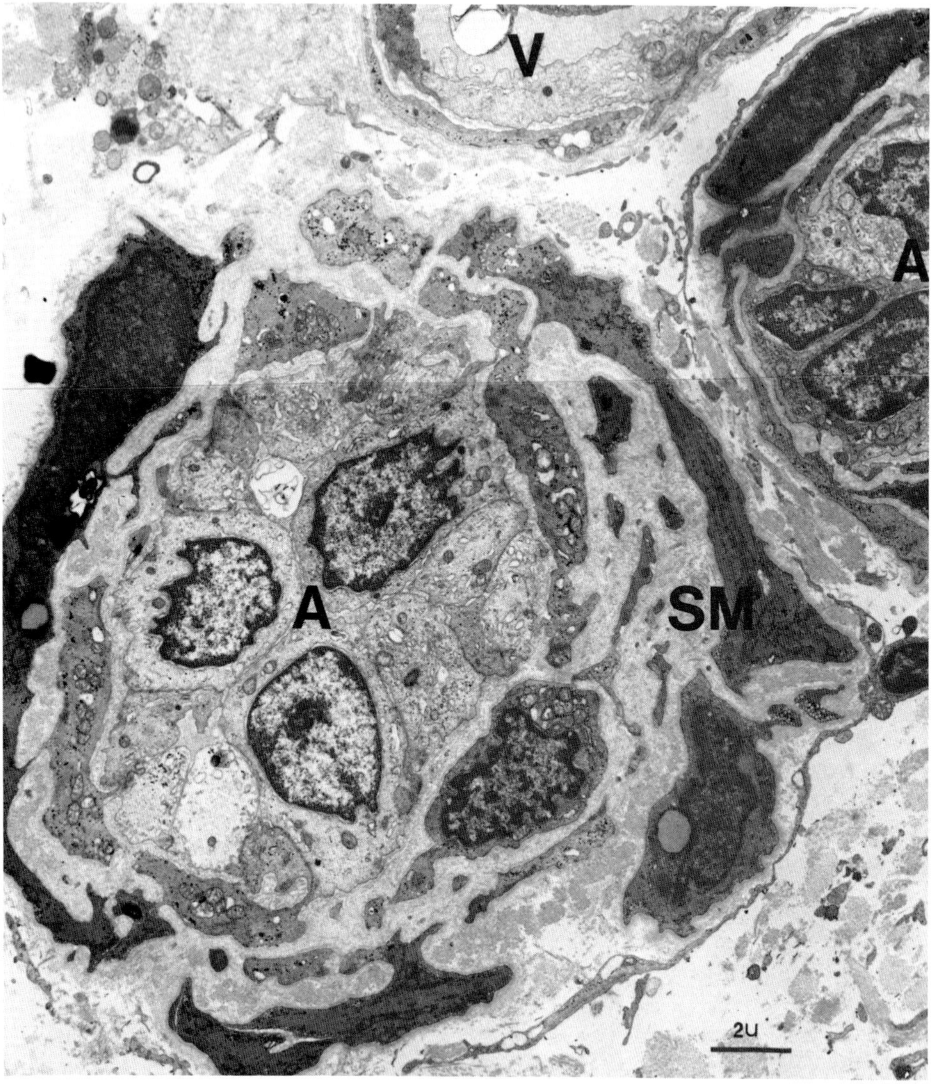

Figure 6 Transmission electron micrograph of human airway segmental bronchus. Two small arterioles (A) are seen in the airway mucosa. The smooth muscle cells (SM) in the tunica media of the vascular walls make membrane-to-membrane contacts with the endothelial cells. Magnification × 7800. Bar = 2 μm.

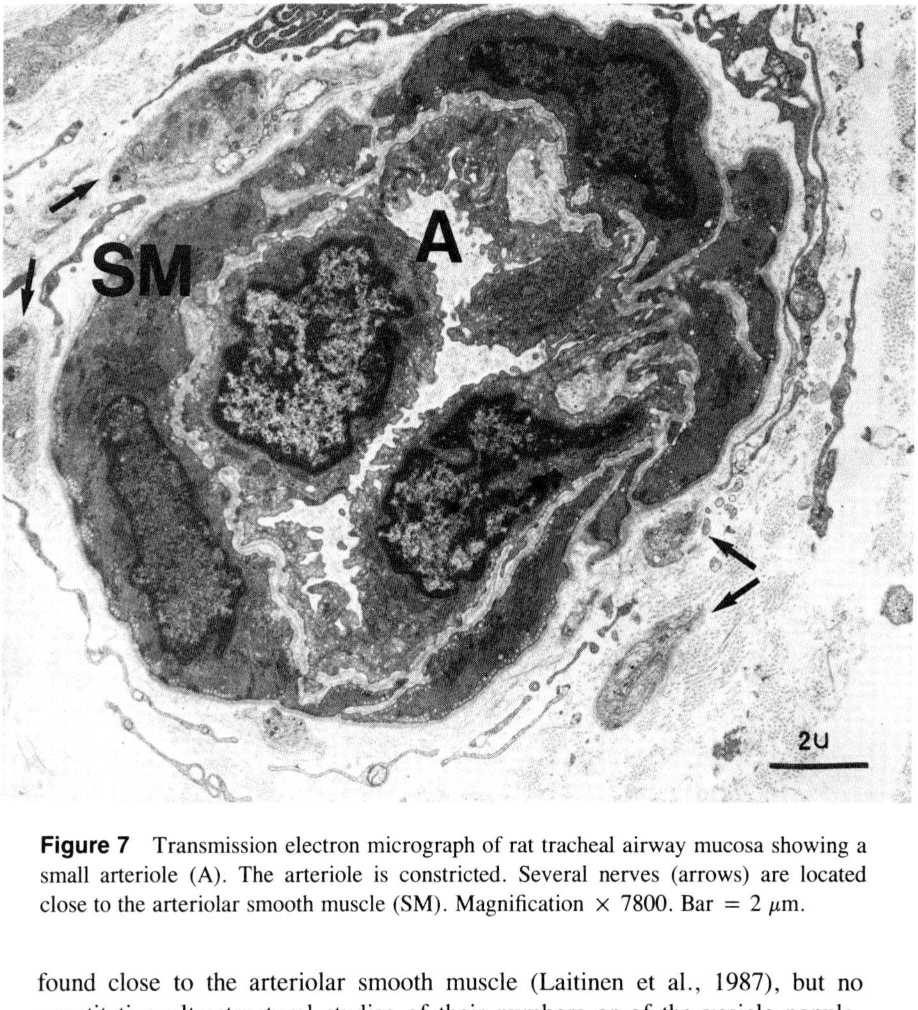

Figure 7 Transmission electron micrograph of rat tracheal airway mucosa showing a small arteriole (A). The arteriole is constricted. Several nerves (arrows) are located close to the arteriolar smooth muscle (SM). Magnification × 7800. Bar = 2 μm.

found close to the arteriolar smooth muscle (Laitinen et al., 1987), but no quantitative ultrastructural studies of their numbers or of the vesicle populations of their axons exist. Histochemical data suggest that the airway vascular bed in the human is innervated by adrenergic and peptidergic nerves. Adrenergic nerves are found in close association with the bronchial vessels (Partanen et al., 1982). Vasoactive intestinal peptide (VIP)-containing nerves (Dey et al., 1981; Laitinen et al., 1985) have been identified close to the airway vasculature.

B. Capillovenular Plexus

The terminal arterioles give rise to capillaries. They are located just beneath the epithelial basement membrane and tend to run parallel to the long axis of the airway (Hughes, 1965).

The numbers of the vessels vary to some extent between different species when counted in a cross section by light microscopy. Capillovenular structures show a density of approximately 84 ±8 vessels per mm^2 in dog tracheal mucosa between the epithelium and cartilage. When counted within a distance of 100 μm from the epithelium and basement membrane, the vessels have a much higher density of 289 ±29 vessels per mm^2 (Laitinen et al., 1989). This suggests that the microvessels are mainly concentrated beneath the basement membrane.

In human airways, the total number of vessels lying in the submucosa within 200 μm of the bronchial epithelial basement membrane has been counted using light microscopy. About 120 vessels per mm^2 was the density reported by Beasley et al. (1989). However, they did not further analyze the vessels in different groups. The difference in numbers of the vessels reported in different studies seems to be related to the different distances of the mucosa from the epithelium in the sections used for the enumerations.

To determine the percentage of the mucosa occupied by the microvasculature, the total volume fraction of the microvasculature has been measured. In sheep bronchi 1 mm in diameter the total microvascular volume fraction was measured within a 50 μm depth of the epithelial basement membrane. It forms about 5% of the subepithelial tissue, which is a somewhat smaller volume than that in the same tissue in the trachea and smaller bronchioles (Mariassy et al., 1989).

The mucosal capillaries have diameters of about 7–10 μm depending on the animal species examined (McDonald et al., 1988; Laitinen et al., 1989; see Leak, 1980). The capillary wall consists of a single layer of flattened endothelial cells surrounded by a continuous basal lamina and an incomplete layer of pericytes. The classification of different kinds of capillaries is usually based on the completeness of the endothelium (Rhodin, 1962). Airway mucosal capillaries show species-related variation in the structure of the endothelium. Some animals show continuous endothelium; others, for example the human, show capillaries with fenestrations (Laitinen, 1988).

Both along the basal and apical surfaces of the capillary endothelium and in the cell cytoplasm, there are numerous small vesicular invaginations approximately 500–700 Å in diameter. It has been suggested that these vesicles may account for fluid movement from one side of the cell to the other (Florey, 1966). The endothelial cells are connected to each other by occluding junctions. Using a freeze-fracture technique, these occluding junctions appear to consist of several ridges or shallow grooves that form a continuous network, or they look like a maze in which the grooves are staggered in parallel fashion (Simionescu et al., 1975).

The capillaries give rise to a network of postcapillary venules of approximately 10–30 μm. These venules are situated deeper in the mucosa than the capillaries. The postcapillary venules receive connections from the capillaries and other postcapillary venules and join larger collecting venules. The postcapillary venules have a continuous endothelium surrounded by a continuous basal lamina and a varying number of pericytes. The number of pericytes increases with increasing vessel diameter, and they form a continuous layer around larger (30–50 μm) venules. In postcapillary venules, the intercellular junctions between endothelial cells are loosely organized compared with the junctions between the endothelial cells of the capillary wall (Simionescu et al., 1975; Bartels, 1982). In freeze-fracture replicas, the junctions between the venular endothelial cells are found to consist of discontinuous strands of intramembranous particles (Bartels, 1982). The loose arrangement of the endothelial cell junctions facilitates the separation of the adjacent cells and may contribute to making these vessels more susceptible to the effects of various kinds of inflammatory mediators. In contrast to the bronchial vessels, the pulmonary vessels, which do not respond to inflammatory mediators in the same way, have a somewhat different vascular wall structure. The endothelium is thicker, and there are more surrounding pericytes (Pietra et al., 1971). With increasing vessel diameter, cells with ultrastructural features of smooth muscle begin to appear in the periendothelial layer of the venules. Venous return from the larger bronchi is via bronchial veins to the azygos and hemiazygos veins. From the more peripheral airways, bronchial blood is drained by tributaries of the pulmonary veins (Miller, 1947; Pietra and Magno, 1978; Deffebach et al., 1987).

Very little quantitative information is available about the lymphatic vessels of the airway mucosa. These differ from venules in having a thin endothelium, a discontinuous basal lamina, and no surrounding pericytes.

IV. Special Ultrastructural Features of the Bronchial Vessels

A. Fenestrated Capillaries

In addition to the human, the capillaries of the endothelium beneath the respiratory epithelium of the rat, guinea pig, and hamster often contains fenestrations (Hirabayashi and Yamamoto, 1984). The endothelial cells of fenestrated capillaries are punctured by rounded windows or fenestrations approximately 50 nm in diameter. The fenestrations are bridged by thin diaphragms having an average thickness of 60 Å (Fig. 8). In the human the fenestrated capillaries in the mucosa arc often seen beneath neuroendocrinelike cells (APUD cells) in the airway epithelium (Laitinen, 1988). These neuroendocrinelike cells (NE) may extend up to the airway lumen. Because these neu-

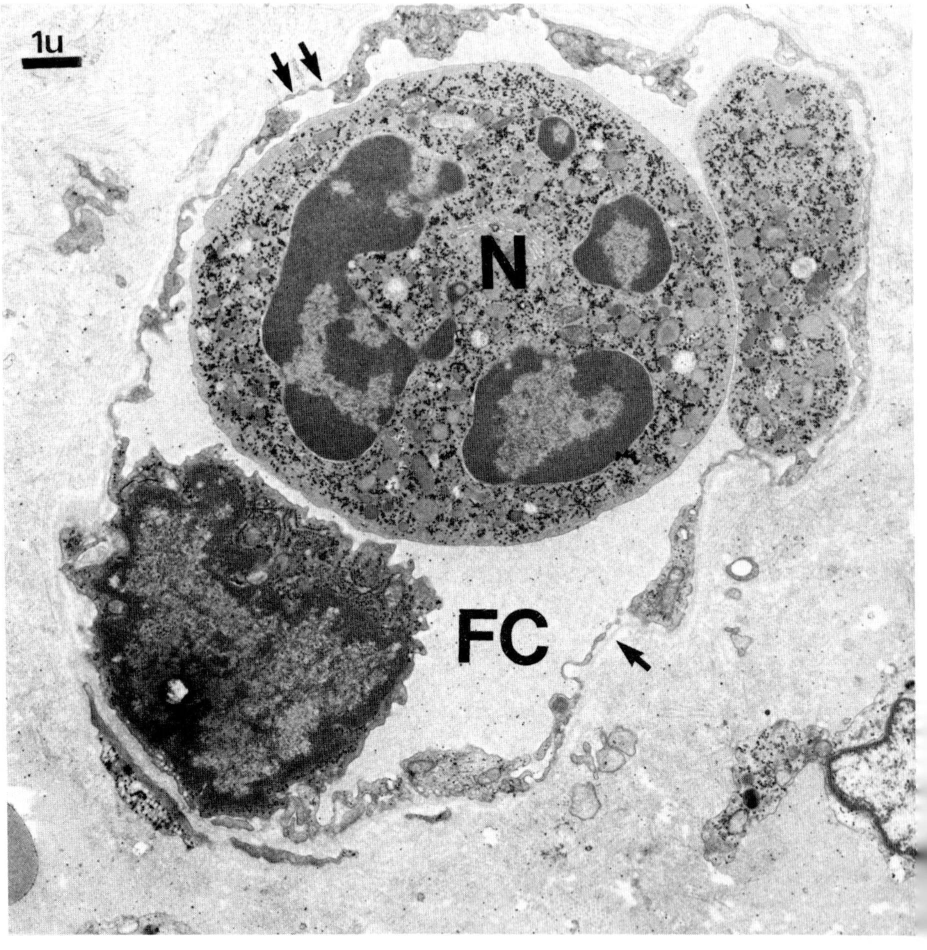

Figure 8 Electron micrograph from the airway mucosa of a clinically severe asthmatic patient shows a fenestrated capillary (FC) located beneath the epithelial basement membrane. A neutrophilic leukocyte (N) is seen in its lumen. Several fenestrations closed by diaphragms (arrows) are seen in the capillary endothelial wall. Magnification × 10,400. Bar = 1 μm.

roendocrinelike cells also contain high numbers of secretory vesicles in their basal cytoplasm, they may form a link between airway lumen and bronchial vasculature. The released mediators may reach the circulation by the fenestrated capillaries close to the epithelium and extend widespread effects via the circulation, and vice versa: circulating mediators may stimulate the release of secretory vesicles from NE cells to the epithelium. NE cells are closely innervated by afferentlike nerves (Lauweryns et al., 1983, 1985) that may be stimulated by NE cells, leading to airway reflex effects. Thus, the possibility exists of circulatory mechanisms, such as inflammatory responses, participating in neurally mediated reflexes.

B. Endothelial Gap Formation

The endothelium of bronchial postcapillary venules in asthmatic individuals may have wide, unclosed gaps (Fig. 9). Another typical finding in the bronchial mucosal microvasculature in asthmatic subjects is the adherence of inflammatory cells. The most common cells in asthmatic bronchial vessels are eosinophils and neutrophils. These inflammatory cells can be seen free in the vascular lumen, in close contact to the vessel wall, or penetrating through the vessel wall. Also, red blood cells may be located close to the gaps in the endothelial wall or penetrating through the vessel wall (Laitinen and Laitinen, 1990). These features are seldom seen in normal healthy airways.

Using Monastral blue as a tracer, McDonald and coworkers (1988) have shown in rat airways that sensory nerve stimulation or exposure to histamine produces an increase in vascular permeability, but only in postcapillary and collecting venules. This increase in vascular permeability is thought to be due to the formation of endothelial gaps in the postcapillary venules. Gaps as wide as 1.5 μm have been seen. A contractionlike change in the shape of the endothelial cells was also described in the venules with the gaps (McDonald et al., 1988). Endothelial gap formation is thought to result from an active change in the configuration of the endothelial cells rather than from passive distention due to increased venous pressure (Majno and Leventhal, 1967).

The endothelial gaps in postcapillary venules in asthmatic airways look morphologically similar to those experimentally induced gaps in rat airways described by McDonald and coworkers (1988). The gap formation may be relevant to the pathogenesis of asthma. The neurogenic inflammation caused by irritation of nerve endings in the damaged airway epithelium (Laitinen et al., 1985; Barnes, 1986) and the resulting increase in plasma exudation (Persson, 1986) may be important contributing factors to the development of the special cellular features in human asthma.

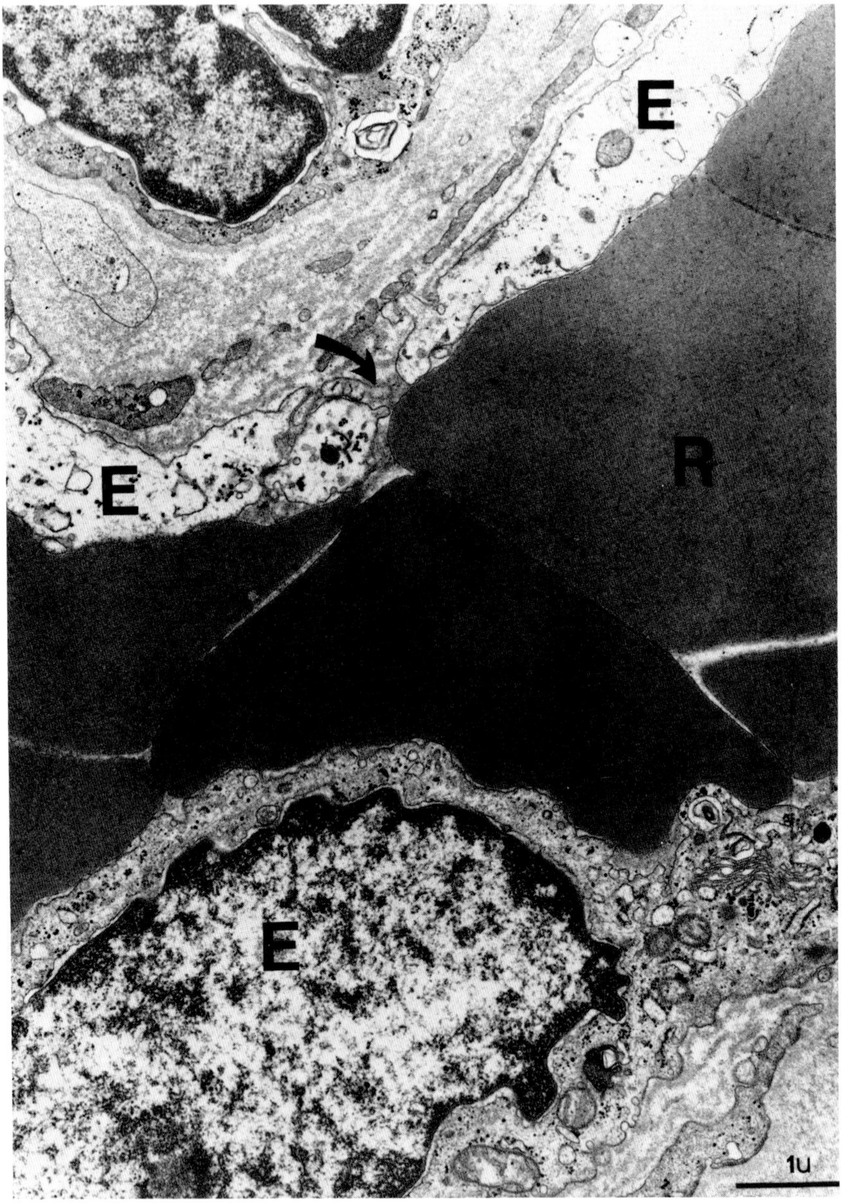

Figure 9 Transmission electron micrograph. The specimen was taken during rigid tube bronchoscopy from a patient with moderately severe asthma. The picture shows a longitudinally cut postcapillary venule. An endothelial gap (arrow) has been formed between two endothelial cells (E). R = red blood cell. Magnification × 19,500. Bar = 1 μm.

V. Conclusions

Scanning electron microscopy of the bronchial vasculature shows species differences, but similarities between human and dog allow extrapolations. In general there is a lack of information concerning the bronchial vessels in the normal human.

As the arteriole becomes progressively smaller in diameter, there is a corresponding decrease in the thickness of its three tunicae: intima, media, and adventitia. In arterioles of 100 μm there is usually a tunica media of two or more layers of smooth muscle cells. In the terminal arteriole the tunica media contains only a single layer of smooth muscle cells.

Histochemical data suggest that the airway vascular bed in the human is innervated by adrenergic and peptidergic nerves. Adrenergic and vasoactive intestinal peptide containing nerves are found in close association with the bronchial vessels.

Very little quantitative information is available about the airway mucosal lymphatic vessels. These differ from venules in having a thin endothelium, a discontinuous basal lamina, and no surrounding pericytes.

There are special ultrastructural features in the bronchial vessels: (1) fenestrated capillaries; and (2) endothelial gap formation in postcapillary venules, especially evident in asthmatic patients.

References

Baier, H., Long, W. M., and Wanner, A. (1985). Bronchial circulation in asthma. *Respiration* **48**:199–205.

Barnes, P. J. (1986). Asthma as an axon reflex. *Lancet* **1**:242–245.

Bartels, H. (1982). Open junctions in the venular plexuses of the bronchial microcirculation. *J. Submicrosc. Cytol.* **14**:93–97.

Beasley, R., Roche, W. R., Roberts, J. A., and Holgate, S. T. (1989). Cellular events in the bronchi in mild asthma and after bronchial provocation. *Am. Rev. Respir. Dis.* **139**:806–817.

Castenholtz, A. (1983). The outer surface morphology of blood vessels as revealed in scanning electron microscopy in resin casts and non-corroded tissue specimens. *Scanning Electron Microsc.* **4**:1955–1962.

Castenholtz, A. (1989). Interpretation of structural patterns appearing on corrosion casts of small blood and initial lymphatic vessels. *Scanning Electron Microsc.* **3**(1):315–325.

Charan, N. B., Turk, G., and Dhand, R. (1984). Gross and subgross anatomy of bronchial circulation in sheep. *J. Appl. Physiol.* **57**:658–664.

Charan, N. B., Turk, G. M., Czartolomny, J., and Andreazuk, T. (1987). Systemic arterial blood supply to the trachea and lung in the sheep. *J. Appl. Physiol.* **62**:2283–2287.

Cudkowicz, L. (1979). Bronchial arterial circulation in man: Normal anatomy and response to disease. In *Lung Biology in Health and Disease*. Edited by K. M. Moser. New York, Marcel Dekker, Vol. 14, *Pulmonary Vascular Diseases*, pp. 111–232.

Cudkowicz, L., and Armstrong, J. B. (1951). Observations on the normal anatomy of the bronchial arteries. *Thorax* **6**:343–358.

Daly, M. de B., and Hebb, C. (1966). *Pulmonary and Bronchial Vascular System*. London, Edward Arnold.

Deffebach, M. E., Charan, N. B., Lakshminarayan, S., and Butler, J. (1987). The bronchial circulation: Small but vital attribute of the lung. *Am. Rev. Respir. Dis.* **135**:463–481.

Dey, R. D., Shannon, W. A. Jr., and Said, S. I. (1981). Localization of VIP-immunoreactive nerves in airways and pulmonary vessels of dogs, cats, and human subjects. *Cell Tissue Res.* **220**:231–238.

Florey, H. W. (1966). The endothelial cell. *Br. Med. J.* **2**:2512.

Hebb, C. (1969). Motor innervation of the pulmonary blood vessels of mammals. In *The Pulmonary Circulation and Interstitial space*. Edited by A. P. Fishman and H. H. Hecht. Chicago, University of Chicago Press, pp. 195–222.

Hill, P., Goulding, D., Webber, S. E., and Widdicombe, J. G. (1989). Blood sinuses in the submucosa of the large airways of the sheep. *J Anat.* **162**:235–247.

Hirabayashi, M., and Yamamoto, T. (1984). An electron-microscopic study of the endothelium in mammalian bronchial microvasculature. *Cell Tissue Res.* **236**:19–25.

Hughes, T. (1965). Microcirculation of the tracheobronchial tree. *Nature (Lond.)* **206**:425–426.

Laitinen, A., and Laitinen, L. A. (1990). Vascular beds in the airways of normal subjects and asthmatics. *Eur. Respir. J.* **12**(3. Suppl):659–662.

Laitinen, A., Partanen, M., Hervonen, A., Pelto-Huikko, M., and Laitinen, L. A. (1985). VIP like immunoreactive nerves in the human lower respiratory tract: Light and electron microscopic study. *Histochemistry* **82**:313–319.

Laitinen, A., Laitinen, L. A., Moss, R., and Widdicombe, J. G. (1989). Organization and structure of the tracheal and bronchial blood vessels in the dog. *J. Anat* **166**:133–140.

Laitinen, L. A. (1988). Detailed analysis of neural elements in human airways. In *The Airways: Neural Control in Health and Disease*. Edited by M. A. Kaliner and P. J. Barnes. New York, Marcel Dekker, pp. 35–56.

Laitinen, L. A., and Laitinen, A. (1991). Overview of the pathology of asthma. In *Pharmacology of Asthma, Handbook of Experimental Phar-*

macology. Edited by C. P. Page and P. J. Barnes. New York, Springer-Verlag, pp. 1–25.

Laitinen, L. A., Heino, M., Laitinen, A., Kava, T., and Haahtela, T. (1985). Damage of the airway epithelium and bronchial reactivity in patients with asthma. *Am. Rev. Respir. Dis.* **131**:599–606.

Laitinen, L. A., Laitinen, A., Salonen, R. O., and Widdicombe, J. G. (1987). Vascular actions of airway neuropeptides. *Am. Rev. Respir. Dis.* **136**:S59–S64.

Lauweryns, J. M., de Boc, V., Guelinckx, P., and Decamer, M. (1983). Effects of unilateral hypoxia on neuroepithelial bodes in rabbit lungs. *J. Appl. Physiol.* **55**:1665–1668.

Lauweryns, J. M., Van Lommer, A. T., and Dom, R. J. (1985). Innervation of rabbit intrapulmonary neuroepithelial bodies. Quantitative and qualitative ultrastructural study after vagotomy. *J. Neurol. Sci* **67**:81–92.

Leak, L. V. (1980). Blood vessels. In *Electron Microscopy in Human Medicine*, Vol 5, *Cardiovascular System, Lymphoreticular and Hematopoietic System*. Edited by J. V. Johannessen. London, McGraw-Hill International. pp. 87–197.

Lundberg, J. M., Hokfelt, T., Martling, C. R., Saria, A., and Cuello, C. (1984). Substance P-immunoreactive sensory nerves in the lower respiratory tract of various mammals including man. *Cell Tissue Res.* **235**:251–261.

Magno, M. G., and Fishman, A. P. (1982). Origin, distribution, and blood flow of bronchial circulation in anesthesized sheep. *J. Appl. Physiol.* **53**:272–279.

Majno, G., and Leventhal, M. (1967). Pathogenesis of histamine-type vascular leakage. *Lancet* **8**:99–100.

Mann, S. P. (1971). The innervation of mammalian bronchial smooth muscle: The localization of catecholamines and cholinesterases. *Histochem J.* **3**:319–331.

Marchand, P., Gilroy J. C., and Wilson, V. H. (1950). An anatomical study of the bronchial vascular system and its variations in disease. *Thorax* **5**:207–221.

Mariassy, A. T., Gazeroglu, H., and Wanner, A. (1989). Morphometry of the subepithelial circulation in the sheep airways: Effect of vascular congestion. *Am. Rev. Respir. Dis.* **139**(4):A452.

McDonald, D. M. (1988). Respiratory tract infections increase susceptibility to neurogenic inflammation in the rat trachea. *Am. Rev. Respir. Dis.* **137**:1432–1440.

McDonald, D. M., Mitchell, R. A., Gabella, G., and Haskell, A. (1988). Neurogenic inflammation in the rat trachea. II. Identity and distribution of nerves mediating the increase in vascular permeability. *J. Neurocytol.* **17**:605–628.

McLaughlin, R. F., Jr. (1983). Bronchial artery distribution in various mammals and humans. *Am. Rev. Respir. Dis.* **128**:S57–58.

McLaughlin, R. F., Tyler, W. S., and Canada, R. O. (1966). Subgross pulmonary anatomy of the rabbit, rat and guinea pig, with additional notes on the human lung. *Am. Rev. Respir. Dis.* **94**:380–387.

Miller, S. W. (1947). *The Lung*, 2nd ed. Springfield, Illinois: Charles C. Thomas.

Murakami, T. (1971). Application of the SEM to the study of the fine distribution of the blood vessels. *Arch. Histol. Jpn.* **32**:445–454.

Partanen, M., Laitinen, A., Hervonen, A., Toivanen, M., and Laitinen, L. A. (1982). Catecholamine- and acetylcholinesterase containing nerves in human lower respiratory tract. *Histochemistry* **76**:175–188.

Persson, C. G. A. (1986). Role of plasma exudation in asthmatic airways. *Lancet* **2**:1126–1129.

Pietra, G. G., and Magno, M. (1978). Pharmacologic factors influencing permeability of the bronchial microcirculation. *Fed Proc.* **37**:2466–2470.

Pietra, G. G., Szidon, J. P., Leventhal, M. M., and Fisherman, A. P. (1971). Histamine and interstitial pulmonary edema in the dog. *Circ. Res.* **29**:323–337.

Pump, K. K. (1972). Distribution of bronchial arteries in the human lung. *Chest* **62**:447–451.

Rhodin, J. A. G. (1962). The diaphragm of capillary endothelial fenestrations. *J. Ultrastruct. Res.* **6**:171.

Simionescu, M., Simionescu, N., and Palade, G. E. (1975). Segmental differentiations of the cell junctions in the vascular endothelium. The microvasculature. *J. Cell Biol.* **67**:863.

Sobin, S. S., Frasher, W. G., Tremer, H. M., and Hadley, G. G. (1963). The microcirculation of the tracheal mucosa. *Angiology* **14**:165–170.

Springall, D. R., Bloom, S. R., and Polak, J. M. (1988). Distribution, nature, and origin of peptide containing nerves in mammalian airways. In *The Airways*. Edited by M. A. Kaliner and P. J. Barnes. New York, Marcel Dekker, pp. 299–342.

Wanner, A. (1989). Circulation of the airway mucosa. *J. Appl. Physiol.* **67**:917–925.

Zweifach, B. W. (1957). General principles governing behavior of the microcirculation. *Am. J. Med.* **23**:684.

Part III

MEASUREMENT

4

Methods of Measuring Bronchial Blood Flow

ELISABETH M. BAILE and PETER D. PARÉ

University of British Columbia
St. Paul's Hospital
Vancouver, British Columbia, Canada

I. Introduction

The first measurements of bronchial blood flow were made by Berry and Daly in 1931. Since that time a wide variety of techniques have been devised in an attempt to quantitate the blood flow to this diminutive and elusive circulation. That such a wide variety of techniques have been used to measure bronchial arterial blood flow is indicative of the technical difficulties encountered. There are several reasons for these difficulties: under normal physiological conditions the total bronchial blood flow is only about 1% of the cardiac output; the bronchial vessels themselves are small and are located deep within the thorax adjacent to vital structures; there may be multiple sites of origin of the bronchial vessels; the bronchial vessels supply collateral blood flow to the mediastinum, pleura, pericardium, and other structures, and the bronchial circulation has a dual venous drainage so that a proportion of the blood drains into the right side of the heart via the azygos and hemiazygos veins and the remainder drains into the left side of the heart via the pulmonary veins.

Despite the ingenious and imaginative techniques that have been devised to measure bronchial blood flow, there are frequently problems associated with measuring the two components of bronchial blood flow draining into the left and right heart, respectively; in some cases the values obtained may represent either an overestimation or an underestimation of the true flow. For instance, when "total" bronchial blood flow is measured by isolating a single bronchial vessel, a substantial proportion of flow supplied by collateral vessels may be missed; on the other hand, a significant percentage of the flow in the isolated vessel may be directed to nonpulmonary structures, such as the pericardium and mediastinal lymph nodes. A variety of hemodynamic parameters can affect the amount and distribution of bronchial flow. Systemic and pulmonary arterial and venous pressures as well as airway pressure and lung inflation may all affect bronchial blood flow in a complex manner.

Many of the methods devised to measure bronchial blood flow necessitate extensive surgical preparation, which in itself can affect the measurements by changing the normal physiological control by causing release of vasodilatory prostaglandins. Inadequate control of inspired air conditions, humidity and temperature, and the thermal environment of open-chested preparations can also affect normal physiological measurements of bronchial blood flow because the bronchial vasculature is extremely temperature sensitive.

Another confounding feature of the bronchial vasculature is the potentially different responses of the systemic and systemic-to-pulmonary components to stimuli, such as neural and inflammatory mediators and hypoxia. It is not known at what anatomic level the systemic-to-pulmonary anastomatic bronchial vessels start to respond, physiologically, as pulmonary vessels. The diversity of the bronchial vasculature creates the additional challenge of devising techniques to measure blood flow to different regions of the airways and lung parenchyma, and within these regions there may be large differences in flow to the various tissues, such as cartilage, mucosa, and muscularis.

In summary, measurements of bronchial blood flow represent a real and continuous challenge to the investigator. Values may vary depending on the technique and the species used as well as the relative vascular pressures of the two systems, the extent of the surgery, the temperature and humidity of the environment, and the ingenuity of the investigator.

In this chapter, the various techniques used to measure bronchial blood flow are reviewed in some detail. For each technique a description of the methodology is given followed by data for measurements of blood flow obtained during baseline conditions. The applications of the technique and its advantages and disadvantages relative to other methods of measurement are also presented.

An overview of the methods that have been devised to measure bronchial arterial blood flow is shown in Tables 1, 2, and 3. These methods can be divided into three major categories. First, those in which total bronchial arterial blood flow (i.e., blood returning to the right and left atrium) is meas-

Table 1 Total Bronchial Arterial Blood Flow[a]

Method	Species	Values	Reference
Isolated aortic pouch and rotameter			
Rotameter	Dog	12 ml/min; range 3–35 ml/min	Horisberger and Rodbard, 1960
Rotameter	Dog	29.8 ml/min; range 11–42 ml/min	Martinez L. De Latona et al., 1961
Flowmeter	Dog	49 ml/min (arterial) 21 ml/min (Venous)	Aramendia et al. 1962
	Dog	21 ml/min; range 1–45 ml/min	Murao, 1965
	Sheep	39 ±3.1 ml/min	Zapata-Ortiz et al., 1967
Measurements in single vessels: flow probes			
Bubble flowmeter	Dog	4.8 ±2.5 ml/min (right lung); range 1–12 ml/min	Bruner and Schmidt, 1947
EMFP	Sheep	19.9 ±18.3 ml/min; range 5–90 ml/min; 3.97 ±1.6 ml/min/100g wet lung wt; 0.46 ±0.37 ml/min/kg body wt	Magno and Fishman, 1982
EMFP	Sheep	30.7 ±7.4 ml/min; 1.06% CO; range 0.33–3.3%	Long et al., 1985
EMPF	Sheep	1.2 ±0.9% CO	Baier et al., 1985
Ultrasonic flow probe	Horse	0.09–0.33 ml/min/kg body wt (awake) 0.01–0.7 ml/min/kg body wt (anesthetized)	Gleed et al., 1990

Table 1 (Continued)

Method	Species	Values	Reference
Perfusion of a bronchial artery			
Const flow	Dogs	% Change from baseline	Lung et al., 1976
Const press	Dogs	9.7 ±0.5 ml/min	Yanaura et al., 1981
Const press	Sheep	34.1 ±2.9 ml/min; 0.62 ml/min/kg body wt; BVR 3.9 ±0.5 cmH_2O/ml/min	Charan et al., 1985
Pba change	Sheep	12.3 ±1.1 ml/min 0.48 ml/min/kg body wt; BVR, 6.1 ±0.6 mmHg/ml/min	Wagner et al., 1987
Pba change	Sheep	22 ±2 ml/min; 0.7 ml/min/kg body wt; BVR 3.8 ±0.4 mmHg/ml/min	Wagner and Mitzner, 1988
Videodensitometry			
	Sheep	28.5 ±7 ml/min; 0.62 ±0.2% CO; 0.71 ±0.17 ml/min/kg	Link et al., 1985
	Sheep	32 ±19 ml/min; 0.6 ±2% CO	Parsons et al., 1985
	Sheep	35.3 ±8.4 ml/min	Parsons et al., 1987
Radioactive microspheres			
Ref flow	Dogs	31.2 ±6.2 ml/min; 83.4 ±23.1 ml/min/100 g dry lung; 1.6 ±0.5% CO	Malik and Tracy, 1980

Ref flow	Dogs	8.3 ±1.1 ml/min; 0.4% CO left lung, trachea, mainstem bronchus	Baile et al., 1982
Ref flow	Dogs	6.1 ±1.6 ml/min; 0.3 ±0.1% CO left lung, trachea, mainstem bronchus	Baile and Paré, 1983
Ref flow	Dogs	Trachea, left lung, 7.8 ±0.8 ml/min; 0.4 ±0.04% CO	Baile et al., 1985a
Ref flow	Dogs	2.8 ±0.3 ml/min trachea and LL bronchi	Baile et al., 1986b
Ref flow	Dogs	3.6 ml/min; 0.2% CO	Baile et al., 1987a
Ref flow	Sheep	7.6 ±3.5 ml/min trachea 9.0 ±5.4 LL bronchi 9.0 ±6.5 LL parenchyma	Parsons et al., 1989
PaO DMT	sheep	16.8 ±2.1 ml/min/100 g LL bronchi 15.1 ±2.5 ml/min/100 g	Wu et al., 1988
PaO DMT	sheep	1.52 ±0.98% CO 1.39 ±0.88% CO	Wu et al., 1988

[a] EMFP, electromagnetic flow probe; CO, cardiac output; const flow, constant flow; const press, constant pressure; BVR, Bronchial vascular resistance; Pba, bronchial arterial pressure; Ref flow, reference flow; PaO, pulmonary artery occlusion; LL, left lung; DMT, double-microsphere technique; wt, weight.

Table 2 Bronchial Systemic-to-Pulmonary Blood Flow[a]

Method	Species	Values	Reference
Isolated Lobe			
No Pa			
Perfusion: arterial and/or venous collection	Dogs	4.4–9 ml/min	Williams and Towbin, 1955
	Dogs	4.4 ml/min; range 2.1–7.7 ml/min; 0.1–0.4 ml/min/kg	Aviado et al., 1961
	Sheep	48.6 ±7.8 ml/min	Zapata-Ortiz et al., 1967
	Dogs	2.3 to 5.3 ml/min	Modell et al., 1981
Pa perfusion: lobar weight change	Dogs	24.4 ±0.9 ml/min/100 g dry lobe wt/100 mmHg Psa	Jindal et al., 1984
	Dogs	31 ±10 ml/min/100 g dry lobe wt/100 mmHg Psa	Jindal et al., 1985
	Dogs	23.7 ±3.0 ml/min/100 g dry lobe 24.5 ±6.4 ml/min/100 g dry lobe	Deffebach et al., 1987
	Dogs	73.0 ±21.4 ml/min/100 g dry lobe wt/100 mmHg Psa	Agostoni et al., 1987c
Cardiopulmonary bypass			
	Dogs (4)	44 ml/min; range 3.5–250 (La outflow when Pa inflow = 0)	Berry and Daly, 1931
	Dogs (2)	21 ml/min; range 13–33 ml/min (aortic inflow—azygos vein outflow)	

	Dog (1)	19 ml/min, range 9–38 ml/min (La outflow—Pa inflow)	
	Dogs	0.5–1.05% total arterial blood flow	State et al., 1957
	Dogs	2–12 ml/min	Auld et al., 1960
	Dogs	5–60 ml/min	Goetz and Rohman, 1965
	Dogs	8.8 ±4.9 ml/min; range 2.4–19 ml/min	Cartwright et al., 1962
	Dogs	52.3 ±16.3 ml/min; range 18–108 ml/min	Warren and Powell, 1986
	Humans	15 ±6 ml/min	Lajos and Glicken, 1980
	Humans	140 ±182 ml/min; 3.2 ±4.15% pump flow; range 8–1043 ml/min	Baile et al., 1985b
	Humans	65 ±35 ml/min; 1.6 ±0.84% pump flow	Baile et al., 1986a
	Humans	0.32–2.76% pump flow	Agostoni et al., 1989
Difference between left and right ventricular output			
	Dogs	65 ±49 ml/min (indirect);	Cudkowicz et al., 1959a
	Humans	mean 90 ml/min; 1.5% of right ventricular output	Cudkowicz et al., 1959b
Chronic Pa ligation	Dogs	660 ml/min direct; 640 ml/min indirect	Cudkowicz et al., 1960
	Humans	70 ml/min	Cudkowicz et al., 1960
	Humans	540 ml/min direct; 510 ml/min indirect	
	Dogs	6–9% CO; mean 8.2% CO	Aramendia et al., 1962

Table 2 (Continued)

Method	Species	Values	Reference
Fick principle and bronchospirometry			
Oxygen			
	Dogs	Range 700–2233 ml/min	Bloomer et al., 1949
	Humans	950 ml/min or 17% CO	Madoff et al., 1952
	Humans	Range 860–350 ml/min	Fishman et al., 1958
Carbon dioxide			
Bypass	Humans	112 ml/min; range 11–311 ml/min	Deal et al., 1968
Chronic Pa ligation LL	Dogs	94 ±34ml/min	Lilker and Nagy, 1975
Carbon monoxide, left lung			
	Dogs	8 ±2 ml/min; range 5–10 ml/min	Fisher et al., 1970
Earpiece dye dilution			
	Humans	Increased in 18 of 67 patients	Katori et al., 1970b

[a] Pa, pulmonary artery; Psa, mean systemic arterial pressure; CO, cardiac output.

Table 3 Tracheal Blood Flow

Method	Species	Values	Reference
Tracheal perfusion			
	Dogs	9.5 ±0.5 ml/min	Himori and Taira, 1976
	Dogs	8.7 ±1.1 ml/min	Himori and Taira, 1978
Hydrogen Clearance			
	Dogs	31 ±3.8 (SEM) ml/min/100 g	Joh 1986
	Dogs	30 ±6.5 (SEM) ml/min/100 g	Joh et al., 1987
Inert soluble gas			
	Sheep	1.2 ml/min; range 0.9–1.7 ml/min	Wanner et al., 1988
Laser Doppler flowmetry			
	Cats	All values reported as % change	Martling et al., 1987
	Dogs		Godden et al., 1991a
	Sheep		Godden et al., 1991b
	Humans		Baile et al., 1988

ured. These techniques include those that provide direct and continuous measurements, usually by application of some form of flow probe to a vessel, or indirect and discrete measurements involving the injection of markers or indicators of flow.

The second major category includes those techniques designed to measure the bronchial systemic-to-pulmonary blood flow $\dot{Q}Br(s\text{-}p)$ and may involve collection of the systemic contribution to pulmonary venous blood flow in intact lobes or lungs or a more indirect approach, such as application of the Fick principle and bronchospirometry.

The third category includes techniques that allow measurement of blood flow to the airway mucosa. These techniques are usually much less invasive, and one of them (laser Doppler velocimetry) has recently been applied to human studies. However, they provide data for only a very limited portion of the total airway flow and often allow measurements of only relative blood flow to be made.

The earlier methods of measuring tracheobronchial blood flow were invariably invasive, and consequently experimentation was confined to animals (mainly the dog). More recently, as a result of the advent of more sophisticated technology, such as videodensitometry and laser Doppler flowmetry, the potential is there to make noninvasive, real-time, continuous measurements of tracheobronchial blood flow in human subjects.

II. Total Bronchial Arterial Blood Flow

A. Direct and Continuous Measurement

This category includes techniques that require the isolation of a systemic vessel or vessels that supply the airways and lung. All these techniques are invasive, since they involve a thoracotomy to provide access to the vessel being studied, and they are therefore confined to animal experimentation. Because in all species there is more than one systemic vessel supplying the airways and lung, these techniques tend to underestimate "total" bronchial blood flow, despite including portions of the bronchial flow that return to the right and left sides of the heart. These techniques could also overestimate "total" flow in that the bronchial arteries may supply structures other than the lungs and airways.

Isolated Aortic Pouch and Rotameter

Horisberger and Rodbard (1960) devised a method for measuring bronchial arterial blood flow continuously and directly in open-chested, anesthetized dogs. The method involves isolation of a small segment of the descending aorta from the second to the fourth intercostal artery to form a small vascular sac containing the vessels to the mediastinum, pleura, and bronchial tree. Other vessels originating from this segment (intercostal and esophageal vessels) are ligated. A T tube is then inserted into the aorta to bypass the isolated segment, and one arm is connected to a previously calibrated rotameter and then to the isolated aortic segment for measurement of the bronchial flow (Fig. 1). In addition to measuring changes in flow, these investigators also determined changes in bronchovascular resistance, which was calculated as the pressure drop between the aorta and pulmonary vein divided by the bronchial blood flow. In seven dogs baseline values for bronchial blood flow averaged 12 ml/min, ranging from 3 to 35 ml/min. In addition, measurements of bronchial blood flow were obtained after increasing and decreasing airway pressure, vagotomy, and administration of pharmacological agents, such as *l*-epinephrine and serotonin.

It should be noted that the measurements just described overestimated the total bronchial arterial blood flow because some of the vessels in the isolated aortic segment supplied the pleura and mediastinum.

The technique of Horisberger and Rodbard was used by Martinez L. De Latona et al. to compare "total" bronchial arterial blood flow and bronchial systemic-to-pulmonary blood flow (1961). They reported a mean value for bronchial arterial flow obtained from 15 dogs during baseline conditions of 29.8ml/min and values ranging from 11 to 42 ml/min. In the same dogs in which the pouch technique was used they collected pulmonary venous blood

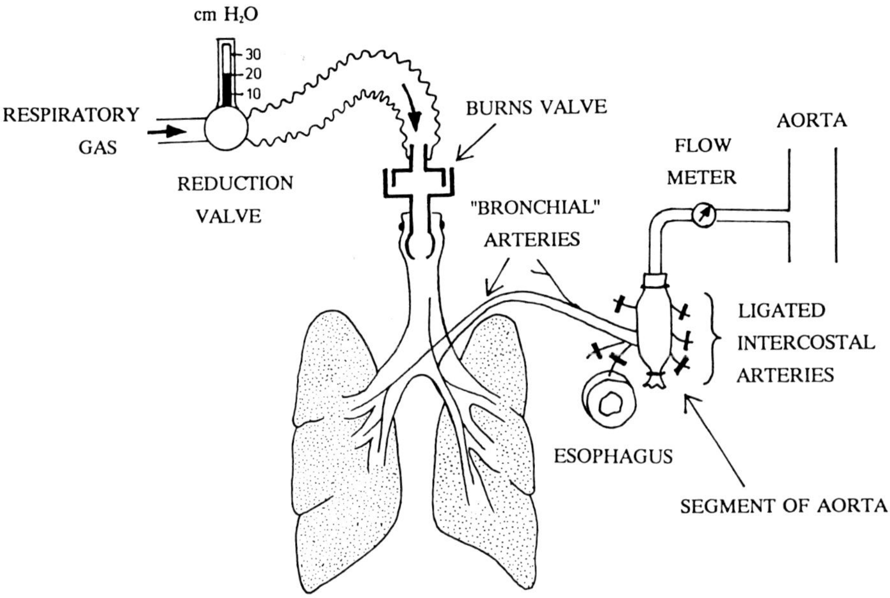

Figure 1 Essentials of the preparation. Respiratory gases were supplied from commercial cylinders to a series of reduction valves (upper left), which lowered the insufflation pressure to a selected value. The gas then passed through a Burns valve to the trachea. The bronchial blood supply is shown at right. Aortic blood passes through a flowmeter to the isolated aortic segment from which the branches to the bronchial arteries originate. The crossmarks on the lines to the esophagus and intercostals indicate that these vessels have been ligated. The "bronchial" arteries supply the bronchial tree and both lungs, as well as the mediastinum. (Adapted from Horisberger and Rodbard, 1960, by permission of the American Heart Association, Inc.)

from the left lung after ligation of the left main pulmonary artery to allow calculation of the systemic-to-pulmonary fraction of bronchial blood flow. Because some of the anastomotic flow reaching the pulmonary veins comes from vessels that did not originate in the pouch, they devised a technique to subtract this flow from the total pulmonary venous return. The blood flow from the major bronchial arteries originating from the pouch was temporarily interrupted, and the persisting pulmonary venous flow (which averaged 5 ml/min) was subtracted from the total systemic-to-pulmonary flow. To estimate a value for flow to the right lung they multiplied the left lung bronchial systemic-to-pulmonary flow by 1.26 (a factor derived experimentally by

Bruner and Schmidt (1947) to correct for the greater mass of the right lung). The bronchial systemic-to-pulmonary blood flow for both lungs averaged 67% of the total bronchial flow from the aortic pouch; presumably the remaining 33% of flow drained to the bronchial veins. In this study the role of sympathetic control of the bronchial circulation was also examined by comparing sympathetic nerve stimulation with injection of vasodilating (epinephrine, norepinephrine, and isoproterenol) and vasoconstricting (histamine, acetylcholine, and serotonin) pharmacological agents.

To determine what fraction of the total bronchial blood flow returned to the right heart via the bronchial veins, Aramendia et al. used an adaptation of the aortic pouch technique in anesthetized, open-chested dogs (1962). The bronchial circulation was perfused with blood from the aorta, and the bronchial arterial flow was measured using a flowmeter attached to the aortic pouch. The azygos vein was cannulated and ligated just above the diaphragm. Its blood flow, which represented the bronchial venous flow, was measured using another flowmeter. The bronchial arterial and venous blood was drained into a reservoir and returned to the circulation via the inferior vena cava using a pump. In six dogs the average bronchial arterial blood flow was 49 ml/min and the azygos venous flow was 21 ml/min (45% of the arterial flow). Further mechanical and pharmacological interventions were carried out to assess their effects on bronchial venous blood flow.

A different modification of the aortic pouch technique was later made by Murao (1965). Arterial blood was shunted from the ascending to the descending aorta as before, but instead of remaining connected to the aorta, the pouch was perfused from a reservoir of physiological saline kept at a constant pressure. The inflow to the pouch, measured using an electromagnetic flowmeter, represented the bronchial arterial flow (Fig. 2). At constant perfusion pressure, any changes in flow were interpreted as reflecting changes in bronchomotor tone. Bronchial vascular resistance was calculated as the difference between bronchial arterial pressure (pouch pressure) and left atrial pressure divided by bronchial arterial flow. The mean baseline value of bronchial blood flow for 50 measurements from 24 dogs was 21 ml/min, ranging from 1 to 45 ml/min. In this extensive series of experiments, these investigators also examined the effect on bronchovascular resistance of stimulating the sympathetic nerve, vagosympathetic trunk, and carotid sinus nerve. The advantage of this modification is that changes in bronchial arterial blood flow are not influenced by interventions that change perfusion pressure. One weakness of this study is the use of normal saline rather than blood as a perfusion medium. The pressure-flow characteristics of the bronchial circulation are altered by perfusing with saline, which has a different viscosity from that of blood.

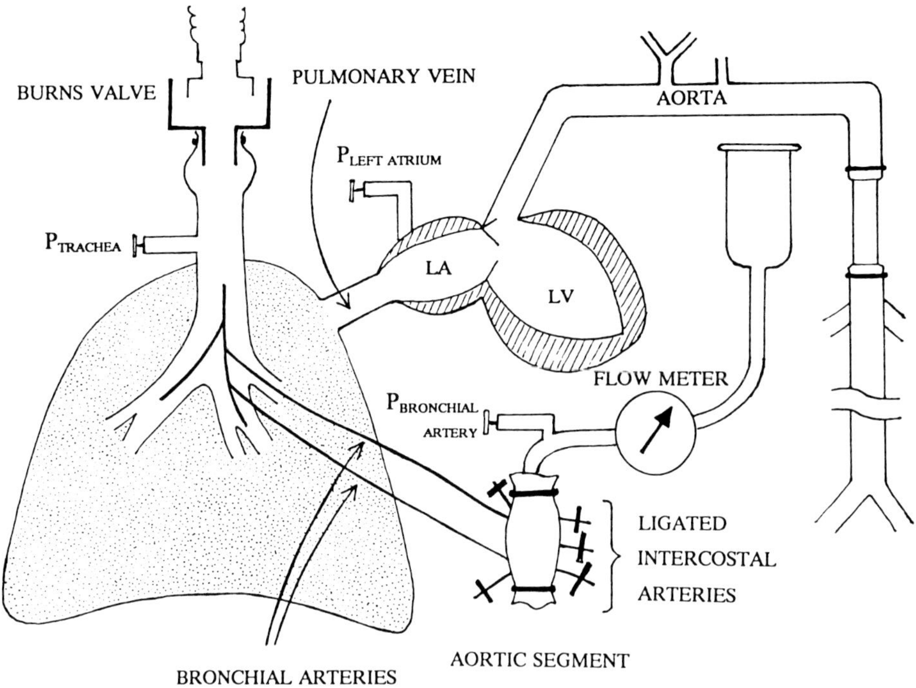

Figure 2 The preparation: $P_{LEFT\ ATRIUM}$, left atrial pressure; $P_{TRACHEA}$, tracheal pressure; LA, left atrium; LV, left ventricle; $P_{BRONCHIAL\ ARTERY}$, bronchial arterial pressure. (Adapted from Murao, 1965.)

The aortic pouch technique (Horisberger and Rodbard, 1960) was also slightly modified for use in sheep by Zapata-Ortiz et al. (1967). In retrospect, the use of this technique in the sheep was perhaps unnecessary, since unlike the dog the sheep has one main bronchial artery, the common bronchial artery (ramus bronchialis communis), originating from the bronchoesophageal artery (arteria bronchoesophagea) (Magno et al., 1987) between the fifth and sixth intercostal spaces; this vessel accounts for at least 50% of the total intrathoracic tracheobronchial blood flow (Charan et al., 1987). As subsequent investigators have shown, this vessel can readily be isolated and cannulated to make more direct measurements. The mean baseline value for bronchial arterial flow in eight sheep using the pouch technique was 39.0 ±3.1 ml/min. These investigators also examined the effects on bronchial arterial blood flow of raising sheep at high altitude under conditions of chronic hypoxia.

An ingenious modification of the technique of Horisberger and Rodbard (1960) was devised to obviate the need for thoracotomy at the time of the experiment (DeKock et al., 1966). A stainless steel tube with a balloon at each end was inserted through the abdominal aorta into the segment of the thoracic aorta containing the origin of the bronchial arteries (Fig. 3). This aortic seg-

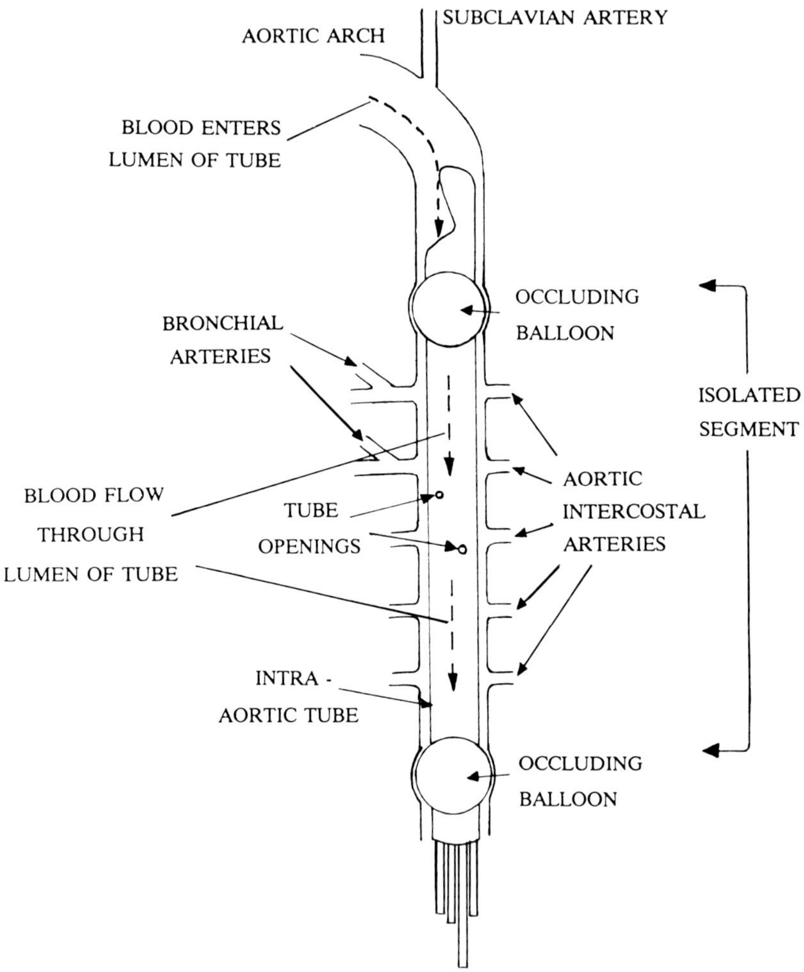

Figure 3 The aortic tube properly palced in the thoracic aorta. By inflating the ballons, the segment of aorta including the first five intercostal arteries was isolated, but blood flowed from the descending thoracic aorta through the tube to the abdominal aorta. (Adapted from DeKock et al., 1966, with permission from the *Journal of Applied Physiology.)*

ment could be isolated by inflating the balloons. A side cannula in the tube allowed perfusion of the segment and injection of various drugs, and flow could also be measured. Although this technique allowed the measurement of bronchial arterial flow, it was designed primarily to examine the effects of bronchial arterial injection of various pharmacological agents on lung mechanics: values for flow were therefore not reported in the original article. However, using the same technique, Zwi, Karp, and Nadel recorded measurements of bronchial blood flow in a group of eight dogs. The mean baseline value was 29 $\pm$13 ml/min (standard deviation, SD). Injection of histamine into the isolated segment produced a fivefold increase in blood flow while systemic pressure remained constant (personal communication, Dr. Saul Zwi, 1990).

The most obvious advantage of the aortic pouch technique compared with techniques that were previously developed for measuring bronchial arterial blood flow (see Table 1) was that it provided a continuous and direct measurement of flow in a species (the dog) in which it was extremely difficult to isolate the bronchial arteries because of their multiple and variable origin (Notkovitch, 1957). A slight modification of this preparation allows bronchial arterial pressure to be controlled during interventions that may change systemic arterial pressure (Murao, 1965). Another possible advantage is that it measures the "total" bronchial arterial blood flow (i.e., blood flow returning to the right and left heart). Some disadvantages are that it can overestimate the total flow if any of the extrabronchial vessels are not isolated and ligated. For instance, Bruner and Schmidt estimated that about 30% of the bronchial arterial flow supplied mediastinal structures (1947). It is also possible that flow may be underestimated if some of the bronchial arteries do not originate from the aortic pouch. These methods do not measure any contribution of "retrograde" pulmonary vascular-to-bronchial flow, which may be present (Barman et al., 1988). In addition, this technique necessitates extensive surgery, which may affect the normal physiological values for flow and pressure as well as requiring considerable technical expertise. Obviously it is not suited to chronic experimentation, and finally, it does not allow separation of bronchial systemic-to-pulmonary or bronchial venous flow from total bronchial blood flow.

Single Vessels

Various methods have been devised to make direct and continuous measurements of flow in single bronchial vessels: these include the bubble flowmeter, electromagnetic flow probe, transit-time flow probe, ultrasonic pulsed or continuous-wave Doppler flow probe, and cannulation and perfusion of a bronchial artery at either constant perfusion pressure or at a constant flow. These methods obviously require extensive surgery to isolate the bronchial vessel or its "parent" intercostal artery (in the case of the dog) to allow cannulation or placement of the probe.

Bubble Flowmeter

Early studies were carried out by Bruner and Schmidt (1947) in an attempt to evaluate bronchial arterial flow in the etiology of pulmonary edema. In an initial study involving more than 75 dogs, they established that 60% of the time the right bronchial artery was the major artery, branching from the fifth or sixth right intercostal artery. In further studies on anesthetized dogs, after the initial thoracotomy the sixth rib was partially resected and the parent intercostal was isolated and ligated. A cannula was then introduced into the origin of the right bronchial artery, and it was perfused with blood from the femoral artery (Fig. 4). Blood flow through the vessel was measured by a small bubble flowmeter, designed previously by Dumke and Schmidt (1943). In 50 dogs, they recorded a mean baseline value of bronchial arterial blood flow to the right lung of 4.8 ±2.5 ml/min (range 1–12 ml/min). These two investigators also examined the role of the sympathetic and parasympathetic nervous systems in altering bronchial arterial blood flow and the effect on the bronchial vasculature of administering various pharmacological agents and increasing intratracheal pressure.

One of the limitations of this technique is that it allows measurement of blood flow only to the right lung and does not include that fraction originating from minor bronchial arteries. Further experiments in which red blood cells labeled with ^{32}P were injected showed that about 70% of the flow in the bronchial artery supplied the right lung and about 30% supplied mediastinal structures. Thus this technique may simultaneously overestimate and underestimate total bronchial blood flow! An additional problem is the reduction in systemic arterial blood pressure and blood flow observed over time, even when no experimental procedure had been carried out; this was considered a consequence of the extensive surgery.

Electromagnetic Flow Probe

The first measurements of bronchial arterial blood flow to be made using an electromagnetic flow probe were in the sheep. This species was chosen because it had been shown to have one main bronchial artery (Fig. 5) (Magno and Fishman, 1982), as opposed to the dog, which was a variable and inconsistent number (Notkovitch, 1957). Since then a number of investigators have used this technique to measure bronchial arterial blood flow in the sheep (see Table 1). To allow placement of the flow probe a left thoracotomy is done, the common bronchial artery is exposed, and its esophageal branch (or branches) is ligated. A previously calibrated electromagnetic flow probe is carefully placed around the common bronchial branch of the bronchoesophageal artery

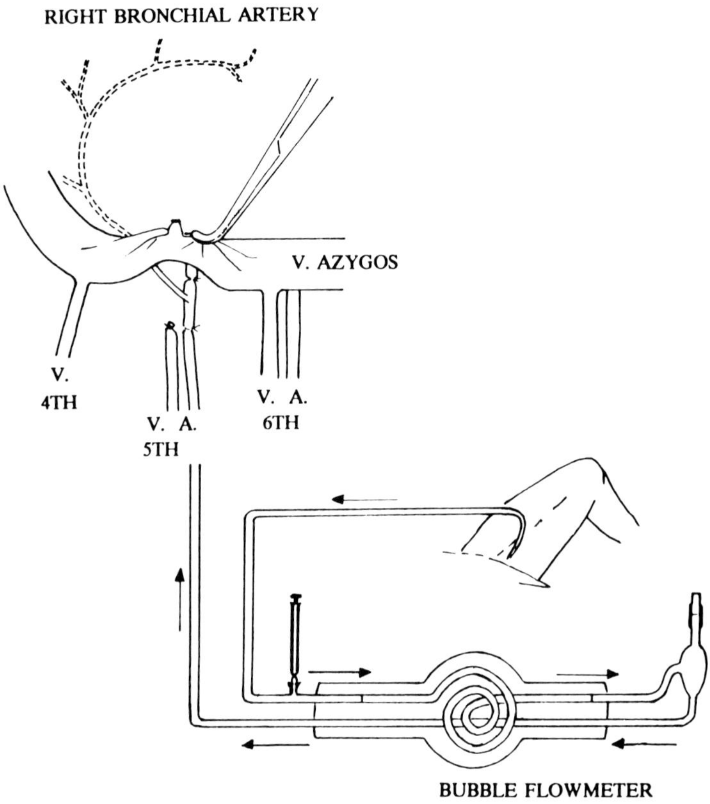

Figure 4 The usual origin of the right posterior bronchial artery of the dog and the circuit containing the bubble flow meter. V, vein; A, artery; 4TH, 5TH, and 6TH refer to intercostal veins and arteries. (Adapted from Bruner and Schmidt, 1947, with permission from the *American Journal of Physiology.*)

to avoid kinking or occlusion of the vessel, and the probe is then connected to a flowmeter. In the initial studies (Magno and Fishman, 1982) the mean bronchial arterial blood flow was 19.9 ±18.3 ml/min (range 5–90 ml/min). Flow was also expressed per 100 g wet lung, and the mean value was 3.97 ±1.6 ml/min per 100 g; when normalized for body weight the mean flow was 0.46 ±0.37 ml/min/kg.

Later studies were carried out by Long et al. (1985) using this technique, and they obtained a mean baseline value for bronchial arterial blood flow of 30.7 ±7.4 ml/min or 1.06% of the cardiac output, ranging from 0.33 to 3.33%. The effects of aerosolized histamine on bronchial arterial blood flow

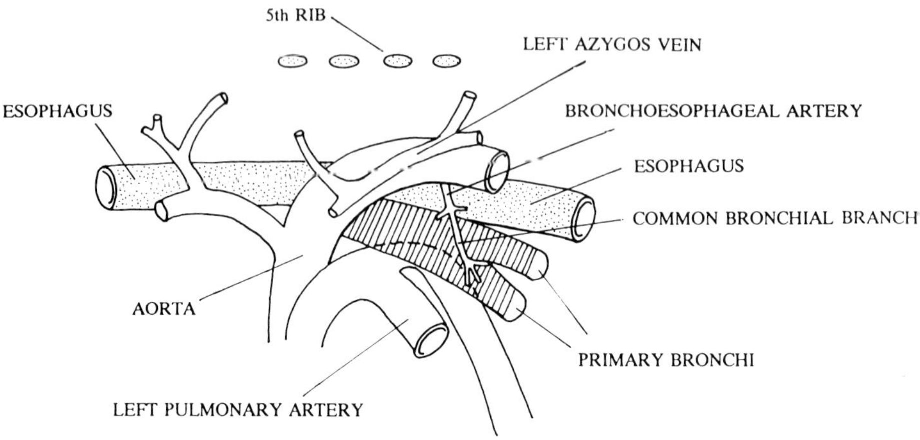

Figure 5 The left thoracic cavity showing the location of the common bronchial branch of the bronchoesophageal artery in the sheep. For clarity the azygos vein is shown transsected. (Adapted from Magno and Fishman, 1982, with permission from the *Journal of Applied Physiology*.)

and bronchomotor tone were also examined. This preparation was reported to be stable for as long as 8–12 h. Sheep were excluded from the study if they had bronchoesophageal arteries that had multiple origins (5%) or a circumference of less than 3.0 mm (10%).

Baier et al. (1985) also used an electromagnetic flow probe to measure bronchial arterial blood flow in anesthetized sheep in a study designed to examine the effect of endogenous cyclooxygenase products on pulmonary and bronchial hemodynamics and pulmonary resistance and elasticity during lung inflation. The mean baseline value for bronchial blood flow, expressed as a percentage of cardiac output, was 1.2 ±0.9%. They also demonstrated a reduction in bronchial blood flow during the application of positive end-expiratory pressure.

It has been suggested that about 88% of the bronchial blood flow in the sheep is supplied by the common bronchial branch of the bronchoesophageal artery (Magno and Fishman, 1982). However, this may be an overestimation because the sheep has since been shown to have multiple systemic arteries to the lung (Charan et al., 1987), and the common bronchial branch probably supplies only about 50% of the intrathoracic tracheobronchial blood flow. The major advantages of using the electromagnetic flow probe is that relatively stable measurements of blood flow can be made continuously and in real time. The obvious disadvantages are that it is invasive and is, of course, confined to sheep and those species having one major bronchial artery. Like the aortic pouch technique in the dog, some of the flow may supply mediastinal structures, such as the pericardium and lymph nodes, in addition to the airways and lung.

Ultrasonic Transit-Time Volume Flowmetry

The ultrasonic flow probe has been developed and validated over the past decade and has been used to measure volume flow in a wide variety of animals and organs (Canty and Brooks, 1985; Sellers et al., 1982; Shimura et al., 1986; Barnes et al., 1983).

Ultrasonic transit-time flowmetry is based on the principle of acoustic reflection. The flow probe has two ultrasonic transducers, situated so that they are located upstream and downstream on the vessel; a fixed acoustic reflector is positioned halfway between the two transducers on the opposite side of the vessel. The two transducers pass ultrasonic signals back and forth, alternately crossing the flowing liquid in the upstream and downstream directions. The difference in travel time between the upstream and downstream signals is an accurate measure of volume flow.

Gleed and associates (1990) have recently used a chronically implanted 4 mm cuff-type ultrasonic transit-time flow probe to measure bronchial arterial blood flow in six standardbred horses before and during halothane anesthesia. The horses were anesthetized 6 weeks or more before the experimental study and a thoracotomy performed by resecting the left seventh rib. The probe was then placed around the bronchial artery, the chest closed, and the horses allowed to recover. On the study day measurements of bronchial arterial flow were recorded before and at 15, 30, 45, 60, and 75 min after induction of anesthesia. In the awake horses the flow varied between 0.09 and 0.33 ml/min/kg body weight. During anesthesia values for bronchial arterial flow were lower and varied between 0.01 and 0.07 ml/min/kg.

The advantage of this technique over the electromagnetic flow probe is that it does not require precise fitting of the probe to the vessel since the sensor requires only acoustic contact with the vessel and a loose fit is acceptable (Drost, 1978). Indeed, it has been shown that its stability improves with time after implantation as the probe becomes encapsulated (Drost et al., 1979). Other advantages are, of course, that it can be used for repeated studies. Its disadvantages are similar to those cited for the electromagnetic flow probe.

Ultrasonic Pulsed Doppler Flow Probe

This is another technique that has recently been applied to the measurement of bronchial arterial blood flow in sheep. Ultrasonic pulsed or continuous-wave Doppler flow crystals are implanted chronically on the common bronchial branch of the bronchoesophageal artery in sheep. After the sheep have recovered from the surgery, real-time, continuous measurements of bronchial blood flow can be made in awake, bleating, eating sheep (Parsons, personal communication, 1989).

Briefly, the principle of this technique is that sound is continuously directed from an emitter crystal through a vessel wall, reflected off moving particles, detected by a sensor crystal, and shifted in frequency by an amount proportional to the velocity of blood flow (Angelsen et al., 1985; Hartley et al., 1978; Vatner et al., 1985; White et al., 1974).

Bronchial Arterial Perfusion

Methods of perfusing the bronchial artery have been devised in which either the bronchial arterial pressure or the flow is kept constant.

Constant Flow

A technique of constant flow autoperfusion of the bronchial artery of dogs was devised by Lung and her colleagues (1976) in an attempt to characterize the vasomotor activity of the bronchial vasculature in response to autonomic agonists. In this preparation the bronchoesophageal artery, which usually arises from the fifth right intercostal artery, was cannulated retrogradely via its parent intercostal artery and perfused with blood from a femoral artery using a pump. Femoral and bronchial arterial pressures were measured, and a cannulating electromagnetic flow probe was used to measure bronchial arterial blood flow. Using this method, under conditions of constant flow, vasomotion of the bronchial vasculature is observed as a change in perfusion pressure. Because of this, the results were reported as changes in perfusion pressure in response to various pharmacological interventions, and no baseline value for bronchial arterial blood flow was provided.

One advantage of this technique, unlike several of the earlier perfusion methods (Bruner and Schmidt, 1947; Horisberger and Rodbard, 1960; Martinez L. De Latona et al., 1961), is that the pressure changes are independent of any cardiac activity. In addition, according to these investigators (Lung et al., 1976), maintaining constant flow, as opposed to constant pressure (Murao, 1965), prevents critical closure of vessels. The disadvantages of this method are that it is invasive and that there is no means of determining what the bronchial arterial flow might be in the presence of physiological driving pressures; changes in vascular caliber are represented as changes in bronchial arterial pressure.

Constant Perfusion Pressure

A very similar technique to the one already described (Lung et al., 1976) was used by Yamatake and Yanaura to evaluate the pharmacological action of drugs on the bronchial vasculature in dogs (Yamatake and Yanaura, 1978;

Yanaura et al., 1981). However, in this study constant perfusion pressure, as opposed to constant flow, was maintained by means of a Starling pneumatic resistance and peristaltic pump. The perfusion pressure was initially adjusted to equal the mean systemic arterial blood pressure, and an electromagnetic flow probe was used to measure blood flow through the (right) bronchial artery (Fig 6). Dye was injected post-mortem to ascertain that the cannulated bronchial artery in fact supplied the bronchi and bronchioles of the right lung and right main bronchus. The mean baseline value for this partial right lung blood flow in 24 dogs was 9.7 ±0.5 ml/min. Values are also given for bronchial blood flow after administration of histamine and H_1 and H_2 receptor antagonists.

A variation of the constant perfusion pressure method has also been used in the sheep by Charan et al. (1985) to make direct measurements of bronchial arterial blood flow and downstream bronchial arterial pressure, thereby allow-

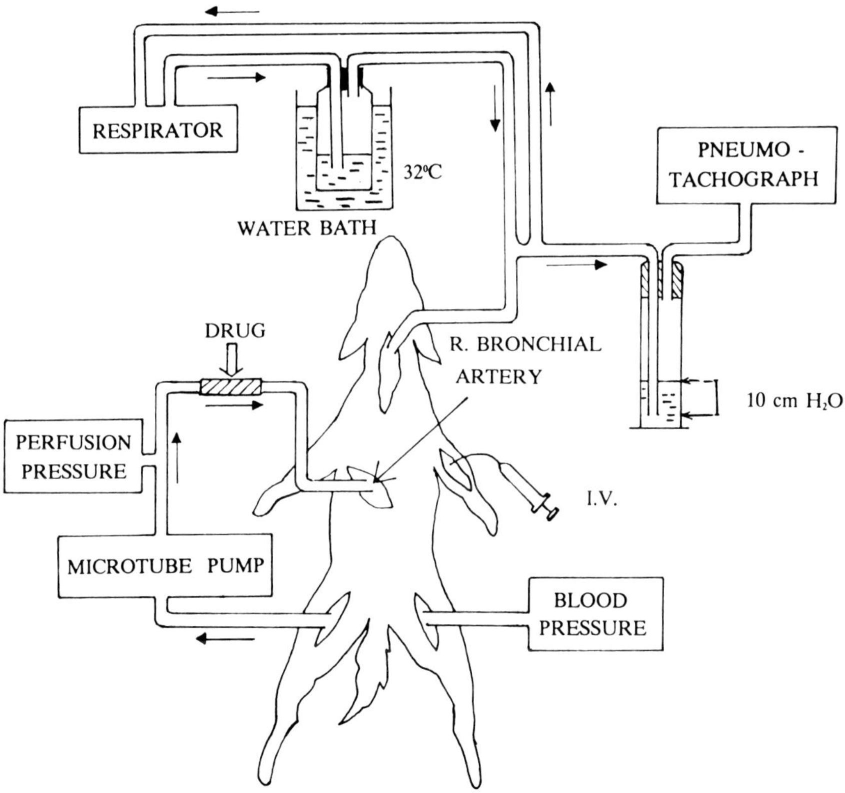

Figure 6 The preparation for perfusing the right bronchial artery. (Adapted from Yamatake and Yanaura, 1978.)

ing calculation of bronchovascular resistance. In this preparation, a carotid-to-bronchial artery shunt was formed by introducing a Teflon-tipped silastic catheter into the common bronchial branch of the bronchoesophageal artery. The proximal end of the catheter was brought out through the sheep's chest wall and introduced into the carotid artery, enabling blood to be shunted from the carotid to the bronchial artery between experimental measurements (Fig. 7). A side arm was connected to the shunt and led to a reservoir filled with warmed blood. Constant pressure was maintained by setting the reservoir height at 150 cm above the level of the left atrium (upstream pressure). Bronchial blood flow was measured, after occluding the carotid-to-bronchial artery shunt, by recording the change in reservoir volume against time. The downstream or backpressure in the bronchial artery was measured directly by occluding both carotid and reservoir flow and measuring the pressure in the system. This pressure represents a combined intravascular pressure at the sites of junction of bronchial-venous and systemic-venous circulations and the junction of bronchial-pulmonary anastomoses. In addition, this pressure could be influenced by precapillary anastomoses with other systemic vessels supplying the lung. In this study the backpressure was between about 17 and 25 cmH_2O, which was higher than the pulmonary capillary wedge pressure measured

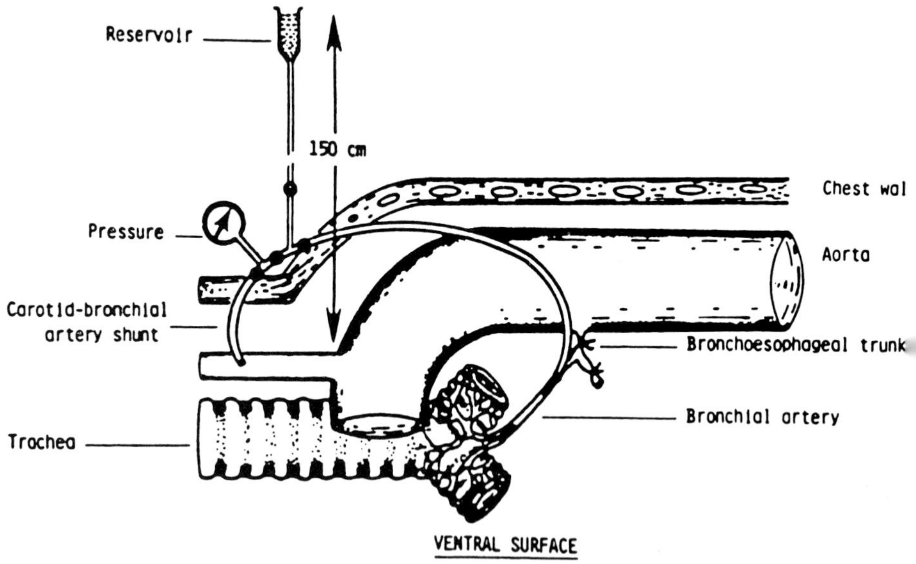

Figure 7 Carotid-to-bronchial artery shunt model in the sheep. (From Charan et al., 1985, with permission from the *Journal of Applied Physiology*.)

simultaneously but was closely related to the pulmonary arterial pressure. It was concluded that the backpressure was mainly a reflection of precapillary anastomoses between the bronchial and pulmonary circulations. Bronchial arterial resistance was calculated as the difference between the upstream and downstream bronchial arterial pressures, divided by the bronchial arterial blood flow. The mean baseline value for bronchial blood flow and bronchovascular resistance in nine sheep was 34.1 ±2.9 ml/min (0.62 ±0.06 ml/min/kg) and 3.9 ±0.5 cmH_2O/ml/min, respectively. Bronchial blood flow and vascular resistance were also measured after increasing left atrial pressure and administering histamine and epinephrine directly into the bronchial artery.

Using a somewhat different approach, Wagner et al. (1987) studied the effects of increasing airway pressure on the bronchial arterial pressure-flow relationships. In anesthetized sheep, the common bronchial artery was exposed and isolated, similarly to the procedure described by Magno and Fishman (1982), and the esophageal and tracheal branches were ligated. The common bronchial branch was cannulated and perfused with blood from the femoral artery using a variable-speed roller pump. Inflow pressure was measured at a side arm of the bronchial artery catheter (Fig. 8). Characterization of the bronchovascular pressure-flow relationship allows calculation of an "incremental" bronchovascular resistance and an intercept when flow is set to zero, which represents the functional downstream pressure (arterial closing pressure). Incremental resistance is the slope of the actual pressure-flow curve. When vascular resistance is calculated using the "ordinary" equation, the assumption is made that zero flow occurs at zero pressure. Using the technique of Wagner et al. (1987), changes in bronchial blood flow can be precisely controlled and varied in a stepwise fashion to values above and below physiological norms. Normal baseline flow was defined as the flow that resulted in a bronchial arterial pressure equal to mean systemic pressure; under these conditions the mean bronchial blood flow in eight sheep was 12.3 ±1.1 ml/min or 0.48 ml/min/kg body weight and bronchovascular resistance was 6.1 ±0.6 mmHg/ml/min at a mean airway pressure of 4.8 cmH_2O.

In a further series of experiments, using an identical technique Wagner and Mitzner examined the effects of systemic hypoxia on the bronchial vascular pressure-flow relationship (1988). The mean baseline bronchial blood flow in 25 sheep was 22 ±2 ml/min (0.7 ml/min/kg body weight) and bronchovascular resistance was 3.8 ±0.4 mmHg/ml/min. They found that the pressure at zero flow was consistently less than the pulmonary arterial pressure when it was measured simultaneously and was unaffected by hypoxia, which substantially increased the pulmonary arterial pressure. They concluded that the downstream pressure was a reflection of the pulmonary capillary pressure and that the main site of anastomoses was at the capillary level.

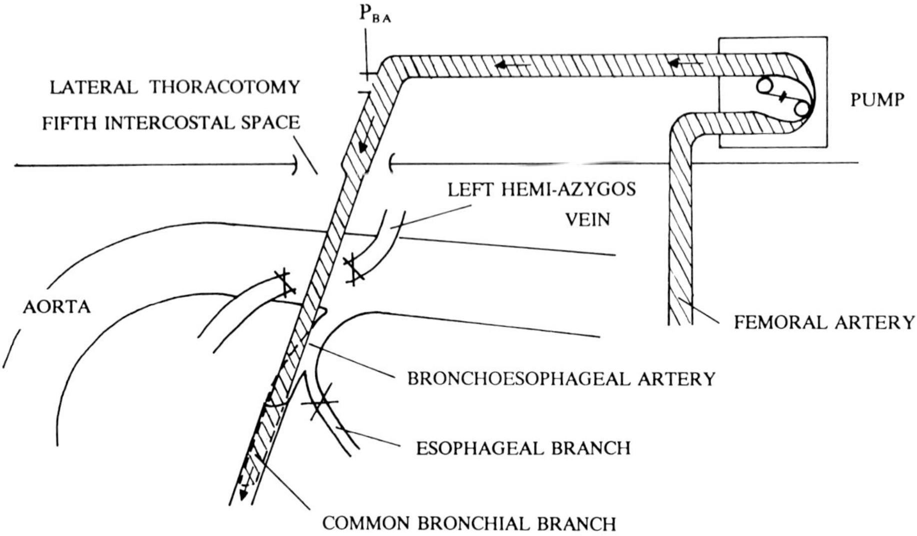

Figure 8 The bronchial arterial perfusion circuit. The common bronchial artery, a branch of the bronchoesophageal artery, is cannulated and perfused with blood from the femoral artery. Bronchial arterial pressure (P_{BA}) is measured at the inflow port of the cannula. (From Wagner et al., 1987, with permission from the *Journal of Applied Physiology*.)

A theoretical advantage of the constant flow system, according to Lung and her colleagues (1976), is that by maintaining a constant flow, critical closure of the vasculature cannot occur even when a considerable increase in bronchial vascular tone occurs, since pressure invariably rises to maintain flow and vascular patency. However, a constant pressure system seems to be a more appropriate model to use in the study of a relatively small vascular bed, such as the bronchial circulation. Vasodilatation or constriction of the bronchial vasculature, in vivo, has little effect on systemic hemodynamics, and the driving pressure for flow, the mean aortic pressure, remains relatively constant despite major acute changes in bronchial vascular caliber. One also expects larger changes in vascular resistance for the same stimulus in the constant pressure system. In the constant flow method, vasoconstriction is accompanied by an increase in intravascular pressure, which tends to counteract the increase in vascular smooth muscle tone and attenuate the vascular narrowing. Similarly, during vasodilatation, the pressure decreases so that the increase in flow is less than if perfusion pressure is constant. Additionally, the determinants of a critical closing pressure in a vascular bed may vary independently of changes in the pressure-flow relationship. Certain drugs, for example, may alter the critical closing pressure or the slope of the vascular pressure-flow curve. Neither the constant flow nor the constant pressure techniques allow these effects to be separated, but the modification of Wagner and Mitzner (1988), in which the entire pressure-flow curve is described, provides data on both aspects of vascular resistance.

The advantages of the carotid-to-bronchial artery shunt preparation (Charan et al., 1985) is that it provides controlled measurements of bronchial blood flow and allows calculation of bronchovascular resistance. A potential advantage is that a chronic carotid-to-bronchial arterial shunt could be established, thereby allowing measurements of bronchial vascular dynamics to be made over time. Some disadvantages are that it is invasive and is technically demanding and the use of an open reservoir could result in fluctuations in blood temperature and gas tensions, possibly resulting in locally mediated changes in bronchovascular resistance.

The cannulated, perfused bronchial artery preparation of Wagner et al. (1987) requires fairly extensive surgery and considerable expertise and is limited to acute studies. However, its advantages are that it avoids the problems inherent in the constant pressure or constant flow methods; although the flow rate is set it can be varied, and it is possible to examine bronchial vascular pressure-flow relationships under different physiological conditions. Both methods suffer from the drawback of measuring only a portion of total systemic arterial supply to the lung.

B. Indirect and Discrete Measurement

Two very different techniques have been used to make indirect and discrete measurements of bronchial blood flow. One of these is videodensitometry, and the other is the radioactive microsphere technique.

Videodensitometry

Videodensitometry is an indicator dilution technique that uses angiographic contrast medium as the flow indicator and was originally applied to the measurement of blood flow in larger arteries. The theory and validation of the technique and its applications have been clearly described in a series of papers (Lantz et al., 1980; Lantz, 1974, 1983, 1984), and the technique has been successfully adapted for the measurement of blood flow in small vessels (Lantz et al., 1980; Parsons et al., 1987). It was first validated for measurement of bronchial arterial blood flow in the sheep (Parsons et al., 1987) because the bronchoesophageal artery in this species is known to supply a large proportion of the total lung mass (Magno and Fishman, 1982; Charan et al., 1987) and can be catheterized under fluoroscopic control.

The principals of measuring blood flow using videodensitometry are outlined, briefly, as follows. Radiopaque dye is injected into an artery, and an electronic window, placed over a downstream vessel, measures the dye concentration within the window over time, thereby generating a dye mass versus time curve. The area under the curve is proportional to the injected dye volume, inversely proportional to flow at the site of dye injection, and independent of the distance from the injection point to the recording site or the size of the vessel at the injection site (Lantz, 1974). Absolute flow is equal to the mass of dye injected M divided by the area A under the dye mass versus time curve and multiplied by a factor K:

$$\dot{Q} = K \frac{M}{A} \tag{1}$$

where K is a radiographic and electronic conversion factor that corrects M and A to equivalent units. As it turns out, K is dependent on a whole host of factors that are difficult or impossible to measure. However, even without knowing the precise value for K the technique can be used to calculate bronchial blood flow as a fraction of cardiac output (Link et al., 1985) or to calculate relative bronchial blood flow (Parsons et al., 1985, 1987).

To calculate flow as a percentage of cardiac output, a second, larger volume of dye is injected into the aortic root and the mass-time curve over the identical window is measured. The ratio of the two mass-time curves gives the flow as a percentage of the cardiac output:

$$\frac{\dot{Q}_1}{\dot{Q}_2} = \frac{M_1 A_2}{M_2 A_1} \tag{2}$$

where $\dot{Q}_1$ and $\dot{Q}_2$ are the flows at the two injection sites, M_1 is the mass of dye injected into the bronchial artery, M_2 the mass of dye injected into the aortic root. A_1 and A_2 are the integrated areas under the mass-time curve recorded at the identical site, the bronchoesophageal artery. If cardiac output is measured by the thermal dilution technique immediately before the two injections of dye, then flow can be expressed in absolute units.

Using repeated injections of dye into the same blood vessel, relative blood flow can be determined provided none of the factors that affect K change between making two dye injections; K can be made to cancel by measuring over the identical videodensitometric window, using the same fluoroscopic settings, so that the second flow can be calculated as a percentage of the first flow:

$$\frac{\dot{Q}_2}{\dot{Q}_1} = \frac{KM_2/A_2}{KM_1/A_1} 100 \tag{3}$$

Initial studies in sheep demonstrated the feasibility of using videodensitometry to make reliable measurements of bronchial arterial blood flow (Link et al., 1985; Parsons et al., 1985, 1987). Measurements of bronchial arterial flow were made in anesthetized sheep as follows (Parsons et al., 1987). A bronchial arterial catheter with a specifically designed tip was introduced into the femoral artery and advanced to the thoracic aorta, where, using fluoroscopy, it was guided into the bronchoesophageal artery. Another catheter was introduced into the thoracic aorta. A videodensitometer and a videotape replay of the fluoroscopic image of dye moving through the common bronchial artery (the major branch of the bronchoesophageal artery) are used to construct dye mass versus time curves. The areas under the curves are inversely proportional to flow in the bronchoesophageal artery. To validate the technique these sheep were also subjected to a thoracotomy to place an electromagnetic flow probe on the common bronchial artery to enable measurements to be made simultaneously using both techniques (Fig 9). During spontaneous and pharmacologically induced changes in bronchial arterial flow, there was a close correlation between the percentage change in flow obtained by the two techniques ($R = 0.96$, slope $= 0.96$, and standard error of the mean, SEM, $\pm 15\%$; Fig.

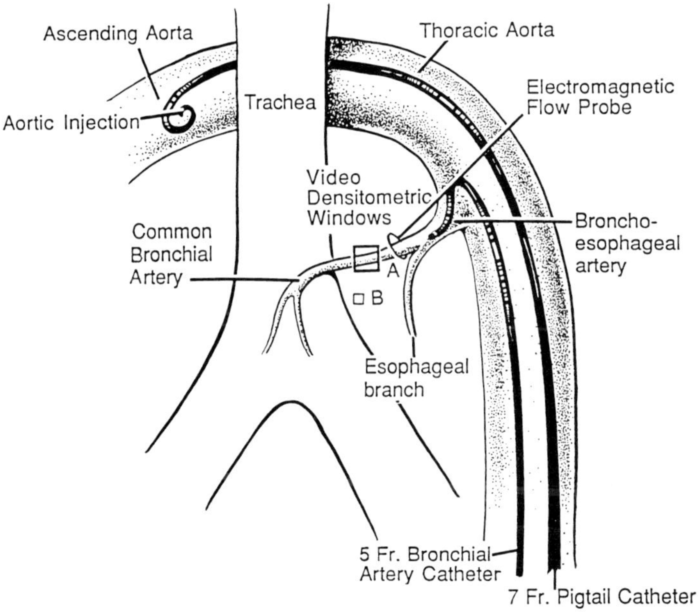

Figure 9 The relative position (from left side) of the bronchoesophageal artery and location of the catheters and electromagnetic flow probe and approximate position of the videodensitometric windows A and B. (Adapted from Parsons et al., 1987.)

10). In a previous study in which measurements of bronchial arterial blood flow were made in five sheep using videodensitometry (but not compared with another technique), the average bronchial arterial blood flow was 28.5 ±7.0 ml/min, 0.62 ±0.2% of cardiac output or 0.71 ±0.17 ml/min/kg (Link et al., 1985). Further measurements were made after injection of histamine and histamine plus methacholine directly into the bronchial artery. In another nine sheep baseline values of 32 ±19 ml/min or 0.6 ±0.2% cardiac output were obtained (Parsons et al., 1985).

The major advantages of this technique are that it is relatively noninvasive, requiring catheterization of only the bronchial and a systemic artery, and is therefore suitable for chronic studies. Measurements have been found to be relatively stable over a 2 h period. Some of the more negative aspects are the initial cost of the equipment; measurements of flow are not continuous and

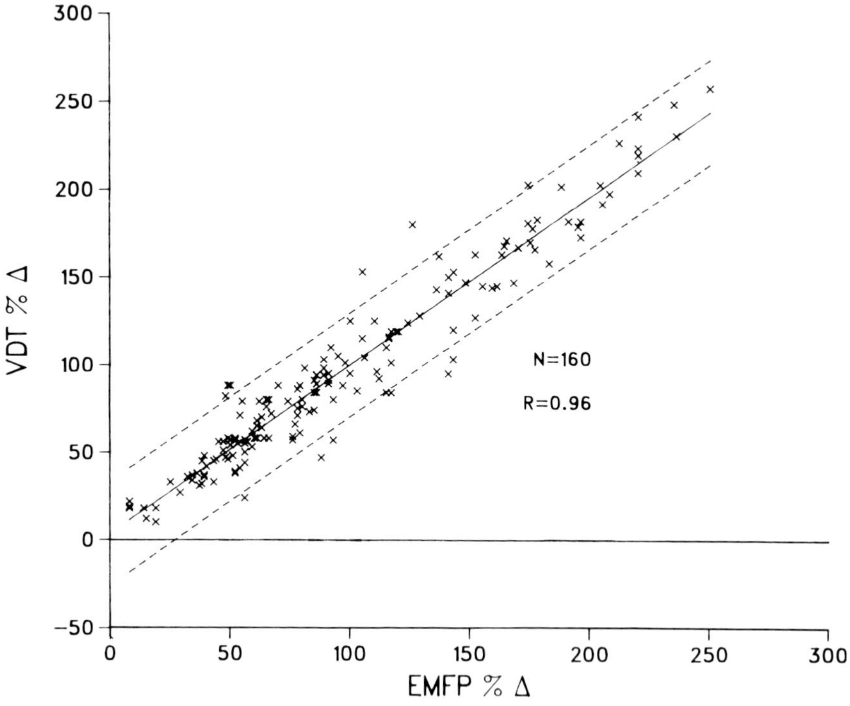

Figure 10 Linear regression and 95% confidence bands of 28 simultaneous measurements (five sheep) when flow was changed by aortic pressure variations (9 observations) or pharmacological intervention (19 observations). VDT, videodensitometry; EMFP, electromagnetic flow probe. (From Parsons et al., 1987.)

must be calculated after the actual measurements are made; and finally, even in the sheep only a portion of the total bronchial blood flow is measured. A potential concern is that the hypertonic bolus of contrast media could in itself alter the vascular resistance in the vessel being studied.

Radioactive Microspheres

The use of radioactive microspheres as a measure of regional or organ blood flow has been established for over 20 years (Rudolph and Heyman, 1967). In their original study, Rudolph and Heyman demonstrated that 50 μm diameter radioactive microspheres, injected into the circulation, became trapped in small peripheral vessels in proportion to the regional blood flow; they also confirmed that there was no recirculation of the spheres and that repeated measurements could be made without changing the circulatory physiology by using different nuclides and subsequently separating them by gamma spectrometry. An excellent review of the theoretical and practical aspects of the radioactive microsphere technique has been written by Wagner et al. (1969), and recently Austin et al. (1989) have reviewed the sources of error of this technique.

There are three assumptions that must be fulfilled to measure regional or organ blood flow accurately using radioactive microspheres. First, the spheres must be well mixed at the site of injection before their dispersal; second, they should be distributed in proportion to regional blood flow; and third, there should be no recirculation. If these assumptions are met, the fractional distribution of the spheres to the organs is in proportion to the fraction of cardiac output to the organs. The fractional distribution of cardiac output is obtained by measuring the proportion of the radioactivity of each organ or tissue of interest relative to the injected dose of microspheres. If the cardiac output is also obtained independently at the time of microsphere injection, then blood flow (ml/min) to any organ or region can be obtained:

$$\text{Flow (ml/min)} = \frac{\text{organ counts}}{\text{total injected counts}} \times \text{Cardiac Output} \tag{4}$$

The flow can also be calculated for any organ X if the radioactivity and flow to another organ Y is known because the method implies that the ratio of flow and radioactivity is the same in all organs. Thus flow X = flow Y (counts X/counts Y).

Cardiac output (CO) can be measured by injecting a known amount of radioactive microspheres into the left side of the heart and sampling arterial blood at a constant rate:

$$\text{CO} = \text{flow rate of pump (ml/min)} \frac{\text{total counts injected}}{\text{counts in arterial sample}} \tag{5}$$

This method of measuring organ flow was later simplified (Domenech et al., 1969; Makowski et al., 1968) so that the flow to any organ could be determined by withdrawing a known quantity of arterial blood (reference sample) at a constant rate ($\dot{Q}_{ref}$, ml/min), measuring its radioactivity (counts X) and that of the organ to which the flow was required (counts Y), and then calculating the flow to that organ:

$$\text{Flow X} = \frac{\text{counts X}}{\text{counts Y}} \dot{Q}_{ref} \tag{6}$$

The accuracy of the technique is related both to the actual blood flow to the region of interest and to the number of spheres injected (Buckberg et al., 1971). The lower the blood flow being measured, the greater is the number of spheres that must be injected. Because the bronchial circulation forms such a small percentage of the total blood flow and because investigators frequently try to portion blood flow into even smaller anatomic compartments within the lung, these considerations regarding accuracy are of particular concern. Practically speaking, the accuracy relates to the absolute number of spheres that lodge in the region of interest. The relationship between confidence intervals and precision of the microsphere technique with varying numbers of spheres is shown in Fig. 11. The confidence interval denotes the statistical likelihood that a difference that one detects is real, and precision is an indication of the magnitude of the difference that can be detected. For example, if one wants to be 95% confident of detecting a real change in flow at a precision level of ±10%,then it is necessary to have at least 400 spheres in the region of interest. If a greater degree of accuracy is required then a 99% confidence level can be chosen with a ±1% precision; in this case 68,000 spheres are required in the region of interest.

The use of the reference flow technique in measuring bronchial blood flow had to be modified, however, because a proportion of the injected microspheres are shunted through peripheral arteriovenous anastomoses and recirculate to the lung capillaries; the amount of recirculating spheres is about 1% of the cardiac output, which is equivalent to the bronchial flow being measured. In addition, the degree of peripheral arteriovenous shunting is very variable and can be affected by body temperature.

To overcome the problem of recirculating spheres, three modifications of the reference flow technique have been developed. One modification entails correcting for recirculating spheres by the simultaneous withdrawal of reference flow blood samples at a constant rate from a systemic artery (femoral) and the pulmonary artery after injection of the spheres into the left atrium. The activity of the radionuclide in the lung due to shunted microspheres (As) is equal to the ratio of the pulmonary blood flow ($\dot{Q}_L$) to pulmonary reference

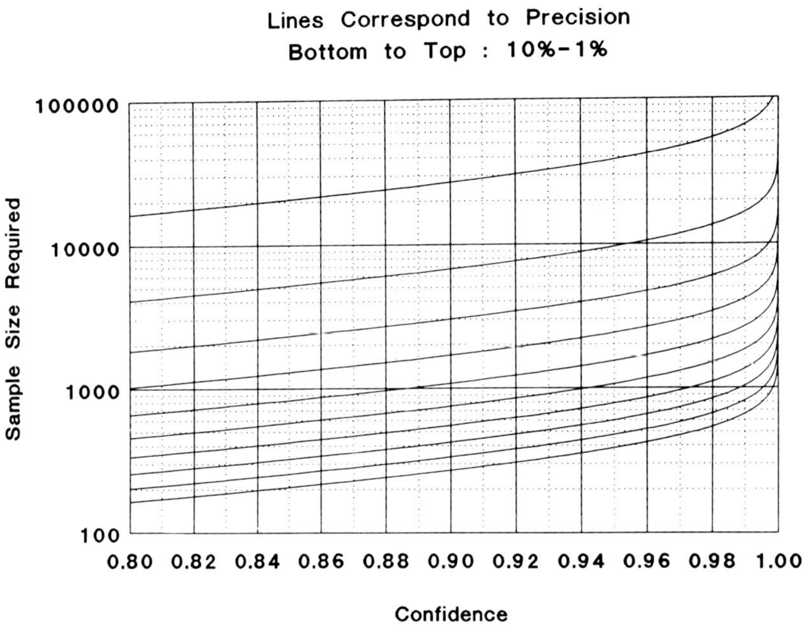

Figure 11 Relationship between confidence intervals and precision of the microsphere technique using varying numbers of microspheres (sample size). See text for explanation.

flow ($\dot{Q}L_{ref}$) multiplied by the radioactivity in the pulmonary reference flow blood sample (AL_{ref}):

$$As = \frac{\dot{Q}L}{\dot{Q}L_{ref}} AL_{ref} \tag{7}$$

The activity in the lung attributable to the bronchial blood flow (Ab) is obtained by subtracting the radioactivity in the lung due to shunted spheres (As) from the total radioactivity in the lung (AL):

$$Ab = AL - As \tag{8}$$

$$\text{Bronchial blood flow } \dot{Q}br = \frac{Ab}{Afa_{ref}} \dot{Q}fa_{ref} \tag{9}$$

where Afa_{ref} is the activity in the femoral artery reference flow sample and $\dot{Q}fa_{ref}$ is the femoral artery reference flow rate.

This modification of the microsphere method was used by Malik and Tracy (1980) in a study of anesthetized dogs in which they examined the immediate and long-term effects of pulmonary artery embolization on bronchial arterial blood flow. Measurements of bronchial blood flow were made by injecting 15 μm diameter microspheres, labeled with different nuclides, into the left atrium over 20 s while reference flow blood samples were withdrawn simultaneously for 2 min from the femoral arterial and pulmonary arterial catheters. At the end of the experiment the dogs were killed, the lungs excised, and the radioactivity in the tissue samples and the reference flow blood samples counted. The mean baseline value for bronchial arterial blood flow for 14 dogs was 31.2 ±6.2 ml/min (1.6 ±0.5% cardiac output or 83.4 ±23.1 ml/min per 100 g dry lung). The extraparenchymal airway blood flow was also measured using the standard equation (6) since it was assumed that there is no shunting of spheres to this region. The mean baseline value was 33.6 ±6.8 ml/min per 100 g dry weight.

Cassidy and Haynes (1986) also used this method to account for the recirculating microspheres in dogs in which one lung was first injured by temporary occlusion of one pulmonary artery and then the dogs were ventilated using 10 cmH_2O positive end-expiratory pressure to determine whether this would enhance the injury. The baseline value for bronchial blood flow to the occluded lung was 9.9 ml/min or 0.12 ml/min/g wet weight.

A disadvantage of this method of calculating the contribution of recirculating microspheres is that only a single value for systemic blood flow to the lung can be derived. The regional distribution of the recirculating microspheres, which is dependent on the regional pulmonary artery blood flow, is unknown so that regional bronchial blood flow cannot be determined.

The second modification of the reference flow technique, which was developed to overcome the problem of recirculating spheres, is achieved by temporarily occluding the pulmonary artery to one lung, thereby preventing the accumulation of peripherally shunted spheres in this lung. This modification was devised by Baile and her colleagues and has been used in a series of experiments in anesthetized dogs and sheep (Baile et al., 1982, 1984, 1985a, 1986b, 1987a; Baile and Paré, 1983; Parsons et al., 1989). The first studies were done to assess the reproducibility and reliability of serial and simultaneous measurements of bronchial blood flow using this modification (Fig. 12) (Baile et al., 1982). The basic protocol was described as follows: a femoral arterial reference flow blood sample was withdrawn at a constant rate, and 15 μm diameter microspheres were injected into the left atrium. The left main pulmonary artery was temporarily occluded 5 s after their injection to prevent recirculation of peripherally shunted spheres. At 2 min the withdrawal pump was stopped and the pulmonary artery ligature loosened. In initial pilot

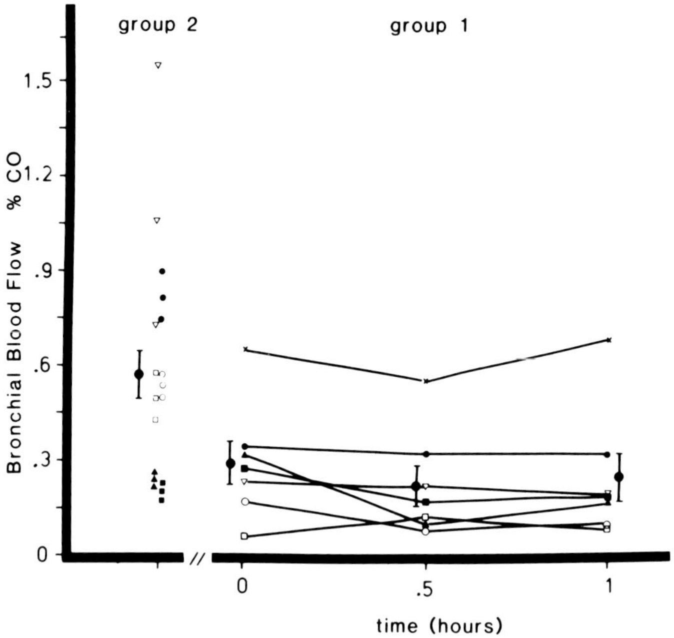

Figure 12 Individual values of left lung bronchial arterial blood flow (% cardiac output, CO) for each dog (represented by different symbols). Mean values ±SEM are shown for groups 1 and 2. In group 1, three different measurements of blood flow were made at 0.5 h intervals, and in group 2 they were made simultaneously. (From Baile et al., 1982, with permission from the *Journal of Applied Physiology*.)

studies it was determined that the appearance time for microspheres injected into the left atrium and sampled serially in the right atrium was at least 8 s. It was assumed that, because the bronchial vessels originate in the proximal aorta, the blood going to this circulation would have reached the origin of the bronchial arteries before occluding the pulmonary artery 5 s after injection of the spheres. The assumption is therefore that downstream vascular pressures at sites of bronchopulmonary anastomoses are physiological at the time of the initial distribution of the microspheres. Using this technique it is possible to make four to five separate measurements of bronchial blood flow; the number of discrete measurements that can be made is dependent on how successfully the various isotope peaks can be separated by gamma spectroscopy. At the end of the experiments the animal is killed and the lungs and trachea excised for measurement of the radioactivity in the tissues of interest. Blood flow to the region of interest is calculated using the standard equation (6).

This technique permits the measurement of regional blood flow to one lung and the trachea. Bronchial blood flow to both lungs can be derived by assuming that blood flow to the left lung represents 45% of the total flow (Bruner and Schmidt, 1947). Mean baseline values from this series of studies for tracheal and left lung bronchial and parenchymal blood flow are shown in Table 1.

A variation of the pulmonary artery occlusion technique has been described by Wu et al. (1988) in which the pulmonary artery is occluded before the microspheres are injected, over a 15 s period, into the left atrium. However, this was found to yield values for blood flow that were significantly higher (15%) than if the pulmonary artery had been occluded 5 s after injection of the spheres, and it was recommended, as originally proposed, that the spheres be injected as a bolus before pulmonary artery occlusion. These investigators have also used the occlusion technique to allow measurements to be made in awake sheep (Wu et al., 1988) by placing a vascular occluder cuff around the left main pulmonary artery during a preliminary thoracotomy and, in subsequent studies, inflating the cuff transiently to occlude this vessel.

Wu et al. have recently described a third modification of the reference flow method, to account for recirculating spheres, in which two nuclides are injected simultaneously into the right and left heart (1988). The separate injection of an additional, differently labeled bolus of microspheres into the right heart allows not only the total amount of recirculating spheres to be calculated but also allows the fraction of radioactivity due to recirculating spheres to any piece of tissue to be determined. Like the pulmonary artery occlusion method, this modification allows the distribution of regional bronchial blood flow to be measured. In contrast to the pulmonary artery occlusion method, measurements of systemic blood flow to both lungs can be calculated. Regional pulmonary blood flow ($\dot{Q}L_{reg}$, ml/min) is determined by injecting a second nuclide (N_2) into the right atrium and collecting a pulmonary arterial reference flow blood sample. Regional pulmonary blood flow is calculated using the standard equation (6):

$$\dot{Q}L_{reg} = At(N_2)\,\frac{\dot{Q}L_{ref}}{AL_{ref}\,N_2}$$

where $\dot{Q}L_{ref}$ is the pulmonary arterial reference flow rate (ml/min) and $AL_{ref}\,N_2$ is the activity in the pulmonary arterial reference flow blood sample of the nuclide N_2 injected into the right atrium. To calculate the systemic blood flow to any tissue sample the radioactivity due to the recirculation of the microspheres injected into the left atrium ($A_{recirc}\,N_1$) is obtained using a rearrangement of the standard equation (6):

$$A_{recirc}\,N_1 = \dot{Q}L_{reg}\,\frac{(A_{ref\text{-}recirc}\,N_1)}{\dot{Q}L_{ref}}$$

where $A_{ref\text{-}recirc}\,N_1$ is the radioactivity in the pulmonary arterial reference flow blood sample of the nuclide injected into the left atrium. The radioactivity due to recirculation is then subtracted from the total radioactivity for each tissue sample ($A_{tot}\,N_1$) to give the correct counts $A_{OK}N_1$:

$$A_{OK}\,N_1 = A_{tot}\,N_1 - A_{recirc}\,N_1$$

These corrected counts are then used to calculate the true systemic blood flow to the lung using the standard equation (6) (Fig. 13).

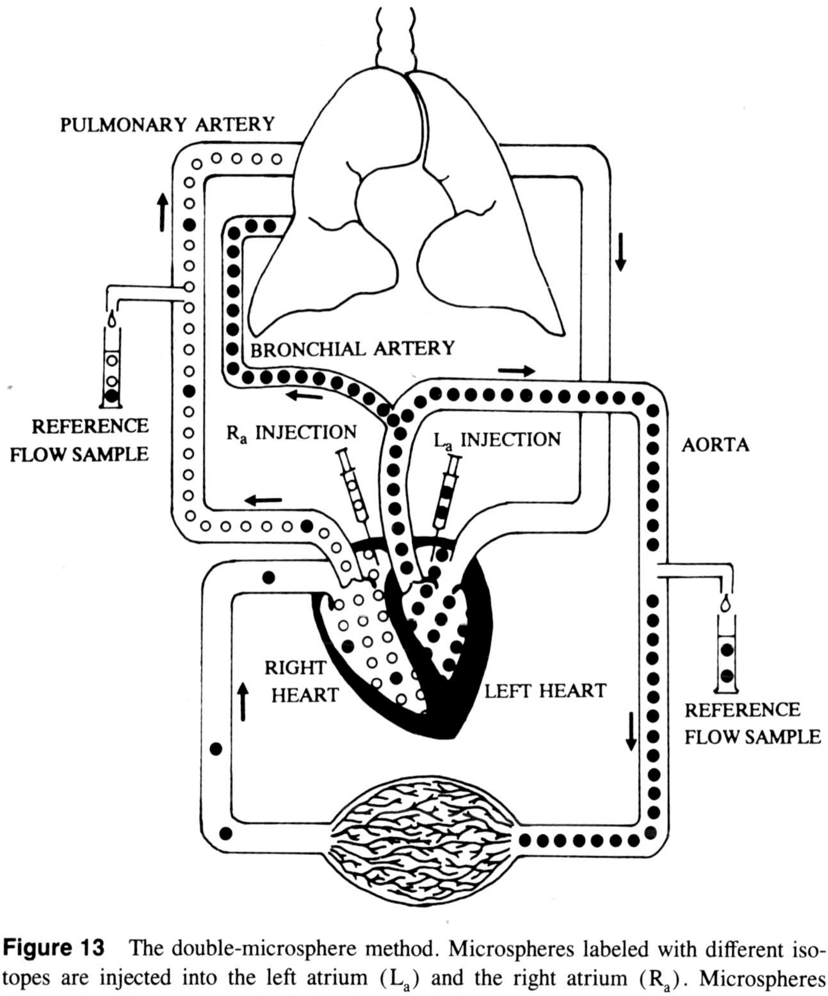

Figure 13 The double-microsphere method. Microspheres labeled with different isotopes are injected into the left atrium (L_a) and the right atrium (R_a). Microspheres delivered to the lung from the left atrium result from bronchial blood flow and systemic arteriovenous shunting with subsequent trapping in the pulmonary circulation. (Adapted from Wu et al., 1988, with permission from the *Journal of Applied Physiology*.)

In 5 sheep Wu et al. (1988) compared measurements of bronchial blood flow to the left lung, using the pulmonary artery occlusion method, with the double-microsphere method. They reported mean values of 16.8 ±2.1 and 15.1 ±2.5 ml/min per 100 g, respectively. In nine sheep total bronchial blood flow measured using the pulmonary artery occlusion method was 1.52 ±0.98% of cardiac output, and using the double-microsphere method it was 1.39 ±0.88% of cardiac output.

Some of the disadvantages of the radioactive microsphere technique are that the animal must be killed at the end of the experiment to calculate the amount of radioactivity in the tissue samples; only an average flow can be obtained at one instant in time, and the number of measurements that can be made is limited to the number of isotopes that can be separated by gamma emission spectroscopy; radiolabeled microspheres are relatively expensive, and disposal of the radioactive carcass may also be expensive and/or difficult; knowledge of the safe use and disposal of the isotopes is essential. Another potentially serious drawback, which was suggested in one study (Baile et al., 1987a), is that 15 μm diameter microspheres may fail to lodge in the lung, passing through pathways that are larger than 15 μm. If one is not too discouraged by these problems, the advantages of the method are that it is the only reliable method that allows repeated measurements of total and regional bronchial blood flow to be made relatively noninvasively and that, using modifications, the technique can be applied to make measurements in awake animals. If measurements are limited to the extraparenchymal airways, where it is assumed there is no recirculation, the experimental protocol is considerably simplified.

There are advantages and disadvantages of each of these three modifications of the reference flow technique. The first modification (Malik and Tracy, 1980) precludes the measurement of regional blood flow since it does not allow the calculation of the percentage of shunted spheres in a lung region. In addition there is the potential inaccuracy involved in calculating the amount of radioactivity due solely to the bronchial blood flow because a small error in measuring the radioactivity of the shunt flow may result in a negative value for the calculated bronchial blood flow. The potential for error is always large when "noise," represented by the circulating spheres, is large in relation to the "signal," represented by the systemically delivered microspheres. The double-microsphere method requires two different radiolabels for one measurement of flow and is therefore expensive, and if, as is not unusual, the separation of isotopes by gamma spectroscopy is limited to four isotopes, then it is possible to obtain only two measurements of flow. Pulmonary artery occlusion seems to be the method of choice. It is less expensive than the double-microsphere method, and it is possible to make twice the number of flow measurements for the same cost. Fewer calculations and procedures are required than for either of the other two methods, so that there are fewer chances of making experimental errors. In general, one possible disadvantage of using 15 μm diameter spheres is that under some circumstances measurements of the systemic blood flow to the lung parenchyma may not be reliable because shunting of 15 μm diameter microspheres can occur (Baile et al., 1987a).

III. Bronchial Systemic-to-Pulmonary Blood Flow

The bronchial systemic-to-pulmonary blood flow $\dot{Q}$br(s-p) is often referred to as bronchopulmonary anastomotic blood flow and sometimes as pulmonary collateral blood flow. It is that fraction of the systemic circulation to the lungs that anastomoses with the pulmonary circulation and drains into the left atrium through the pulmonary veins.

Like the total bronchial blood flow, the bronchial systemic-to-pulmonary blood flow has been measured both directly and indirectly using a wide variety of techniques.

A. Direct Continuous Measurement

Methods that measure $\dot{Q}$br(s-p) directly involve isolation of the pulmonary vasculature. Such measurements have been made in isolated lobes of animals whose systemic circulation remains intact. Measurements of $\dot{Q}$br(s-p) from isolated lobes have been made with and without perfusion of the pulmonary artery ("overflow technique"). When the pulmonary artery is perfused, flow is measured as a change in volume in the pulmonary perfusion circuit (Jindal et al., 1984), and when it is not perfused $\dot{Q}$br(s-p) is measured by collecting the flow from the cannulated pulmonary artery and vein (Baile et al., 1984; Modell et al., 1981; Zapata-Ortiz et al., 1967; Aviado et al., 1961; Williams and Towbin, 1955). Measurements of $\dot{Q}$br(s-p) have also been made directly in intact lungs of humans and other animals during total cardiopulmonary bypass (Aramendia et al., 1962; State et al., 1957; Auld et al., 1960; Mandelbaum et al., 1966; Goetz and Rohman, 1965; Warren and Powell, 1986; Baile et al., 1985b, 1986a; Aviado et al., 1961; Agostoni et al., 1989).

Isolated Lobe

No Pulmonary Perfusion

A number of investigators have measured $\dot{Q}$br(s-p) by isolating one lobe (or lung), ligating the lobar pulmonary artery and vein, and collecting the blood from the cannulated artery and/or vein. Because the pulmonary artery and vein are obstructed, any blood reaching the lung must be arriving via the systemic vessels to the lung.

Early studies were carried out by Shedd et al. (1951), who ligated the left lower lobe pulmonary artery and vein in anesthetized, closed-chested dogs using snare cannulas. They observed that if the cannula upstream of the occlusion in the pulmonary vein was opened there was a flow of blood of about 6–8 drops per min, although the outflow end of the catheter was situated 40 cm above the pulmonary vein!

Williams and Towbin (1955) improved this basic technique and cannulated the left lower lobe pulmonary artery distal to the ligature and also ligated the pulmonary vein in anesthetized, open-chested dogs. The cannula tip was open to atmosphere and placed about 5 cm below the level of the pulmonary artery. The blood flow was collected in a graduated cylinder. In five dogs they recorded a flow of 4.4–9 ml/min immediately after pulmonary artery ligation, which decreased over time in each dog and also varied with systemic arterial pressure. $\dot{Q}$br(s-p) was also measured in another 26 dogs at intervals varying from 3 days to 12 months after ligation of the pulmonary artery. Chronic ligation was associated with a progressive increase in $\dot{Q}$br(s-p) to the lung.

A slightly different approach was taken by Aviado et al. (1961), who ligated and cannulated both the left lower lobe pulmonary artery and vein and kept both the cannula tips at the same level as the lobar vessels. $\dot{Q}$br(s-p) was measured by collecting the lobar blood in graduated cylinders, and it was then returned to the systemic circulation via a femoral vein. In 3 dogs the chest was closed and the dogs were allowed to breathe spontaneously. In 6 open-chested dogs the combined flow from the pulmonary artery and vein averaged 4.4 ml/min (ranging from 2.1 to 7.7 ml/min, or 0.11–0.36 ml/min/kg body weight); there was no difference between these values and those from the spontaneously breathing dogs (5.3 ml/min). In yet another 10 dogs $\dot{Q}$br(s-p) was collected from either the pulmonary artery or the pulmonary vein. The vessel that was not cannulated was ligated. Again, values for $\dot{Q}$br(s-p) were similar to those from both the artery and vein (mean 5.0 ml/min; range 2.4–8.5 ml/min). The overall flow for all 19 dogs averaged 4.8 ml/min. These investigators concluded that in a normally perfused lobe the overall flow was the same whether it was collected from the pulmonary artery or vein or both, indicating that the bronchial systemic-to-pulmonary blood can flow in either direction.

A further modification of this technique was used to measure $\dot{Q}$br(s-p) in the ubiquitous Peruvian sheep (Zapata-Ortiz et al., 1967). The pulmonary veins and artery of the left lung were ligated intrapericardially, and the pulmonary artery was cannulated distal to the ligature. $\dot{Q}$br(s-p) from the cannulated pulmonary artery was measured using a rotameter and the blood then reinfused into a peripheral vein. Baseline values for $\dot{Q}$br(s-p) in nine sheep were 48.6 ±7.8 ml/min. Similar measurements were made in another group of Andean sheep resident at more than 4000 m above sea level. Values for $\dot{Q}$br(s-p) were lower in the Andean than in the Peruvian sheep.

Modell and associates chose to use a modified, isolated left lower lobe preparation to evaluate the influence of changes in systemic arterial pressure, lung volume, and transpulmonary pressure on bronchial-pulmonary vascular communications (Modell et al., 1981). In this preparation (Fig. 14), a balloon-tipped, double-lumen cannula was used to cannulate the lobar pulmonary artery, and a double-lumen cannula was tied into the pulmonary vein. The lobar venous blood drained into a reservoir and was reinfused using a roller pump. The left apical and cardiac lobes were removed, and a warmed, humidified tent was placed over the open chest. Unlike previous studies, lobar perfusion could be stopped transiently either by tightening a ligature around the pulmonary artery or by inflating the balloon of the pulmonary arterial cannula, or both. Perfusion of the left lower lobe was interrupted only while an experimental run was being made. Blood for measurement of $\dot{Q}$br(s-p) could be collected from both the arterial and the venous cannulas. To compare the relative distribution of bronchial drainage within the lobe, the flow collected from the lobar pulmonary artery was expressed as a percentage of the total flow collected. Total lobar flows ranged from 2.3 to 5.3 ml/min and 43–61% of the flow drained via the arterial side. It was also shown that decreased sys-

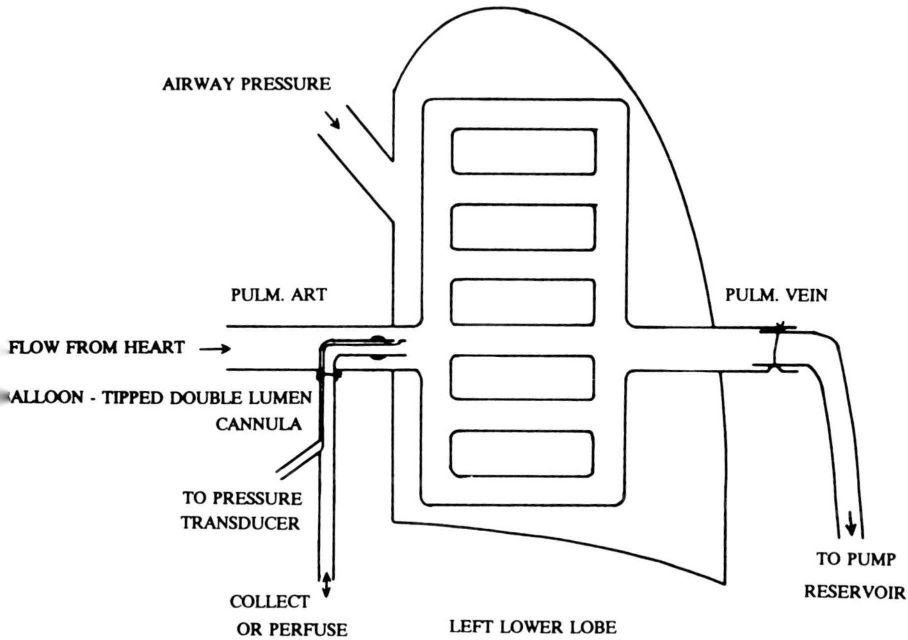

Figure 14 The isolated left lower lobe preparation. (From Modell et al., 1981, with permission from the *Journal of Applied Physiology*.)

temic arterial pressure, increased transpulmonary pressure, and increased lung volume resulted in a reduction in $\dot{Q}br(s\text{-}p)$.

In a collaborative study (Baile et al., 1984), measurements of Qbr(s-p) were made using the isolated left lower lobe preparation and were compared with measurements made using radioactive microspheres and a modification of the reference flow technique (Baile et al., 1982). Measurements of bronchial blood flow, using the two different methods (microspheres and left lower lobe overflow) were compared during increases in positive end-expiratory pressure while pulmonary venous pressure was kept at 0 cmH_2O. The baseline value for bronchial blood flow (microspheres) in four dogs was 4.9 ±2 ml/min and was only slightly greater than that measured simultaneously using the left lower lobe overflow technique. Both flows decreased during the application of positive end-expiratory pressure (Fig. 15). At low levels of positive end-expiratory pressure there was no difference between measurements of bronchial blood flow using either technique.

A potential problem regarding the use of the isolated lobe preparation is that by occluding the pulmonary artery and vein the downstream pressure in the pulmonary vasculature at the site of anastomoses may be changed; consequently it is impossible to extrapolate values of flow to a more physiological state. This method was therefore modified to make measurements of $\dot{Q}br(s\text{-}p)$ during pulmonary perfusion.

Pulmonary Perfusion

To date all the studies using the isolated, perfused lobe technique for measuring $\dot{Q}br(s\text{-}p)$ have been carried out in dogs. The reason that only the dog has been studied is probably because, in this species, the left lower lobe is separated from the right upper lobe by a complete fissure and the lobar artery and vein can easily be cannulated. The methods used by different investigators are very similar, and the basic technique is adapted appropriately to address each particular problem.

In open-chested, anesthetized dogs, the lingular lobe is excised and the left lower lobe pulmonary artery and vein cannulated and perfused with autologous blood using a roller pump set at a predetermined flow rate. The right lung and left lower lobe are ventilated separately using different gas mixtures. The right lung is ventilated appropriately to keep the systemic acid-base status constant (usually 100% oxygen), and the left lower lobe is ventilated with 5% CO_2 in air during baseline conditions and thereafter the inspired gas composition may be varied according to the experimental protocol. In some applications the azygos vein is snared. Since the bronchial veins drain to the right side of the heart via the azygos, this allows interruption of the nonanastomotic component of bronchial blood flow. The left lower lobe is supported in a net and suspended from a strain gauge that provides an accurate record of the

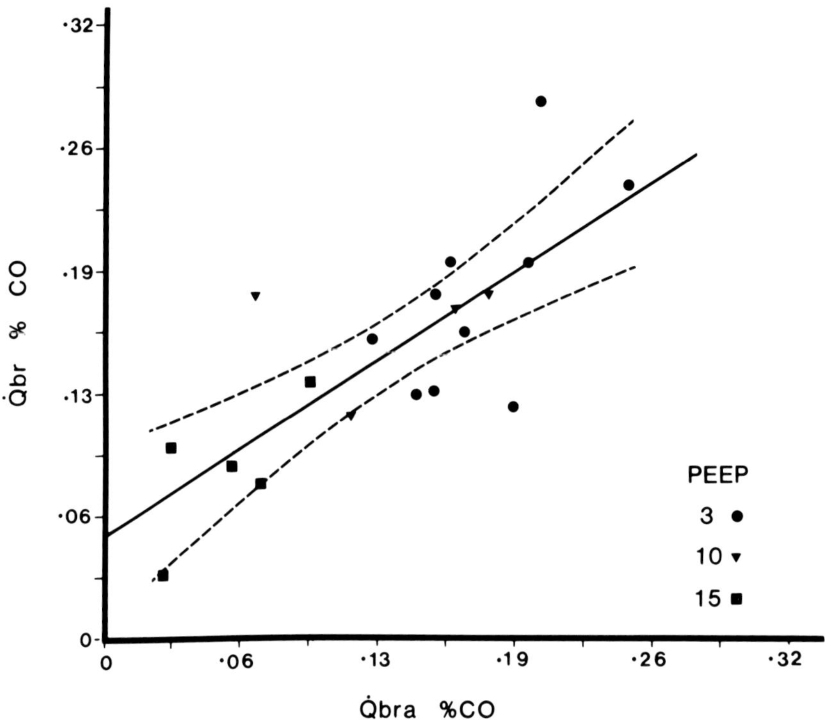

Figure 15 Correlation between sum of bronchial and parenchymal fractions of bronchial blood flow to the left lower lobe measured by the microsphere technique (Q̇br) and anastomotic (systemic-to-pumonary) bronchial blood flow (Q̇bra). Flows are expressed as percentage cardiac output (CO). Broken lines indicate 95% confidence interval. Measurements of Q̇br were made at 3 (●), 10 (▼), and 15 (■) cmH_2O positive end-expiratory pressure. (From Baile et al., 1984, with permission from the *Journal of Applied Physiology*.)

change in lobar weight. Q̇br(s-p) is measured as the flow of blood into the left lower lobe perfusion circuit. The change in the lobar circuit volume is measured as the overflow of blood from the constant-volume perfusion circuit, which is collected in a graduated cylinder. Changes in the lobar weight may be due to changes in lobar blood volume, extravascular leakage from the pulmonary or bronchial circulation, or reabsorption of fluid from the interstitium of the lobe. When the changes accompanied step changes in intravascular pressures, they were assumed to represent step changes in lobar blood volume and were added to or subtracted from the measured overflow volume (Fig. 16).

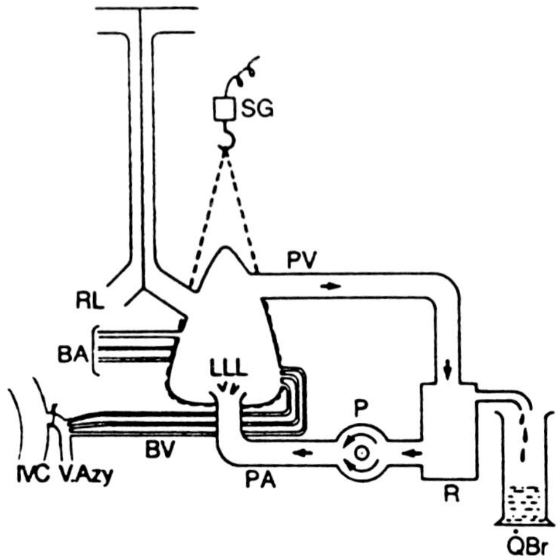

Figure 16 Experimental lobe. Pulmonary circulation is perfused from pump (P) via pulmonary artery (PA) and back by pulmonary vein (PV) in the intact continuously weighed left lower lobe (LLL). Overflow from closed circuit is due to bronchial blood flow ($\dot{Q}$Br). SG, strain gauge; RL, right lung; BA, bronchial arteries; BV, bronchial veins; IVC, inferior vena cava; V. Azy, vena azygos; R, reservoir. (From Jindal et al., 1984, with permission from the *Journal of Applied Physiology*.)

Jindal et al. used this method to examine the acute changes in $\dot{Q}$br(s-p) during the first hour after pulmonary arterial obstruction and following subsequent lobar reprefusion (1984). In six control dogs in which the test lobe was in zone II conditions (pulmonary artery pressure > alveolar pressure > pulmonary venous pressure), $\dot{Q}$br(s-p) was stable for 2 h and the lobar weight was constant. In three dogs the mean baseline values for $\dot{Q}$br(s-p) was 24.4 $\pm$0.9 ml/min per 100 g dry lobe weight per 100 mmHg (mean systemic arterial pressure) when the test lobe was ventilated with room air and did not change when ventilated with 5% CO_2 in air. $\dot{Q}$br(s-p) was expressed as flow per 100 mmHg mean systemic arterial pressure to adjust for variations in mean systemic pressure between dogs because $\dot{Q}$br(s-p) has been shown to be influenced by the mean systemic blood pressure (Modell et al., 1981; Auld et al., 1960; State et al., 1957).

In a further series of experiments (Jindal et al., 1985) that were designed to examine the mechanism of the increase in $\dot{Q}$br(s-p) after acute pulmonary artery occlusion, the mean baseline value for nine dogs was 31 $\pm$10 ml/min per 100 g dry lobe weight per 100 mmHg.

Discrepancies in the results of measurements of bronchial blood flow from different laboratories using either open- (Jindal et al., 1984; Baile et al., 1982) or closed-chested conditions (Malik and Tracy, 1980) have been reported. Because it was hypothesized that the variability may have been a result of the varying thermal conditions, certain modifications were made to the isolated lobe technique to stabilize and maintain a constant thermal environment. Agostoni et al. (1987a) controlled the thermal environment by warming and humidifying the inspired gases to the test lobes and right lung and enclosed the thorax of the dog in a plexiglass box in which the air was humidified and the temperature controlled. In addition, the temperature of the autologous blood perfusing the lobe was controlled by means of a water bath (Fig. 17). In five dogs the mean value for $\dot{Q}br(s\text{-}p)$, measured at physiological temperatures (before pulmonary artery obstruction), was 73.0 ±21.4 ml/min per 100 g dry lobe weight per 100 torr (mean systemic arterial pressure), which was considerably higher than flow measurements recorded in preparations in which temperature and humidity were not controlled.

To further investigate the influence of temperature on the bronchial vasculature, Agostoni et al. again used the thermally controlled left lower lobe preparation to record $\dot{Q}br(s\text{-}p)$; by injecting 15 μm diameter radiolabeled microspheres, they simultaneously measured total lobar flow $\dot{Q}br$ as well as cardiac, tracheal, and esophageal blood flow (1987b). The dog's core temperature was kept constant, as was the humidified air surrounding the left lower lobe. The pulmonary circulation of the lobe was perfused with blood of different temperatures, varying from 30 to 42°C. At temperatures above or below 36°C lobar bronchial blood flow decreased, whereas there was no change in flow to the other tissues even when they were supplied by the bronchial vasculature. $\dot{Q}br(s\text{-}p)$ correlated closely with $\dot{Q}br$: $\dot{Q}br = 2.75 \pm 0.94\ \dot{Q}br(s\text{-}p)$; $r = 0.90$.

Agostoni and colleagues also examined the influence of temperature on the bronchial vasculature before and after pulmonary artery occlusion, using the thermally controlled, isolated left lower lobe technique as well as the radioactive microsphere technique (Agostoni et al., 1987c). To simulate pulmonary artery obstruction, the lobar circuit pump was turned off for 30 min. In five dogs the mean value for $\dot{Q}br(s\text{-}p)$, measured at physiological temperatures before pulmonary artery obstruction, was 73.0 ±21.4 ml/min per 100 g dry weight per 100 torr (mean systemic arterial pressure). There was also a close correlation between measurements of $\dot{Q}br(s\text{-}p)$ and $\dot{Q}br$ (microspheres) regardless of whether the pulmonary artery was obstructed [$\dot{Q}br$, ml/min = $1.12 \pm 0.98\dot{Q}br(s\text{-}p)$; $r = 0.91$].

Deffebach et al. (1987) examined the role of cyclooxygenase products in the response of the bronchial circulation to acute lung injury using the isolated

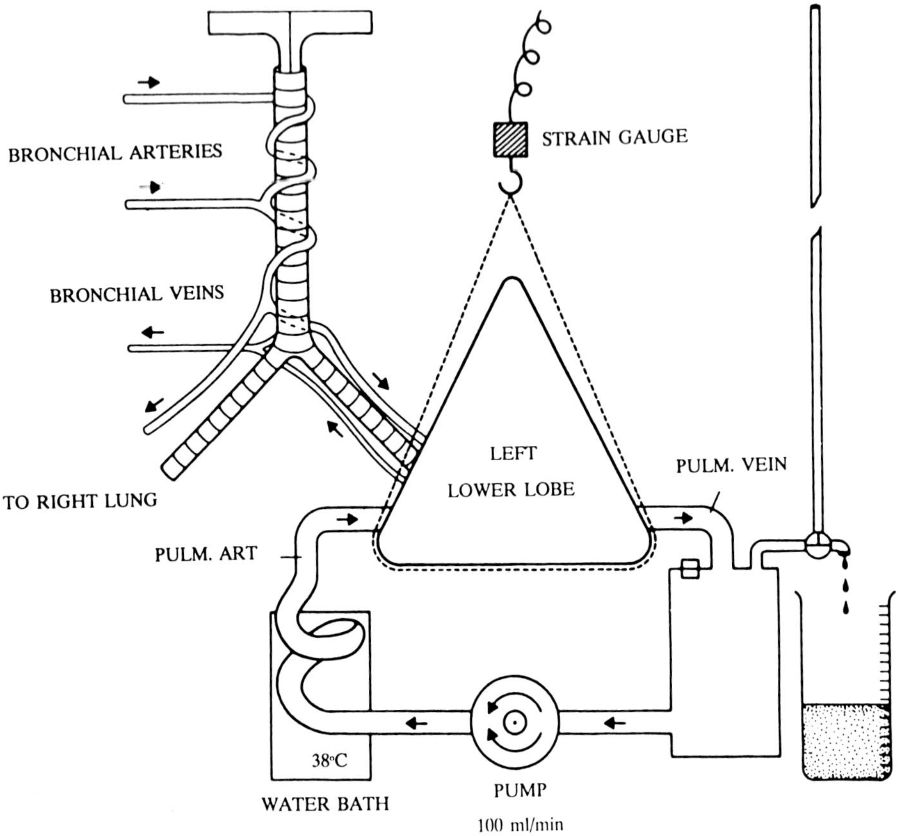

Figure 17 Isolated left lower lobe preparation. Bronchial systemic-to-pulmonary flow was measured as the volume of blood that overflowed from left lower lobe vascular circuit plus left lower lobe weight changes. A water bath is used to control temperature of blood perfusing the lobe. A vertical column was used to observe pressure in the overflow cannula. (From Agostoni et al., 1987a, with permission from the *Journal of Applied Physiology.)*

left lower lobe preparation and maintaining a thermally stable environment. In two groups of 10 and 6 dogs the mean baseline values for $\dot{Q}br(s\text{-}p)$ were 23.7 ±3.0 and 24.5 ±6.4 ml/min per 100 g dry lobe weight, respectively. When cyclooxygenase inhibitors were given before surgery the mean baseline value for $\dot{Q}br(s\text{-}p)$ in another two groups of 4 and 10 dogs was substantially reduced to 5.2 ±1.8 and 9.6 ±1.6 ml/min per 100 g dry lobe weight, respectively. The authors suggested that the extensive surgery required to isolate the left lower lobe caused the release of vasodilator prostaglandins, resulting in a three- to fivefold increase in the baseline values for bronchial blood flow.

Agostoni and collaborators (1987a) measured the upstream pressure for $\dot{Q}br(s\text{-}p)$ using a modification of the left lower lobe perfusion method. This was achieved by adding a side arm and cannula to the pulmonary venous reservoir so that by raising or lowering the cannula the pulmonary venous pressure could be controlled. Pulmonary venous pressure was increased until the bronchial systemic-to-pulmonary flow stopped; this pressure at zero flow was equated with the effective upstream pressure for systemic-to-pulmonary flow. The venous pressure at which $\dot{Q}br(s\text{-}p)$ stopped was 44 $\pm$6 cmH_2O and was directly related to the systemic arterial pressure. They found that the decrease in $\dot{Q}br(s\text{-}p)$ was related to the increase in pulmonary venous pressure according to the equation $\dot{Q}br(s\text{-}p) = 34.4 \pm (-0.78Ppv)$ ml/min per 100 g dry lobe weight.

The disadvantages of the left lower lobe preparation is that it is invasive and must be maintained in a thermally stable environment to obtain reliable and reproducible measurements; the extensive surgery may precipitate the release of vasodilatory prostaglandins, thereby affecting the baseline values of bronchial blood flow. Blood flow leaving the lobe via the bronchial veins to the azygos is not measured. However, if the azygos vein is snared so that bronchial blood cannot return to the systemic circulation, $\dot{Q}br(s\text{-}p)$ is probably equal to total bronchial blood flow. Some advantages of this method included the fact that continuous and repeated measurements of $\dot{Q}br(s\text{-}p)$ can be easily made; there is independent access to both the pulmonary and the bronchial circulation, which allows separate control of vascular pressures and precise control of the zonal conditions; and pulmonary perfusion may be continuous or intermittent, and any fluid shifts within the test lobe can readily be assessed by changes in lobar weight.

Separate Perfusion of the Pulmonary and Systemic Circulations

Cardiopulmonary Bypass

A direct, albeit invasive, method of measuring $\dot{Q}br(s\text{-}p)$ is by separate perfusion of the systemic and pulmonary circulations. Under these circumstances any increase in the volume of blood in the pulmonary circuit must occur by way of anastomoses between the systemic and pulmonary circulations. The majority of the studies using this method have been done in dogs, although measurements of $\dot{Q}br(s\text{-}p)$ have also been made in humans during cardiopulmonary surgery.

The basic technique for separate perfusion of the pulmonary and systemic circulations used by different investigators is similar. Improvements and refinements have been made as a result of the advent of newer technology, such as the use of more sophisticated oxygenators and perfusion pumps. In this preparation, dogs are anesthetized and a thoracotomy is performed. Separate perfusion of the pulmonary and systemic circulations is maintained using two pumps. Both perfusion circuits are primed using heparinized donor blood. The superior and inferior vena cavae are cannulated and the venous blood diverted through an oxygenator and pump (heart-lung machine) and returned to the systemic circulation through a femoral or carotid artery. The pulmonary venous blood is drained via a left ventricular cannula into a graduated reservoir and pumped back through the pulmonary perfusion circuitry into the cannulated pulmonary artery.

The first, and historic, measurements of bronchial blood flow were made by Berry and Daly in 1931. They used a modification of the technique just described in an attempt to determine what fraction of the bronchial circulation anastomoses with the pulmonary circulation. Figure 18 is included to illustrate just how extraordinarily complex and demanding these first measurements of bronchial blood flow must have been!

These initial studies were carried out on anesthetized dogs and, briefly, entailed separate perfusion of the pulmonary and systemic circulations, perfusion of the bronchial arteries, and collection of the blood from the left atrium and cannulated azygos vein. The pressures in the perfusion circuits were kept at physiological values. In four dogs the anastomotic fraction was determined by measuring the left atrial outflow when the pulmonary arterial inflow was stopped; in these dogs the average blood flow was 44 ml/min and values varied widely from 3.5 to 250 ml/min. In two other dogs in which $\dot{Q}br(s\text{-}p)$ was calculated by subtracting azygos vein outflow from aortic inflow, the average value was 21 ml/min and varied from 13 to 33 ml/min. In the one dog in which pulmonary arterial inflow was subtracted from left atrial outflow the average value for $\dot{Q}br(s\text{-}p)$ was 19 ml/min and varied from 9 to 38 ml/min.

With the advent of the pump oxygenator the measurement of Qbr(s-p) became more feasible. Using a somewhat simpler aproach to that of Berry and Daly (1931), State and colleagues (1957) studied 25 anesthetized dogs. After a thoracotomy cannulas were inserted into the right ventricle and into the superior vena cava. The pulmonary artery was ligated so that the venous blood from the right heart was passed through an oxygenator and pumped back to the systemic circulation via a femoral artery. The left ventricle was cannulated and the blood allowed to drain into a reservoir. This blood was then pumped into the pulmonary artery through a cannula placed distal to the ligature. Under steady-state conditions, the volume of blood pumped into the pulmonary artery was known, and when the volume collected in the cylinder exceeded the pulmonary arterial flow, this was confirmed to be the $\dot{Q}br(s\text{-}p)$. The aorta was

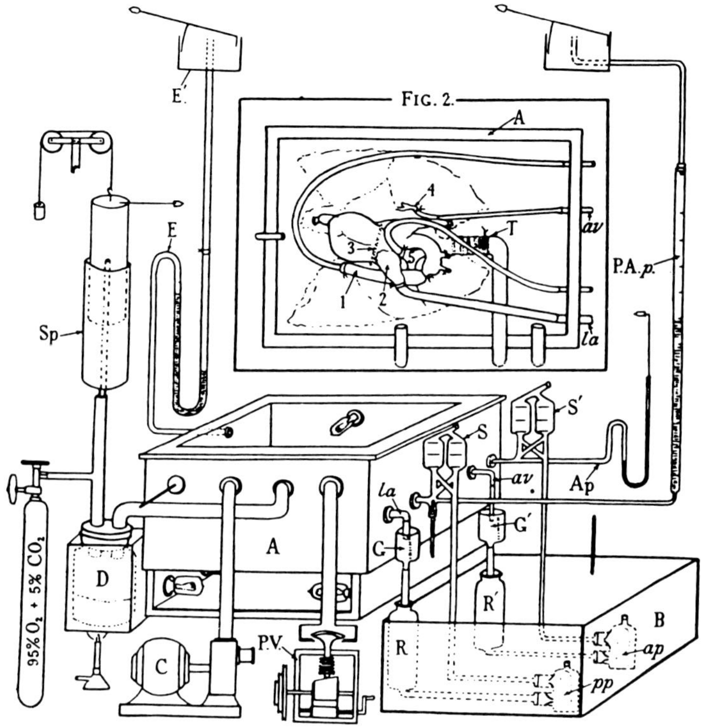

Figure 18 Apparatus used for simultaneous perfusion of the pulmonary and bronchial vascular systems in lungs under negative pressure ventilation. A, respiratory chamber; Ap, aortic pressure manometer; B, Dale and Schuster pump; C, Cenco exhauster; D, bottle for rendering inspired gas warm and moist; E, E′, manometer and recorder for respiratory pressure; G, G′, graduated cylinders; P. A. *p*., pulmonary arterial pressure manometer; P. V., poppet valve; R, R′, venous reservoirs; Sp, spirometer; S, S′, stromhurs; T, trachea; *ap*, aortic pump; *av*, azygos vein outlet; *la*, left auricular outlet; *pp*, pulmonary pump; 1, thoracic aorta, 2, left auricle; 3, clamp at auriculoventricular groove; 4, superior azygos vein; 5, pulmonary artery. (From Berry and Daly, 1931, with permission of the *Proceedings of the Royal Society of London*.)

cross-clamped to prevent blood entering the left ventricle from the coronaries or passing through the aortic valve. Results from these studies showed that there was a direct relationship between mean systemic arterial pressure and $\dot{Q}$br(s-p). When the systolic pressure was between 90 and 120 mmHg, $\dot{Q}$br(s-p) ranged from 0.5 to 1% of the total arterial blood flow, which was comparable to values obtained using other, previously described, techniques

(Bloomer et al., 1949; Bruner and Schmidt, 1947). In this extensive study they also examined the effect of changing systemic arterial pressure, venous pressure, and pulmonary artery flow rate on $\dot{Q}br(s\text{-}p)$ and also examined the effect of deflation, ventilation using an increased CO_2 content (10%), administration of serotonin, and the effect of air embolism.

Using a similar technique, Auld and his colleagues (1960) conducted a series of experiments on anesthetized dogs and examined the mechanical factors that influence $\dot{Q}br(s\text{-}p)$. They found that there was little variation in $\dot{Q}br(s\text{-}p)$ when the mean systemic blood pressure was between 70 and 100 mmHg; values for individual dogs ranged between 2 and 12 ml/min. They also examined the influence of increasing systemic and pulmonary arterial and venous pressures.

Goetz and Rohman (1965) used this technique to measure $\dot{Q}br(s\text{-}p)$ in normal dogs and those subjected to chronic ligation of the left main pulmonary artery. The change in volume of blood in the reservoir [$\dot{Q}br(s\text{-}p)$] was constantly recorded using a strain gauge, and the pump flow rate was recorded using a rotameter. Results from their study showed considerable variation between measurements of $\dot{Q}br(s\text{-}p)$; values ranged from 5 to 60 ml/min in normal dogs, and in several dogs flow could not be recorded. Changes in $\dot{Q}br(s\text{-}p)$ were also examined during variations in pulmonary, left atrial, and systemic pressure and acute and chronic pulmonary artery ligation and changes in lung volume.

Cartwright et al. (1962) carried out a study using this basic technique to examine the most physiological method of maintaining the lungs during cardiopulmonary bypass. In 10 dogs the mean value for $\dot{Q}br(s\text{-}p)$, measured as the left ventricular vent flow, was 8.8 ±4.9 ml/min (range 2.4–19.0 ml/min, or 0.7% of the pump flow), and the measured oxygen consumption of the lungs was 1.6 ml/min. The effect of varying superior vena caval pressure on $\dot{Q}br(s\text{-}p)$ was also examined.

More recently, Warren and Powell (1986) have examined the effects of alveolar hypoxia on $\dot{Q}br(s\text{-}p)$ using pulmonary perfusion in a biventricular bypass preparation (Fig. 19). $\dot{Q}br(s\text{-}p)$ was measured somewhat differently than in the Cartwright study. The blood from the right atrium and ventricle was drained by gravity into a reservoir (nonoxygenated) and was pumped, at a constant rate, back into the pulmonary artery. The pulmonary venous return was drained from the left atrium into a tall, narrow cylinder, and this blood was pumped from a side hole in the bottom of the cylinder into a reservoir, where it was oxygenated, and was returned via the femoral arteries using yet another pump. The hydrostatic pressure of the column of blood in the cylinder was measured continuously using a pressure transducer located near the bottom of the column, providing a measure of the change in blood volume in the column. The change in pulmonary venous return was determined by changes

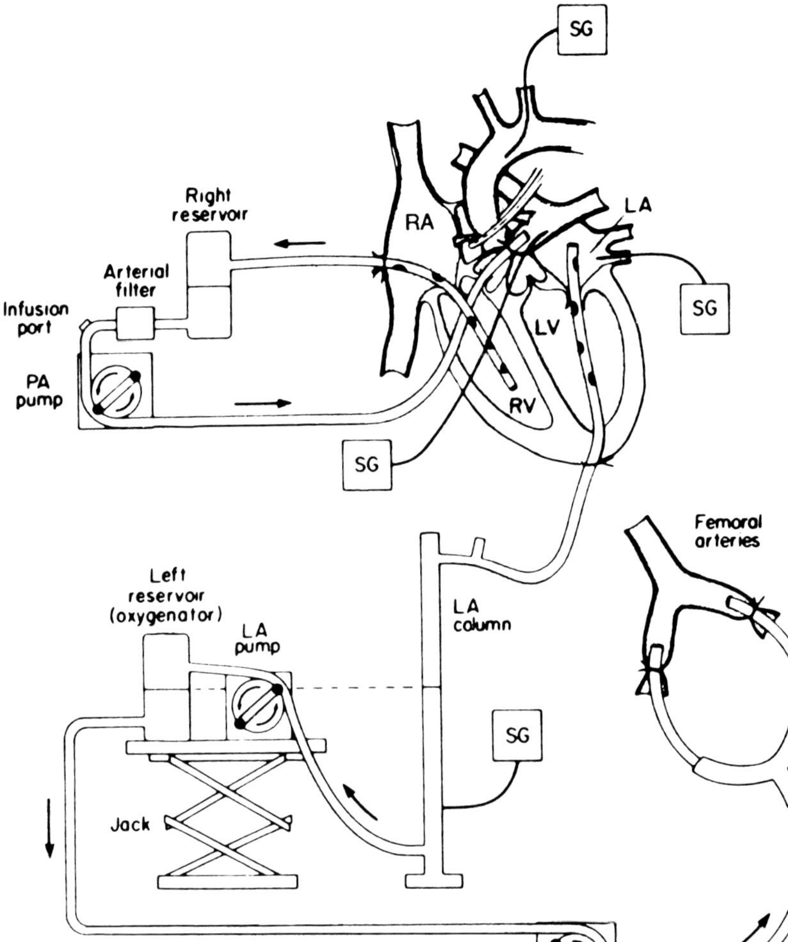

Figure 19 The experimental preparation. LA, left atrium; LV, left ventricle; PA, pulmonary artery; RA, right atrium; RV, right ventricle; SG, strain gauge pressure transducer. (Reproduced from the *Journal of Clinical Investigation* **77**:1515–1524, 1986; by copyright permission of the American Society of Clinical Investigation.)

in $\dot{Q}$br(s-p), changes in pulmonary intravascular blood volume, and changes in pulmonary extravascular fluid content. In five dogs baseline measurements of $\dot{Q}$br(s-p) were 52.3 ±16.3 ml/min (range 18–108 ml/min). When alveolar hypoxia was induced $\dot{Q}$br(s-p) increased, and this was thought to be related to the release of vasodilatory prostaglandins.

A disadvantage of this method is that the technical skill required to carry out a double-cardiac bypass may well be beyond the expertise of the average investigator. Given that it is not, then the surgery itself is invasive and conditions during measurement of $\dot{Q}$br(s-p) could be far from physiological. On the brighter side is that precise and independent control of factors affecting the systemic and pulmonary circulations is possible.

Although $\dot{Q}$br(s-p) had been measured relatively frequently in dogs, it was some time before these measurements were made in pateints undergoing routine cardiopulmonary bypass (Lajos and Glicken, 1980; Baile et al 1985b; Agostoni et al., 1989). Under these conditions, when the only flow returning to the left atrium is $\dot{Q}$br(s-p), it can be repeatedly and accurately measured during the operative procedure with no additional surgical intervention.

Lajos and Glicken (1980) measured $\dot{Q}$br(s-p) in 10 patients undergoing routine cardiopulmonary bypass surgery. In these patients both the pulmonary artery and aorta were cross-clamped, and blood and cardioplegic solution returning to the left ventricle was drained by gravity. Corrections were made for dilution by the cardioplegic solution, and $\dot{Q}$br(s-p) was calculated as total bronchial flow/cross-clamp time. Values ranged from 11 to 28 ml/min, with a mean value of 15 ±6 ml/min.

Baile et al. (1985b), using a somewhat different method, measured $\dot{Q}$br(s-p) in 40 patients undergoing routine cardiopulmonary bypass surgery for grafting of coronary arteries. After full bypass had been instituted, a drainage sump was placed into the apex of the left ventricle via the right superior pulmonary vein. During anastomosis of the distal vein grafts, when the aorta is cross-clamped, the only blood returning to the left ventricle should be $\dot{Q}$br(s-p), and this is vented and returned to the main circuitry, usually via a cardiotomy reservoir (Fig. 20). $\dot{Q}$br(s-p) was readily measured by clamping the precalibrated tubing leaving the cardiotomy reservoir and recording the time taken to fill a given length of tubing. In this study, in addition to measuring $\dot{Q}$br(s-p), the noncoronary collateral blood flow was also measured. This is blood that originates from bronchial, esophageal, pleural, and pericardial vessels and anastomoses with the coronaries. The blood drains into the right atrium and may reach the left atrium via the intact pulmonary circulation, contributing to the apparent $\dot{Q}$br(s-p). However, if the pulmonary artery trunk is clamped or a separate drain is placed in the right atrium, then the noncoronary collateral flow does not contribute to the $\dot{Q}$br(s-p) (Baile et al., 1986a).

Baile et al. (1985b) measured noncoronary collateral blood flow by inserting a cannula into the right atrium and diverting the blood either to the cardiotomy reservoir or directly back to the main pump circuitry (Fig. 20). If the flow is diverted to the cardiotomy reservoir, then the sum of $\dot{Q}$br(s-p) and

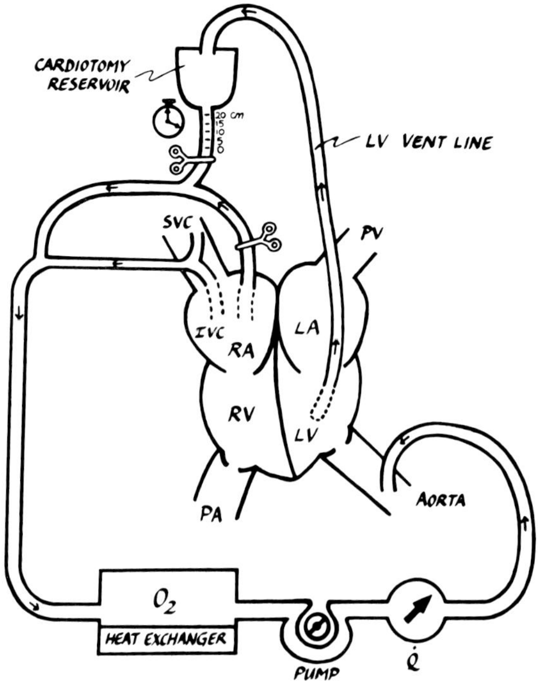

Figure 20 The circuitry used during cardiopulmonary bypass surgery. IVC, inferior vena cava; SVC, superior vena cava; RA, right atrium; LA, left atrium; RV, right ventricle; LV, left ventricle; PA, pulmonary artery; PV, pulmonary vein; $\dot{Q}$, pump flow. (From Baile et al., 1985.)

noncoronary collateral flow is obtained, and if the flow is directed back to the main pump circuitry, then only $\dot{Q}$br(s-p) is measured. In the 40 patients studied, values for $\dot{Q}$br(s-p) were extremely variable. The mean value was 140 ± 182 ml/min (3.2 ±4.2% of pump flow) and ranged from as low as 8 ml/min to higher than 1 L/min. Although high, this mean value is close to that reported by Deal et al. (1968), who used an application of the Fick principle based on CO_2 to measure $\dot{Q}$br(s-p). The highest values were found in patients who had various forms of lung disease, including cryptogenic fibrosing alveolitis and asbestosis associated with pleural plaques.

In another study of 20 patients undergoing routine cardiopulmonary bypass, Baile et al. (1986a) reported a somewhat lower mean value for $\dot{Q}$br(s-p) of 65 ±35 ml/min (1.6 ±0.8% of the pump flow).

Agostoni et al. recently examined the effect of positive alveolar pressure on $\dot{Q}$br(s-p) in 20 patients during routine cardiopulmonary bypass (1989).

$\dot{Q}br(s\text{-}p)$ was drained by gravity from the left ventricle into a calibrated cylinder in which timed collections were made. The tubing from the cylinder was connected to a pump and the blood was returned to the cardiotomy reservoir. In 10 patients in whom alveolar pressure was kept constant, $\dot{Q}br(s\text{-}p)$ ranged from 0.32 to 2.76% of the pump flow and was constant over time. Increasing alveolar pressure by about 10 cmH_2O caused a 40% reduction in $\dot{Q}br(s\text{-}p)$.

One advantage of measuring $\dot{Q}br(s\text{-}p)$ in patients during cardiopulmonary bypass is that it is a unique experience for the investigator since it is probably the one time when there is virtually no preparation before the study and no cleaning up afterward: the entire operating room staff takes care of this! Another advantage is that precise and independent control of physiological factors, such as vascular pressures, airway pressure, and blood gas tensions, which affect the systemic and pulmonary circulations, is possible. However, some of the potential problems are that values obtained for $\dot{Q}br(s\text{-}p)$ during bypass may be different from those occurring during normal physiological conditions: during bypass, there is no pulmonary circulation so that the downstream pressure at the site of systemic bronchopulmonary anastomoses is different from the pressure normally present at this site. The surgery itself could affect $\dot{Q}br(s\text{-}p)$ through the release of vasodilatory prostaglandins, and if measurements are not made during stable thermal conditions this could influence $\dot{Q}br(s\text{-}p)$ since the bronchovasculature is known to be temperature sensitive. Other factors that may affect $\dot{Q}br(s\text{-}p)$ are the use of nonpulsatile flow and, in some cases, the absence of ventilation of the lungs.

B. Indirect and Discrete Measurement

Several methods were devised in the 1950s and 1960s in an attempt to quantitate the bronchial systemic-to-pulmonary blood flow. These included the combined use of bronchospirometry and the Fick principle (Bloomer et al., 1949; Madoff et al., 1952; Fishman et al. 1958), the simultaneous estimation of the right and left ventricular output by the indicator dilution technique (Nakamura et al., 1960, 1961; Cudkowicz, 1959a,b; Cudkowicz, 1965; Fritts et al., 1957, 1961), and a more direct estimation obtained by making simultaneous dilution curves recorded from the left atrium and a systemic artery after dye injection into the ascending aorta (Cudkowicz et al., 1960; Nakamura et al., 1968). More recently, a simpler method has been devised in which a dye curve is obtained using two earpieces and a densitometer after injection of dye into a femoral vein (Katori et al., 1970a).

Difference Between Left and Right Ventricular Output

Cudkowicz et al. (1959a) were the first to suggest that the difference between the outputs of the left and right ventricles should provide an indirect estimate of the bronchial arterial blood flow returning to the left heart via the pulmonary veins, provided there were no other "obvious arteriovenous anomalies." Bronchial venous flow was not included in this estimate, although pulmonary collateral flow from other systemic arteries was included but was considered insignificant.

In this study the simultaneous output of both ventricles was obtained in anesthetized, spontaneously breathing dogs by injecting radioiodinated serum albumin indicator close to the right atrium. Reference blood samples of 1.1 ml were withdrawn simultaneously each second for half a minute from pulmonary artery and femoral artery catheters, and the radioactivity was counted in each of the sampled fractions. The outputs of the left $\dot{Q}_{LV}$ and right $\dot{Q}_{RV}$ ventricles were calculated using standard indicator dilution methods; the difference between the left and right ventricular output was considered an estimate of $\dot{Q}br(s\text{-}p)$:

$$\dot{Q}br(s\text{-}p) = \dot{Q}_{LV} - \dot{Q}_{RV}$$

In the first study the mean value for $\dot{Q}br(s\text{-}p)$ in six control dogs was 65 $\pm$49 ml/min, and in five of six dogs the left ventricular output was higher than the right ventricular output. In the dogs that had one pulmonary artery permanently ligated, large differences were observed between the left and right ventricular outputs, suggesting the presence of an enlarged bronchial vasculature. The validity of this method was tested using in vitro glass model experiments.

Having validated this method, Cudkowicz and colleagues measured $\dot{Q}br(s\text{-}p)$ in 13 patients (1959a). In 4 patients, who had no known lung disease, an average flow of 90 ml./min was measured, which was 1.5% of the right ventricular output.

Other investigators found similar results using the indicator dilution technique to estimate the difference in output between the right and left heart (Fritts et al., 1957; Nakamura, 1956, 1958).

Cudkowicz et al. (1960) soon devised a more direct method for estimating $\dot{Q}br(s\text{-}p)$. They reasoned that if the dye is injected into the aorta or left ventricle, as opposed to the right atrium, some of the indicator traversing through the shorter, bronchial circulatory pathways would appear in the left atrium before the dye recirculating via the systemic pathway and therefore estimates of $\dot{Q}br(s\text{-}p)$ could be made from this left atrial dye curve. In the application of this method, timed samples are withdrawn from the left atrium and a femoral artery after an aortic injection of radiolabeled, iodinated serum albumin, and the area under the initial left atrial curve was taken to represent $\dot{Q}br(s\text{-}p)$ that had made the rapid transit through bronchial vessels and returned directly to the left side of the heart. This technique was used to study two normal dogs and six dogs in which one pulmonary artery had been ligated for 10 months. Values for $\dot{Q}br(s\text{-}p)$ were compared with those obtained by estimating the simultaneous output of the left and right ventricles (Fig. 21). In

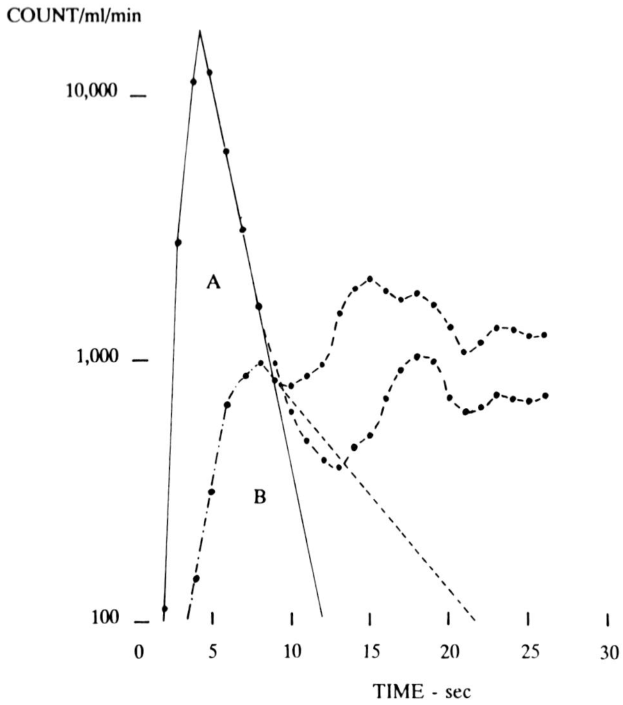

Figure 21 Example of a left atrial indicator dilution curve obtained 10 months after left pulmonary artery ligation. A, Aortic flow area; B, bronchial flow area. (From Cudkowicz et al., 1960.)

the six dogs that were subjected to chronic pulmonary artery ligation, $\dot{Q}$br(s-p) was 660 ml/min (aortic injection, the direct method) and 640 ml/min (right atrial injection, the indirect method). However, for the two normal dogs no $\dot{Q}$br(s-p) could be measured using the aortic injection curves, although values of approximately 50 ml/min were obtained using right atrial injection.

A similar comparison of the direct and indirect methods was also made in 10 patients undergoing routine left and right heart catheterization for diagnosis of suspected cardiopulmonary disease (Cudkowicz et al., 1960). Evans blue dye (T-1824) was used as the indicator and rapidly injected into the ascending aorta while blood samples were obtained simultaneously from the left atrium and a brachial artery. In 4 patients who had no significant cardiopulmonary disease, $\dot{Q}$br(s-p) was not detected using the aortic injection in 2 and was very low in the other 2, whereas the value obtained using the direct method was 70 ml/min. In 4 of the other 6 patients the mean values for $\dot{Q}$br(s-p) were 540 ml/min using the direct method and 510 ml/min using the indirect method, although in the 2 remaining patients negative values were obtained using the indirect method and flows of only 20 and 40 ml/min were measured using the direct method.

The dye dilution technique was subsequently modified by Aramendia et al. (1962) in an attempt to measure bidirectional bronchial blood flow (i.e., bronchial-to-pulmonary and pulmonary-to-bronchial) in anesthetized, open-chested dogs. Catheters were introduced into the azygos vein, pulmonary artery, left atrium, left ventricle, and femoral arteries. To detect a shunt from pulmonary artery to bronchial vein, Cardio-Green dye (indocyanine green) was injected into the pulmonary artery while a sample was withdrawn simultaneously from the azygos vein and passed through a cuvette densitometer for continuous recording of the dye concentration. This curve was then compared with that obtained by injecting dye into the left ventricle. It was reasoned that injection of dye into the left ventricle would bypass any pulmonary artery-to-bronchial shunt so that a difference between these two curves would indicate the presence of a right-to-left shunt. After pulmonary arterial injection, a double peak, which would have confirmed the presence of a shunt, was not detected in the azygos vein dye concentration curve. However, these results do not necessarily exclude a shunt since it is possible that the flow of dye may take longer to reach the bronchial veins from the pulmonary artery than from the bronchial artery. $\dot{Q}$br(s-p) (left-to-left shunt) was measured using the direct method, as described by Cudkowicz et al. (1960), except for the substitution of Cardio-Green dye and use of a continuously recording densitometer to sample blood alternately between the left atrium and the femoral artery. To achieve better mixing, the dye was injected into the left ventricle. In five normal dogs $\dot{Q}$br(s-p) ranged from 6 to 9% of cardiac output (mean 8.2%). Although of historical interest, the calculation of $\dot{Q}$br(s-p) by comparing the outputs of the two ventricles is not accurate or practical. In addition to the bronchial anastomotic flow there are other left-to-left shunts, such as the portion of the coronary blood flow that returns to the left heart via the Thebesian veins. In addition, the technique is inherently inaccurate because it involves the subtraction of two large numbers to derive a small number. Errors represent the compounded errors of measuring the cardiac output of both ventricles. It is possible that the techniques may give estimates of the magnitude of increase in $\dot{Q}$br(s-p) under pathological conditions in which flow is usually augmented, but the frequent negative values obtained during normal physiological conditions illustrates its inherent inaccuracy.

Fick Principle and Bronchospirometry

Techniques that use the uptake of gas in the lungs to measure the systemic blood supply to the lung measure that portion of the bronchial circulation involved in gas exchange, the "effective" blood flow, and do not take into account the blood flow that bypasses the gas-exchanging units.

Fick Principle Based on Oxygen

In an ingenious study, Bloomer et al. (1949) used an indirect application of the Fick principle and bronchospirometry to measure the effective systemic blood supply to the left lung in dogs whose left main pulmonary artery had been previously ligated. The "effective" bronchial arterial flow to the lung is the flow that takes part in gas exchange, and it was calculated as follows:

$$\text{Bronchial blood flow (ml/min)} = \frac{a}{c - b} \times 100$$

where a is the oxygen uptake of the left lung, obtained using bronchospirometry (ml/min); b is the oxygen content of the systemic arterial blood reaching the left lung (ml/100 ml); and c is the oxygen content of blood leaving the left lung (ml/100 ml). Because the systemically perfused left lung would only have a net absorption of oxygen under conditions of systemic hypoxemia and/or local hyperoxia, the value for c, the oxygen content of the blood leaving the lung, was assigned the value of the arterial oxygen content when both lungs were ventilated with 100% oxygen, and the value for b, the content of blood reaching the lung, was the measured arterial content while the left lung received 100% oxygen and the right lung room air. In this study it was demonstrated that the flow to these lungs increased considerably with time after ligation. In the 10 dogs that were studied it was reported that in 16 measurements blood flow was more than 700 $ml/min/m^2$; in 12 it was more than 1 $L/min/m^2$, and in 4 it was more than 1500 $ml/min/m^2$; the highest flow was 2233 $ml/min/m^2$.

Madoff et al. (1952) reported a healthy 14-year-old girl who had congenital absence of the right branch of the pulmonary artery. By the application of the Fick principle to one lung, as just described, they estimated that the "effective bronchial arterial flow" was around 950 ml/min, or about 17% of the cardiac output.

Fishman et al. (1958) used a more direct approach to measure the systemic blood supply to the lungs in 12 patients who had various types of pulmonary and cardiac abnormalities. The patients were divided into three groups according to their abnormalities, and the Fick principle was applied to the measurement of $\dot{Q}br(s\text{-}p)$ and adapted to the special anatomic circumstances of each group. Bronchospirometry was used to obtain gas samples for the calculation of oxygen uptake and the respiratory exchange ratio for each lung independently, and peripheral arterial blood samples were taken for estimation of the oxygen content of the pulmonary capillary blood of the affected lung. Values obtained for $\dot{Q}br(s\text{-}p)$ were extremely variable, ranging from 860 ml/

min in 1 patient who had chronic occlusion of one pulmonary artery to about 350 ml/min in 3 patients who had bronchiectasis. In 4 patients the oxygen uptake was too low to allow calculation of blood flow using the Fick principle. Using the same technique, Viola and Abbate also reported an inordinately high flow of 1160 ml/min in a young man 21 years old who had his left pulmonary artery ligated 8 years before (1973).

The application of the Fick principle based on oxygen has several disadvantages that have limited its use (Bloomer et al., (1949). Serial as opposed to simultaneous sampling of blood and gas contents must be used, and the calculations are subject to the compounded errors in the measurement of oxygen content and uptake. Although the measurement is relatively noninvasive and is repeatable, it is not sufficiently sensitive to measure $\dot{Q}br(s\text{-}p)$ under normal conditions of "low flow."

Fick Principle Based on Carbon Dioxide

Gases other than oxygen can be used in the measurement of $\dot{Q}br(s\text{-}p)$ using an application of the Fick principle. Deal et al. (1968) used CO_2 as the test gas to measure the effective $\dot{Q}br(s\text{-}p)$ in patients undergoing routine cardiopulmonary bypass. As these investigators pointed out, under these conditions (when the pulmonary valve is competent and there is no contribution from the right ventricle) the only blood to supply the pulmonary circulation is bronchial systemic-to-pulmonary blood. During measurements of $\dot{Q}br(s\text{-}p)$ the P_{CO_2} of the arterial blood leaving the oxygenator was kept constant and was measured using the Astrup technique. The percentage of end-expiratory CO_2 was assumed to be in equilibrium with the blood leaving the alveoli. The product of respiratory ventilation and the percentage of CO_2 gave the volume of CO_2 excreted. By means of the CO_2 dissociation curve for oxygenated blood, the CO_2 content of blood entering and leaving the lung was derived from the P_{CO_2} values. $\dot{Q}br(s\text{-}p)$ is obtained by subtracting these values and dividing the difference into the volume of CO_2 excreted. In 23 patients they found an average value for flow of 114 ml/min (range 11–311), which is similar to the values obtained by Baile et al. (1985b), who measured $\dot{Q}br(s\text{-}p)$ in a similar group of patients by collecting the left ventricular return during cardiopulmonary bypass (range 8 ml/min to over 1 L/min).

In another study using the Fick principle and carbon dioxide as the test gas, Lilker and Nagy (1975) examined the effect of hypoxemia and alveolar hypoxia on $\dot{Q}br(s\text{-}p)$ in anesthetized dogs in which the left pulmonary artery had been chronically ligated to produce enlargement of the systemic circulation to the left lung. In seven dogs ventilated with room air, $\dot{Q}br(s\text{-}p)$ to the obstructed left lung was 94 ±34 ml/min. When the normal right lung was ventilated with a hypoxemic mixture, $\dot{Q}br(s\text{-}p)$ to the left lung increased to

194 ml/min, and when the left lung was ventilated with a hypoxemic mixture, $\dot{Q}$br(s-p) in that lung increased to 136 ml/min.

Fick Principle Using Carbon Monoxide

Another gas that has been substituted for oxygen when measuring $\dot{Q}$br(s-p) using the Fick principle is carbon monoxide. Fisher et al. (1970) used a modification of the method of Bloomer et al. (1949) and chose carbon monoxide as the test gas since they anticipated a low rate of uptake. The objective of this study was to determine the time course of regeneration of the systemic blood supply to the lung in 14 dogs at intervals after transection and reanastomosis of the left mainstem bronchus and stripping of the bronchial vessels from the hilum. $\dot{Q}$br(s-p) to the gas-exchanging vessels of the left lung ["effective" $\dot{Q}$br(s-p)] was measured by determining the increase in carboxyhemoglobin in the arterial blood during transient occlusion of the left pulmonary artery. Because the left pulmonary artery was occluded, the uptake of carbon monoxide was proportional to the systemic blood flow through the gas-exchanging vessels. Using this technique, $\dot{Q}$br(s-p) to the left lung was 8 ±2 ml/min (range 5–10 ml/min) in 5 control dogs. Serial measurements of $\dot{Q}$br(s-p) in the experimental dogs showed that the systemic blood supply to the lungs was reestablished within 1 month of its interruption.

The advantage of using carbon monoxide as the test gas, as opposed to oxygen, is that normal or decreased rates of bronchial blood flow can be detected. However, when bronchial blood flow is higher than normal the use of this gas can lead to systemic carbon monoxide poisoning. For this reason, this gas has not been used in making measurements in humans. A major disadvantage of all the techniques that rely on the Fick principle is that $\dot{Q}$br(s-p) to only one lung can be measured and only during cessation of the pulmonary blood flow to that lung. Because it is likely that there are acute as well as chronic changes in systemic blood flow to a lung in which the pulmonary blood flow has been interrupted, the value of these measurements must be questioned.

Earpiece Dye Dilution

Nakamura et al. (1967) have shown that it is possible to estimate a left-to-right shunt using a single earpiece and densitometer to record the dye curve. Subsequently, Katori et al. (1970a) postulated that since it had been shown that aortic root injection of dye results in the early appearance of dye in the left atrium as a result of the contribution of $\dot{Q}$br(s-p), then an increase in bronchial blood flow, as has been shown to occur in various disease states, would result in a distortion of the peripheral dye dilution curve as well as of the left atrial dye curve. This study was designed to investigate the distortion of downslope of the earpiece dye dilution curve to detect an increase in bronchial blood flow in patients who had lung disease and to compare these results with those obtained previously using a somewhat different (direct) method (Nakamura et al., 1968). A group of 20 patients who had pulmonary disease were studied. Ear-piece dye dilution curves were obtained after injecting dye (30 mg Coomassie blue) into the femoral vein, main pulmonary artery, left atrium, or aortic root. A significant correlation was observed between this method and the direct method regardless of where the dye was injected.

Using the method already described, Katori et al. attempted to measure an increase in $\dot{Q}br(s\text{-}p)$ in 67 patients who had pulmonary tuberculosis; they reported an increase in $\dot{Q}br(s\text{-}p)$ in 18 of the 67 patients studied (1970b).

The major limitation of such techniques is their inaccuracy and nonquantitative nature. Although it may be possible to detect an increase in $\dot{Q}br(s\text{-}p)$, it is not possible to measure the actual amount by which the flow may have increased. Because normal or decreased values for $\dot{Q}br(s\text{-}p)$ cannot be measured, these techniques are now really only of historical interest.

IV. Tracheal Blood Flow

Techniques that are used to measure tracheal blood flow are in general different from those used to measure bronchial blood flow and, not surprisingly, are considerably less invasive because the tracheal vasculature is relatively accessible compared with the rest of the bronchial vasculature. Despite this, only one of the techniques has been applied to the measurement of blood flow in humans. Tracheal blood flow can be measured using tracheal perfusion, radioactive microspheres, hydrogen clearance, inert soluble gas uptake, and laser Doppler flowmetry.

A. Tracheal Perfusion

Himori and Taira (1976) devised an in vivo preparation for measuring tracheal blood flow and changes in tracheal smooth muscle tone in anesthetized dogs. A midline incision was made in the upper cervical region, and the tracheal branch of the cranial thyroid artery was isolated. All other branches of the cranial thyroid arteries were ligated, and the right and left cranial thyroid arteries were cannulated using the two ends of a Y-shaped cannula (Fig. 22). The vessels were perfused with blood from the femoral artery using a peristaltic pump at constant perfusion pressure, set so that the pressure was similar to the mean systemic arterial pressure. Tracheal blood flow was measured by an electromagnetic flowmeter placed just proximal to the Y-shaped cannula. Changes in the tone of the tracheal smooth muscle were measured as changes in the intraluminal pressure of a water-filled cuff, which encircled the endotra-

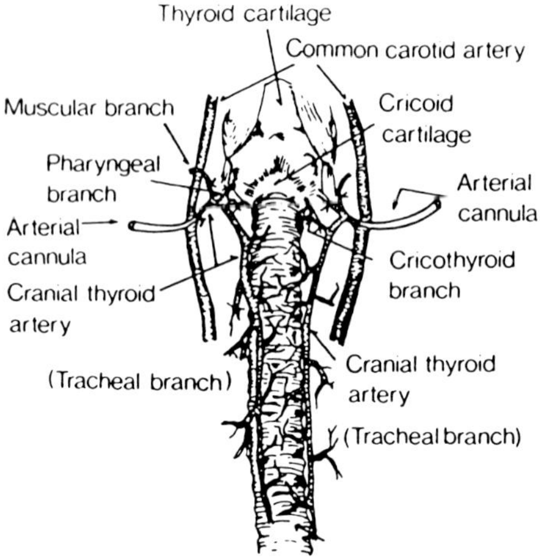

Figure 22 Arterial supply of the trachea of the dog. Cannulae are inserted into the cranial thyroid arteries on both sides. [From Himori, N., and Taira, N. (1976). A method for recording smooth muscle and vascular responses of the blood-perfused dog trachea in situ. *Br. J. Pharmacol.* **56**:293–299.]

cheal tube and was situated 3–8 cm caudal to the larynx. The cuff was connected to a pressure transducer, allowing measurement of constriction and dilation of the trachea. During baseline conditions the blood flow, measured at constant perfusion pressure (130 mmHg) in 38 dogs, was 9.5 ±0.5 ml/min. Measurements of tracheal blood flow were also made after various pharmacological interventions.

In a subsequent study (Himori and Taira, 1978), designed to examine the role of histamine H_1 and H_2 receptors in the tracheal vasculature and musculature, these investigators, using the same technique of tracheal perfusion, obtained a mean baseline value of 8.7 ±1.1 ml/min, which was similar to that of their previous study (Himori and Taira, 1976).

In a series of studies using anesthetized greyhounds, Laitinen and colleagues have used a similar technique to isolate the tracheal perfusion circuit from the systemic circulation (1986a, b, 1987). In this preparation, the tracheal branches of the cranial thyroid arteries were perfused on both sides with blood from a reservoir supplied by the femoral arteries. The preparation was perfused by two peristaltic pumps, and the flow was adjusted so that the tracheal perfusion pressure was similar to the systemic arterial pressure. Tracheal vascular resistance was calculated as the tracheal arterial (inflow) pressure divided by the flow. The results obtained after the interventions were expressed as the percentage change in resistance from the baseline value; however, baseline values for resistance are not reported so that it is not possible to provide values for tracheal blood flow.

B. Radioactive Microspheres

The radioactive microsphere technique, which is described in the first section of this chapter, has been used to make measurements of blood flow specifically to the tracheal mucosa in several different species of animals, including rabbits (Nordin et al., 1977), cats (Martling et al., 1985), dogs (Baile et al., 1987b), and sheep (Wu et al., 1988). Baseline values for tracheal mucosal blood flow from these studies are given in Table 3. Of interest is that when the mucosal blood flow is expressed as ml/min per 100 g tissue, values are three to eight times higher than values for the whole tracheobronchial tree. Because there is no problem of recirculating microspheres in the trachea, measurements are considerably easier to make, requiring only the injection of radiolabeled microspheres into the left atrium or ventricle and the simultaneous collection of a reference flow blood sample from a systemic artery.

C. Hydrogen Clearance

The hydrogen clearance method for measuring local blood flow involves the local generation of hydrogen by an electrode or the washout after the addition of hydrogen to the inspired gas and continuous recording of tissue hydrogen concentration using a platinum electrode implanted in the tissue of interest. The rate at which the hydrogen is washed out of the tissue is proportional to the blood flow through the tissue. This technique was validated experimentally for measurement of blood flow to the myocardium, skeletal muscle, and renal cortex (Aukland et al., 1964) and was found suitable for measurements of cerebral blood flow (Pasztor et al., 1973; Doyle et al., 1975).

This technique was first used by Joh (Joh, 1986; Joh et al., 1987) to examine the effects of endotracheal cuff pressure on canine tracheal mucosal blood flow. In this study the dogs were anesthetized and the trachea exposed through a median incision and a platinum wire hydrogen electrode inserted into the mucosal layer covering the tracheal cartilage (Fig. 23). A second, reference electrode was then placed under the cutaneous layer close to the measuring electrode. Hydrogen gas was passed through a side arm of the endotracheal tube. Under stable conditions, a hydrogen clearance curve may be obtained as a measure of tracheal mucosal blood flow:

$$\dot{Q}\text{muc (ml/min per 100 g)} = \lambda \frac{0.693 \times 100}{T_{1/2}}$$

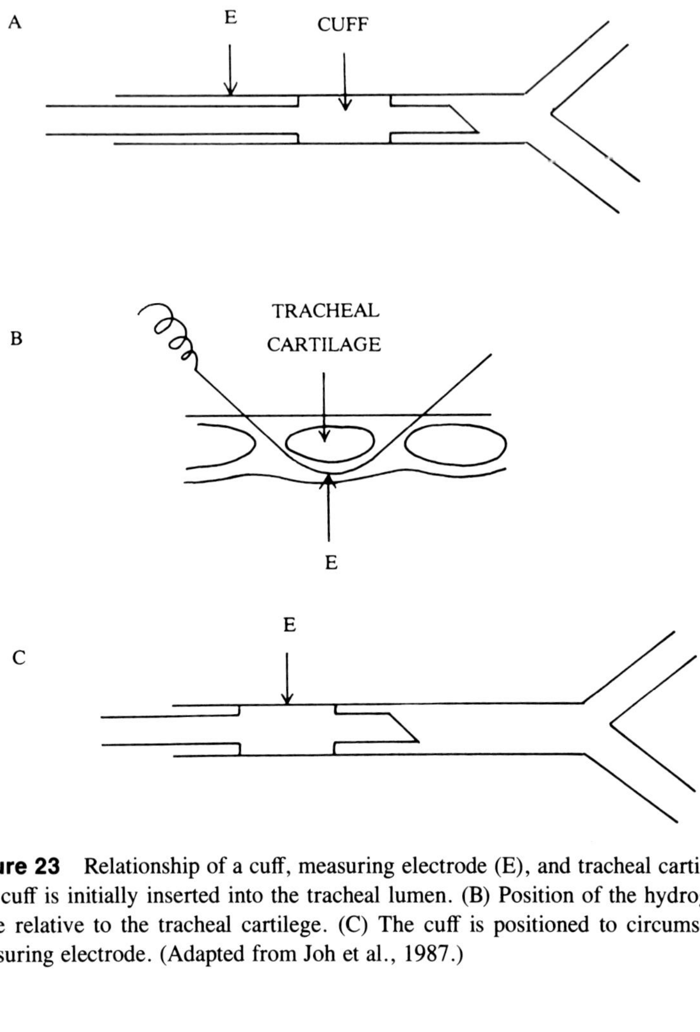

Figure 23 Relationship of a cuff, measuring electrode (E), and tracheal cartilage. (A) The cuff is initially inserted into the tracheal lumen. (B) Position of the hydrogen electrode relative to the tracheal cartilege. (C) The cuff is positioned to circumscribe the measuring electrode. (Adapted from Joh et al., 1987.)

where λ is the tissue-to-blood partition coefficient for hydrogen, and $T_{1/2}$ is the time taken, in minutes (after stopping the hydrogen delivery), for tissue hydrogen concentration to be reduced to half its numerical value. The $T_{1/2}$ is obtained from the slope of the tissue hydrogen decay curve plotted on a semilogarithmic scale (Fig. 24). Using standard formulas, the half-time of the clearance curve can be expressed in ml/min per 100 g. If we assume that tissue is in instantaneous diffusion equilibrium with local venous blood with respect to hydrogen, then the local blood flow per volume of tissue can be calculated according to the Fick principle (Aukland et al., 1964).

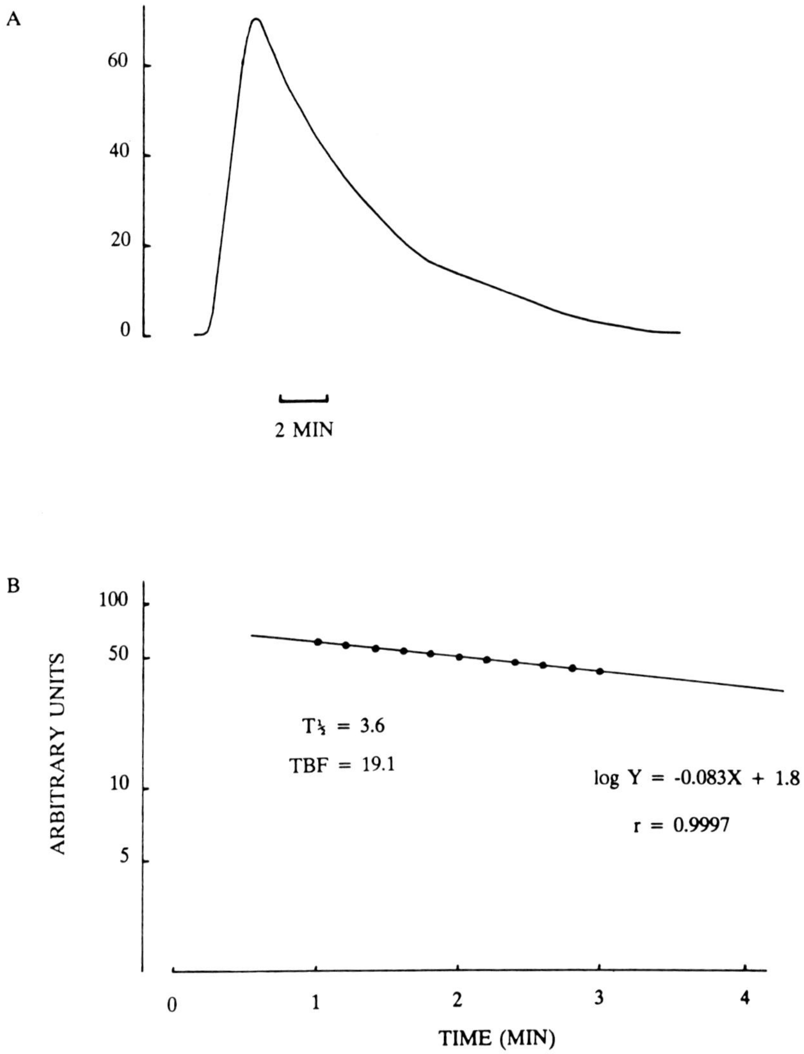

Figure 24 (A) Typical hydrogen clearance curve obtained from tracheal mucosa; (B) a desaturation curve plotted on semilogarithmic axes. (From Joh et al., 1987.)

In his first study Joh (1986) made baseline measurements of tracheal mucosal blood flow in seven dogs at a tracheal wall pressure of 10 mmHg. The mean value for flow was 30.5 ±3.8 ml/min per 100 g. Similar values were obtained for tracheal mucosal blood flow in another study (Joh et al.,

1987) also designed to examine the effect of tracheal cuff pressure on tracheal mucosal blood flow. The mean baseline value for seven dogs was 31 ±17 ml/min per 100 g. Measurements were also obtained during inflation of the endotracheal cuff to produce increases in tracheal wall pressure of up to 6 kPa.

One of the potential problems related to this technique, when hydrogen is given by inhalation, is the early recirculation of hydrogen. However, this is usually evident within the first 40 s of the clearance curve, so that if the analysis is made after this time a uniform rate of blood flow can be obtained. The advantages of this technique are that it is well suited to measurements of regional blood flow in small areas. Although it is slightly invasive, repeated measurements of local blood flow can be made without arterial or venous sampling and measurements require a steady state of only 2 min, so that it is suitable for looking at changes in blood flow.

D. Inert Soluble Gas

Wanner et al. have recently adapted a technique to measure tracheal mucosal blood flow and tissue volume from the transient state and steady-state uptake of a soluble inert gas (1988). Briefly, the theory states that if vascular tissue is exposed to an inert gas that is soluble in tissue and blood, then the uptake of that gas is determined by the volume of tissue with which the gas equilibrates and by the blood flow through the capillaries (Cander and Forster, 1959; Begin et al., 1976). For a given length of trachea, the disappearance of an inert soluble gas from the lumen must therefore reflect the volume of tracheal wall tissue to a certain depth and the capillary blood flow within that tissue. The blood flow and tissue volume were arbitrarily termed tracheal mucosal blood flow and tissue volume.

This study was done on sedated, adult ewes. The upper airway was anesthetized with topical lidocaine, and using a fiberoptic bronchoscope, a nasotracheal tube equipped with two inflatable cuffs, a known distance apart, was inserted; the sheep were ventilated to maintain physiological blood gas tensions. When the cuffs were inflated a chamber was created consisting of the outer wall of the tube, the two cuffs at either end, and the tracheal mucosa between them (Fig. 25). To measure mucosal blood flow the chamber was filled with an inert soluble gas (dimethyl ether, DME) via a catheter situated at one end of the chamber and vented via a catheter at the other end of the chamber. The flow of air or gas through the chamber was measured using a pneumotachograph. The uptake of gas from the chamber by the mucosa is initially high because the inert gas equilibrates with the tracheal mucosal tissue volume and then decreases to a steady state that is dependent on the mucosal blood flow. Calculation of tracheal mucosal blood flow is based on the Bronstein modification of the Fick principle (Sackner, 1987):

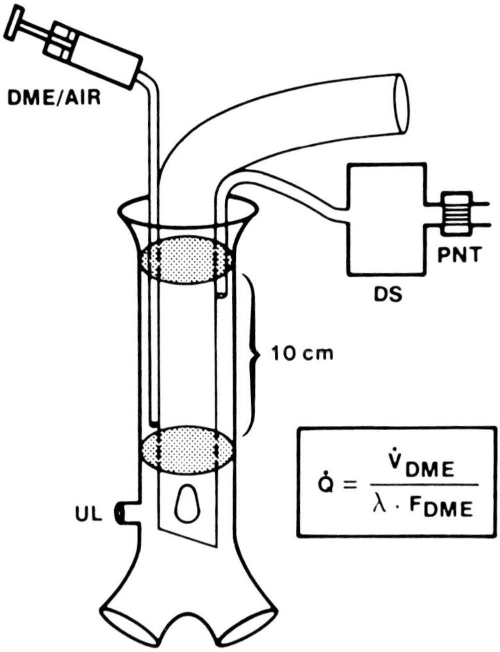

Figure 25 Experimental preparation for measuring tracheal mucosal blood flow ($\dot{Q}$), tissue volume, and dead space. DME, dimethyl ether; UL, upper lobe orifice; DS, external dead space; PNT, pneumotachometer; $\dot{V}_{DME}$, uptake of DME measured by PNT; λ, solubility coefficient for DME in tissue and blood; F_{DME}, fractional DME concentration in tracheal chamber. In this example, the length of the tracheal chamber is 10 cm. (From Wanner et al., 1988, with permission of the *Journal of Applied Physiology*.)

$$\text{Tracheal mucosal flow} = \frac{\dot{V}_{DME}}{\lambda \cdot F_{DME}}$$

where V_{DME} is the steady-state uptake of DME from the tracheal chamber, λ is the Bunsen solubility coefficient for DME in tissue and blood, and F_{DME} is the DME concentration in the tracheal chamber, which in this preparation remained constant throughout the measurement. The validity of this technique is based on several assumptions: to calculate tracheal blood flow, the concentration of DME in the blood leaving the capillaries should be uniform throughout the mucosal vascular bed; there should be no gradient in partial pressure for DME between the tracheal chamber, the mucosal tissue, and the capillary blood; and the tracheal arterial blood should contain no DME. In addition, the depth of the tracheal wall accessible to the inert gas may influence the measurements since it is likely that there is a gradient in DME concentration from luminal to serosal surface. Consequently, measurements could be more influenced by the blood flowing to the superficial layers of tissue.

The mean baseline value for tracheal mucosal blood flow obtained in nine ewes was 1.2 ml/min and ranged from 0.87 to 1.73 ml/min. This was calculated to be about 52 ml/min per 100 g wet tissue. To validate this technique, measurements of tracheal mucosal blood flow made in five ewes were compared with measurements made using the radioactive microsphere technique. Using the soluble inert gas method, tracheal mucosal blood flow was 80% of that measured using radioactive microspheres. The response of the tracheal vasculature to various pharmacological agents was also examined.

An advantage of this technique is that it is relatively noninvasive and can be carried out in sedated animals so that numerous measurements could theoretically be made in the same animal over a period of time, although it is possible that in high concentrations DME may itself produce some vascular effects. This technique is potentially applicable to measurement of blood flow in humans. Perhaps the main disadvantage is that an expensive mass spectrometer is required; however, the savings made by being able to restudy each sheep could soon recover this initial cost.

E. Laser Doppler Flowmetry

Of all the techniques that have been developed to measure airway blood flow, laser Doppler flowmetry is probably the least invasive. It was first applied to a biological system in 1972 by Riva et al. (1972). They measured the flow of 0.56 μm polystyrene beads and blood through 200 μm diameter glass tubes.

To measure microvascular blood flow using laser Doppler flowmetry, laser light is directed by an optical fiber into the tissue and illuminates a volume that contains both moving red blood cells and stationary tissue cells. Photons are scattered randomly by the tissue and red blood cells. Those photons that strike moving red blood cells in the microvascular bed undergo a frequency shift according to the Doppler principle. An increase or decrease in the number of moving red cells in the tissue causes an increase or decrease in the number of shifted photons, whereas an increase or decrease in red cell velocity causes an increase or decrease in the magnitude of the Doppler shift. The photons that are scattered by moving red blood cells are Doppler shifted in the same way in which sound is Doppler shifted. Part of this scattered light is collected by returning optical fibers coupled to a photodetector, and the shifted and unshifted light mixes on the photodetector, producing Doppler beat frequencies, similar to a beat frequency in music. The photodetector converts the light into electronic signals that contain the same Doppler information. Using electronic processing, the product of the velocity and volume produces a signal that is proportional to blood flow, or rather flux, since the laser light within the tissue becomes completely randomized within a few micrometers and it is not possible to obtain information regarding the direction of flow (Bonner and Nossal, 1981). The spatial resolution of laser Doppler flowmetry is approximately a hemisphere with a radius of about 1 mm, although this has been shown to vary in different tissues (Johansson et al., 1987). An extensive and excellent review by Oberg on the principles, applications, and pitfalls of laser Doppler flowmetry has recently been published (1990).

Because laser Doppler flowmetry is noninvasive and is capable of making measurements of microvascular blood flow continuously and in real time, its applications are rapidly becoming more numerous and it has been used to measure blood flow to a wide variety of organs and tissues, including the skin, gastric mucosa, cochlea, and nasal mucosa (Taylor et al., 1988; Ahn et al., 1986; Hultcrantz and Nuttall, 1987; Olsson and Bende, 1986). However, until recently it had not been applied to the measurement of airway blood flow, which is obviously inherently difficult because of movement produced by the lungs and heart.

The first measurements of bronchial mucosal blood flow, using laser Doppler flowmetry, were made by Aoki et al. (1986) in anesthetized dogs undergoing bronchoplasty of the right main bronchus. A close relationship was found between the healing of the anastomotic site and the regional blood flow measured using laser Doppler flowmetry.

Soon after, Martling and colleagues (1987) measured tracheal blood flow in the anesthetized cat in an attempt to characterize the nervous control of tracheal blood flow. In this preparation the cats were breathing spontaneously and the trachea was exposed from the larynx to the sternum. The laser flow probe was inserted into the tracheal lumen through a small hole in the anterior tracheal wall and positioned either at the second tracheal cartilage or just above the sternum for measurement of mucosal blood flow during stimulation of the superior laryngeal nerve or the vagus nerve. Because laser Doppler flowmetry does not provide values for blood flow in absolute units (unless it is precalibrated using another technique), in this study flow was expressed as the percentage maximal change in the output signal (volts) or as a percentage of the baseline value. In support of the accuracy of the method, a direct relationship was observed between systemic arterial blood pressure and the laser Doppler signal. It was also found that stimulation of the sympathetic trunk or application of epinephrine to the tracheal mucosa (both of which are expected to decrease mucosal blood flow) was associated with a decrease in the laser Doppler signal. Measurements of changes in mucosal blood flow were also made after stimulation of the superior laryngeal and the vagal nerve at different voltages and frequencies and before and after various pharmacological interventions. However, these investigators did not carry out a systematic validation of the technique for the specific measurement of tracheobronchial blood flow.

More recently, measurements of tracheal and bronchial blood flow have been made in anesthetized dogs (Godden et al., 1991a), sheep (Godden et al., 1991b) and awake human volunteer subjects (Baile et al., 1988) using laser Doppler flowmetry. Because the laser light can be transmitted to the tissue through a fiberoptic probe (2 mm), it is possible to make measurements in the trachea and bronchi by introducing the probe down the suction channel of a flexible bronchoscope, advancing the probe tip about 3 cm beyond the tip of the bronchoscope and allowing it to rest lightly against the tracheal mucosa. Readings were obtained only during cessation of ventilation to avoid the problem of artifactual signals due to respiratory movement. In the animal studies this was achieved by briefly turning off the ventilator, and in the human study the subjects were asked to hold their breath for 5–10 s. In the animal studies it was possible to make comparisons of measurements of tracheal wall blood flow using laser Doppler flowmetry with those made using a previously validated technique.

Godden et al. (1991b) made measurements of airway wall blood flow in four different regions in both alive and dead sheep using the laser Doppler flow probe and compared the laser Doppler signals with measurements made by perfusing the common bronchial artery at blood flow rates varying from zero to 1.2 ml/min/kg body weight, as described by Wagner et al. (1987). In the live sheep variations in bronchial arterial blood flow resulted in variations in laser Doppler signals in the principal bronchus and in lobar and segmental bronchi, but not in the lower trachea, presumably because this area of the tracheal mucosa is supplied by vessels other than the common bronchial artery. In the dead sheep, variations in bronchial arterial blood flow resulted in variations in the laser Doppler signal in all four regions, which suggests that there are anastomoses between the various systemic arteries supplying the mucosa and that when the systemic vascular pressure decreases (i.e., after death) blood from the common bronchial artery perfuses a larger region. Within a region the average laser Doppler signal was linearly related to the bronchial arterial flow in both live and dead sheep; however, changes in the laser Doppler signal during life were proportionally less than the changes in the flow through the common bronchial artery and there was a site-to-site variation in the slope relating these two measurements. Interestingly, while the sheep were alive a substantial laser Doppler signal persisted even when bronchial arterial flow was set to zero. However, in the dead sheep this signal was close to zero. A smaller signal was observed in the live sheep when the bronchial artery was perfused with dextran solution (Fig. 26), which in theory is expected to pro-

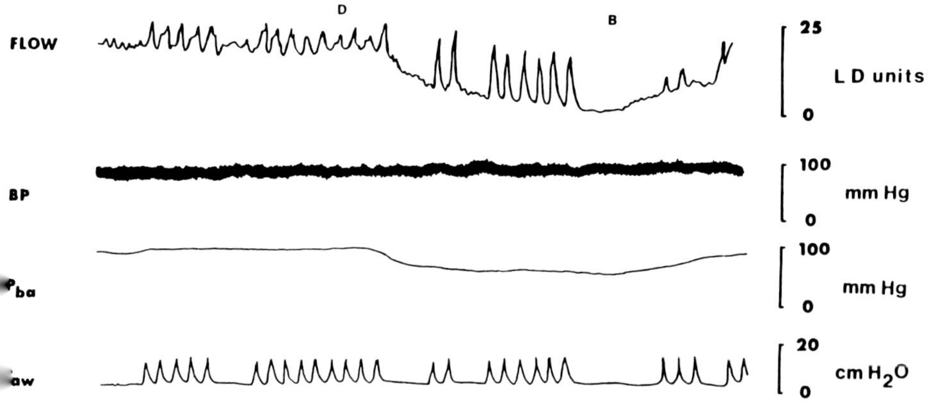

Figure 26 The effects in one sheep of perfusing the bronchial artery with dextran solution. D, dextran perfusion; B, blood perfusion. BP, systemic arterial blood pressure; P_{ba}, bronchial arterial pressure; P_{aw}, airway pressure. Measurements using laser Doppler flowmetry (in arbitrary LD units) were made during brief cessation of ventilation, as indicated from the P_{aw} signal.

duce no laser Doppler signal since it contains no cells. It was suggested that, as well as detecting blood flow from the bronchial artery, laser Dopler flowmetery also detected background noise and/or collateral circulation.

Godden et al. (1991a) have made measurements of tracheal wall blood flow in anesthetized dogs using laser Doppler flowmetry. Measurements were obtained from different sites of the tracheal mucosa before and after the application of 12 cm H_2O positive end-expiratory pressure and eucapnic hyperventilation of dry air and were compared with sequential measurements made using radioactive microspheres and the reference flow technique (Baile et al., 1982). The results showed comparable decreases in the overall laser Doppler signals and the overall microsphere flow during application of positive end-expiratory pressure. There was no correlation between the regional changes in the two signals, however, probably because the laser Doppler probe measures flow to such a small volume of tissue, and consequently there are insufficient numbers of microspheres within this region to be able to make an accurate assessment of blood flow (Fig. 27). The laser Doppler technique was unable to detect the increase in blood flow during hyperventilation. Mucosal blood flow increased an average of 87% as measured with microspheres but decreased 12% as measured by laser Doppler flowmetry.

Baile et al. (1988) also made measurements of tracheal wall blood flow using laser Doppler flowmetry and fiberoptic bronchoscopy in five normal,

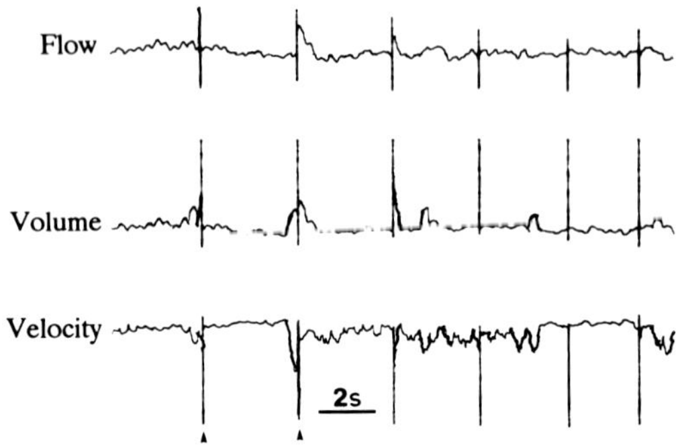

Figure 27 Recording of laser Doppler signals of flow, volume, and velocity from one subject during baseline conditions. Measurements obtained during breathholding. Arrows indicate where breathing recommenced and the chart recorder was turned off.

volunteer subjects aged 19–47 years (Fig. 28). The study was done on two different occasions, and measurements were obtained during baseline conditions while the subjects were breathing room air. Results showed that there was considerable variability in tracheal wall blood flow both within and between measurements. The coefficient of variation between subjects was 51%

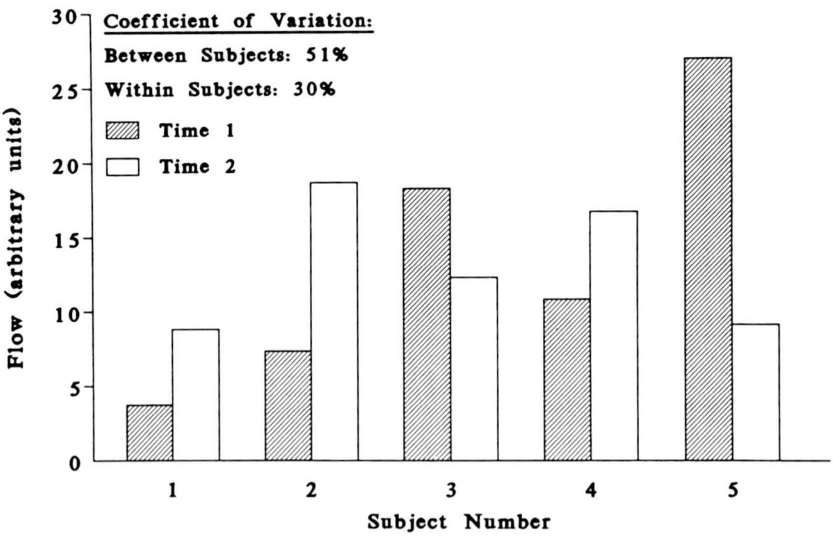

Figure 28 Measurements of airway wall blood flow (arbitrary units) in five subjects recorded on two different occasions (time 1 and time 2).

and that within subjects was 30%. A more detailed account of this study is given in Chap. 5.

One problem associated with using the laser Doppler flow probe in making measurements of blood flow is that any movement of the tissue relative to the probe is interpreted as a signal. Therefore, measurements of tracheal wall blood flow were always made during temporary cessation of respiration. However, cardiac movement caused significant problems when measurements were recorded closer to the main carina and the major bronchi. Artifactual signals could also be caused by incorrect positioning of the probe relative to the airway mucosa and to accumulation of mucous secretions between the probe tip and the mucosa. Other problems associated with measuring airway blood flow have recently been discussed by Godden et al. (1991b).

V. Conclusion

In this chapter many different methods have been described, all of which were designed to measure various components of blood flow in the bronchial vasculature—a bronchial circulation that is diminutive, elusive, and capricious. These very qualities have stimulated investigators, who have devised a variety of ingenious techniques in the attempt to capture the nature of the bronchial circulation and to record it in concrete terms of pressures and flows. Sixty years have now passed since the first measurements of bronchial blood flow were recorded, and despite the advent of sophisticated techniques, such as laser Doppler flowmetry, we still do not have a simple, reliable method of measuring bronchial blood flow in humans. The challenge remains!

References

Agostoni, P. G., Deffebach, M. E., Kirk, W., Lakshminarayan, S., and Butler, J. (1987a). Upstream pressure for systemic to pulmonary flow from bronchial circulation in dogs. *J. Appl. Physiol.* **63**:485–491.

Agostoni, P. G., Deffebach, M. E., Kirk, W., and Brengelmann, G. L. (1987b). Temperature dependence of intraparenchymal bronchial blood flow. *Respir. Physiol.* **68**:259–267.

Agostoni, P. G., Deffebach, M. E., Kirk, W., Mendenhall, J. M., Albert, R. K., and Butler, J. (1987c). Temperature alters bronchial blood flow response to pulmonary arterial obstruction. *J. Appl. Physiol.* **62**:1907–1911.

Agostoni, P. G., Arena, V., Biglioli, P., Doria, E., Sola, A., and Susini, G. (1989). Increase of alveolar pressure reduces systemic-to-pulmonary bronchial blood flow in humans. *Chest* **96**:1081–1085.

Ahn, H., Lindhagen, J., Nilsson, G. E., Oberg, P. A., and Lundgren, O. (1986). Assessment of blood flow in the small intestine with laser Doppler flowmetry. *Scand. J. Gastroenterol.* **21**:863–870.

Angelsen, B. A. J., Kristofersen, K., and Torp, H. (1985). On measurement of maximum velocity in blood jets in the heart. In *Cardiovascular Ultrasonic Flowmetry*, Third Lovelace Medical Foundation Research Symposium, Albuquerque, New Mexico. Edited by S. A. Altobelli, W. F. Voyles, and E. R. Green. New York, Elsevier.

Aoki, M., Wada, H., Inui, K., Yamazaki, H., and Hitomi, S. (1986). Measurement of bronchial mucosal blood flow by laser Doppler velocimetry in the dog. *J. Jpn. Soc. Bronchol.* **8**:622–629.

Aramendia, P., Martinez, L., De Letona, J., and Aviado, D. M. (1962). Exchange of blood between pulmonary and systemic circulations via bronchopulmonary anastomoses. *Circ. Res.* **11**:870–879.

Aukland, K., Bower, B. F., and Berliner, R. W. (1964). Measurement of local blood flow with hydrogen gas. *Circ. Res.* **14**:164–187.

Auld, P. A. M., Rudolph, A. M., and Golinko, R. J. (1960). Factors affecting bronchial collateral flow in the dog. *Am. J. Physiol.* **198**:1166–1170.

Austin, R. E., Jr., Hauck, W. W., Aldea, G. S., Flynn, A. E., Coggins, D. E., and Hoffman, J. I. E. (1989). Quantitating error in blood flow measurements with radioactive microspheres. *Am. J. Physiol.* **257**:H280–H288.

Aviado, D. M., De Burgh Daly, M., Lee, C. Y., and Schmidt, C. F. (1961). The contribution of the bronchial circulation to the venous admixture in pulmonary venous blood. *J. Physiol. (Lond.)* **155**:602–622.

Baier, H., Yerger, L., Moas, R., and Wanner, A. (1985). Vascular and airway effects of indogenous cyclooxygenase products during lung inflation. *J. Appl. Physiol.* **59**:884–889.

Baile, E. M., and Paré, P. D. (1983). Response of the bronchial circulation to acute hypoxemia and hypercarbia in the dog. *J. Appl. Physiol.* **55**:1474–1479.

Baile, E. M., Nelems, J. M. B., Schulzer, M., and Paré, P. (1982). Measurement of regional bronchial arterial blood flow and bronchovascular resistance in dogs. *J. Appl. Physiol.* **53**:1044–1049.

Baile, E. M., Albert, R., Kirk, W., Lakshaminarayan, S., Wiggs, B. J., and Paré, P. D. (1984). Positive end-expiratory pressure decreases bronchial blood flow in the dog. *J. Appl. Physiol.* **56**:1289–1293.

Baile, E. M., Dahlby, R. W., Wiggs, B. R., and Paré, P. D. (1985a). Role of tracheal and bronchial circulation in respiratory heat exchange. *J. Appl. Physiol.* **58**:217–222.

Baile, E. M., Ling, H., Heyworth, J. R., Hogg, J. C., and Paré, P. D. (1985b). Bronchopulmonary anastomotic and noncoronary collateral blood flow in humans during cardiopulmonary bypass. *Chest* **87**:749–754.

Baile, E. M., Ling, H., Miyagishima, R. T., Kronhardt, H., and Paré, P. D. (1986a). Cardiac temperature and cardioplegic volume during cardiopulmonary bypass. *J. Surg. Res.* **41**:388–393.

Baile, E. M., Osborne, S., and Paré, P. D. (1986b). Effect of autonomic blockade on tracheobronchial blood flow. *J. Appl. Physiol.* **62**:520–525.

Baile, E. M., Dahlby, R. W., Wiggs, B. R., Parsons, G. H., and Paré, P. D. (1987a). Effect of cold and warm dry air hyperventilation on canine airway blood flow. *J. Appl. Physiol.* **62**:526–532.

Baile, E. M., Guillemi, S., and Paré, P. D. (1987b). Tracheobronchial and upper airway blood flow in dogs during thermally-induced panting. *J. Appl. Physiol.* **63**:2240–2246.

Baile, E. M., Godden, D. J., and Paré, P. D. (1988). Non-invasive, real-time measurement of tracheal blood flow in humans. *Clin. Invest. Med.* **11**:C110.

Barman, S. A., Ardell, J. L., Parker, J. C., Perry, M. L., and Taylor, A. E. (1988). Pulmonary and systemic blood flow contributions to upper airways in canine lung. *Am. J. Physiol.* **255**:H1130–H1135.

Barnes, R. J., Comline, R. S., Dobson, A., and Drost, C. J. (1983). An implantable transit-time ultrasonic blood flow meter. *J. Physiol. (Lond.)* **35**:2–3.

Begin, R., Dougherty, R., Michaelson, E. D., and Sacker, M. A. (1976). Effect of sequential anti-G suit inflation on pulmonary capillary blood flow in man. *Aviat. Space Environ. Med.* **47**:937–941.

Berry, J. L., and Daly, I. De B. (1931). The relation between the pulmonary and bronchial vascular systems. *Proc. R. Lond. [Biol.]* **109**:319–336.

Bloomer, W. E., Harrison, W., Lindskog, G. E., and Liebow, A. A. (1949). Respiratory function and blood flow in the bronchial aratery after ligation of the pulmonary artery. *Am. J. Physiol.* **157**:317–328.

Bonner, R., and Nossal, R. (1981). Model for laser Doppler measurements of blood flow in tissue. *Appl. Optics* **20**:2097–2107.

Bruner, H. D., and Schmidt, C. R. (1947). Blood flow in the bronchial artery of the anesthetized dog. *Am. J. Physiol.* **148**:648–666.

Buckberg, G. D., Luck, J. C., Payne, D. B., Hoffman, J. I. E., Archie, J. P., and Fixler, D. E. (1971). Some sources of error in measuring regional blood flow with radioactive microspheres. *J. Appl. Physiol.* **31**:598–604.

Cander, L., and Forster, R. E. (1959). Determination of pulmonary parenchymal tissue volume and pulmonary capillary blood flow in man. *J. Appl. Physiol.* **14**:541–551.

Canty, J. M., Jr., and Brooks, A. (1985). Characterization of coronary venous outflow in conscious dogs using a volumetric ultrasonic flowmeter. *Physiologist* **28**:316.

Cartwright, R. S., Lim, T. P. K., Luft, U. C., and Palich, W. E. (1962). Pathophysiological changes in the lungs during extracorporeal circulation. *Circ. Res.* **10**:131–141.

Cassidy, S. S., and Haynes, M. S. (1986). The effects of ventilation with positive end-expiratory pressure on the bronchial circulation. *Respir. Physiol.* **66**:269–278.

Charan, N. B., Turk, G. M., and Ripley, R. (1985). Measurement of bronchial arterial blood flow and bronchovascular resistance in sheep. *J. Appl. Physiol.* **59**:305–308.

Charan, N. B., Turk, G. M., Czartolomny, J., and Andreazuk, T. (1987). Systemic arterial blood supply to the trachea and lung in sheep. *J. Appl. Physiol.* **62**:2283–2287.

Cudkowicz, L., (1965). Cardiorespiratory studies in patients with pulmonary tuberculosis. *Can. Med. Assoc. J.* **92**:111–115.

Cudkowicz, L., Calabresi, M., Nims, R. G., and Gray, F. D., Jr. (1959a). The simultaneous estimation of right and left ventricular outputs applied to a study of the bronchial circulation in dogs. *Am. Heart J.* **58**:732–742.

Cudkowicz, L., Calabresi, M., Nims, R. G., and Gray, F. D., Jr. (1959b). The simultaneous estimation of right and left ventricular outputs applied to a study of the bronchial circulation in patients with chronic lung disease. *Am. Heart J.* **58**:743–749.

Cudkowicz, L., Abelmann, W. H., Levinson, G. E., Katznelson, G., and Jreissaty, R. M. (1960). Bronchial arterial blood flow. *Clin. Sci.* **19**:1–15.

Deal, C. W., Louis, E., Kerth, W. J., Osborn, J. J., and Gerbode, F. G. (1968). Bronchopulmonary precapillary blood flow during cardiopulmonary bypass. *Am. Heart J.* **75**:43–48.

Deffebach, M. E., Lakshminarayan, S., Kirk, W., and Butler, J. (1987). Bronchial circulation and cyclooxygenase products in acute lung injury. *J. Appl. Physiol.* **63**:1083–1088.

DeKock, M. A., Nadel, J. A., Zwi, S., Colebatch, H. J. H., and Olsen, C. R. (1966). New method for perfusing bronchial arteries: Histamine bronchoconstriction and apnea. *J. Appl. Physiol.* **21**:185–194.

Domenech, R. J., Hoffman, J. I. E., Noble, M. I., Saunders, K. B., Henson, J. R., and Subijanto, S. (1969). Total and regional coronary blood flow measured by radioactive microspheres in conscious and anesthetized dogs. *Circ. Res.* **25**:581–596.

Doyle, T. F., Martins, A. N., and Kobrine, A. I. (1975). Estimating total cerebral blood flow from the initial slope of hydrogen washout curves. *Stroke* **6**:149–152.

Drost, C. J. (1978). Vessel diameter-independent volume flow measurement using ultrasound. In *Proceedings of the San Diego Biomedical Symposium*, San Diego CA. *San Diego Biomed. Soc.* **17**:299–302.

Drost, C. J., Thomas, G. G., and Sellers, A. F. (1979). In vivo validation of the transit time volume flow meter. In *Proceedings of the 7th New England (NE) Bioengineering Conference*, Troy, New York, pp. 220–223.

Dumke, P. R., and Schmidt, C. F. (1943). Quantitative measurements of cerebral blood flow in the macacque monkey. *Am. J. Physiol.* **138**:421–431.

Fisher, A. B., Kollmeier, H., Brody, J. S., Hyde, R. W., Hansell, J., Friedman, J. N., and Waldhausen, J. A. (1970). Restoration of systemic blood flow to the lung after division of bronchial arteries. *J. Appl. Physiol.* **29**:839–846.

Fishman, A. P., Turino, G., Brandfonbrener, M., and Himmelstein, A. (1958). The "effective" pulmonary collateral blood flow in man. *J. Clin. Invest.* **37**:1071–1086.

Fritts, H. W., Jr., Harris, P., Chidsey, C. A., Clauss, R. H., and Cournand, A. (1957). Validation of a method for measuring the output of the right ventricle in man by inscription of dye-dilution curves from the pulmonary artery. *J. Appl. Physiol.* **11**:362–364.

Fritts, H. W., Jr., Harris, P., Chidsey, C.A., Clauss, R. H., and Cournand, A. (1961). Estimation of flow through bronchial-pulmonary vascular anastomoses with use of T-1824 dye. *Circulation* **23**:390–398.

Gleed, R. D., Dobson, A., and Hacket, R. P. (1990). Pulmonary shunting by the bronchoid artery in the anesthetized horse. *Exp. Physiol.* **75**:115–118.

Godden, D. J., Baile, E. M., and Paré, P. D. (1991a). A comparison of laser Doppler flowmetry with the radiolabelled microsphere reference flow technique to measure trachael blood flow in dogs. *Acta Physiol. Scand.* **142**:49–57.

Godden, D. J., Wagner, E. M., Paré, P. D., Mitzner, W., and Baile, E. M. (1991b). Measurement of airway blood flow in sheep by laser Doppler flowmetry: interpretation and problems. *J. Appl. Physiol.* **70**:641–649.

Goetz, R. H., and Rohman, M. (1965). The hemodynamics of bronchopulmonary anastomoses. *Surg. Gynecol. Obstet.* **120**:517–529.

Hartley, C. J., Hanley, H. G., Lewis, R. M., and Cole, J. S. (1978). Synchronized pulsed Doppler blood flow and ultrasonic dimension measurement in conscious dogs. *Ultrasound Med. Biol.* **4**:99–110.

Himori, N., and Taira, N. (1976). A method for recording smooth muscle and vascular responses of the blood-perfused dog trachea in situ. *Br. J. Pharmacol.* **56**:293–299.

Himori, N., and Taira, N. (1978). Pharmacological analysis of histamine receptors in musculature and vasculature of the dog trachea in situ *Br. J. Pharmacol.* **64**:553–558.

Horisberger, B., and Rodbard, S. (1960). Direct measurement of bronchial arterial flow. *Circ. Res.* **8**:1149–1156.

Hultcrantz, E., and Nuttall, A. L. (1987). Effect of hemodilution on cochlear blood flow measured by laser Doppler flowmetry. *Am. J. Otolaryngol.* **8**:16–22.

Jindal, S. K., Lakshminarayan, S., Kirk, W., and Butler, J. (1984). Acute increase in anastomotic bronchial blood flow after pulmonary arterial obstruction. *J. Appl. Physiol* **57**:424–428.

Jindal, S. K., Lakshminarayanan, S., Kirk, W., and Butler, J. (1985). Regulation of increase in anastomotic blood flow following pulmonary arterial occlusion. *J. Appl. Physiol.* **59**:180–182.

Joh, S. (1986). Impairment of tracheal mucosal blood flow by endotracheal tube cuffs and its recovery. *J. Osaka Univ. Dent. Soc.* **31**:334–350.

Joh, S., Matsuura, H., Kotani, J., Hirota, Y., Kiyomitsu, Y., and Kubota, Y. (1987). Changes in tracheal blood flow during endotracheal intubation. *Acta Anaesthesiol. Scand.* **31**:300–304.

Johansson, K., Ahn, H., Lindhagen, J., and Lundgren, O. (1987). Tissue penetration and measuring depth of laser Doppler flowmetry in the gastrointestinal application. *Scand. J. Gastroenterol.* **22**:1081–1088.

Katori, R., Miyazawa, K., Ishikawa, K., and Nakamura, T. (1970a). Detection of bronchial blood flow from earpiece dye-dilution curve. *Tohoku J. Exp. Med.* **100**:127–133.

Katori, R., Miyazawa, K., Ishikawa, K., Yamaki, M., Kobayashi, Y., Sendo, Y., and Nakamura, T. (1970b). Bronchial blood flow in pulmonary tuberculosis. *Tohoku J. Exp. Med.* **100**:135–142.

Laitinen, L. A., Robinson, N. P., Laitinen, A., and Widdicombe, J. G. (1986). Relationship between tracheal mucosal thickness and vascular resistance in dogs. *J. Appl. Physiol.* **61**:2186–2193.

Laitinen, L. A., Laitinen, A., and Widdicombe, J. G. (1987a). Parasympathetic nervous control of tracheal vascular resistance in the dog. *J Physiol (Lond.)* **385**:135–146.

Laitinen, L. A., Laitinen, A., and Widdicombe, J. G. (1987b). Effects of inflammatory and other mediators on airway vascular beds. *Am. Rev. Respir. Dis.* **135**:S67–S70.

Lajos, T. Z., and Glicken, D. (1980). Metabolic measurements in the human heart-lung preparation during hypothermic cardioplegia. *Thorac. Cardiovasc. Surg.* **28**:34–41.

Lantz, B. M. T. (1974). *A Methodologic Investigation of Roentgen Videodensitometric Measurements of Relative Flow*. Berkeley, University of California Press.

Lantz, B. M. T. (1983). Videodilution technique: A new approach to vascular physiology. *Int. Angiol.* **2**:329–336.

Lantz, B M. T. (1984). Quantitative angiography by video dilution technique. *Appl. Radiol.* **10**:447–471.

Lantz, B. M. T., Foerster, J. M., Link, D. P., and Holcroft, J. W. (1980). Determination of relative blood flow in single arteries: New videodilution technique. *Am. J. Roentgenol.* **134**:1161–1168.

Lilker, E. S., and Nagy, E. J. (1975). Gas exchange in the pulmonary collateral circulation of dogs. *Am. Rev. Respir. Dis.* **112**:615–620.

Link, D. P., Parsons, G. H., Lantz, B. M. T., Gunther, R. A., Green, J. F., and Cross, C. E. (1985). Measurement of bronchial blood flow in sheep by videodilution technique. *Thorax* **40**:143–149.

Long, W. M., Sprung, C. L., El Fawal, H., Yerger, L. D., Eyre, P., Abraham, W. M., and Wanner, A. (1985). Effects of histamine on bronchial artery blood flow and bronchomotor tone. *J. Appl. Physiol.* **59**:254–261.

Lung, M. A., Wang, J. C. C., and Cheng, K. K. (1976). Bronchial circulation: An auto-perfusion method for assessing its vasomotor activity and the study of alpha and beta-adrenoceptors in the bronchial artery. *Life Sci.* **19**:577–580.

Madoff, I. M., Gaensler, E. A., and Strieder, J. W. (1952). Congenital absence of the right pulmonary artery. *N. Engl. J. Med.* **247**:149–157.

Magno, M. G., and Fishman, A. P. (1982). Origin, distribution, and blood flow of bronchial circulation in anesthetized sheep. *J. Appl. Physiol.* **53**:272–279.

Magno, M. G., Charan, N., Parsons, G. H., Baile, E. M., Albertine, K. H., and Butler, J. (1987). Nomenclature for the bronchial circulation. *J. Appl. Physiol.* **62**:2512.

Makowski, E. L., Meschia, G., Droegemueller, G. W., and Battaglia, F. C. (1968). Measurement of umbilical arterial blood flow to the sheep placenta and fetus in utero. *Circ. Res.* **23**:623–631.

Malik, A. B., and Tracy, S. E. (1980). Bronchovascular adjustments after pulmonary embolism. *J. Appl. Physiol.* **49**:476–481.

Mandelbaum, I., and Giammona, S. T. (1966). Bronchial circulation during cardiopulmonary bypass. *Ann. Surg.* **164**:985–989.

Martinez L. De Latona, J., Castro De La Mata, R., and Aviado, D. M. (1961). Local and reflex effects of bronchial arterial injection of drugs. *J. Pharmacol. Exp. Ther.* **133**:295–303.

Martling, C.-R., Anggard, A., and Lundberg, J. M. (1985). Non-cholinergic vasodilation in the tracheobronchial tree of the cat induced by vagal nerve stimulation. *Acta Physiol. Scand.* **125**:343–346.

Martling, C.-R., Gazelius, B., and Lundberg, J. M. (1987). Nervous control of tracheal blood flow in the cat measured by the laser Doppler technique. *Acta Physiol. Scand.* **130**:409–417.

Modell, H. I., Beck, K., and Butler, J. (1981). Functional aspects of canine bronchial-pulmonary vascular communications. *J. Appl. Physiol.* **50**:1045–1051.

Murao, H. (1965). Nervous regulation of the bronchial vascular system. *Jpn. Circ. J.* **29**:855–865.

Nakamura, T. (1956). Pulmonary circulation in silicosis. *Jpn. Circ. J.* **19**: 513–531.

Nakamura, T. (1958). Broncho-pulmonary circulation. Its system and functional implications. *Jpn. Circ. J.* **22**:427–442.

Nakamura, T., Katori, R., Miyazawa, K., Ohtomo, S., Watanabe, Ta, and Watanabe, Te (1960). Proposal of a method for estimating bronchial blood flow by simultaneous measurements of the left and right ventricular outputs with the dye dilution technique. *Dis. Chest* **37**:680–686.

Nakamura, T., Katori, R., Miyasawa, K., Ohtomo, S., Watanabe, Ta, Watanabe, Te, Miura, Y., and Takizawa, T. (1961). Bronchial blood flow in patients with chronic pulmonary disease and its influence upon respiration and circulation. *Dis. Chest* **39**:193–206.

Nakamura, T., Katori, R., Watanabe, T., Watanabe, T., Miyazawa, K., Murao, M., Oda, J., and Ishikawa, K. (1967). Quantitation of left-to-right shunt from a single earpiece dye-dilution curve. *J. Appl. Physiol.* **22**:1156–1160.

Nakamura, T., Katori, R., Mayazawa, K., Ishikawa, K., Yamaki, M., and Kobayashi, Y. (1968). Aortopulmonary collateral flow in patients with pulmonary disease. *Am. Rev. Respir. Dis.* **93**:464–473.

Nordin, U., Lindholm, C.-E., and Wolgast, M. (1977). Blood flow in the rabbit tracheal mucosa under normal conditions and under the influence of tracheal intubation. *Acta Anaesthesiol. Scand.* **21**:81–94.

Notkovich, H. (1957). The anatomy of the bronchial arteries of the dog. *J. Thorac. Surg.* **33**:242–253.

Öberg, P. Å. (1990). Laser-Doppler flowmetry. *Crit. Rev. Biomed. Eng.* **18**:125–163.

Olsson, P., and Bende, M. (1986). Sympathetic neurogenic control of blood flow in human nasal mucosa. *Acta Otolaryngol.* **102**:482–487.

Parsons, G. H., Kramer, G. C., Link, D. P., Lantz, B. M. T., Gunther, R. A., Green, J. F., and Cross, C. E. (1985). Studies of reactivity and distribution of bronchial blood flow in sheep. *Chest* **87**:180S–182S.

Parsons, G. H., Link, D. P., Greenberg, D., Lantz, B. M. T., and Cross, C. E. (1987). Bronchial blood flow measured by videodilation technique in sheep. *Invest. Radiol.* **22**:544–549.

Parsons, G. H., Paré, P. D., White, D. A., and Baile, E. M. (1989). Airway blood flow response to eucapnic dry air hyperventilation in sheep. *J. Appl. Physiol.* **66**:1443–1447.

Pasztor, E., Symon, L., Dorsch, C., and Branston, N. M. (1973). The hydrogen clearance method in assessment of blood flow in cortex, white matter and deep nuclei of baboons. *Stroke* **4**:556–567.

Riva, C., Ross, B., and Benedeck, G. B. (1972). laser Doppler measurements in blood flow in capillary tubes and retinal arteries. *Invest. Opthalmol.* **11**:936–944.

Rudoph, A. M., and Heyman, M. A. (1967). The circulation of the fetus in utero. Methods for studying distribution of blood flow, cardiac output and organ blood flow. *Circ. Res.* **21**:163–184.

Sackner, M. A. (1987). Measurement of cardiac output by alveolar gas exchange. In *Handbook of Physiology. The Respiratory System. Gas Exchange*, Sect. 3, Vol 1V, Chapter 13. Bethesda, M. American Physiology Society, pp. 233–255.

Sellers, A. F., Lowe, J. E., Drost, C. J., Rendano, V. T., Georgi, J. R., and Roberts, M. C. (1982). Rctropulsion-propulsion in equine large colon. *Am. J. Vet. Res.* **43**:390–396.

Shedd, D. P., Alley, R. D., and Lindskog, G. E. (1951). Observations on the hemodynamics of bronchial-pulmonary vascular communications. *J. Thorac. Surg.* **22**:537–548.

Shimura, H., Watanabe, Y., Imanishi, N., and Shibuya, T. (1986). A new simultaneous method for measuring the blood flow in small experimental animals using the transit-time ultrasonic volume flowmeter. *Jpn. J. Pharmacol.* **40**:s101.

State, D., Salisbury, P. F., and Weil, P. (1957). Histologic and pharmacologic studies of collateral pulmonary flow. *J. Thorac. Surg.* **34**:599–608.

Taylor, W.F., Johnson, J. M., Kosiba, W. A., and Kwan, C. M. (1988). Graded cutaneous vascular responses to dynamic leg exercise. *J. Appl. Physiol.* **64**:1803–1809.

Vatner, S. F., Young, M., and Patrick, T. A. (1985). Measurement of coronary blood flow in conscious animals. In *Cardiovascular Ultrasonic Flowmetry*, 3rd Lovelace Medical Foundation Research Symposium, Albuquerque, New Mexico. Edited by S. A. Altobelli, W. F. Voyles, and E. R. Green. New York, Elsevier.

Viola, A. R., and Abbate, E. (1973). Respiratory function and effective collateral flow 8 years after ligation of the left pulmonary artery. *Am. Rev. Respir. Dis.* **108**:1216–1220.

Wagner, E. M., and Mitzner, W. A. (1988). Effect of hypoxia on bronchial circulation. *J. Appl. Physiol.* **65**:1627–1633.

Wagner, H. N., Jr., Rhodes, B. A., Sasaki, Y., and Ryan, J. P. (1969). Studies of the circulation with radioactive microspheres. *Invest. Radiol.* **4**:374–386.

Wagner, E. M., Mitzner, W. A., and Bleecker, E. R. (1987). Effects of airway pressure on bronchial blood flow. *J. Appl. Physiol.* **62**:561–566.

Wanner, A., Barker, J. A., Long, W., Mariassy, A. T., and Chediak, A. D. (1988). Measurement of airway mucosal perfusion and water volume with an inert soluble gas. *J. Appl. Physiol.* **65**:264–271.

Warren, R. L., and Powell, W. J., Jr. (1986). Acute alveolar hypoxia increases bronchopulmonary shunt flow in the dog. *J. Clin. Invest.* **77**:1515–1524.

White, S. W., Angus, J. A., McRitchie, R. J., and Porges, W. L. (1974). Evaluation of the Doppler flowmeter for measurement of blood flow in small vessels of ananesthetized animals. *Clin. Exp. Pharmacol. Physiol. (Suppl)* 79–92.

Williams, H. M., and Towbin, E. J. (1955). Magnitude and time of development of the collateral circulation to the lung after occlusion of the left pulmonary artery. *Circ. Res.* **3**:422–424.

Wu, C.-H., Lindsey, D. C., Traber, D. L., Cross, C. E., Herndon, D. N., and Kramer, G. C. (1988). Measurement of bronchial blood flow with radioactive microspheres in awake sheep. *J. Appl. Physiol.* **65**:1131–1139.

Yamatake, Y., and Yanaura, S. (1978). New method for evaluating bronchomotor and bronchosecretory activities: Effects of prostoglandins and antigen. *Jpn. J. Pharmacol.* **28**:391–402.

Yanaura, S., Hosokawa, T., Goto, K., and Misawa, M. (1981). Histamine receptors in the bronchial musculature and vasculature of the dog. *J. Pharm. Dyn.* **4**:85–90.

Zapata-Ortiz, V., Castro de la Mata, R., Fernandez, E., Geu, A., and Batalla, L. (1967). Bronchial circulation in high altitudes. *Am. J. Physiol.* **212**:1464–1468.

5

Measurement of Bronchial Blood Flow in Humans

PIERGIUSEPPE AGOSTONI

University of Milan
Milan, Italy

DAVID JOHN GODDEN

University of Aberdeen
Aberdeen, Scotland

ELISABETH M. BAILE

University of British Columbia
St. Paul's Hospital
Vancouver, British Columbia, Canada

I. Introduction

Bronchial blood flow is technically extremely difficult to measure, largely because of the anatomic arrangement of the bronchial vasculature but also because it represents such a small proportion of the cardiac output. In humans, as in many other animal species, the bronchial arteries have multiple sites of origin. They usually stem directly from the aorta or from the intercostal arteries but may occasionally originate from the subclavian and the innominate arteries (Pump, 1963). This means that techniques such as the electromagnetic flow probe, which are used to measure blood flow through a single bronchial vessel and are often used for the measurement of bronchial blood flow in such animals as the sheep, are not suitable for use in humans (see Chapter 4). Even if it were possible to use a single bronchial artery, there remains the difficulty that in addition to supplying the airways the bronchial arteries also supply the mediastinal lymph nodes, the lower third of the esophagus, the visceral pleura, and the vasa vasorum of the pulmonary arteries and veins.

Another technique that is often used to measure regional systemic flow to the lungs in experimental animals is the radioactive microsphere technique;

however, this necessitates killing the animal at the end of the experiment and excision of the tissue under study.

Indirect measurements of bronchial blood flow have been made previously in humans using different techniques, such as indirect application of the Fick principle and bronchospirometry (Madoff et al., 1952; Fishman et al., 1958) and dye dilution curves using an earpiece and densitometer (Katori et al., 1970). However, these techniques are no longer used, largely because of their inaccuracy and inability to measure normal or decreased values for bronchial blood flow. More recently, systemic-to-pulmonary bronchial blood flow has been measured in patients during cardiopulmonary bypass surgery and measurements of tracheal wall blood flow have been made using the relatively noninvasive technique of laser Doppler flowmetry. In this chapter the methodology, results from, and associated advantages and disadvantages of these two widely differing techniques are discussed.

II. Systemic-to-Pulmonary Bronchial Blood Flow

A. Cardiopulmonary Bypass

Cudkowicz and colleagues (1959) were the first to attempt to measure systemic-to-pulmonary bronchial blood flow $\dot{Q}br(s\text{-}p)$ in humans by subtracting the right from the left ventricular output. However, because $\dot{Q}br(s\text{-}p)$ is normally so minute, only about 1% of the cardiac output, this technique allows reliable measurements to be made only when $\dot{Q}br(s\text{-}p)$ is considerably augmented, as in people who have chronic lung infection, pulmonary vascular obstruction, or congenital heart disease. In 1968, Deal and coworkers realized that it was possible to measure $\dot{Q}br(s\text{-}p)$ in humans under conditions of total cardiopulmonary bypass. When there is no pulmonary blood flow, the only blood flowing through the pulmonary circulation is $\dot{Q}br(s\text{-}p)$. These investigators measured $\dot{Q}br(s\text{-}p)$ by applying the Fick principle to carbon dioxide production (see Chap. 4). Almost 20 years later Baile and colleagues (1985) made the first direct measurements of $\dot{Q}br(s\text{-}p)$ in humans during total cardiopulmonary bypass surgery by venting $\dot{Q}br(s\text{-}p)$ from the apex of the left ventricle. This technique was later slightly modified by Agostoni and associates (1989), who also measured $\dot{Q}br(s\text{-}p)$ during total cardiopulmonary bypass as the volume of blood returning to the left heart in the absence of pulmonary and coronary flows. However, unlike Baile et al., Agostoni and colleagues introduced a second cannula, open to atmosphere, into the left heart and also clamped the pulmonary artery (Fig. 1). This second cannula guaranteed a left heart pressure of zero and therefore avoided any possible vacuum effect of the left ventricular vent. The pulmonary artery clamp prevented blood leaking through the pulmonary valve and flowing from the right to the left heart. In

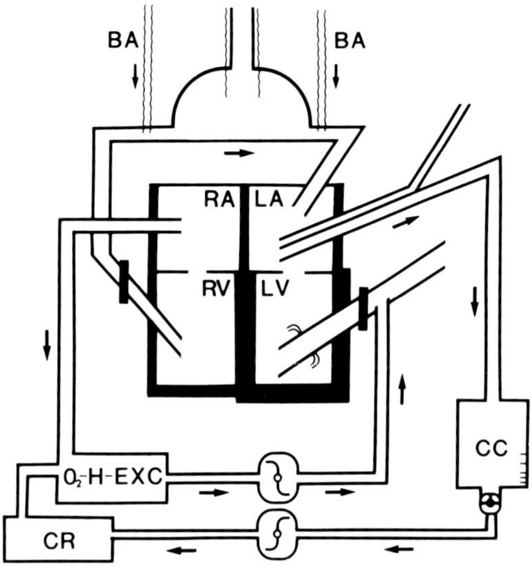

Figure 1 The circuit used to measure systemic-to-pulmonary bronchial blood flow $\dot{Q}$br(s-p) in humans during total cardiopulmonary bypass. BA, bronchial artery; RA, right atrium; LA, left atrium; RV, right ventricle; LV, left ventricle; CC, calibrated cylinder; CR, extracorporeal circuit reservoir; O_2 – H – EXC, oxygen heat exchanger; (▌) aortic and pulmonary artery clamps.

theory this could happen as a consequence of increased right heart pressures due to incomplete drainage of blood from the right atrium.

B. Problems

Technical Problems

Although these changes, introduced by Agostini and colleagues (1989), improved the technique for measuring $\dot{Q}$br(s-p), a few problems remained unresolved. Drainage of the left ventricular vent flow should be continuous. However, inadequate venting may occur periodically when the surgeon turns the heart, resulting in accumulation of blood in the lowermost portion of the left heart. This can be prevented if it is recognized and the position of the left ventricular vent is readjusted.

Administration of the cardioplegic solution can be a potential problem when measuring $\dot{Q}$br(s-p). This solution, which is necessary to cool and arrest the heart, is injected into the aortic root, flows through the coronary arteries, and may reach the left heart chambers via the Thebesian veins. Usually a single injection (~1000 ml) of cardioplegic solution is given at the beginning of cardiopulmonary bypass. However, sometimes repeated or even continuous infusions of cardioplegic solution are given, in which case $\dot{Q}$br(s-p) cannot be measured.

Potentially, some bronchial blood flow can accumulate in the lungs without reaching the left heart. In fact, when $\dot{Q}$br(s-p) is measured in experimental animals using a similar technique, lung weight changes are considered in the calculation of $\dot{Q}$br(s-p) (Jindal et al., 1984; Charan et al., 1986). Although it is not possible to measure lung weight changes in patients during total cardiopulmonary bypass, it is reasonable to assume that no major changes in pulmonary blood volume occur during cardiopulmonary bypass because the lungs are in zone 1 (alveolar pressure > pulmonary vascular pressure). It has been shown by Charan and coworkers (1986) in experimental animals that lung weight is constant during the measurement of $\dot{Q}$br(s-p) as long as the lungs are in zone 1, even if alveolar pressure is increased to 15 cmH_20.

Unphysiological Conditions

Besides the technical difficulties associated with measuring $\dot{Q}$br(s-p), there are also problems related to the unphysiological conditions necessarily encountered during cardiopulmonary bypass, which may directly or indirectly affect $\dot{Q}$br(s-p). Body temperature is reduced during bypass because the patients are cooled systemically, and this may affect $\dot{Q}$br(s-p), as has been recently shown in experimental animals, (Agostoni et al., (1987a). Also, the downstream vascular (left ventricular vent) pressures during cardiopulmonary bypass are always zero and therefore, obviously, less than physiological. Studies by Agostoni and colleagues (1987b) have shown that decreases in pulmonary vascular pressure increase $\dot{Q}$br(s-p). The absence of pulmonary blood flow during cardiopulmonary bypass may also affect $\dot{Q}$br(s-p): Agostoni et al., (1987a) and Malik and Tracy (1980) measured a reduction in bronchial arterial blood flow in experimental animals after cessation of pulmonary arterial blood flow. Other factors that could affect $\dot{Q}$br(s-p) are the use of nonpulsatile flow and, in some cases, the absence of ventilation of the lungs.

C. Results

It is clear that the $\dot{Q}$br(s-p) in humans undergoing bypass surgery is extremely variable. However, $\dot{Q}$br(s-p) seems to be higher in those patients who have severe chronic lung diseases.

Chronic Disease

Baile and colleagues (1985) have reported one patient who had severe asbestosis in whom $\dot{Q}$br(s-p) was 24% of cardiac output (extracorporeal circulation pump flow). It was also observed that there was a tendency for $\dot{Q}br(s\text{-}p)$ to be higher in smokers than in nonsmokers. This has been noted by Agostoni et al. (1990b), who observed that without humidification of the inspired gas (see later) $\dot{Q}br(s\text{-}p)$ was more than twice as high in chronic cigarette smokers (43 ±3 ml/min, n = 17) than in nonsmokers (19 ±3 ml/min, n = 7, $p < 0.05$).

$\dot{Q}br(s\text{-}p)$ has also been shown to be higher in patients who have chronically elevated pulmonary venous pressure due to mitral stenosis. Agostoni et al. (1991) studied two groups of patients during cardiopulmonary bypass who were matched for age and smoking habits. One group had mitral stenosis and elevated pulmonary wedge pressure (22 ±1 mmHg) and the other, the control group, had mitral stenosis and a normal pulmonary wedge pressure. They observed that during mitral valve replacement, $\dot{Q}br(s\text{-}p)$ was 76 ±4 ml/min in the high wedge pressure group and 22 ±1 ml/min in the control group. It should be emphasized that during the measurement pulmonary vascular pressure is always reduced to zero, as described earlier, and that, under physiological conditions when pulmonary vascular pressures are normal, $\dot{Q}br(s\text{-}p)$ may be different. However, these data suggest that in patients who have mitral stenosis and an elevated pulmonary wedge pressure the resistance to blood flow through the $\dot{Q}br(s\text{-}p)$ anastomotic channels is reduced, implying a larger number or dimension of these channels. This observation may have clinical relevance: it is possible that when there is an increase in pulmonary venous pressure in the presence of such a decrease in the resistance of the anastomotic channels, a reversal of blood flow may occur. Such a reversal of flow, from pulmonary to systemic circulations, when pulmonary vascular pressure is increased has been described in studies using experimental animals (Auld et al., 1960; Goetz and Rohman, 1965; Agostoni et al., 1987b). It has even been postulated that the $\dot{Q}br(s\text{-}p)$ channels act as a "safety valve" for the pulmonary circulation, allowing a reduction in pulmonary blood and vascular pressure at a time when this is most needed, such as during the formation of pulmonary edema, although the rate of even an augmented anastomotic flow relative to the pulmonary flow must make this unlikely. However, dilation of anastomotic channels and reversal of flow could decrease the formation of airway edema.

Acute Conditions

To examine the effect of changing the relative humidity of the inspired gas on $\dot{Q}br(s\text{-}p)$, Agostini et al. (1990b) recently studied 50 patients who were free of lung disease and heart failure while undergoing coronary artery surgery. The patients were randomly assigned to one of two groups: group A, in whom the relative humidity of the inspired gas was less than 20%, or group B, in whom the relative humidity was over 85%. The lungs were kept inflated by a constant flow of gas (10 L/min), and the inspired gas temperature was 24° C in both groups. There was no difference between groups in bypass duration, body temperature, or magnitude of extracorporeal circulation pump flow. The results from this study showed that $\dot{Q}br(s\text{-}p)$ was greater in the group who received the drier air (group A), (Fig. 2). This observation is in accordance with the findings of Baile et al. in the dog (1987) and Parsons et al. in the sheep (1989). Although the physiological implications of this study may be diminished because of the unphysiological experimental conditions, the results suggest that humidification of the inspired air is important, although this is not usually done when assisted ventilation is maintained for short periods. Indeed, an increase in the anastomotic bronchial blood returning to the left heart is undesirable for the surgeon because this blood may distend the left ventricle or flow retrogradely through the coronary arteries, thereby complicating the surgery, or possibly also induce an undesirable rewarming of the heart.

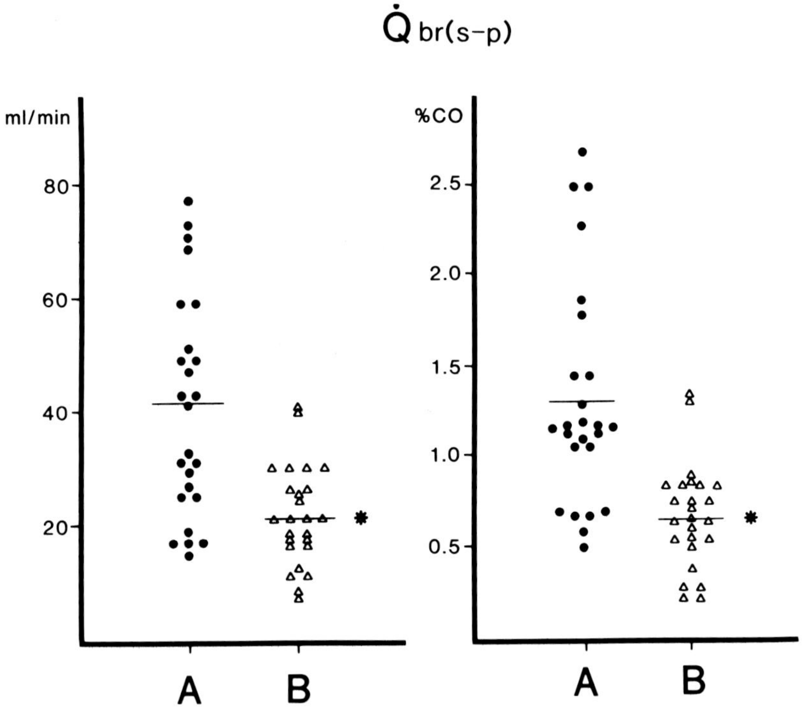

Figure 2 Effects of relative humidity of the inspired gas on systemic-to-pulmonary bronchial blood flow $\dot{Q}br(s\text{-}p)$ reported as absolute flow (left) and as a percentage of cardiac output (CO) from the extracorporeal circulation pump flow (right). (A) Inspired gas relative humidity $< 20\%$; (B) inspired gas relative humidity $> 85\%$. $^*P < 0.01$, A versus B.

The effect of increased alveolar pressure on $\dot{Q}br(s\text{-}p)$ in humans undergoing bypass surgery has also been examined by Agostoni and colleagues (1989). The results from their study are similar to those of other investigators (Baile et al., 1984; Charan et al., 1986; Cassidy and Haynes, 1987), who demonstrated in dogs that positive alveolar pressure reduces bronchial blood flow to the lung. In humans a 40% reduction in $\dot{Q}br(s\text{-}p)$ was obtained when alveolar pressure was increased from 4 to 14 cmH_20 (Fig. 3)

This study also has clinical implications because positive end-expiratory pressure is frequently applied, often over-applied, in medical practice. A reduction in bronchial blood flow could be deleterious for the survival of the lung parenchyma in some circumstances; for example after a pulmonary arterial obstruction, when the bronchial blood flow to the lung parenchyma downstream from the embolus is important for the nutrition of the alveolar as well as the bronchial tissue. In the adult respiratory distress syndrome, when pulmonary blood flow to the diseased region is reduced, the bronchial blood flow increases, allowing inflammation to go on to repair. Its reduction by

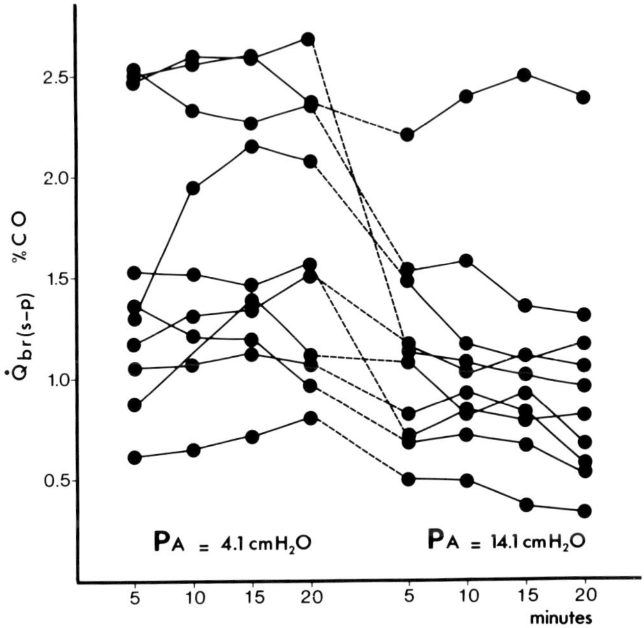

Figure 3 Increases in alveolar pressure (PA) from 4.1 cmH_20 (left) to 14.1 cmH_20 (right) reduce systemic-to-pulmonary bronchial blood flow $\dot{Q}br(s\text{-}p)$, here reported as a percentage of cardiac output (CO) from the extracorporeal circulation pump flow.

excessive alveolar pressures could delay this process or lead to abnormal healing.

III. Airway Wall Blood Flow

For a more detailed account of the principles of laser Doppler flowmetry and some of its associated problems, see Chap. 4.

Briefly, laser Doppler flowmetry is a technique based on the observation that, when laser light is shone into tissue, photons that strike moving red blood cells undergo a frequency shift according to the Doppler principle. Light backscattered from the tissue is therefore comprised of an unshifted component derived from static tissues and a shifted component derived from moving red blood cells (Stern, 1975). The number of photons shifted is related to the volume of flowing blood in the tissue, and the magnitude of the frequency shift is related to the blood velocity. By appropriate signal processing (Bonner and Nossal, 1981; Nilsson et al., 1980), a blood flow signal can be determined. All signals are expressed as arbitrary laser Doppler units (LD units). Absolute flow cannot be determined without in vivo calibration by an independent method, but relative changes in flow can be detected.

Because laser Doppler flowmetry is a relatively noninvasive technique and provides a continuous measurement, it has been used to measure microvascular blood flow in humans in a variety of organs, including skin (Holloway and Watkins, 1977; Johnson et al., 1984), nasal mucosa (Druce et al., 1984; Olsson et al., 1985), stomach (Ahn et al., 1986a; Kvernebo et al., 1986), and intestine (Ahn et al., 1986b, c) Only recently however, have attempts been made to apply this technique to the measurement of airway blood flow. This is an inherently difficult undertaking because of the persistent movements of the lungs and heart. Any movement of the tissue relative to the flow probe is interpreted as a signal, since all currently available laser Doppler flowmeters are essentially extremely sensitive movement detectors. They derive signals from a small but incompletely defined tissue volume, so the interpretation of the measurements is complicated by both extraneous movements and by spatial and temporal variation in the sources of the signals. Movement of the probe during recording may also introduce a fiber movement artifact (Newsom et al., 1987). In the airways, interpretation of measurements is further complicated by the complex anatomy of the microvascular bed because of the multiple sources of inflow to, and outflow from, this bed.

Despite the potential difficulties, attempts have recently been made to measure airway wall blood flow in humans using a laser Doppler flowmeter (Baile et al., 1989). Measurements were made in two groups of subjects, one group undergoing coronary artery bypass surgery under general anesthesia and a second group of awake, spontaneously breathing volunteers.

In the first group, eight patients were studied during cardiopulmonary bypass. To minimize artifactual signals due to repiratory and cardiac movement, all laser Doppler measurements were recorded when the heart was arrested and ventilation was stopped, and a constant airway pressure of 3–5 cm H_20 was maintained. Blood was perfused into the aorta using a non-pulsatile pump. A flexible bonchoscope was introduced into the airway via the endotracheal tube, and a laser Doppler flow probe with a prismatic tip was allowed to rest, under direct vision, on the airway mucosa. Four laser Doppler flow measurements were made, each lasting about 5 s, in each of four regions: the posterior and the lateral walls of the trachea and the right and left mainstem bronchi.

In the group of six awake volunteer subjects, laser Doppler flow measurements similar to those in the bypass patients were again made in the trachea using a flexible bronchoscope. Before bronchoscopy each subject was given 0.6 mg atropine IV to minimize secretions, and the nasopharynx, larynx, and trachea were anesthetized using topical anesthesia. Each measurement was obtained during a 5–10 s voluntary breathhold. A total of 15 such measurements were made on the lateral wall of the trachea on two separate occasions at least 1 week apart.

Typical flow, volume, and velocity recordings are shown in Fig. 4. In the cardiopulmonary bypass patients, the flow tracing was relatively flat and the volume signal from the mucosal blood was high in relation to the velocity signal. In contrast, in the awake subjects there was a prominent oscillation related to cardiac pulsation and the velocity signal was high in relation to the volume signal. However, the average level of flow recorded on the lateral tracheal wall of both groups was similar. Values for flow, expressed in arbitrary units, for individual patients and subjects are shown in Fig. 5. Mean ±SD (standard deviation) flow values were 16 ±11 units for the bypass patients, 17 ±11 units for the awake subjects on the first occasion, and 16 ±7 units on the second occasion. There was substantial inter-person variation in flow signals, the coefficient of variation between patients being 66% for the bypass group and 78% for the awake subjects. In the bypass group there was also a considerable variation between regions, the mean coefficient of variation being 51 ±12%. More importantly, within each region there was a considerable site-to-site variation in the flow signals. The mean coefficient of variation between sites in the bypass group was 20 ±14% and, in the awake group, 23 ±14%. Finally, for the awake subjects who underwent repeated studies, the coefficient of variation between the two occasions was 43 ±22%.

The most important sources of artifact in the laser Doppler signals were movement due to respiration, which was eliminated by breathholding during measurements, and cardiac motion, which varied between regions of the airways. This obviously cannot be avoided in noninvasive measurements. How-

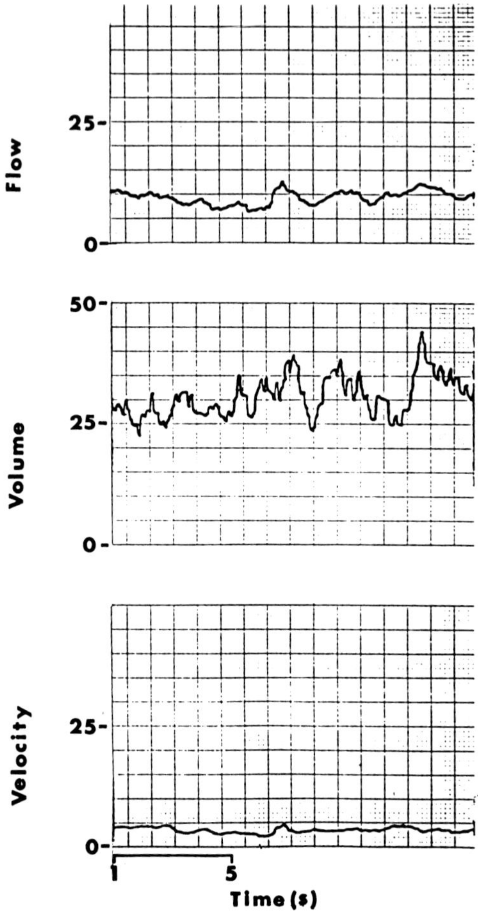

(A)

Figure 4 Specimen laser Doppler recordings from the midtracheal region in (A) a patient undergoing cardiopulmonary bypass, and (B) an awake subject. In A the flow tracing is smooth and the velocity signal is small. In B there is pronouned cardiac pulsation and the velocity signal is higher.

ever, even in the absence of respiratory and cardiac motion, as was the case during cardiopulmonary bypass, site-to-site and region-to-region variation in signals was considerable. A similar spatial variation in laser Doppler signals has been observed in other biological systems. For example, the coefficient of variation between sites is reported to be 25% for skin (Swanson Beck and Spence, 1986) and 33–39% for stomach (Kvernebo et al., 1986). This variation is probably attributable to local variation in capillary density and nonuni-

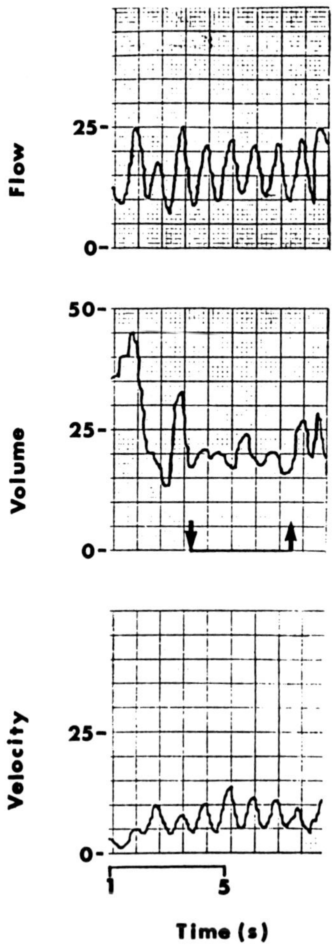

(B)

formity of blood flow pattern. The practical importance of this observation is that relative changes in blood flow can only be reliably detected if the probe is maintained at a single site throughout the recording period. This is a substantial limitation for measurements within the airways, especially when the probe is introduced endoscopically. Furthermore, the behavior of the small portion of the microvasculature "seen" by the laser Doppler flow probe may not be representative of the organ as a whole.

Even when the probe is held at one position during a series of recordings, there is a possibility that the airway mucosal thickness at that site and

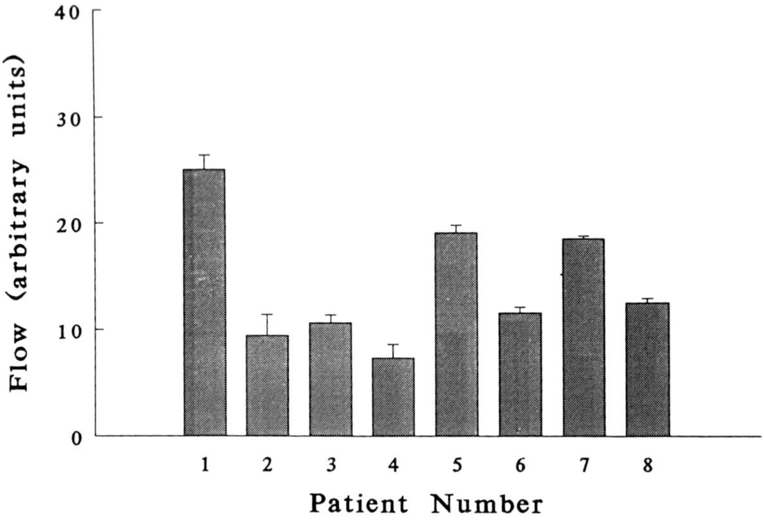

(A)

Figure 5 Tracheal wall blood flow (arbitrary units): (A) Eight patients during cardiopulmonary bypass; (B) Six subjects, recorded on two different occasions (time 1 and time 2). Values are mean ± SD.

therefore the distance between the probe and the flowing blood may undergo dynamic changes. This has been demonstrated in animal airways (Laitinen et al., 1986) and may in turn alter the relative proportions of mucosa, submucosa, and cartilage in the tissue volume sampled by the laser Doppler probe. The absolute depth of tissue sampled by the laser Doppler probe remains uncertain and is the subject of controversy (Shepherd and Oberg, 1990).

Although the laser Doppler technique is noninvasive, introduction of the flow probe requires endoscopy, which necessitates at least topical anesthesia of the airways. Topical anesthetic agents may themselves affect the responses of the airway vasculature, as has been shown in animals (Baile et al., 1990), and this must be borne in mind when interpreting physiological events studied by laser Doppler flowmetry.

Several potential future refinements of laser Doppler flowmetry may pemit more meaningful measurements to be obtained in humans. Probes have been designed that contain a reference fiber from which a signal can be detected related to fiber movement (Newsom et al., 1987). This signal can then be subtracted from the flow signal to correct for fiber-movement artifact. A probe has been developed for use in the skin that will sample seven sites

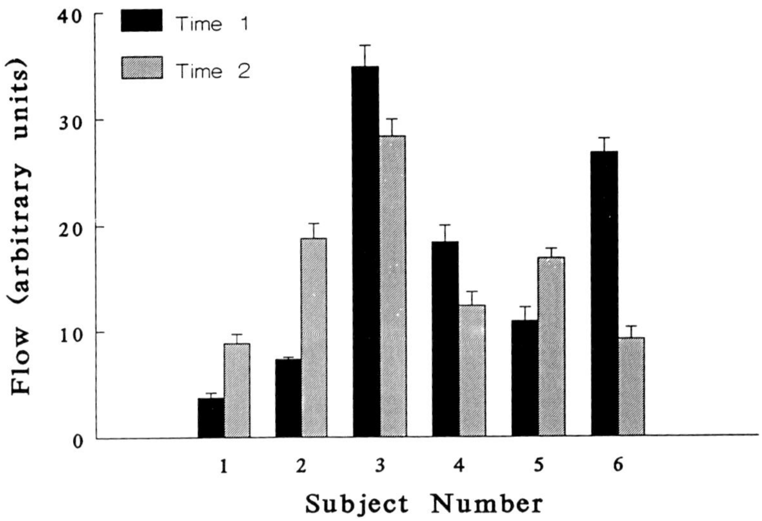

(B)

simultaneously and produce an integrated value for flow (Salerud and Nilsson, 1986). This therefore reduces reduces the spatial variation in signals obtained by the probe. In an attempt to obtain an *in vitro* calibration of the laser Doppler signals, a hybrid probe has been developed that combines laser Doppler optical fibers and platinum electrodes, which allow intermittent measurements of blood flow to be derived by the hydrogen clearance technique (DiResta et al., 1987). These measurements can then be used as point calibrations for the laser Doppler instrument. At present, however, the size of these probes would preclude their use in the human airways.

The potential value of a technique that would provide continuous measurements of airway wall blood flow in humans is obvious. Research applications would include investigation of the role of the airway vasculature in the pathogenesis of airways obstruction and examination of the blood supply around endobronchial tumors. Clinical applications could include monitoring of blood flow to bronchial anastomoses in lung transplantation; a preliminary study of this type has been done in animals (Inui et al., 1990). However, improved laser Doppler flowmeters will have to be developed and tested in relation to established techniques before this technology can be further exploited in human airways.

References

Agostoni, P. G., Deffebach, M. E., Kirk, W. Mendenhall, J. M., Albert, R. K., and Butler, J. (1987a). Temperature alters bronchial blood flow response to pulmonary artery obstruction. *J. Appl. Physiol.* **62**:1907–1911.

Agostoni, P. G., Deffebach, M. E., Kirk, W., Lakshminarayan, S., and Butler, J. (1987b). Upstream pressure for systemic-to-pulmonary bronchial blood flow in dogs. *J. Appl Physiol* **63**:485–491.

Agostoni, P. G., Arena, V., Biglioli, P., Doria, E., Sala, A., and Susini, G. (1989). Increase of alveolar pressure reduces systemic-to-pulmonary bronchial blood flow in humans. *Chest* **96**:1081–1085.

Agostoni, P. G., Agrifoglio, M., Arena, V., Doria, E., Sala, A., and Susini, G. (1991). Systemic-to-pulmonary bronchial blood flow in mitral stenosis. *Chest* **99**:642–645.

Agostoni, P. G., Arena, V., Doria, E., and Susini, G. (1990b). Inspired gas relative humidity affects systemic-to-pulmonary bronchial blood flow in humans. *Chest* **97**:1377–1380.

Ahn, H., Johansson, K. and Lindhagen, J. (1986a). Local blood flow changes in association with proximal gastric vagotomy. *Scand. J. Gastroenterol.* **21**:961–964.

Ahn, H., Lindhagen, J., and Lundgren, O. (1986b). Measurement of colonic blood flow with laser Doppler flowmetry. *Scand. J. Gastroenterol.* **21**:871–880.

Ahn, H., Lindhagen, J., Nilsson, G. E., Oberg, P.A., and Lundgren, O. (1986c). Assessment of blood flow in the small intestine with laser Doppler flowmetry. *Scand. J. Gastroenterol* **21**:863–870.

Auld, P. A. M., Rudolph, A. M., and Golinko, R. J. (1960). Factors affecting bronchial collateral flow in the dog. *Am. J. Physiol.* **198**:1166–1170.

Baile, E. M., Albert, R. K., Kirk, W., Lakshminarayan, S., Wiggs, B. J. R., and Pare, P. D. (1984). Positive end-expiratory pressure decreases bronchial blood flow in the dog. *J. Appl. Physiol.* **5**:1289–1293.

Baile, E. M., Ling, H., Heyworth, J., Hogg, J. C., and Pare, P. D. (1985). Bronchopulmonary anastomotic and noncoronary collateral blood flow in humans during total cardiopulmonary bypass. *Chest* **6**:749–754.

Baile, E. M., Dahlby, R. W., Wiggs, B. R., Parsons, G. H., and Pare, P. D. (1987). Effect of cold and warm dry air hyperventilation on canine airway blood flow. *J. Appl. Physiol.* **62**:526–532.

Baile, E. M., Godden, D. J., and Pare, P. D. (1989). Effect of cold dry and warm humid air hyperventilation on tracheal wall blood flow in humans. *Am. Rev. Respir. Dis.* **139**(4):A63.

Baile, E. M., Godden, D. J., and Pare, P. D. (1990). Mechanism for the increase in tracheobronchial blood flow induced by hyperventilation of dry air in dogs. *J. Appl. Physiol.* **68**:105–112.

Bonner, R., and Nossal, R. (1981). Model for laser Doppler measurements of blood flow in tissue. *Appl. Optics* **20**:2097–2107.

Cassidy, S. S., and Haynes, M. S. (1987). The effects of ventilation with positive end-expiratory pressure on the bronchial circulation. *Respir. Physiol.* **66**:269–278.

Charan, N. B., Albert, R. K., Lakshminarayan, S., Kirk, W., and Butler, J. (1986). Factors affecting bronchial blood flow through bronchopulmonary anastomoses in dogs. *Am. Rev. Respir. Dis.* **134**:85–88.

Cudkowicz, L., Calabresi, M., Nims, R. G., and Gray, F. D. (1959). The simultaneous estimation of right and left ventricular outputs applied to a study of the bronchial circulation in patients with chronic lung diseases. *Am. Heart J.* **58**:743–749.

Deal, C. W., Louis, E., Kerth, W. J., Osborn, J. J., and Gerbode, F. (1968). Bronchopulmonary precapillary blood flow during cardiopulmonary bypass. *Am. Heart J.* **75**:43–48.

DiResta, G. R., Kiel, J. W., Riedel, G. L., Kaplan, P., and Shepherd, A. P. (1987). Hybrid blood flow probe for simultaneous H_2 clearance and laser Doppler velocimetry. *Am. J. Physiol.* **253**(16):G573–581.

Druce, H. M., Bonner, R. F., Patow, C., Choo, P., Summers, R. J., and Kaliner, M. A. (1984). Response of nasal blood flow to neurohormones as measured by laser Doppler velocimetry. *J. Appl. Physiol.* **57**:1276–1283.

Fishman, A. P., Turino, G. M., Brandfonbrener, M., and Himmelstein, A. (1958). The "effective" pulmonary collateral blood flow in man. *J. Clin. Invest.* **37**:1071–1086.

Goetz, R. H., and Rohman, M. (1965). The hemodynamics of bronchopulmonary anastomoses. *Surg. Gynecol. Obstet.* **120**:517–529.

Holloway, G. A., and Wakins, D. W. (1977). Laser Doppler measurement of cutaneous blood flow. *J. Invest. Dermatol.* **69**:306–309.

Inui, K., Wada, H., Yokomise, H., Lee, M., Yamazaki, F., Aoki, M., and Hitomi, S. (1990). Evaluation of a bronchial anastomosis by laser Doppler velocimetry. *J. Thorac. Cardiovasc. Surg.* **99**:614–619.

Jindal, S. K., Lakshminarayan, S., Kirk, W., and Butler, J. (1984). Acute increase in anastomotic bronchial blood flow after pulmonary arterial obstruction. *J. Appl. Physiol.* **57**:424–428.

Johnson, J. M., Taylor, W. F., Shepherd, A. P., and Park, M. K. (1984). Laser Doppler measurement of skin blood flow: Comparison with plethysmography. *J. Appl. Physiol.* **56**:798–803.

Katori, R., Miyazawa, K., Ishikawa, K., Yamaki, M., Kobayashi, Y., Sendo, Y., and Nakamura, T. (1970). Bronchial blood flow in pulmonary tuberculosis. *Tohoku J Exp. Ed.* **100**:135–142.

Kvernebo, K., Lunde, O. C., Stranden, E., and Larsen, S. (1986). Human gastric blood circulation evaluated by endoscopic laser Doppler flowmetry. *Scand. J. Gastroenterol.* **21**:685–692.

Laitinen, L. A., Robinson, N. P., Laitinen, A., and Widdicombe, J. G. (1986). Relationship between tracheal mucosal thickness and vascular resistance in dogs. *J. Appl. Physiol.* **61**:2186–2193.

Madoff, I. M., Gaensler, E. A., and Strieder, J. W. (1952). Congenital absence of the right pulmonary artery. *N. Engl. J. Med.* **247**:149–157.

Malik, A. B., and Tracy, S. E. (1980). Bronchovascular adjustments after pulmonary embolism. *J. Appl. Physiol.* **49**:476–481.

Newsom, T. P., Obeid, A., Wolton, R. S., Boggett, D., and Rolfe, P. (1987). Laser Doppler velocimetry: The problem of fiber movement artefact. *J. Biomed. Eng.*.**9**:169–172.

Nilsson, G. E., Tenland, T., and Oberg, P. A. (1980). Evaluation of a laser Doppler flowmeter for measurement of tissue blood flow. *IEEE Trans. Biomed. Eng.* **27**:597–604.

Olsson, P., Bende, M., and Ohlin, P. (1985). The laser Doppler flowmeter for measuring microcirculation in human nasal mucosa. *Acta Otolaryngol. (Stockh.)* **99**:133–139.

Parsons, G. H., Pare, P. D., White, D. A., and Baile, E. M. (1989). Airway blood flow response to eucapnic dry air hyperventilation in the sheep. *J. Appl. Physiol.* **66**:1443–1447.

Pump, K. K. (1963). Distribution of bronchial arteries in human lungs. *Dis. Chest* **43**:245–255.

Salerud, E. G., and Nilsson, G. E. (1986). Integrating probe for laser Doppler flowmeters. *Med. Biol. Eng. Comput.* **24**:415–419.

Shepherd, A. P., and P. A. Oberg, eds. (1990). *Laser Doppler Blood Flowmetry*. Dordrecht, Kluwerr Academic Publishers.

Stern, M. D. (1975). In vivo evaluation of microcirculation by coherent light scattering. *Nature* **254**:56–58.

Swanson Beck, J., and Spence, V. A. (1986). Patterns of blood flow in the microcirculation of the skin during the course of the tuberculin reaction in normal human subjects. *Immunology* **58**:209–215.

Part IV

REGULATION

6

Pulmonary and Bronchial Contributions to Airway Blood Flow

SCOTT A. BARMAN

Medical College of Georgia
Augusta, Georgia

JEFFREY L. ARDELL and AUBREY E. TAYLOR

University of South Alabama
College of Medicine
Mobile, Alabama

I. Introduction

Since the time of Galen (129–190), it has been known that lung tissue receives blood flow from two distinct circulations: the pulmonary circulation, which was originally thought to act only as a vehicle for gas exchange, not to provide nutrients to airway structures; and the bronchial (systemic) circulation, which was thought to be the only blood supply to all of the airways. The interactions that occur between the pulmonary and bronchial circulations in regard to fluid balance, delivery of metabolites, and removal of end products of metabolism in the airway tissue were not well understood.

The pulmonary circulation is now known to provide nutrients for the alveolar tissues, but little information is available concerning the contribution of the pulmonary and bronchial blood flows to the lower trachea and airway nutrition. Available information indicates that the trachea receives its blood flow predominantly from the systemic circulation (termed "bronchial" within the chest), but the pulmonary and bronchial circulations both contribute to the blood supply of the intrathoracic airways. Surprisingly, it seems that arterial inflow from either circulation can be obstructed without dire consequences for the airways. This could be explained by the relationship between the two supplies of blood. Thus this chapter focuses on the contribution from each circulation to the different parts of the airways and the interactions between them.

II. Airway Blood Flow

Until the last few years it was thought that the pulmonary circulation provided no blood flow to the tracheobronchial structures. We discuss here, however, recent studies that have shown that the pulmonary circulation is also a source of tracheobronchial and small airway blood flows (Michelassi et al., 1987; Barman et al., 1988).

A. Anatomic Systemic-to-Pulmonary Vascular Anastomoses

Depending on the particular animal species, anastomoses between the bronchial and pulmonary circulations exist at the precapillary, capillary, and postcapillary levels. The presence of bronchopulmonary connections was first observed by Ruyisch in 1721 and subsequently by many investigators (Verloop, 1949; Marchand et al., 1950; Tobin, 1952). McLaughlin and coworkers (1961) observed that bronchial artery–pulmonary artery shunts were present in cow and horse lungs, and similar anastomoses are also present in sheep lungs (Charan, et al., 1984, 1985). Although the systemic-to-pulmonary circulation has been studied extensively in an *in situ* dog lung preparation in which the pulmonary circulation is eliminated by ligation, conflicting evidence exists about the exact location of the bronchopulmonary anastomoses that produce the measured flow. Miller (1906) performed extensive anatomic studies of anastomotic connections in dog lungs and found that the bronchial circulation drains into the pulmonary circulation at the capillary level. Subsequent studies have revealed that bronchopulmonary connections are present at both the precapillary (Modell et al., 1981; Hyman et al., 1975; Auld et al., 1960) and postcapillary levels (Baile et al., 1985; Berry and Daly, 1931). In addition, communications exist between the bronchial artery and the pulmonary vein (Tobin, 1952), and Hyman et al. (1975) found that bronchial arteries supply the vasa vasorum of pulmonary arteries greater than 200 μm in diameter. In human lungs, "bronchopulmonary arteries" are commonly seen in neonates but appear less frequently in the lungs of children and adults (Wagenvoort and Wagenvoort, 1967).

In some species, a portion of the bronchial blood flow draining the extrapulmonary tracheobronchial tree flows into the hemiazygos and azygos veins, but the intrapulmonary bronchial blood flow drains directly into the pulmonary venous system (Marchand et al., 1950). This drainage pattern is seen in the dog lung, with the extrapulmonary portion of the airway venous blood flow draining via the azygos veins into the right atrium and the other bronchial veins emptying into the pulmonary veins (Marchand et al., 1950).

B. Physiological Functions

The tracheobronchial circulation is involved in many physiological functions, which include warming and moistening of inspired air (Baile et al., 1985; Cole, 1954; Webb, 1951), airway tissue fluid balance (Pietra et al., 1971), airway clearance of particles (Rizk et al., 1984), and airway nourishment (Baier et al., 1986). The bronchial circulation supplies nutrients to the metabolically active epithelial cells and the mucous and serous glands of the airways (Deffebach et al., 1987a). In addition, the airway circulation provides the fluid and electrolytes for the active transport processes responsible for solute and water movement across the mucosal epithelial membrane (Nathanson and Nadel, 1984). Rizk et al. (1984) examined airway clearance of inhaled aerosols and found that both the bronchial and pulmonary circulations were involved in the clearance of particles less than 2 μm in diameter.

C. Bronchial (Systemic) and Pulmonary Anastomotic Flows

Blood flow to the trachea is almost entirely from the systemic circulation (Baile et al., 1982; Michelassi et al., 1987; Barman et al., 1988); the pulmonary circulation contributes less than 5% to the total tracheal blood flow (Fig. 6.1) (Barman et al., 1988). Recent studies indicate that the pulmonary

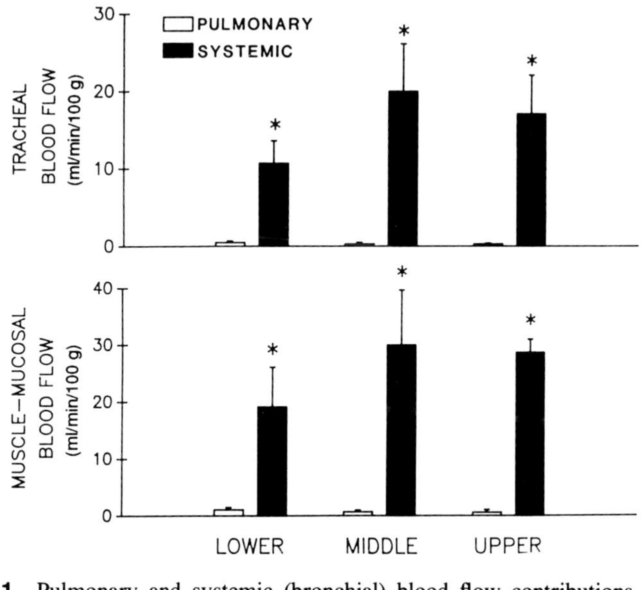

Figure 1 Pulmonary and systemic (bronchial) blood flow contributions to regional tracheal cartilage and muscle-mucosa. Values are mean ±standard error of the mean (SEM) *$P < 0.05$, pulmonary versus systemic. (From Barman et al., 1988.)

circulation contributes a substantial amount of the blood flow to the main bronchi in the dog lung (Fig. 6.2) (Barman et al., 1988). Michelassi et al. (1987) found a smaller contribution, but their values may be low because they did not assess lung contamination from the recirculation of radiolabeled microspheres. Control measurements of tracheobronchial blood flow from several research laboratories using different techniques of measurement, the most common being radiolabeled microspheres (Table 1) (Rudolph and Heymann, 1967), show values ranging from 30 to 95 ml/min per 100 g wet weight, depending on species and experimental technique. Normal tracheal mucosal blood flow is approximately 24 ml/min per 100 g wet weight in the dog lung (Barman et al., 1988). In the sheep lung, tracheal muscle-mucosal blood flow is somewhat higher, ranging from 45 ml/min per 100 g wet weight in lightly anesthetized sheep (Barker et al., 1988) to 143 ml/min per 100 g wet weight in unanesthetized sheep (Wu et al., 1988). Tracheal cartilage blood flow is only 14 ml/min per 100 g wet weight, indicating that the muscle-mucosa receives the highest flow per tissue mass in the trachea, although in terms of absolute flow, the muscle-mucosa has the lowest blood flow because of its low tissue mass. Studies have shown that the bronchial blood flow to the main bronchi alone ranges from 13 to 18 ml/min per 100 g wet weight, although **both** tracheal and main bronchial blood flows range from 9 to 16 ml/min per 100 g wet tissue weight (Malik and Tracy, 1980; Baile et al., 1982; Michelassi et al., 1987).

The effect of various perturbations on bronchial (systemic) blood flow to the upper and lower airways is shown in Tables 2 and 3. The airway vascular bed responds to adrenergic (α and β) compounds by decreasing (α) or increasing (β) upper airway blood flow (Table 2). Baile and Paré (1983) observed that hypercarbia (high blood CO_2 tension) greatly increased bronchial blood flow. The increased blood flow response seen with hypercarbia

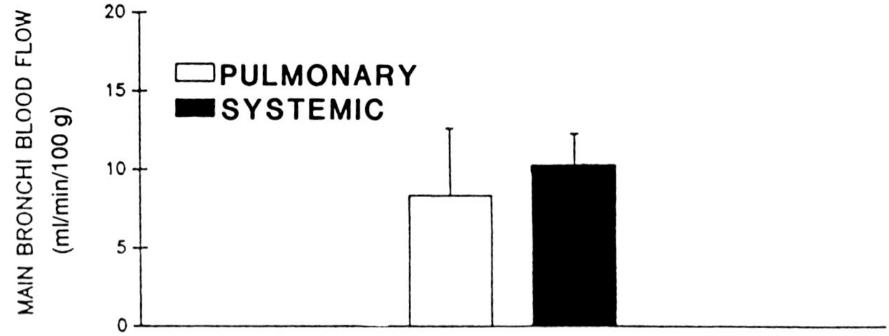

Figure 2 Pulmonary and systemic (bronchial) blood flow contributions to main bronchial blood flow. Values are mean ±SEM (From Barman et al., 1988.)

Table 1 Systemic Tracheobronchial Blood Flow

Source	Species	Method	Conditions	Tissue[a]	Blood flow (ml/min per 100 g)[b]	Total blood flow (ml/min)
Michelassi et al., 1987	Dog	Microsphere	Control	Upper trachea;	—	2.5
				lower trachea	—	0.7
Agostoni et al., 1987	Dog	Microsphere	Control	Trachea	70[c] (18)	2.9
Baile et al., 1982	Dog	Microsphere	Control	T-MB	62[c] (16)	2.6
Barman et al., 1988	Dog	Microsphere	Control	T-MM	24	0.13
Barman et al., 1988	Dog	Microsphere	Control	T-C	14	2.1
Michelassi et al., 1987	Dog	Microsphere	Control	Main bronchi	—	0.1–0.3
Barman et al., 1988	Dog	Microsphere	Control	Main bronchi	13	0.03
Malik and Tracy, 1980	Dog	Microsphere	Control	T-MB	34[c] (9)	1.5
Barker et al., 1988	Sheep	Soluble Gas	Control	T-MM	45	0.3
Parsons et al., 1985	Sheep	Microsphere	Control	Trachea	95	15.2
Wanner et al., 1988	Sheep	Soluble Gas	Control	Trachea	52	8.3
Wu et al., 1988	Sheep	Microsphere	Control	Trachea	32	5.1
Wu et al., 1988	Sheep	Microsphere	Control	T-MM	143	0.9
Wu et al., 1988	Sheep	Microsphere	Control	Main bronchi	18	0.04
Nordin et al., 1977	Rabbit	Microsphere	Control	Trachea	30	4.8

[a] T-C = tracheal cartilage; T-MM = tracheal muscle-mucosa; T-MB = trachea-main bronchi.

[b] Wet tissue weight unless otherwise indicated.

[c] Dry tissue weight.

Table 2 Effect of Various Treatments on Systemic Tracheobronchial Blood Flow[a]

Source	Species	Treatment	Tissue	Blood flow (ml/min per 100 g)[b]	Total blood flow (ml/min)
Barker et al., 1988	Sheep	α Agonist	Trachea	(45) 14	2.2
Barker et al., 1988	Sheep	β Agonist	Trachea	(45) 59	3.7
Agostoni et al., 1987	Dog	↑ Temperature	Trachea	(70) 75[c] 19	3.0
Baile et al., 1984	Dog	15 cmH_2O PEEP	Trachea	(44) 25[c] 6	0.96
Barman et al., 1989	Dog	15 cmH_2O PEEP	T-MM	(24) 12	0.08
Barman et al., 1989	Dog	↑ LAP	T-MM	(24) 27	0.1
Taylor et al., 1990	Dog	PMA	T-MM	(60) 22	0.14
Barman et al., 1989	Dog	15 cmH_2O PEEP	T-C	(14) 6	0.92
Barman et al., 1989	Dog	↑ LAP	T-C	(14) 9	1.4
Taylor et al., 1990	Dog	PMA	T-C	(28) 10	1.5
Baile and Paré, 1983	Dog	Hypoxemia	T-MB	(90) 48[c] 12	1.9
Baile and Paré, 1983	Dog	Hypercarbia	T-MB	(34) 69[c] 17	2.7
Malik and Tracy, 1980	Dog	Embolization	T-MB	(34) 51[c] 13	2.1
Barman et al., 1989	Dog	15 cm H_2O PEEP	Main bronchi	(13) 5	0.01
Baman et al., 1989	Dog	↑ LAP	Main bronchi	(13) 10	0.02
Taylor et al., 1990	Dog	PMA	Main bronchi	(15) 13	0.03

[a] T-C = tracheal cartilage; T-MM = tracheal muscle-mucosa; T-MB = trachea-main bronchi; PMA = phorbol myristate acetate.

[b] Wet tissue weight unless otherwise indicated. Values in parentheses are control values.

Table 3 Effect of Various Treatments on Systemic Bronchial and Parenchymal Blood Flow

Source	Species	Method	Treatment	Tissue[a]	Blood flow (ml/min per 100 g)[b]	Total blood flow (ml/min)
Baile et al., 1984	Dog	Microsphere	15 cmH_2O PEEP	Bronchi	(176) 70[c] 18	0.04
Baile and Paré, 1983	Dog	Microsphere	Hypoxemia	Bronchi	(191) 75[c] 19	0.04
Baile and Paré, 1983	Dog	Microsphere	Hypercarbia	Bronchi	(82) 183[c] 46	0.11
Taylor et al., 1990	Dog	Microsphere	PMA	2nd bronchi	(12) 10	0.10
Taylor et al., 1990	Dog	Microsphere	PMA	3rd bronchi	(13) 11	0.10
Taylor et al., 1990	Dog	Microsphere	PMA	4th bronchi	(20) 18	0.10
Taylor et al., 1990	Dog	Microsphere	PMA	5th bronchi	(11) 10	0.10
Baile et al., 1984	Dog	Microsphere	15 cmH_2O PEEP	Lung	(37) 7[c] 2	
Baile and Paré, 1983	Dog	Microsphere	Hypoxemia	Lung	(43) 18[c] 5	
Baile and Paré, 1983	Dog	Microsphere	Hypercarbia	Lung	(15) 50[c] 13	

[a] 2nd, 3rd, and so on = second generation, third generation bronchi.

[b] Wet tissue weight unless otherwise indicated. Values in parentheses are control measurements.

[c] Dry tissue weight.

indicates that the bronchial vasculature responds oppositely to the pulmonary circulation, which vasoconstricts when exposed to high blood CO_2 levels (Harris and Heath, 1977).

Only a few studies have tried to measure small airway blood flow (Tables 3 and 4). Barman and coworkers have characterized small airway blood flows from the systemic and pulmonary circulations using the reference flow radioactive microsphere technique (Barman et al., 1988). The protocol for this microsphere injection technique was the following. A femoral and a pulmonary arterial reference flow blood sample was started at zero time using a Harvard withdrawal pump at a flow rate of 7.75 ml/min and continued for 2 min after microsphere injection. Approximately 10 s after starting the blood withdrawal, microspheres suspended in 10% dextran were injected as a bolus into the right or left atrium for measurement of the pulmonary or systemic contribution to airway blood flow. This microsphere technique of assessing airway blood flow from both the systemic and pulmonary circulations is similar to the technique of Wu et al. (1988), who measured bronchial blood flow in unanesthetized sheep using simultaneous left and right atrial microsphere injections.

After the last microsphere injection was completed, the trachea and main bronchi were dissected out for blood flow determination. The procedure for tracheal and main bronchial tissue dissection has been described in detail (Barman et al., 1988). Briefly, the tracheal cartilage and tracheal muscle-mucosa were removed and the main bronchi were collected from the bifurcation to the next airway generation. In addition, the second-generation airways to the fifth airway generation were dissected free of lung parenchyma and also collected. All samples were placed into previously weighed test tubes and again weighed to determine wet tissue weight. These tissue samples were counted in a gamma counter and corrected for gamma spectrum overlap, radioactive decay, and background counts. Regional tissue blood flows ($\dot{Q}_T$) to the airway tissues and lung parenchyma were calculated on a per gram wet weight basis using the equation

$$\dot{Q}_T = R_T \frac{\dot{Q}_{ref}}{R_{ref}}$$

where R_T and R_{ref} are the radioactive counts in the tissue and the reference withdrawal blood flow sample, and $\dot{Q}_{ref}$ is the reference withdrawal blood flow rate.

Calculations and the description for the correction for recirculation of microspheres for the single microsphere injection technique have been described in detail (Barman et al., 1988; Wu et al., 1988). In summary, estimation of microspheres trapped in the lung parenchyma from the left atrial microsphere injection was accomplished by simultaneously withdrawing two

Table 4 Systemic Bronchial and Parenchymal Blood Flow

Source	Species	Method	Conditions	Tissue	Blood flow (ml/min per 100 g)[a]	Total blood flow (ml/min)
Barman et al., 1988	Dog	Microsphere	Control	2nd bronchi	12	0.12
Barman et al., 1988	Dog	Microsphere	Control	3rd bronchi	13	0.12
Barman et al., 1988	Dog	Microsphere	Control	4th bronchi	20	0.12
Barman et al., 1988	Dog	Microsphere	Control	5th bronchi	11	0.12
Barman et al., 1988	Dog	Microsphere	Control	Bronchi	89[b] (22)	
Baile et al., 1982	Dog	Microsphere	Control	Lung	37[b] (9)	
Barman et al., 1988	Dog	Microsphere	Control	Lung	70	
Wu et al., 1988	Sheep	Microsphere	Control	Lung	20	

[a] Wet tissue weight unless otherwise indicated.

[b] Dry tissue weight.

reference flow samples from the pulmonary (microspheres not trapped by the systemic capillaries) and femoral arteries at the same flow rate. The ratio of microsphere counts in these two blood flow samples represents the proportion of microspheres shunted through the systemic circulation. Also, lung parenchymal samples devoid of the larger airways were collected and gamma counted. Flow to the lung from the left atrial injection was calculated using the femoral reference blood flow sample. To measure lung trapping of microspheres injected into the right atrium, pulmonary and femoral reference blood flow samples were again collected. The ratios of the counts in these samples allowed calculation of the proportion of the microspheres lodged in the lung tissue. Lung parenchymal samples were gamma counted, and flow to the lung from the right atrial injection was determined using the pulmonary arterial reference blood flow sample. The actual pulmonary and systemic contributions to blood flow to all the airways were then determined by subtracting the calculated amount of blood flow due to microsphere recirculation to the lungs from the uncorrected values of the pulmonary and systemic blood flows to the airways.

Barman and coworkers (1989) found that the systemic contributions to the lower airway segments remained relatively constant in all segments, averaging 14 ml/min per 100 g or 0.12 ml/min in total blood flow units. Baile et al. (1982) found a similar systemic blood flow to these smaller bronchi at approximately 22 ml/min per 100 g. The pulmonary as well as the systemic blood flow contributions to the lower airway has been measured recently in dog lungs by the radiolabeled microsphere technique (Fig. 6.3) (Barman et al., 1988, 1989). Although the systemic contribution to lower airway blood flow is relatively constant for each airway generation, the pulmonary contribution to

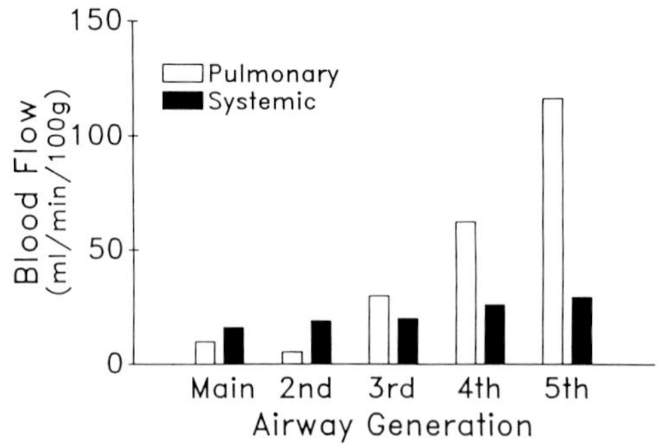

Figure 3 Pulmonary and systemic (bronchial) blood flow contributions to lower airway blood flow.

the lower airways increases in each airway segment to a maximum of over 100 ml/min per 100 g at the fifth generation.

The physiological significance of this phenomena is unknown at present. This pulmonary blood flow pattern may be involved in the regulation of airway temperature and the humidification of inspired air, however. Also, the pulmonary circulation may simply serve as an alternate blood flow pathway that provides additional nutrients to these small airways and their metabolically active epithelium. Other functions of the pulmonary contributions could include water exchange, regulating the thickness of the mucosa, and distributing humoral factors and formed blood elements or removing them from the tissues.

D. Venous Drainage Patterns

The airway circulation has two distinct drainage patterns. In many species, venous blood from the trachea and main bronchi drain via the azygos and hemiazygos veins back into the right atrium (Wanner, 1989). In dog lungs, tracheal blood flow drains primarily into systemic veins, with very little drainage into the pulmonary circulation (Barman et al., 1988). The intrapulmonary portion of the bronchial blood flow drains via broncho-pulmonary anastomoses through the pulmonary veins into the left atrium. In sheep lungs, venous blood from the smaller peripheral airways drains into the pulmonary veins (Wanner, 1989). Many investigators have measured anastomotic blood flow between the bronchial and pulmonary circulations (Table 5), although the exact anatomic location of these bronchopulmonary connections was not determined. In general, anastomotic blood flow between the bronchial and pulmonary circulations [$\dot{Q}$br(s-p)] ranges between 6 and 25 ml/min for the lower left lobe of the dog (Table 5). Various perturbations alter $\dot{Q}$br(s-p) as can be seen. It is difficult to relate $\dot{Q}$br(s-p) to other measurements of airway blood flow. Looking at reversed (pulmonary to systemic) anastomotic blood flow, Barman et al. (1988) measured little blood flow to the trachea of isolated dog lungs perfused in the reverse direction from the pulmonary vein to the pulmonary artery, but a substantial amount of flow occurred to the main bronchi and parenchymal tissues. The same blood flow patterns occurred when the lungs were perfused in the forward direction from the pulmonary artery to the pulmonary vein. Baile et al. (1982) noted that approximately 50% of the systemic blood flow to the lung was to the intrapulmonary bronchi and parenchyma (lower airways). This amounts to approximately 4 ml/min. In the study by Barman et al. (1988), the systemic parenchymal flow was 7 ml/min. It can be inferred that anastomotic systemic-to-pulmonary blood flow is mainly the drainage of the circulation from small airways.

Table 5 Systemic Pulmonary Anastomotic Blood Flow $\dot{Q}br(s\text{-}p)$

Source	Species	Treatment	$\dot{Q}br(s\text{-}p)$ (ml/min per 100 g)
Deffebach et al., 1987a	Dog	Control	24.5
Deffebach et al., 1987b	Dog	Indomethacin	7.3
Charan et al., 1986	Dog	Control	6.3
Charan et al., 1986	Dog	Hypoxemia	8.3
Charan et al., 1986	Dog	Hypercarbia	9.9
Charan et al., 1986	Dog	20 cmH_2O PEEP	2.7
Jindal et al., 1985	Dog	Control	31[a] (8)[b]
Jindal et al., 1985	Dog	Na salicylate	24[a] (6)[b]
Jindal et al., 1985	Dog	Ppa occlusion	43[a] (11)[b]
Jindal et al., 1985	Dog	Reperfusion	67[a] (17)[b]
Jindal et al., 1985	Dog	Indo/occlusion	11[a] (3)[b]
Jindal et al., 1985	Dog	Indo/reperfusion	6[a] (2)[b]

[a] Dry Weight.

[b] Wet weight.

E. Effect of Airway and Left Atrial Pressure on Airway Blood Flow

Increased positive end-expiratory pressures (PEEP) result in increased bronchial (Haynes et al., 1979; Baile et al., 1984) and pulmonary vascular resistances (West et al., 1964; Mitzner, 1983), which cause a decrease in both larger airway blood flow (Pietra and Magno, 1978; Baile et al., 1984) and anastomotic blood flow (Charan et al., 1986). When left atrial pressure is elevated, the bronchial anastomotic flow decreases (Auld et al., 1960; Charan et al., 1985), and drainage can be reversed with outflow to the right atrium if the pulmonary venous pressure exceeds the systemic anastomotic drainage pressure (Goetz et al., 1965; Warren and Powell, 1986). Baile et al. (1984) found that 15 cmH_20 positive end-expiratory pressure lowers both the extrapulmonary and intrapulmonary airway blood flows (Tables 2 and 3), and Wagner et al. (1987) observed that increasing PEEP to 8 mmHg reduced overall bronchial blood flow by 40%, mainly by increasing bronchovascular resistance. Barman et al. (1989) recently reported that the bronchial (systemic) contributions to the tracheal and main bronchial blood flow were decreased by

15 cmH_20 PEEP (Table 2). PEEP also reduced the systemic blood flow to the lower airways (Table 3). The pulmonary component to the main bronchi was reduced (Barman et al., 1989), but the pulmonary component to the lower airways was not altered by PEEP. Barman et al. (1989) showed that elevated left atrial pressures (PLA) attenuated the systemic contributions to the extrapulmonary airways. Like PEEP, elevated PLA also tended to reduce systemic blood flow to the small airways.

Although the exact physiological mechanism explaining these effects on airway blood flow is not known, it is possible that PEEP increases airway systemic vascular resistance as a result of the compression of alveolar vessels upon lung inflation. Horisberger and Rodbard (1960) showed that increasing lung inflation pressures up to 30 cmH_20 greatly increased bronchovascular resistance. A myogenic type of vessel response could also be present in the airway circulation. Wagner and coworkers (1987) hypothesized that the systemic tracheal and small airway blood vessels may constrict in response to an increased lung volume. In contrast, the unaltered pulmonary component of small airway blood flow appears to behave as though regulated by extra alveolar vessels since these expand with PEEP and so would not raise pulmonary vascular resistance to decrease the flow. In addition, as a portion of the airway blood flow drains via bronchial-to-pulmonary anastomotic connections, any condition that raises pulmonary venous pressures would decrease this anastomotic drainage.

F. Effect of Lung Injury on Airway Blood Flow

In many types of airway injury, inflammation of the bronchial wall occurs, which leads to hyperemia, endothelial and epithelial cell damage, and tissue edema (Wanner, 1989). It has been postulated that leukocytes, especially neutrophils, can also be involved in the inflammatory response (Perry and Taylor, 1988; Perry et al., 1990). A recent study by Taylor and coworkers (1990) examined the effect of lung injury on airway blood flow using phorbol myristate acetate (PMA) given intravenously via the femoral vein to activate neutrophils and leukocytes (Tables 2 and 3). PMA causes pulmonary endothelial cell damage by activating neutrophils and monocytes, which results in alveolar flooding (Allison et al., 1988). Taylor and coworkers (1990) observed that PMA greatly decreased systemic blood flow to the trachea (Table 2) and the pulmonary blood flow component to the lower airways, but little effect was observed on the bronchial blood flow to the lower airways (Fig. 6.4). The exact mechanism(s) causing these effects are not known, but it is possible that the increased pulmonary vascular resistance observed with PMA may be due to plugging of pulmonary capillaries by activated plasma cells. It has been shown that PMA increases pulmonary vascular resistance 10-fold (Allison et

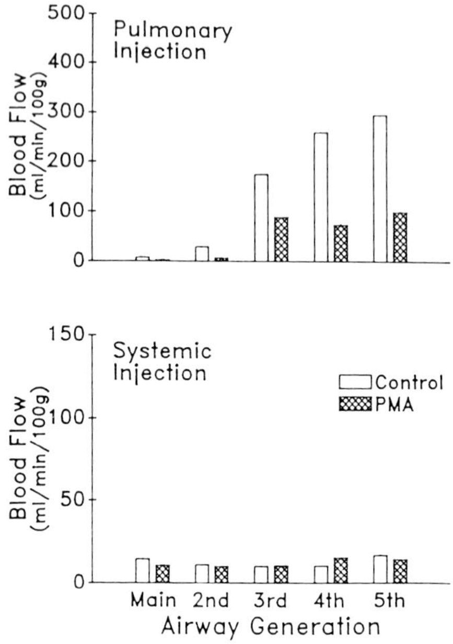

Figure 4 Effect of phorbol myristate acetate (PMA) on pulmonary and systemic (bronchial) lower airway blood flow.

al., 1986; Perry and Taylor, 1988) and causes severe endothelial cell damage resulting in an increased microvascular permeability (Allison et al., 1986, 1988; Perry and Taylor, 1988). The reason that PMA did not affect the bronchial circulation of the lower airways is unknown. It has been reported that total (systemic-to-pulmonary) bronchial and anastomotic blood flow remains constant or increases in lung injury and during prolonged pulmonary arterial obstruction (Malik and Tracy, 1980; Greene et al., 1981; Lakshminarayan et al., 1987). Thus it is possible that the bronchial circulation acts in a manner that assists in both inflammation and the healing process by maintaining or increasing its blood flow contributions to injured tissues when the pulmonary blood flow is compromised. Obviously, further studies must be done to more fully understand the anatomic and physiological interactions that occur between the pulmonary and bronchial circulations in pathophysiological states.

III. Conclusions

Blood flow to the trachea is almost totally provided by the systemic blood supply. However, at the level of the main bronchi and in smaller airways, vascular perfusion is provided by both the pulmonary and bronchial circulations either in an interactive fashion (anastomotic blood flow) or by separate pathways. Many investigators have measured bronchial (systemic) blood flow and ignored the pulmonary contributions to the lower airways (Baile et al., 1982, 1984; Wu et al., 1988). As a result, these studies have underestimated total airway perfusion, especially in the smaller airways. A schematic representation of the possible dual perfusion pattern to the lower airways is shown in Fig. 6.5. In this diagram, both the bronchial and pulmonary circulations are shown perfusing the lower airways down through the terminal bronchioles (TB), which is in keeping with our recent studies in the dog lung. It is obvious that future studies must be done to further evaluate the perfusion patterns of the bronchial and pulmonary circulations to fully determine their importance in airway function. Although past studies have concentrated on total bronchial and pulmonary blood flow, focus should now be directed toward elucidating

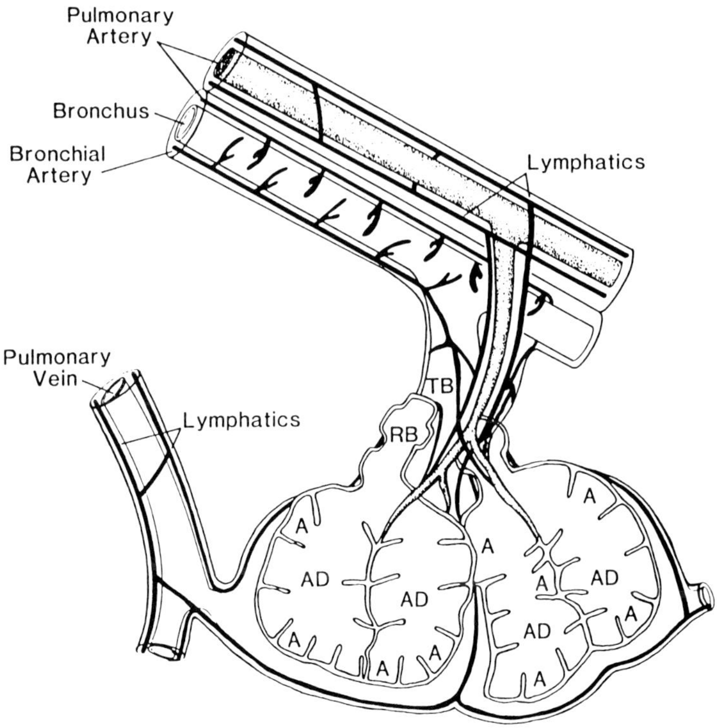

Figure 5 The possible perfusion pattern of the lower airways. TB = terminal bronchiole; RB = respiratory bronchiole; AD = alveolar duct; A = alveoli.

blood flow regulating mechanisms of the muscle-mucosal and subepithelial circulations since airway stress and injury directly affect blood flow patterns in these tissues. An understanding of the airway blood flow patterns in various physiological and pathological conditions should provide new and exciting information in the years to come about how the blood flow is regulated to these airway structures.

References

Agostoni, P. G., Deffebach, M. E., Kirk, W., Lakshminarayan, S., and Butler, J. (1987). Upstream pressure for systemic to pulmonary flow from bronchial circulation in dogs. *J. Appl. Physiol.* **63**:485–491.

Allison, R. C., Marble, K. T., Hernandez, E. M., Townsley, M. I., and Taylor, A. E. (1986). Attenuation of permeability lung injury after phorbol myristate acetate by verapamil and OKY-046. *Am Rev. Respir. Dis.* **134**:93–100.

Allison, R. C., Hernandez, E. M., Prasad, V. R., Grisham, M. B., and Taylor, A. E. (1988). Protective effects of O_2 radical scavengers and adenosine in PMA-induced lung injury. *J. Appl. Physiol.* **64**:2175–2182.

Auld, P. A. M., Rudolph, A. M., and Golinko, R. J. (1960). Factors affecting bronchial collateral flow in the dog. *Am. J. Physiol.* **198:**1166–1170.

Baier, H. (1986). Functional adaptations of the bronchial circulation. *Lung* **164**:247–257.

Baier, H., Moas, R., Yerger, L., and Wanner, A. (1986). In vivo estimation of tracheal wall water: Effects of histamine and carbachol. *J. Appl. Physiol.* **60**:1680–1685.

Baile, E. M., and Paré P. D. (1983). Response of the bronchial circulation to acute hypoxemia and hypercarbia in the dog. *J. Appl. Physiol.* **55**:1474–1479.

Baile, E. M., Nelems, J. M. B., Schulzer, M., and Paré, P. D. (1982). Measurement of regional bronchial arterial flow and bronchovascular resistance in dogs. *J. Appl. Physiol.* **53**:1044–1049.

Baile, E. M., Albert, R. K., Kirk, W., Lakshminarayan, S., Wiggs, B. J. R., and Paré, P. D. (1984). Positive end-expiratory pressure decreases bronchial blood flow in the dog. *J. Appl. Physiol.* **56**:1289–1293.

Baile, E. M., Dalhby, R. W., Wiggs, B. R., and Paré, P. D. (1985). Role of tracheal and bronchial circulation in respiratory heat exchange. *J. Appl. Physiol.* **58**:217–222.

Barker, J. A., Chediak, A. D., Baier, H. J., and Wanner, A. (1988). Tracheal mucosal blood flow responses to autonomic agonists. *J. Appl. Physiol.* **65**:829–834.

Barman, S. A., Ardell, J. L., Parker, J. C., Perry, M. L., and Taylor, A. E. (1988). Pulmonary and systemic blood flow contributions to upper airways in canine lung. *Am. J. Physiol.* **255**:H1130–1135.

Barman, S. A., Ardell, J. L., Townsley, M. I., Beisel, B., and Taylor, A. E. (1989). The effect of pressure gradients on canine airway blood flow. *FASEB J.* **3**:A569.

Berry, J. L., and Daly, I. B. (1931). The relation between the pulmonary and bronchial vascular systems. *Proc. R. Soc. Long. Biol.* **109**:319–336.

Charan, N. B., Turk, G. M., and Dhand, R. (1984). Gross and subgross anatomy of bronchial circulation in sheep. *J. Appl. Physiol.* **57**:658–664.

Charan, N. B., Turk, G. M., and Ripley, R. (1985). Measurement of bronchial arterial blood flow and bronchovascular resistance in sheep. *J. Appl. Physiol.* **59**:305–308.

Charan, N. B., Albert, R. K., Lakshminarayan, S., Kirk, W., and Butler, J. (1986). Factors affecting bronchial blood flow through bronchopulmonary anastomoses in dogs. *Am. Rev. Repir. Dis.* **134**:85–88.

Cole, P. (1954). Recordings of respiratory air temperature. *J. Laryngol. Otol.* **68**:295–307.

Deffebach, M. E., Charan, N. B., Lakshminarayan, S., and Butler, J. (1987a). The bronchial circulation: Small, but vital attribute of the lung. *Am. Rev. Respir. Dis.* **135**:463–681.

Deffebach, M. E., Lakshminarayan, S., Kirk, W., and Butler, J. (1987b). Bronchial circulation and cyclooxygenase products in acute lung injury. *J. Appl. Physiol.* **63**:1083–1088.

Galen, C. (1562). *Tracta Frobenianae*, Book 6. Basel, Switzerland.

Goetz, R. M., Rohman, M., and State, D. (1965). The hemodynamics of bronchopulmonary anastomoses. *Surg. Gynecol. Obstet.* **120**:517–529.

Greene, R., Zapol, W. M., Snider, M. T., Reid, L., Snow, R., O'Connell, R. S., and Novelline, R. A. (1981). Early bedside detection of pulmonary vascular occlusion during acute respiratory failure. *Am. Rev. Respir. Dis.* **124**:593–601.

Harris, P., and Heath, D. (1977). *The Human Pulmonary Circulation*, 2nd ed, New York, Churchill Livingstone, pp. **452–477.**

Haynes, M. S., Cassidy, S. S., and Johnson, R. L. (1979). The effect of PEEP on bronchial blood flow. *Fed. Proc.* **33**:6080.

Horisberger, B., and Rodbard, S. (1960). Direct measurement of bronchial artery flow. *Circ Res.* **8**:1149–1156.

Hyman, A. L., Knight, D. S., Joiner, P. D., and Kadowitz, P. J. (1975). Bronchopulmonary arterial shunting without anatomic anastomosis in the dog. *Circ. Res.* **37**:285–298.

Jindal, S. K., Lakshminarayan, S., Kirk, W., and Butler, J. (1985). Regulation of increase in anastomotic blood flow following pulmonary artery obstruction. *J. Appl. Physiol.* **59**:180–182.

Lakshminarayan, S., Jindal, S. K., Kirk, W., and Butler, J. (1987). Acute increases in anastomotic bronchial systemic to pulmonary blood flow due to generalized lung injury. *J. Appl. Physiol.* **62**:2358–2361.

Malik, A. B., and Tracy, S. E. (1980). Bronchovascular adjustments after pulmonary embolism. *J. Appl. Physiol.* **49**:476–481.

Marchand, P., Gilroy, J. C., and Wilson, N. H. (1950). Anatomical study of the bronchial vascular system and its variations in disease. *Thorax* **5**:207–221.

McLaughlin, R. F., Tyler, W. S., and Canada, R. O. (1961). A study of the subgross pulmonary anatomy in various mammals. *Am. J. Anat.* **108**:149–165.

Michelassi, F., Schuette, A., Landa, L., Zapol, W. M., and Grillo, H. C. (1987). Pulmonary and systemic contribution to canine tracheobronchial blood flow. *Ital. J. Surg. Sci.* **17**:105–112.

Miller, W. S. (1906). The arrangement of bronchial blood vessels. *Anat. Anz.* **28**:432–436.

Mitzner, W. A. (1983). Resistance of the pulmonary circulation. *Clin. Chest Med.* **4**:127–137.

Modell, H. I., Beck, K., and Butler, J. (1981). Functional aspects of canine bronchial-pulmonary vascular connections. *J. Appl. Physiol.* **50**:1045–1051.

Nathanson, I., and Nadel, J. A. (1984). Movement of electrolytes and fluid across airways. *Lung* **162**:125–137.

Nordin, U., Lindholm, C. E., and Wolgast, M. (1977). Blood flow in the rabbit tracheal mucosa under normal conditions and under the influence of tracheal intubation. *Acta Anaesthesiol. Scand.* **21**:81–94.

Parsons, G. H., Kramer, G. C., Link, D. P., Lantz, B. M. T., Gunther, R. A., Green, J. F., and Cross, C. E. (1985). Studies of reactivity and distribution of bronchial blood flow in sheep. *Chest* **87**:180S–184S.

Perry, M. L., and Taylor, A. E. (1988). Phorbol myristate acetate-induced injury of isolated perfused rat lungs: Neutrophil dependence. *J. Appl. Physiol.* **65**:2164–2169.

Perry, M. L., Kayes, S. G., Barnard, J. W., and Taylor, A. E. (1990). Effects of phorbol myristate acetate-stimulated human leukocytes on rat lung. *J. Appl. Physiol.* **68**:235–240.

Pietra, G. G., and Magno, M. (1978). Pharmacological factors influencing permeability of the bronchial circulation. *Fed. Proc.* **37**:2466–2470.

Pietra, G. G., Szidon, J. P., Levanthal, M. M., and Fishman, A. D. (1971). Histamine and interstitial pulmonary edema in the dog. *Circ. Res.* **29**:323–337.

Rizk, N. W., Luce, J. M., Price, D. C., and Murry, J. F. (1984). Site of deposition and factors affecting clearance of aerosolized solute from canine lungs. *J. Appl. Physiol.* **56**:723–729.

Rudolph, A. M., and Heymann, M. A. (1967). Circulation of the fetus in utero: Methods for studying distribution of blood flow, cardiac output, and organ blood flow. *Circ. Res.* **21**:163–184.

Ruyisch, F. (1721). *Opera Omnia.* I. Epistola Anatomica Problematica Sexta. Amtelaedami, apud Janssonio-Walsbergius.

Taylor, A. E., Ardell, J. L., and Barman, S. A. (1990). The effect of phorbol myristate acetate on canine airway blood flow. *FASEB J.* **4**:A575.

Tobin, C. E. (1952). The bronchial arteries and their connections with other vessels in the human lung. *Surg. Gynceol. Obstet.* **95**:741–750.

Verloop, M. C. (1949). On the arteriae bronchioles and their anastomoses, with the arteriae pulmonales in some rodents: A micro-anatomical study. *Acta Anat.* (Basel) **7**:1–32.

Wagenvoort, C. A., and Wagenvoort, N. (1967). Arterial anastomoses, bronchopulmonary arteries, and pulmobronchial arteries in perinatal lungs. *Lab. Invest.* **16**:13–14.

Wagner, E. M., Mitzner, W. A., and Bleecker, E. R. (1987). Effects of airway pressure on bronchial blood flow. *J. Appl. Physiol.* **62**:561–566.

Wanner, A. (1989). Circulation of the airway mucosa. *J. Appl. Physiol.* **67**:917–925.

Wanner, A., Barker, J. A., Long, W. M., Mariassy, A. T., and Chediak, A. D. (1988). Measurement of airway mucosal perfusion and water volume with an inert soluble gas method. *J. Appl. Physiol.* **65**:264–271.

Warren, R. L., and Powell, P. J. (1986). Acute alveolar hypoxia increases bronchopulmonary shunt flow in the dog. *J. Clin. Invest.* **77**:1515–1524.

Webb, P. (1951). Air temperatures in respiratory tracts of resting subjects in cold. *J. Appl. Physiol.* **4**:378–382.

West, J. B., Dollery, C. T., and Naimark, A. (1964). Distribution of blood flow in the isolated lung: Relation of vascular and alveolar pressure. *J. Appl. Physiol.* **19**:713–724.

Wu, C. H., Lindsey, D. C., Traber, D. L., Cross, C. E., Herndon, D. N., and Kramer, G. C. (1988). Measurement of bronchial blood flow with radioactive microspheres in awake sheep. *J. Appl. Physiol.* **65**:1131–1139.

7

Mechanical Aspects of Physiological Regulation of the Bronchial Circulation

ELIZABETH M. WAGNER

John Hopkins Medical Center
Baltimore, Maryland

I. Introduction

The mechanical factors that affect blood flow through the bronchial vasculature make this a unique circulatory bed. Although systemic arterial pressure provides the inflow pressure to this system, it drains predominantly into the low-pressure pulmonary vascular bed. Consequently, bronchial vessels are exposed to the mechanical stresses of ventilation both directly because of their location in airways as well as indirectly through the changes imposed on the pulmonary circulation. An alternate drainage pathway through systemic veins may also be important for blood flow diversion under special circumstances. The existence of these dual drainage pathways complicates the study of the control of this vasculature.

II. Resistive Model

To analyze the mechanical factors that regulate flow through the bronchial vasculature, the resistive model for this circulation proposed for the sheep is used (Wagner et al., 1987). This model (Fig. 1) is based on anatomic descriptions

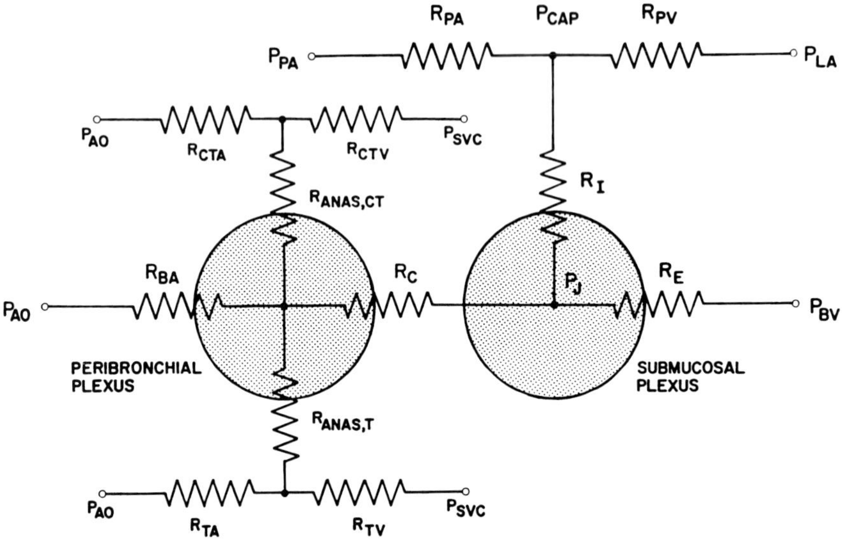

Figure 1 Resistive model of the broncial circulation. P_{AO}, aortic pressure; P_J, junctional pressure, P_{PA}, pulmonary arterial pressure; P_{CAP}, pulmonary capillary pressure; P_{LA}, left atrial pressure; P_{BV}, bronchial venous pressure; P_{SVC}, superior vena cava pressure; R_{BA}, bronchial arterial resistance; R_C, resistance of vessels connecting peribronchial arterial plexus with submucosal plexus; R_{CTA}, resistance of connective tissue arteries; R_{CTV}, resistance of connective tissue veins; R_{TA}, resistance of tracheal arteries; R_{TV}, resistance of tracheal veins; $R_{ANAST,T}$, resistance of anastomotic vessels connecting tracheal vessels with bronchial vessels; $R_{ANAST,CT}$, resistance of anastomic vessels connecting connective tissue vessels with bronchial vessels; R_I, resistance of the intrapulmonary drainage vessels; R_E, resistance of the extrapulmonary drainage vessels; R_{PA}, pulmonary arterial resistance; R_{PV}, pulmonary venous resistance. (Adapted from Wagner et al., 1987 with permission from the *Journal of Applied Physiology.*)

(Magno and Fishman 1982; Charan et al., 1984), and although specific for the sheep, the basic features of systemic arterial inflow, with pulmonary and systemic venous outflow, are similar among all species. This model provides the basis for a more general discussion. Aortic pressure (P_{AO}) provides the inflow pressure for this bed. Blood flowing through small bronchial arteries terminates in the peribronchial arterial plexus. Other small systemic arteries serving the connective tissue or the trachea may also terminate in this plexus as arterial anastomoses. Drainage from the peribronchial plexus is into the submucosal plexus via small connecting vessels (C). The submusocal plexus functions as a capillary plexus, and in intrapulmonary airways, this plexus drains into pulmonary capillaries (CAP) and into the left atrium (LA). Drainage from the extrapulmonary submucosal plexus in the bronchi outside the lung parenchyma is via the bronchial vein (BV) or veins, which empty into the azygos vein and into the right heart. These two outflow drainage pathways are connected by the contiguity of the submucosal plexus along the airway tree.

Blood flow through the bronchial circulation is regulated by the resistance of small bronchial arteries and arterioles (R_{BA}), the resistance of the vessels connecting the peribronchial plexus to the submucosal plexus (R_c), in extrapulmonary airways by the resistance (R_E) of vessels draining into the bronchial veins, and in intrapulmonary airways by the resistance (R_I) of bronchopulmonary anastomotic channels. Because most of the resistance is in the small arteries, changes in the resistance of R_{BA} and/or R_C have major effects on total blood flow through the circuit. Changes in R_I relative to R_E affect the proportion of blood flow through the intrapulmonary versus extrapulmonary drainage pathway. Alterations in inflow pressure (P_{AO}) and outflow pressures (P_{CAP}, P_{LA}, and P_{BV}) affect blood flow through this vasculature. Alterations of these outflow pressures may also result in blood flow diversion. Each of these components is discussed in greater detail in this chapter. Despite the relative simplicity of this model, it can provide a useful basis for examining the effects of physiological alterations of its components as well as the forces imposed on the bronchial circulation with ventilation.

III. Pressure-Flow Characteristics

Bronchial blood flow in humans under baseline conditions has been estimated to be approximately 3% of cardiac output (Baile et al., 1985). However, this baseline value may be an overestimate of actual bronchial blood flow since it was obtained during major surgery and surgery and anesthesia have been shown to increase bronchial blood flow (Deffebach et al., 1987b). In experimental animals, in which measurements can be made with greater precision, values reported range from 0.4 to 4% of cardiac output (Deffebach et al., 1987a). As might be expected, in a vasculature like the bronchial, which shows little evidence of autoregulation, these control values for bronchial blood flow have a direct relationship to the prevailing mean aortic blood pressure (Armendia et al., 1962); Agostoni et al., 1987a). Steady-state measurements of the pressure difference across any vascular bed divided by the blood flow can provide an estimate of vascular resistance and hence the state of vascular tone. However, examination of the pressure-flow relationship obtained by multiple measurements of flow at different inflow pressures can provide considerably more information concerning the mechanisms and site of alterations in vascular tone (Mitzner, 1983). The shape of the pressure-flow curve will provide information concerning the distensibility of the vascular bed and, under steady-state conditions, the degree to which the vascular bed autoregulates. The inverse slope of the pressure (abscissa)-flow (ordinate) curve provides a measure of resistance, and the pressure when flow is zero can provide information about the downstream or backpressure to flow through the vascular bed.

Although the preceding comments can be applied to pressure-flow curves of any vascular bed, the study of pressure-flow relationships in the bronchial circulation is especially interesting because of its dual drainage pathways. Given the complexity of this circulation and the difficulties inherent in measuring bronchial blood flow, it is easy to understand why the pressure-flow characteristics of the entire vasculature, much less each of its components, have not been completely determined. Armendia et al. (1962), in a heart-lung preparation devoid of central neural control, studied the pressure-flow responses of the bronchial vasculature in dogs. Figure 2 (left) shows their

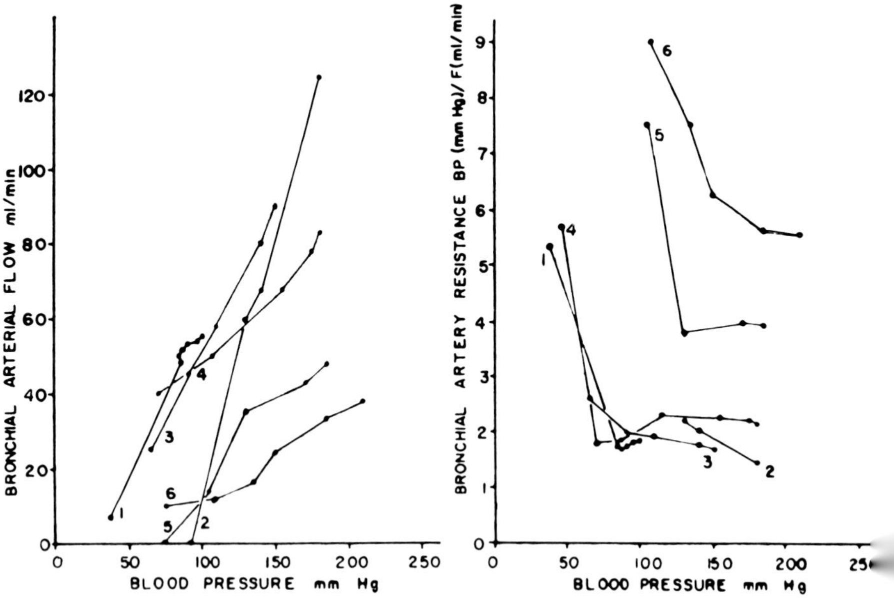

Figure 2 (Left) Pressure-flow relationship of the bronchial vasculature in six dogs. (Right) Effects of increases in inflow pressure on bronchial artery resistance (bronchial artery pressure/bronchial flow). (Reprinted from Armendia et al., 1962).

results. Making step changes in bronchial inflow pressure, they demonstrated proportional steady-state step changes in bronchial arterial inflow. These linear pressure-flow curves in six animals can be interpreted as demonstrating the bronchial vasculature to be relatively nondistensible and nonautoregulating. The pressure at which the relationship intersects the x axis, the zero flow pressure, averages approximately 50 mmHg. Further discussion of the interpretation of this zero flow pressure follows in the discussion of pressure-flow data in context with the proposed resistive model of the bronchial circulation. The right panel in Fig. 2 shows resistance (inflow pressure/flow) presented as a function of arterial pressure. Following the initial sharp decline in this calculated resistance, bronchial vascular resistance remains relatively constant and is unaffected by alterations in pressure.

Further studies in a sheep preparation in which neural control remained intact confirmed the observations of Armendia et al. (1962). In anesthetized sheep, the bronchial artery was cannulated and perfused by a pump with femoral arterial blood (Fig. 3). The esophageal and thoracic tracheal branches of the bronchoesophageal artery were ligated to minimize any nonpulmonary

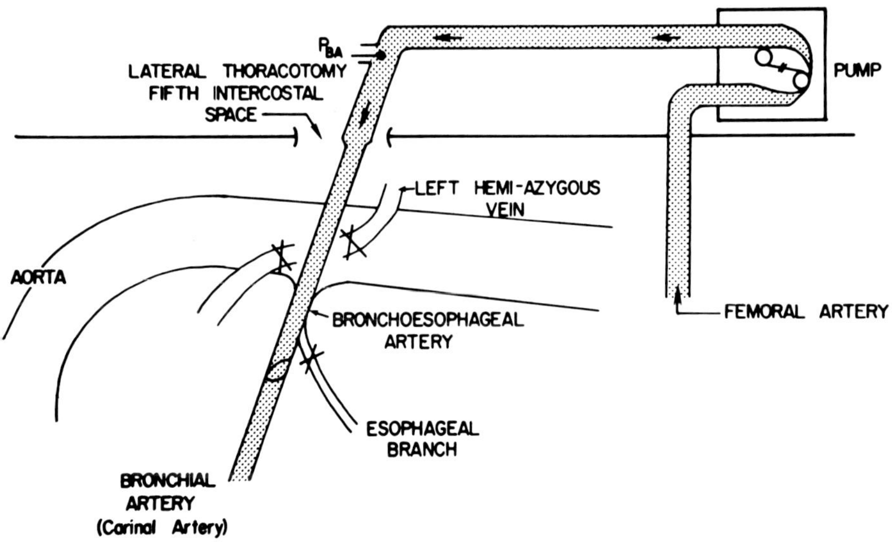

Figure 3 Bronchial artery perfusion circuit. The bronchial artery, a branch of the bronchoesophageal artery, is cannulated and pump perfused with blood from the femoral artery. Bronchial artery pressure (P_{BA}) is measured at the inflow port of the circuit. (Reprinted from Wagner et al., 1987, with permission from the *Journal of Applied Physiology*.)

arterial anastomotic blood flow. Pressure-flow data were obtained by making step decreases in bronchial artery inflow while recording steady-state inflow pressures. All vascular pressures in this preparation are reported relative to atmospheric pressure and referenced to the level of the left atrium. Pressure-flow data from six sheep are presented in Fig. 4. The striking linearity of individual pressure-flow curves again suggests that resistance vessels of this vascular system are fully recruited and distended. These results are consistent with other systemic vascular beds in which linear pressure-flow relationships have been demonstrated (Burton and Stinson, 1960; Girling, 1952). Another possible explanation for the linearity of the bronchial vascular pressure-flow curve is that although they are not fully distended, there is a small degree of active autoregulation to counteract the distensibility of the resistance vessels. Although possible, it is unlikely that this would result in such perfect matching.

Another feature of the bronchial vascular pressure-flow curve is the positive downstream zero flow pressure. This zero flow pressure could conceivably result from smooth muscle tension in bronchial arterial vessels, creating a Starling resistor with an effective downstream pressure (Permutt and Riley, 1963). However, the more likely explanation, consistent with the magnitude of the actual outflow drainage pressures, is that this pressure is the pressure at the junction site in the submucosal plexus, where bronchial blood flow drains either through the intrapulmonary route via pulmonary vessels or through the extrapulmonary route via bronchial veins. Referring back to the resistive model of the bronchial circulation, it can be seen that measurement of the zero flow pressure is a measure of the pressure at the junction of these two drainage sites. However, this junction does not represent a discrete anatomic locus but

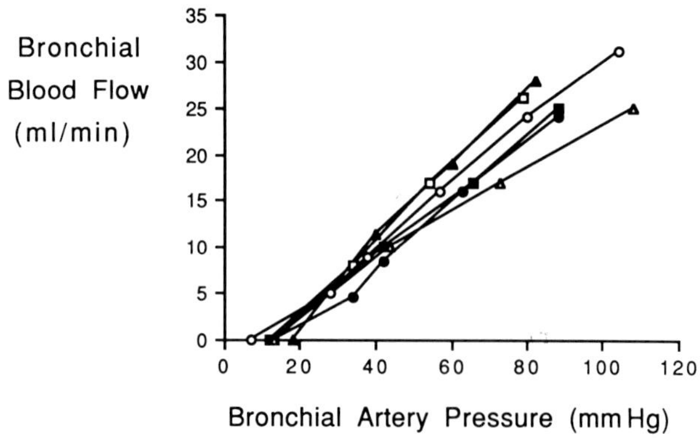

Figure 4 Bronchial vascular pressure-flow relationship in six sheep.

rather is distributed along the length of the airways. Despite this anatomic complexity, we can still define an average junctional pressure P_J measured by the zero flow pressure. In addition, it should be emphasized that the zero flow pressure refers to the pressure measured with zero bronchial arterial inflow. Provided a pressure gradient exists between pulmonary capillary pressure and bronchial venous pressure, flow exists between the pulmonary circulation and bronchial circulation despite there being no bronchial arterial inflow.

Figure 5 shows a Thevenin equivalent electrical circuit (Brenner and Javid, 1959) for the resistive model in Fig. 1. Such equivalent models are useful in simplifying complex resistive networks to provide more intuitive insight into the value of a pressure at a specific locus. The two drainage pathways have been combined into an equivalent resistance R_{EQ} and pressure source P_{EQ}. Calculations show that the P_{EQ} is equal to the zero flow pressure or junctional pressure P_J and

$$P_{J|\dot{Q}=0} = P_{EQ} = P_{CAP}\frac{R_E}{R_I + R_E} + P_{BV}\frac{R_I}{R_I + R_E}$$

As can be seen, the magnitude of P_{EQ} is a resistance weighted sum of the two outflow pressures P_{CAP} and P_{BV}. By rewriting this equation as

$$P_{EQ} = P_{CAP}\frac{1}{1 + R_I/R_E} + P_{BV}\frac{R_I/R_E}{1 + R_I/R_E}$$

it can be appreciated that the magnitude of P_{EQ} depends only on the R_I/R_E ratio, not on the absolute magnitude of either drainage resistance. The absolute magnitude of P_{EQ} should be something less than pulmonary capillary pressure and is within the expected range in the examples in Fig. 4. The R_{EQ} is equal to

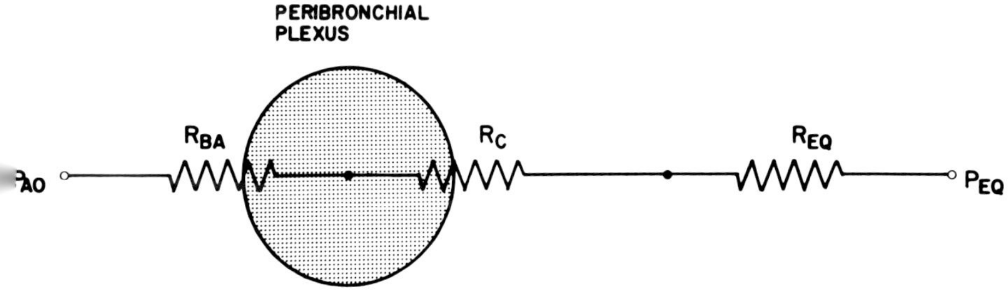

Figure 5 Thevenin equivalent circuit for the resistive model of the bronchial circulation in Fig. 1. R_{EQ} = equivalent resistance, P_{EQ} = equivalent pressure. (Reprinted from Wagner and Mitzner, 1988 with permission from the *Journal of Applied Physiology*).

the parallel resistance of the two venous drainage resistances R_E and R_I, where

$$R_{EQ} = \frac{R_E + R_I}{R_E + R_I}.$$

There is one important feature of the resistive model of Fig. 1 that is brought out by this equivalent circuit. The slope of the pressure-flow curve is equal to the *sum* of the upstream arterial resistance and R_{EQ}. Thus, even though the pressure at zero flow (P_{EQ}) equals the pressure at the junction of the outflow drainage pathways (P_J), the venous resistances contribute to the slope of the pressure-flow relationship.

To summarize, changes in the slope of the pressure-flow relationship reflect a change in bronchial vascular resistance and represent an alteration in R_{BA}, R_C, R_I, or R_E. The measured zero flow pressure is equal to the equivalent downstream pressure for the bronchial vasculature and depends on the magnitude of P_{CAP}, P_{BV}, and R_I/R_E. Although typically this pressure is less than pulmonary arterial pressure, there have been reports of zero flow pressures considerably in excess of pulmonary artery pressure. Magno and Fishman (1982) directed a fluid-filled catheter into the bronchial branch of the bronchoesophageal artery and measured pressures of 30–60 mmHg, Armendia et al. (1962) showed zero flow pressures of approximately 50 mmHg (Fig. 2), and Wagner et al. (1987) showed in a few preparations zero flow pressures of 40 mmHg. These high zero flow pressures are most likely explained by systemic arterial anastomoses with the bronchial circulation (see Fig. 1). Although these arterial anastomotic channels have been described anatomically (Charan et al., 1987), in healthy sheep they appear to provide negligible flow to the airways (Wagner and Mitzner, 1990).

To further extend these pressure-flow observations, several studies have documented the direct relationship between systemic blood pressure and bronchopulmonary anastomotic blood flow (Salisbury et al., 1957; Auld et al., 1960; Modell et al., 1981; Agostoni et al., 1987a). This anastomotic blood flow represents the portion of bronchial blood flow draining intrapulmonary airways from bronchial arteries into pulmonary vessels and into the left atrium. The model in Fig. 1 is shown in simplified form without systemic arterial anastomoses in Fig. 6. The resistive path of bronchial blood flow shown in this figure is designated bronchopulmonary anastomotic flow. Berry and Daly (1931) concluded that this pathyway accounts for approximately two-thirds of total bronchial inflow, and it is generally accepted that this is the major drainage pathway for the bronchial circulation (Deffebach et al., 1987a). Several investigators, using heart-lung preparations and isolating the systemic and pulmonary circulations, measure the overflow volume in the pulmonary

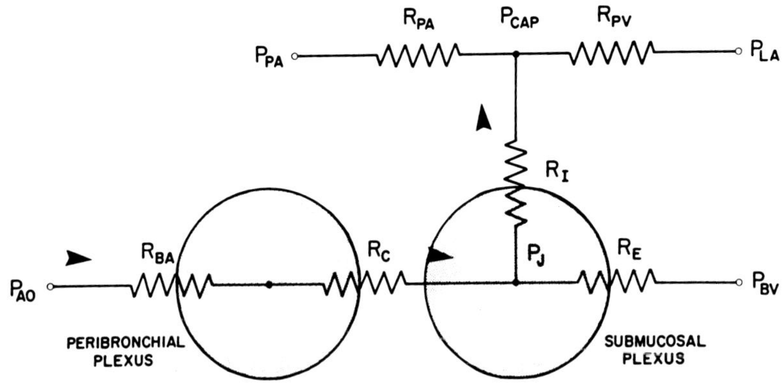

Figure 6 Resistive model of the bronchial circulation without systemic arterial anastomoses. Arrows indicate bronchopulmonary anastomotic flow. (Adapted from Wagner and Mitzner 1988 with permission from the *Journal of Applied Physiology*).

circuit reservoir and designate this the collateral or bronchopulmonary anastomotic blood flow. Salisbury et al. (1957) demonstrated a clear relationship between systemic arterial pressure and collateral outflow (Fig. 7). Auld et al. (1960), as well as Modell et al. (1981), have shown similar relationships between systemic arterial pressure and bronchial flow through the intrapulmonary drainage pathway. It is difficult to make any conclusive statements regarding the control of total bronchial blood flow based on this pressure-flow information, however, since flow through the bronchial veins is not accounted for in these preparations. Armendia et al. (1962) examined the relationship between systemic arterial pressure and bronchial venous outflow. Figure 8 shows their results. In a heart-lung preparation, these investigators demonstrated that bronchial venous outflow as a percentage of total bronchial flow decreased with increases in systemic arterial pressure. As perfusion pressure and inflow increase, bronchial venous outflow does not increase proportionally. Although these results are difficult to interpret given the general lack of information concerning the control of bronchial venous flow, they suggest that the bronchial venous drainage pathway is a high-resistance pathway and can accommodate minimal increases in blood flow. Thus, as bronchial inflow increases, it is likely that most of the outflow is through the low-resistance intrapulmonary drainage pathway. These observations corroborate the earlier findings of Berry and Daly (1931) and emphasize the importance of understanding the effects of alterations of the pulmonary circulation on the bronchial circulation.

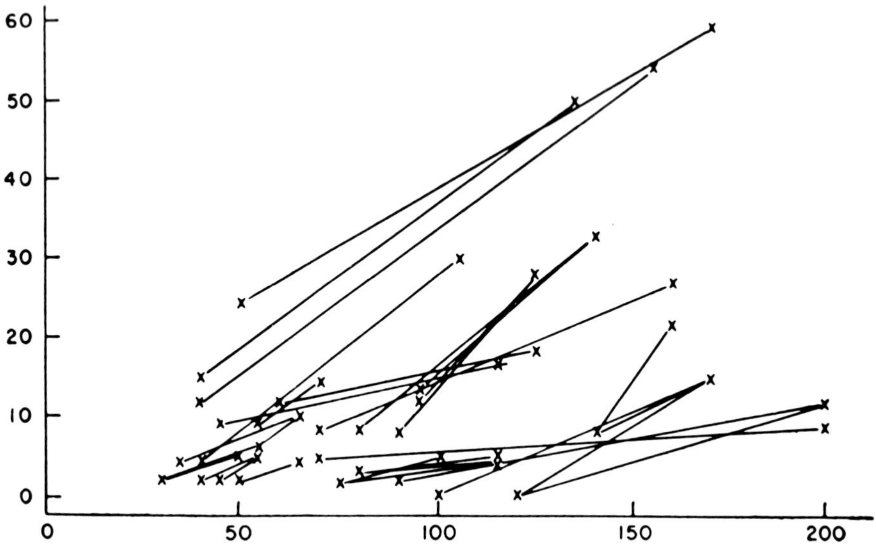

Figure 7 Effect of alterations in systemic arterial pressure (abscissa, mmHg) on bronchopulmonary anastomotic blood flow (ordinate, ml/min); 35 observations in 25 dogs. (Reprinted from Salisbury et al., 1957).

IV. Alteration of Downstream Pressure

The preceding section was concerned with the direct relationship between alteration of inflow pressure and bronchial blood flow. We now consider the effects of alteration in downstream pressure. Since the major portion of bronchial flow drains through the left atrium, it is appropriate to ask how elevations of left atrial pressure affect total bronchial flow. Both passive and active responses to elevations of outflow pressure have been described in different vascular systems. A passive system, like the pulmonary vasculature under zone 3 conditions, shows close to one-for-one increases in inflow pressure with downstream pressure elevations under constant flow conditions. However, blood flow through the liver (Hanson and Johnson, 1966), intestine (Mitzner, 1974), and other vascular beds (Haddy and Gilbert, 1956; Patterson and Shepherd, 1954) demonstrates varying degrees of myogenic regulation; increases in the downstream pressure of these vascular systems result in active smooth muscle constriction and a decrease in blood flow. Thus in these organs at a constant flow, increases in outflow pressure must result in greater than one-for-one increases in inflow pressure. Determination of the effects of alterations in the downstream pressure of the bronchial vasculature is complicated

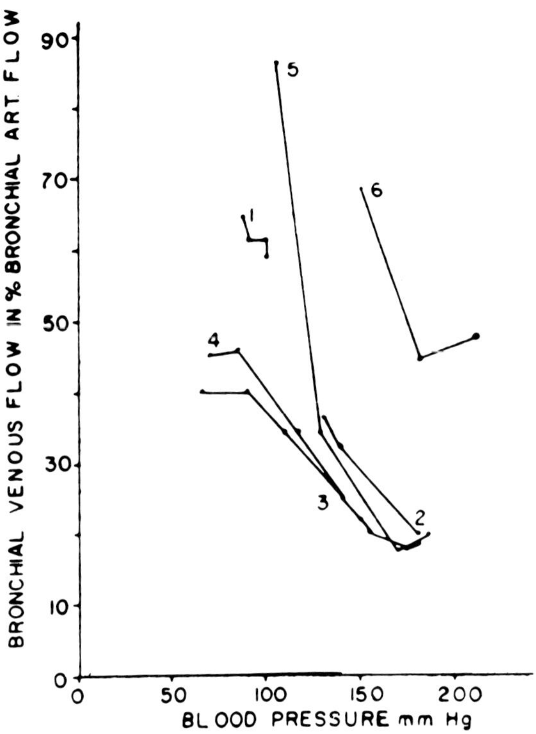

Figure 8 Effect of systemic arterial pressure on bronchial venous outflow as a percentage of total bronchial inflow in six dogs. (Reprinted from Armendia et al., 1962).

by the unique anatomy of this vascular system with its dual drainage pathways. Elevation of only one outflow pressure may result in diversion of outflow through the other drainage path, thereby minimizing the effect on inflow. To determine the effects of left atrial pressure elevation on the bronchial vasculature of sheep, Charan et al. (1985) increased pulmonary capillary wedge pressure from 14 to 25 cmH_2O by inflating a balloon in the left atrium and elicited a 40% increase in bronchial vascular resistance. To determine the mechanism underlying this response, Wagner and Mitzner (1990) used the previously described preparation (Fig. 3) in sheep and generated pressure-flow curves at increasing levels of left atrial pressure elicited by inflating a left atrial balloon. Figure 9 shows a representative example of the response of the bronchial vasculature to three levels of left atrial pressure (P_{LA}). Increasing P_{LA} caused both a rightward shift and a clockwise rotation of the pressure-flow curve. These changes indicate both an increase in the zero-flow pressure as well as an

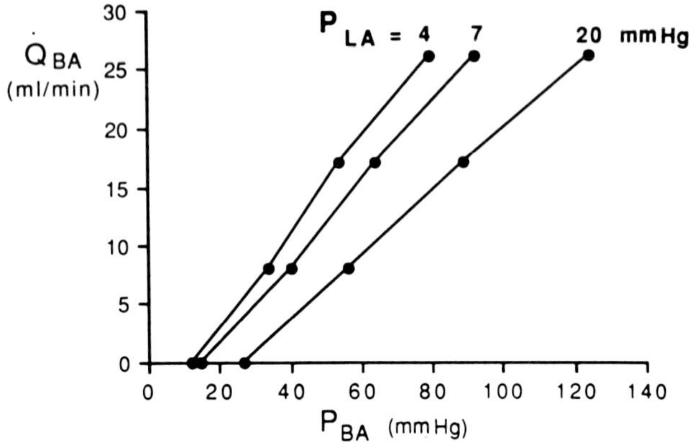

Figure 9 Example of the effect of increasing left atrial pressure (P_{LA}) on the bronchial vascular pressure (P_{BA}) – flow ($\dot{Q}_{BA}$) relationship. (Adapted from Wagner and Mitzner, 1990, with permission from the *Journal of Applied Physiology*).

increase in bronchial vascular resistance calculated as the inverse slope of the pressure-flow relationship. To examine further these pressure-flow data, Fig. 10 shows the effect of left atrial pressure elevation on bronchial artery pressure at constant control flow in seven sheep. Increasing the downstream pres-

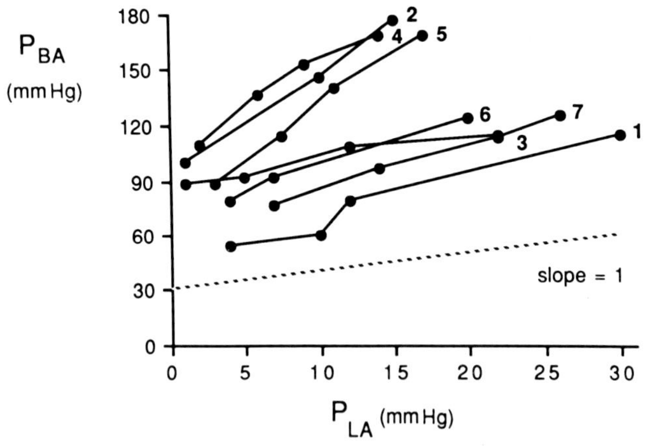

Figure 10 Effect of increases in left atrial pressure (P_{LA}) on bronchial artery pressure (P_{BA}) at control blood flow in seven sheep. Dashed line indicates the line of identity. (Reprinted from Wagner and Mitzner, 1990, with permission from the *Journal of Applied Physiology*.)

sure by increasing P_{LA} resulted in a much greater than one-for-one increase in P_{BA}. The average slope of this linearized relationship between P_{LA} and P_{BA} was 3.5 ±0.7. Thus, the bronchial vascular resistance appears acutely sensitive to changes in left atrial pressure. This work confirms the observations of Charan et al. (1985). The effects of increases in P_{LA} on bronchial artery inflow pressure at zero flow are presented in Fig. 11. At baseline P_{LA} (2.9 ±0.7 mmHg), control zero flow pressure was 11.3 ±0.8 mmHg and control pulmonary artery pressure was 13.0 ±0.8 mmHg. Over the range of P_{LA} studied under zero flow conditions, P_{BA} increased on average 1.3 ±0.2 mmHg for every 1 mmHg increase in P_{LA} (not significantly different from one). The zero flow pressure increases in a manner that might have been predicted based on the effects of increasing a downstream pressure on an inflow pressure in a passive vascular bed.

To determine whether myogenic mechanisms were responsible for the much greater than one-for-one increases in bronchial artery inflow pressure with left atrial pressure elevations at constant flow, the following study was done. Pressure-flow data were obtained with left atrial pressure elevation after pretreatment with the smooth muscle paralytic papaverine. An example of the effects of papaverine on the bronchial artery pressure-flow relationship is presented in Fig. 12. Papaverine caused both a leftward shift and a counterclockwise rotation of the curve, demonstrating both a decrease in the zero flow pressure and a decrease in bronchial vascular resistance (BVR). An example of the effects of P_{LA} elevation on the papaverine-dilated bronchial vasculature in

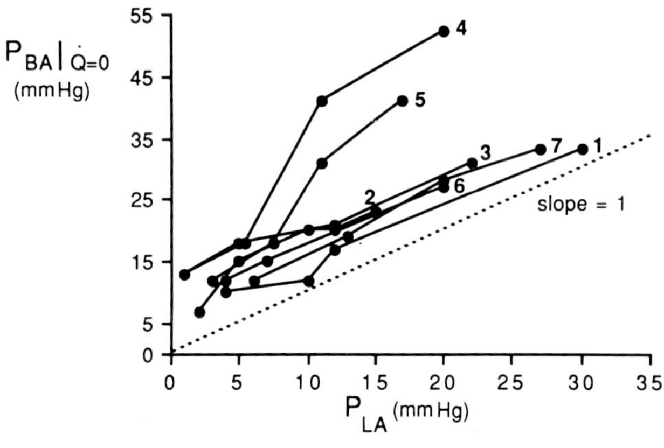

Figure 11 Effect of increases in left atrial pressure (P_{LA}) on bronchial artery pressure at zero flow ($P_{BA|\dot{Q}=0}$) in seven sheep. (Reprinted from Wagner and Mitzner, 1990, with permission from the *Journal of Applied Physiology*.)

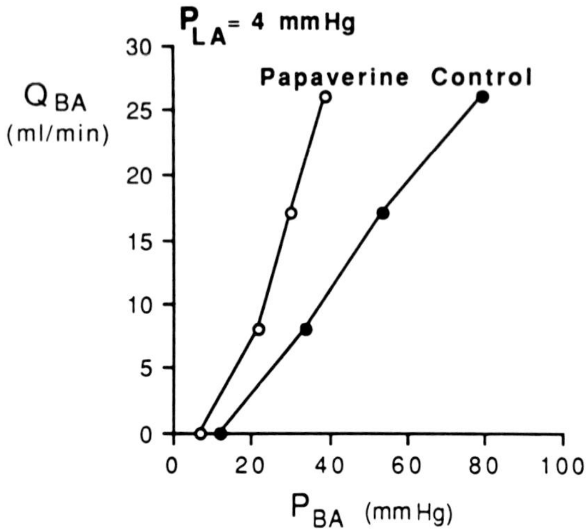

Figure 12 Example of the effect of papaverine on the bronchial vascular pressure (P_{BA}) – flow ($\dot{Q}_{BA}$) relationship at a left atrial pressure (P_{LA}) of 4 mmHg. (Adapted from Wagner and Mitzner, 1990, with permission from the *Journal of Applied Physiology*.)

the same animal can be seen in Fig. 13. In contrast to the results before papaverine (See Fig. 9.) P_{LA} elevation produced a rightward shift of the pressure-flow relationship and a counterclockwise rotation. These results demonstrate an increase in the zero flow pressure; however, in this case, left atrial pressure elevation causes a decrease in the BVR. These findings are consistent with what one might expect of a passive, distensible vasculature; that is, vascular resistance actually decreases as a result of the increased distention brought about by the increased downstream pressure. The average baseline bronchial vascular resistance was 3.2 ±0.3 mmHg/ml/min at a P_{LA} of 2.9 ±0.7 mmHg and decreased significantly after papaverine administration to 1.3 ±0.1 mmHg/ml/min. Figure 14 shows the effects of P_{LA} increases on P_{BA} at constant control flow during papaverine administration for each animal. At control flow and P_{LA}, P_{BA} in this dilated condition was 38 ±2 mmHg for the group of sheep studied. On average, P_{BA} increased 0.9 ±0.1 mmHg for every 1 mmHg increase in P_{LA}. Figure 15 shows the individual zero flow pressures for each animal. Control zero flow pressure at baseline P_{LA} was 8 ±1 mmHg. Under zero flow conditions, P_{BA} increased on average 1.2 ±0.1 mmHg for every 1 mmHg increase in P_{LA}.

To explain these results, let us refer to the resistive model of the bronchial circulation. In these experiments, the outflow pressure through the intra-

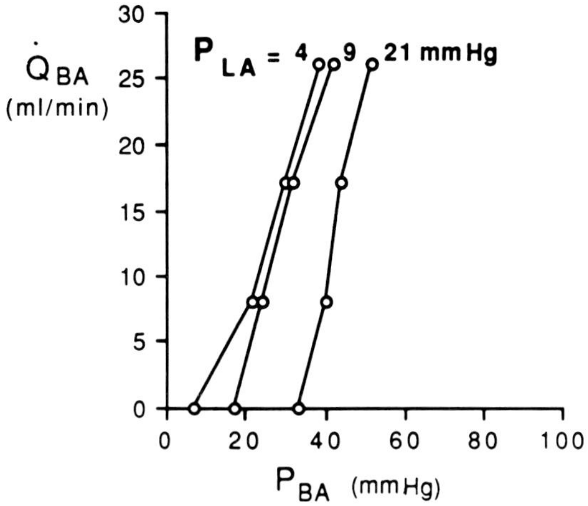

Figure 13 Example of the effect of increases in left atrial pressure (P_{LA}) on the bronchial vascular pressure (P_{BA}) – flow ($\dot{Q}_{BA}$) relationship after papaverine administration. (Reprinted from Wagner and Mitzner, 1990, with permission from the *Journal of Applied Physiology*.)

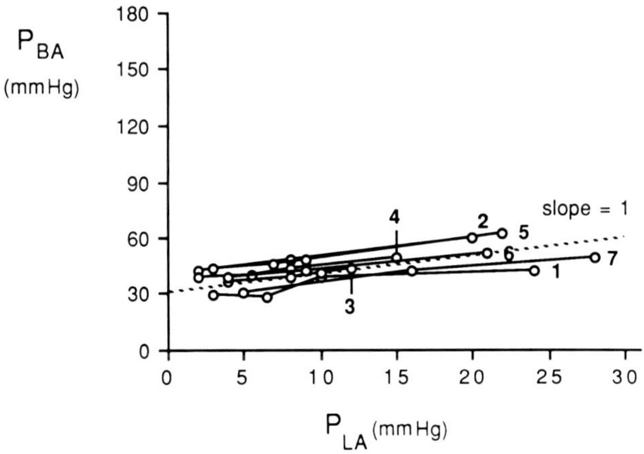

Figure 14 Effect of increases in left atrial pressures (P_{LA}) on bronchial artery inflow pressure (P_{BA}) at control flow after papaverine administration. (Reprinted from Wagner and Mitzner, 1990, with permission from the *Journal of Applied Physiology*.)

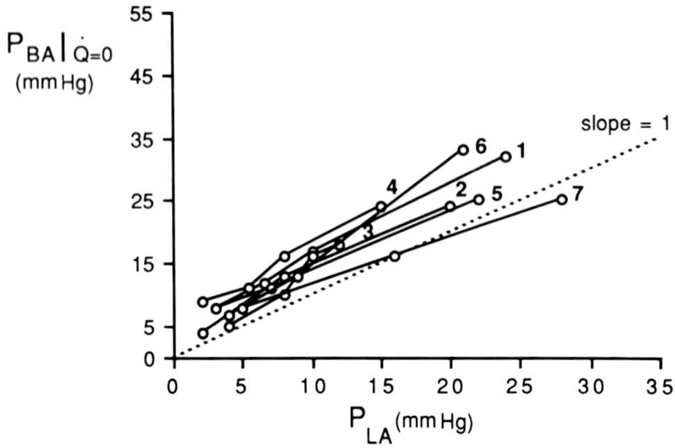

Figure 15 Effect of increase in left atrial pressure (P_{LA}) on bronchial artery pressure at zero flow ($P_{BA|Q=0}$) in seven sheep after papaverine administration. (Reprinted from Wagner and Mitzner, 1990, with permission from the *Journal of Applied Physiology.*)

pulmonary route was increased by left atrial pressure elevations. The results showed that elevations in P_{LA} resulted in approximately one-for-one increases in P_J measured by the zero flow pressure. If we assume that increases in P_{LA} result in very similar increases in the vascular pressure of pulmonary capillaries, venules, and arterioles, then we can use these data to gain insight into the relative magnitudes of the resistances of the intrapulmonary (R_I) and extrapulmonary (R_E) drainage pathways. If the resistances remain relatively constant, the only way for there to be a one-for-one increase in P_J would be if R_E were very much larger than R_I. Thus, it appears that under normal circumstances most of the bronchial venous drainage from bronchial vessels perfused by the bronchoesophageal artery is into the pulmonary vasculature.

In contrast to the nearly one-for-one increase in P_{EQ} with increases in P_{LA}, there was a considerably greater than one-for-one increase in bronchial artery pressure P_{BA}. This result suggested that there was some additional constriction in the vasculature in response to P_{LA} elevation. That papaverine administration resulted in nearly one-for-one changes in P_{BA} in response to increases in P_{LA} suggests that the greater than one-for-one rise normally seen resulted from an active smooth muscle response. The mechanism of this vasospasm resulting in an increased resistance in response to outflow pressure elevation is at present unknown. There may be a central neural reflex, a local venoarteriolar reflex, or a direct myogenic response. Because of the large magnitude of the changes in resistance observed with P_{LA} elevation, it is likely that the resistance changes observed occur in the bronchial arteries upstream from the junction of the bronchial veins. Were they to occur only in R_E or R_I, they would have to be not only large, but also proportionally equal, since if R_I/R_E changed, there would no longer be a one-for-one change in P_{EQ} with P_{LA} elevations. Thus, to summarize, increases in left atrial pressure result in a one-for-one increase in the equivalent downstream pressure of the vasculature and a much greater than one-for-one increase in upstream bronchial artery pressure under constant flow conditions.

Another study that impacts on our understanding of how downstream pressures affect the bronchial vasculature is that of Agostoni et al. (1987a). These investigators measured bronchopulmonary anastomotic blood flow of the left lower lobe in dogs using the pulmonary perfusion circuit overflow method (Modell et al., 1981). They increased pulmonary vascular pressure to determine the pressure at which blood flow through intraparenchymal drainage pathways ceased. The results of their study can be seen in Fig. 16. Anastomotic flow $\dot{Q}$br(s-p) is zero when pulmonary vascular pressure is 44 cmH_2O. According to our resistive model of the bronchial vasculature, the pressure they measured when anastomotic flow was zero could be interpreted as the junctional pressure (P_J). However, it should be emphasized here that the zero flow pressure they refer to is measured only when there is no flow through intraparenchymal drainage vessels. In this case, there remains a much greater than normal flow through the bronchial veins. The zero flow pressure previously described in our resistive model refers to the situation in which there is no arterial inflow, although there can be flow between the two drainage pathways. Although the intent of Agostoni et al. was to determine the upstream pressure for intrapulmonary flow, the method they used necessarily resulted in

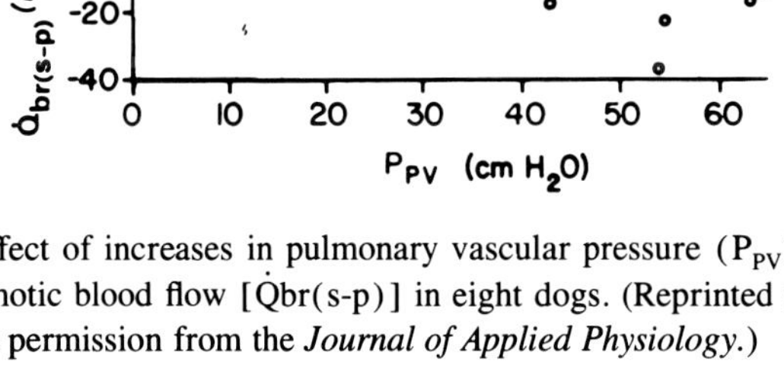

Figure 16 Effect of increases in pulmonary vascular pressure (P_{PV}) on bronchopulmonary anastomotic blood flow [$\dot{Q}$br(s-p)] in eight dogs. (Reprinted from Agostoni et al., 1987a, with permission from the *Journal of Applied Physiology*.)

an elevation of the very upstream pressure that they were trying to measure. Consequently, their measured upstream pressure of 44 cmH_2O is higher than the upstream pressure (P_J) under control conditions with normal flow and a normal left atrial pressure. This conclusion can be demonstrated and quantified based on the following analysis.

To analyze this situation with our resistive model, estimates of all variables must first be provided. It should be emphasized that this analysis is based on available information from work done in dogs and sheep. Responsiveness may be species dependent, and consequently some of the assumptions may not apply. Bronchial vascular resistance in sheep can be estimated to be equal to 3.6 mmHg/ml/min when $P_{AO} = 100$ mmHg, $P_{EQ} = 8$ mmHg, and bronchial blood flow equals 20 ml/min. These values are within the reported range of normal values. If one can assume that bronchial arterial resistance provides the major resistance for flow through this vasculature, then $R_{BA} + R_C$ can be estimated to be approximately 3.3 mmHg/ml/min. Based on information concerning the proportion of drainage through the two pathways, extrapulmonary venous resistance (outflow to the right heart) can be estimated to provide five times the resistance that intrapulmonary drainage pathways offer. Calculation of P_J and anastomotic blood flow through the intraparenchymal drainage pathway ($\dot{Q}_{ANAST}$) based on our resistive model and the variable estimates results in the relationships obtained in Fig. 17 (see the Appendix for details of the calculation). Open symbols show the relationship obtained for P_J (circles) and

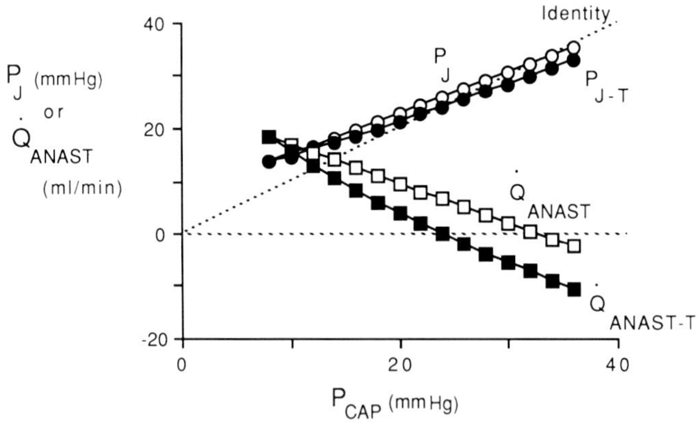

Figure 17 Prediction of the effect of increases in pulmonary capillary pressure (P_{CAP}) on the junctional pressure (P_J) and bronchopulmonary anastomotic blood flow ($\dot{Q}_{ANAST}$). Open symbols indicate responses with no active tone; closed symbols indicate responses with active tone (T). Dashed lines indicate the line of indentity and the zero flow line.

$\dot{Q}_{ANAST}$ (squares) when P_{CAP} is increased when there is no tone in the vasculature. Closed symbols show the same relationships under conditions in which active tone exists. Most significantly, it can be seen that at a normal pulmonary capillary pressure, estimated as 8 mmHg in this example, P_J = 13 mmHg. Thus, under conditions of normal flow the model shows the calculated upstream pressure for anastomotic or collateral flow to be 13 mmHg, not 32.4 mmHg (44 cmH_2O) as suggested by Agostoni et al. (1987a). This analysis can be carried out further to include the condition in which active constriction occurs in response to increases in downstream pressures. Bronchial arterial resistance (R_{BA} + R_C in the electrical model) in sheep is estimated to increase 0.12 mmHg/ml/min for every 1 mmHg increase in P_{LA} (Wagner and Mitzner, 1990). These results show that under conditions of active tone, the P_J when $\dot{Q}_{ANAST}$ is equal to zero is actually somewhat less than under conditions of no tone (23 versus 33 mmHg). This analysis shows that Agostoni's method to measure the upstream pressure for flow would be closer to the calculated upstream pressure if there were active tone in the dog. This model supports the notion that the method used by Agostoni et al. (1987a) to determine the upstream pressure actually provided a stimulus for a myogenic increase in bronchial vascular resistance. However, another possible explanation is that the bronchial arterial circulation of the dog may differ from that of the sheep and may not exhibit myogenic responsiveness to increases in pulmonary venous pressure. The high upstream pressure measured by Agostoni et al. may be related to passive distention of the upstream bronchial vasculature.

Although this discussion is based largely on alterations of pulmonary capillary pressure brought about by increases in left atrial pressure, increases in pulmonary artery inflow pressure may be expected to have similar effects. Decreases in pulmonary capillary pressure induced by pulmonary artery obstruction have been shown in the short term ($<$1 h) to both decrease (Agostoni et al., 1987b; Kowalski et al., 1990) and increase bronchial blood flow (Magno, 1979; Malik and Tracy, 1980). The variability in responses is probably related to the method and portion of pulmonary circulation obstruction, the time of blood flow measurement after obstruction, and the potential alteration of blood gas tensions and temperature (Agostoni et al., 1987b) of the bronchial perfusate. Further studies are needed to determine the effect of hemodynamic alterations in the pulmonary circulation on bronchial blood flow.

Information concerning the effects of elevations of the outflow pressure of the extrapulmonary drainage pathway is relatively scarce. Auld et al. (1960) as well as Salisbury et al. (1957) showed that raising right atrial pressure resulted in an increase in blood flow draining through the intrapulmonary pathway. Results from the study by Salisbury et al. (1957) are presented in Fig. 18. There is a clear increase in the bronchopulmonary anastomotic blood flow in each of the 11 observations from five dogs. However, since the response of

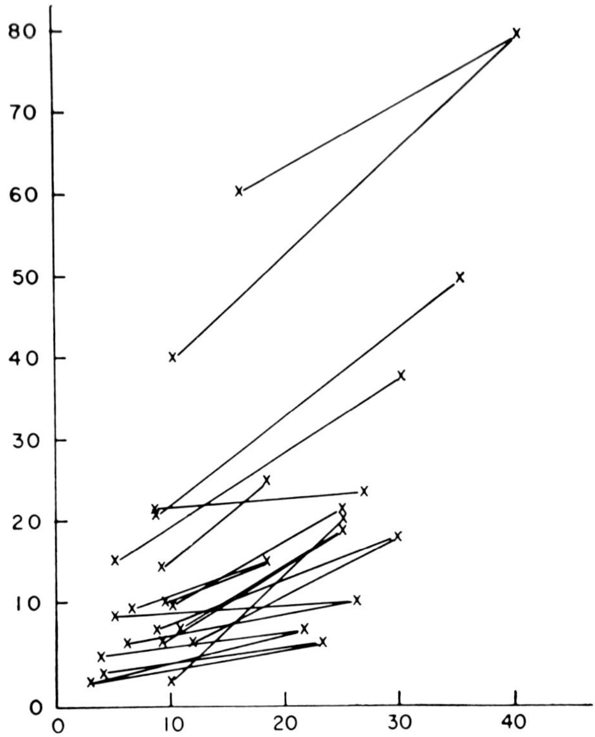

Figure 18 Effects of increases in systemic venous pressure (abscissa, cm saline) on bronchopulmonary anastomotic blood flow (ordinate, ml/min). (Reprinted from Salisbury et al., 1957.)

the total bronchial vasculature is unknown, it is not possible to conclude that there was a diversion of blood flow from extrapulmonary to intrapulmonary pathways with systemic venous pressure elevation. The changes seen in $\dot{Q}_{ANAST}$ may have resulted from changes in flow into the bronchial artery.

V. Alterations in Lung Volume

It is well documented that increases in lung volume and alveolar pressure can result in major changes in the pulmonary circulation (West et al., 1964). Since at least two-thirds of bronchial blood flow drains through the pulmonary circulation, increases in the pressure surrounding pulmonary capillaries result in increases in the outflow pressure of the bronchial vasculature. Several investigators have shown that increases in lung volume and airway pressure with the application of positive end-expiratory pressure (PEEP) cause significant increases in bronchial vascular resistance. Baile et al. (1984) demonstrated that these increases in bronchial vascular resistance were most apparent in lung parenchyma and bronchi and less significant in larger airways outside the lung (Fig. 19). In addition, this study showed that at high levels of PEEP, there is a redistribution of blood flow out the extraparenchymal drainage pathway to the right heart. Cassidy and Haynes (1986) showed that the decrease in bronchial blood flow with the application of PEEP was much greater than what might be expected if the pressure gradient for flow were simply decreased by the increase in alveolar pressure. In this case the downstream pressure for bronchial flow would be comparable to that of the pulmonary circulation in a zone

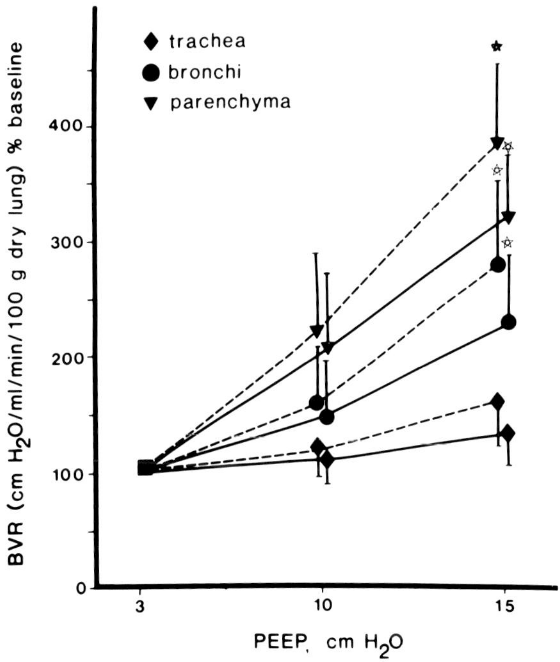

Figure 19 Regional effects of increasing positive end-expiratory pressure (PEEP) on bronchial vascular resistance (BVR) in dogs. Solid lines represent responses with BVR calculated as systemic arterial pressure minus alveolar pressure/bronchial blood flow. Dashed lines indicate responses with BVR calculated as systemic arterial pressure minus venous pressure/bronchial blood flow. (Reprinted from Baile, et al., 1984, with permission from the *Journal of Applied Physiology*.)

2 condition of the lung (West et al., 1964). They suggested some reflex- or mediator-induced response to explain the large increase in bronchial vascular resistance with increased levels of PEEP. Baier et al. (1985) showed that blocking the release of cyclooxygenase products did not significantly modify lung inflation-induced changes in bronchial vascular resistance. Taking advantage of the hysteresis characteristics of the lung, Modell et al. (1981) showed that anastomotic blood flow in the dog decreased both when transpulmonary pressure was increased and lung volume held constant as well as when lung volume was increased and transpulmonary pressure held constant. Wagner et al. (1987) examined the pressure-flow characteristics of the bronchial vascular bed with increases in the level of positive end-expiratory pressure in sheep. Figure 20 shows the typical pressure-flow response of the bronchial circulation to increasing levels of PEEP. Note both the increase in resistance (demonstrated by the decrease in slope) as well as the increase in zero flow pressure with increasing levels of PEEP. Although the level of positive end-expiratory pressure was the controlled variable, if airway pressure per se determines the response, then it is important to consider the average pressure over the entire respiratory cycle. Group data for eight animals are plotted with mean airway pressure as the independent variable. Figure 21 shows the effects of mean airway pressure on bronchial artery pressure at constant control flow. Increasing the mean airway pressure from approximately 4 to 14 mmHg caused the bronchial artery pressure to increase from an average of 91 to 136 mmHg. The

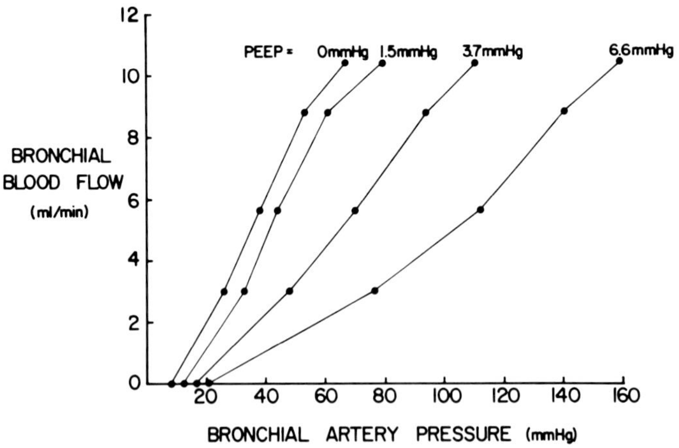

Figure 20 Example of the effects of increasing PEEP on the bronchial vascular pressure-flow relationship. (Reprinted from Wagner et al., 1987, with permission from the *Journal of Applied Physiology*.)

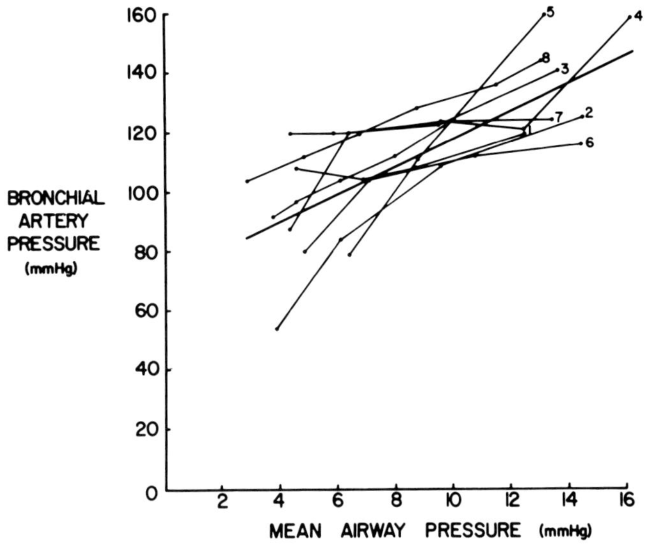

Figure 21 Effects of increasing mean airway pressure on bronchial artery pressure at control flow in eight sheep. (Reprinted from Wagner et al., 1987, with permission from the *Journal of Applied Physiology*.)

slope of the relationship between mean airway pressure and P_{BA} for the group averaged 4.6 ±1.1.

The effects of increasing mean airway pressure on zero flow pressures are presented in Fig. 22. Over a similar range of mean airway pressure, zero flow pressures increased from an average of 21 to 32 mmHg. Slopes of the relationship between mean airway pressure and zero flow pressure obtained by regression analysis gave an average value of 1.2 ±0.1 for the group. Thus, zero flow pressure increased roughly one-for-one with increases in mean airway pressure. Therefore, the predominant reason for the increase in bronchial artery pressure with increases in mean airway pressure was the increase in resistance (from 6.1 to 9.2 mmHg/ml/min), not an alteration of zero flow pressure.

That the zero flow pressure in all animals increased approximately one-for-one with increases in mean airway pressure suggests that most of the drainage from the bronchial circulation perfused in this manner was into the pulmonary capillaries. Since with PEEP and positive pressure ventilation the lungs were predominantly in zone 2, one would expect pulmonary capillary pressure P_{CAP} to increase one-for-one with increases in mean airway pressure. P_{BV} would be unlikely to show this degree of change with lung inflation.

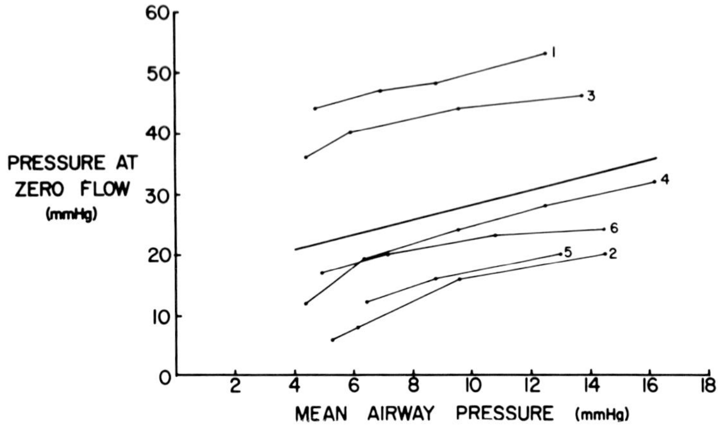

Figure 22 Effects of increasing mean airway pressure on bronchial artery pressure at zero flow. (Reprinted from Wagner et al., 1987, with permission from the *Journal of Applied Physiology*.)

Therefore, if R_E remains relatively constant, the only way for the pressure in the submucosal junction to track capillary pressure would be if R_E were very much greater than R_I.

As can be seen in Fig. 22, the zero flow pressure of two of the animals is much higher than has been shown previously. In these animals arterial anastomoses may have existed between the peribronchial plexus and tracheal and/or connective tissue arteries (see Fig. 1). In this case the zero flow pressure would be a measure of the arterial junction somewhere in the peribronchial plexus or upstream.

Referring to the resistive model of the bronchial vasculature, one can speculate on the anatomic location of the resistance change that occurs with increases in mean airway pressure. Animals with high zero flow pressures (Fig. 22, animals 1 and 3) showed little change in vascular resistance as airway pressure was initially increased (Fig. 23). However, in the other four animals with insignificant arterial anastomoses, the largest increases in resistance were observed as airway pressure initially increased. If the major site of resistance were upstream from the arterial anastomoses, we should also have observed these increases in resistance in sheep 1 and 3. That we did not suggests that the increase in resistance with lung inflation results from vascular changes downstream from the potential arterial anastomoses. The major site of resistance may be in the connecting vessels linking the two plexus. These vessels arise in the peribronchial connective tissue and cross the muscular

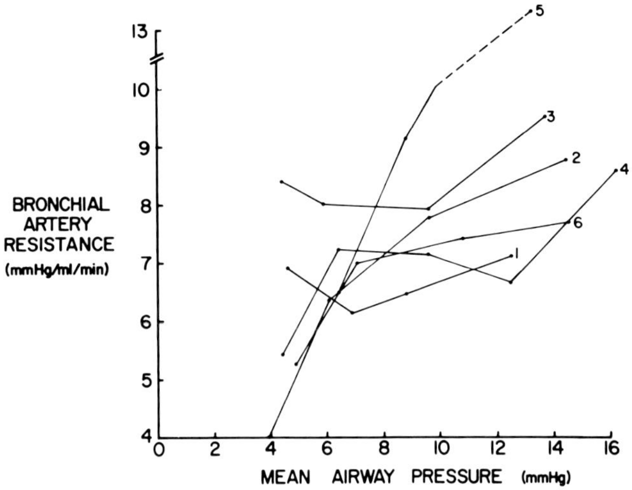

Figure 23 Effects of increasing mean airway pressure on bronchial vascular resistance (calculated as the inverse slope of the pressure-flow relationship) in seven sheep. (Reprinted from Wagner et al., 1987, with permission from the *Journal of Applied Physiology.*)

layer into the bronchial mucosa. Because they run perpendicular to the airway axis, this arrangement may make their resistance more sensitive to the axial stretching of airways that occurs with lung inflation. Another possibility is that stretching of the lung with increases in lung volume results in active constriction of bronchial vessels, as previously suggested.

To test whether active vascular constriction was involved, Wagner and Mitzner (1990) measured bronchial artery inflow pressurc at constant control flow before and after intrabronchial artery infusion of the smooth muscle paralytic papaverine, with the application of PEEP. Figure 24 shows these results. Although baseline bronchial vascular tone decreased significantly with papaverine, the effect of increasing mean airway pressure ($\bar{P}_{AW}$) on inflow pressure was unaltered. In addition, increasing blood flow to establish prepapaverine inflow pressures did not alter the responses of bronchial artery pressure to increases in mean airway pressure.

This result with $\bar{P}_{AW}$ elevation supports the idea that the response of the bronchial circulation to outflow pressure elevation differs depending on how this elevation is affected. With P_{LA} elevation, there is an active muscle constriction that can be abolished with papaverine, but with $\bar{P}_{AW}$ elevation, there must be some mechanical factor that results in an increased resistance. That in

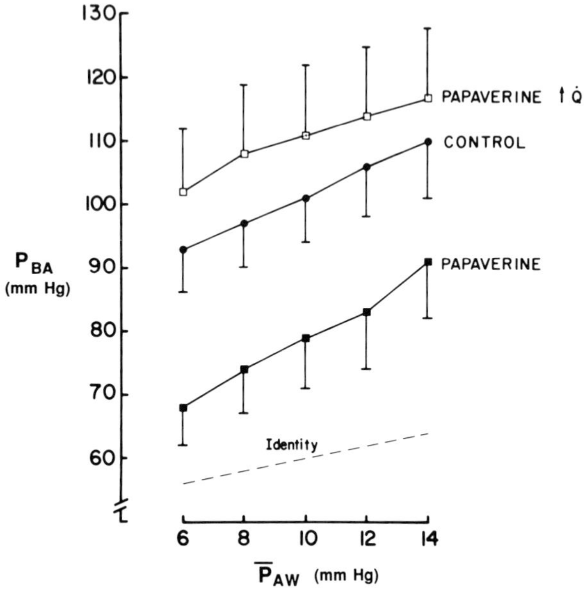

Figure 24 Comparison of the average effects of increasing mean airway pressure on the bronchial artery pressure at constant bronchial blood flow under control conditions (solid circles), after papaverine administration (solid squares), and after papaverine administration with increased bronchial blood flow (open squares).

these studies the lung is inflated with increased $\overline{P}_{AW}$, not with increased P_{LA} may possibly account for this difference. Since the airways are lengthened and dilated with lung inflation, it is not unreasonable to predict that there may be some mechanical distortion of the bronchial vasculature.

VI. Summary

As a result of its anatomic arrangement, the bronchial vasculature is directly exposed to mechanical stresses produced by lung volume changes as well as indirectly through changes in pulmonary vascular pressures. Substantial changes in bronchial vascular resistance can be imposed with the application of positive end-expiratory pressure. Likewise, pathological increases in pulmonary capillary pressure may result in significant decreases in bronchial vascular perfusion. Both situations could impact on airway homeostasis by decreasing bronchial blood flow and hence affect airway reactivity to exogenous substances. These conclusions are based on the described anatomy and physiology of the bronchial circulation. However, a recent study by Barman et al. (1988) suggests that the anatomic descriptions presented in this chapter with the accompanying electrical model may be incomplete. Barman et al. have shown in a dog preparation, using radiolabeled microspheres to measure blood flow, that the pulmonary circulation with normal pressure and flow can provide 50% of the total blood flow to the main bronchi. Thus, the pulmonary circulatory contribution to large airways may be substantial. Further studies are needed to explore the interaction of these two circulatory systems in the maintenance of the nutrition of the lung.

VII. Appendix

The following calculations were made to determine the relationship between pulmonary capillary pressure P_{CAP} and the junctional pressure P_J of the bronchial circulation, as well as anastomotic blood flow $\dot{Q}_{ANAST}$, illustrated in Fig. 17. To simplify, we redefine three resistances, each of which is comprised of the parallel combination of two resistances in Fig. 6. We have also excluded R_C and assumed all resistances upstream from P_J to be represented by R_{BA}.

$$R_1 = \frac{R_{BA}R_I}{R_{BA} + R_I}$$

$$R_2 = \frac{R_{BA}R_E}{R_{BA} + R_E}$$

$$R_3 = \frac{R_I R_E}{R_I + R_E}$$

(*Note*: $R_3 = R_{EQ}$ in Fig. 5.) Algebraic analysis of the resistive model results in the equations

$$P_J = P_{AO}\frac{R_3}{R_3 + R_{BA}} + P_{CAP}\frac{R_2}{R_2 + R_I} + P_{BV}\frac{R_1}{R_1 + R_E} \tag{1}$$

$$\dot{Q}_{ANAST} = \frac{P_J - P_{CAP}}{R_I} \tag{2}$$

and substituting P_J from Eq. (1) and rearranging,

$$\dot{Q}_{ANAST} = P_{AO}\frac{R_3/R_I}{R_3 + R_{BA}} + P_{BV}\frac{R_1/R_I}{R_1 + R_E} + P_{CAP}\frac{1}{R_2 + R_I}$$

Assuming the following variables do not change with increases in P_{CAP}, we have obtained the relationships obtained in Fig. 17 (open symbols): $P_{AO} = 100$mmHg; $P_{BV} = 2$mmHg; $R_E = 1.5$mmHg/ml/min; $R_I = 0.3$mmHg/

ml/min; $R_{BA} = 3.3$mmHg/ml/min. This analysis provides information concerning the effect of increasing P_{CAP} on the junctional pressure P_J and bronchopulmonary anastomotic flow $\dot{Q}_{ANAST}$ when there is no vascular tone. If this analysis is repeated when R_{BA} is allowed to increase because of myogenically induced tone, the relationship displayed in solid symbols in Fig. 17 is obtained. Since it has been shown that R_{BA} increases 0.12 mmHg/ml/min for every 1 mmHg increase in P_{CAP} (Wagner and Mitzner, 1990), this algebraic analysis was repeated with a pressure-sensitive R_{BA} according to the formula $R_{BA} = 3.3 + 0.12P_{CAP}$.

References

Agostoni, P. G., Deffebach, M. E., Kirk, W., Lakshminarayan, S., and Butler, J. (1987a). Upstream pressure for systemic to pulmonary flow from bronchial circulation in dogs. *J. Appl. Physiol.* **63**(2):485–491.

Agostoni, P. G., Deffebach, M. E., Kirk, W., Mendenhall, J. M., Albert, R. K., and Bulter, J. (1987b). Temperature alters bronchial blood flow response to pulmonary artery obstruction. *J. Appl. Physiol.* **62**(5):1907–1911.

Armendia, P., DeLetona, J. M. L., Aviado, D. M. (1962). Responses of the bronchial veins in a heart-lung-bronchial preparation. *Circ. Res.* **10**:3–10.

Auld, P. A., Rudolph, A. M., Golinko, R. J., (1960). Factors affecting bronchial collateral flow in the dog. *Am. J. Physiol.* **198**(6):1166–1170.

Baier, H., Yerger, L., Moas, R., and Wanner, A. (1985). Vascular and airway effects of endogenous cyclooxygenase products during lung inflation. *J. Appl. Physiol.* **59**(3):884–889.

Baile, E. M., Albert, R. K., Kirk, W., Lakshaminarayan, S., Wiggs, B. J. R., and Paré, P. D. (1984). Positive end-expiratory pressure decreases bronchial blood flow in the dog. *J. Appl. Physiol.* **56**(5):1289–1293.

Baile, E. M., Ling, H., Heyworth, J. R., Hogg, J. C., and Paré, P. D. (1985). Bronchopulmonary anastomotic and noncoronary collateral blood flow in humans during cardiopulmonary bypass. *Chest* **87**(6):749–754.

Barman, S. A., Ardell, J. L., Parker, J. C., Perry, M. L., and Taylor, A. E. (1988). Pulmonary and systemic blood flow contributions to upper airways in canine lung. *Am. J. Physiol.* **255**:H1130–H1135.

Berry, J. L., and Daly, I. B. (1931). The relation between the pulmonary and bronchial vascular systems. *Proc. R. Soc. Lond (Biol.)* **109**:319–336.

Brenner, E., and Javid, M. (1959). *Analysis of Electric Circuits*. New York, McGraw Hill, pp. 267–273.

Burton, A. C., and Stinson, R. H. (1960). The measurement of tension in smooth muscle. *J. Physiol. (Lond.)* **153**:290–305.

Cassidy, S. S., and Haynes, M. S. (1986). The effects of ventilation with positive end-expiratory pressure on the bronchial circulation. *Respir. Physiol.* **66**:269–278.

Charan, N. B., Turk, G. M., and Dhand, R. (1984). Gross and subgross anatomy of bronchial circulation in sheep. *J. Appl. Physiol.* **57**(3):658–664.

Charan, N. B., Turk, G. M., and Ripley, R. (1985). Measurement of bronchial arterial blood flow and bronchovascular resistance in sheep. *J. Appl. Physiol.* **59**(2):305–308.

Charan, N. B., Turk, G. M., Czartolomny, J., and Andreazuk, T. (1987). Systemic arterial blood supply to the trachea and lung in sheep. *J. Appl. Physiol.* **62**(6):2283–2287.

Deffebach, M. E., Charan, N. B., Lakshminarayan, S., and Butler, J. (1987a). The bronchial circulation—small, but a vital attribute of the lung. *Am. Rev. Respir. Dis.* **135**:463–481.

Deffebach, M. E., Lakshminarayan, S., Kirk, W., and Butler, J. (1987b). Bronchial circulation and cyclooxygenase products in acute lung injury. *J. Appl. Physiol.* **63**(3):1083–1088.

Girling, F. (1952). Critical closing pressure and venous pressure. *Am. J. Physiol.* **171**:204–207.

Haddy, F. J., and Gilbert, R. P. (1956). The relation of venous-arteriolar reflex to transmural pressure and resistance in small and large systemic vessels. *Circ. Res.* **4**:25–32.

Hanson, K. M., and Johnson, P. C. (1966). Local control of hepatic arterial and portal venous flow in the dog. *Am. J. Physiol.* **211**:712–720.

Kowalski, T. F., Guidotti, S., Deffebach, M., Kubilis, P., and Bishop, M. (1990). Bronchial circulation in pulmonary artery occlusion and reperfusion. *J. Appl. Physiol.* **68**(1):125–129.

Magno, M. (1979). Effect of pulmonary blood flow on the post-occlusion response of the bronchial circulation in anesthesized sheep. *Fed. Proc.* **38**(3):1378.

Magno, M. G., and Fishman, A. P. (1982). Origin, distribution, and blood flow of bronchial circulation in anesthetized sheep. *J. Appl. Physiol.* **53**(1):272–279.

Malik, A. B., and Tracy, S. E. (1980). Bronchovascular adjustments after pulmonary embolism. *J. Appl. Physiol.* **49**(3):476–481.

Mitzner, W. A. (1974). Effect of portal venous pressure on portal venous inflow and splanchnic resistance. *J. Appl. Physiol.* **37**(5):706–711.

Mitzner, W. A. (1983): Resistance of the pulmonary circulation. *Clin. Chest Med.* **4**:127–137.

Modell, H. I., Beck, K., and Butler, J. (1981). Functional aspects of canine bronchial-pulmonary vascular communications. *J. Appl. Physiol.* **50**(5):1045–1051.

Patterson, G. C., and Shepherd, J. T. (1954). The blood flow in the human forearm following venous congestion. *J. Physiol. (Lond.)* **125**:501–507.

Permutt, S., and Riley, R. L. (1963). Hemodynamics of collapsible vessels with tone: The vascular waterfall. *J. Appl. Physiol.* **18**(5):924–932.

Salisbury, P. F., Weil, P., and State, D. (1957). Factors influencing collateral blood flow to the dog's lung. *Circ. Res.* **5**:303–309.

Wagner, E. M., and Mitzner, W. A. (1988) Effect of hypoxia on bronchial circulation. *J. Appl. Physiol.* **65**(4):1627–1633.

Wagner, E. M., and Mitzner, W. A. (1990). Effect of left atrial pressure on bronchial vascular hemodynamics. *J. Appl. Physiol.* **69**(3):837–842.

Wagner, E. M., Mitzner, W. A. and Bleecker, E. R. (1987). Effects of airway pressure on bronchial blood flow. *J. Appl. Physiol.* **62**(2):561–566.

West, J. B., Dollery, C. T., and Naimark, A. (1964). Distribution of blood flow in the isolated lung: Relation of vascular and alveolar pressure. *J. Appl. Physiol.* **19**:713–724.

8

Neuroregulation and Pharmacology of the Tracheobronchial Circulation

JOHN G. WIDDICOMBE and STEPHEN E. WEBBER

St. George's Hospital Medical School
London, England

I. Introduction

In recent years the pharmacology of the tracheobronchial circulation has been extensively studied. It is a subject of considerable basic medical and clinical importance for a number of reasons. Asthma, far and away the most common chronic lower airways disease, is now regarded as primarily an inflammation of the airway mucosa, with secondary smooth muscle changes. Two of its major features are hyperemia and edema of the mucosa. These are caused by the release of many immunological and inflammatory mediators from the airway epithelium and from migratory cells, such as mast cells, eosinophils, and neutrophils. The action of these mediators on the mucosal vascular beds is therefore an important matter for consideration. In addition, the treatment of many airways diseases, including asthma, usually involves inhalation of therapeutic agents. Although many of these are intended primarily to act on airway smooth muscle, nonetheless they may have secondary effects on airway vascular beds and may therefore influence mucosal blood flow and interstitial fluid volume. In assessment of airways hyperresponsiveness, it is common to use aerosols of smooth muscle-contracting agents, such as histamine and methacholine. These may well act on vascular beds during their passage to the smooth muscle and thus change mucosal function and also influence the effectiveness of their penetration through the mucosa.

The airways vasculature is complex (see Chap. 3). Basically it consists of a subepithelial capillary network, with a deeper mucosal system of postcapillary venules, venules, and blood sinuses. The last appear to be a capacitance system, similar to, but less well developed than, that in the nose. The trachea, at least of the sheep, seems to lack arteriovenous anastomoses (Corfield, Webber, and Widdicombe, unpublished observations). Drugs and mediators, whether exogenous or endogenous, may therefore act on many vascular sites. In addition their overall effects include changes in interstitial fluid volume. Nearly all studies of the pharmacology of the airway vasculature have involved assessments of total vascular resistance or total mucosal blood flow, and the precise site of action of drugs, for example, arterioles, venules, or capacitance vessels, has hardly ever been delineated.

A further consideration is that the tracheal circulation has structural and functional features that distinguish it from the bronchial circulation and may be reflected in their respective pharmacologies. The tracheal circulation drains into systemic veins, whereas the bronchial circulation largely drains into the pulmonary vasculature. Not only might one expect differences in the pharmacology of the tracheal and bronchial vessels because of this anatomic distinction, but the bronchial vascular pharmacology may be difficult to distinguish from that of the pulmonary vasculature if drugs and mediators are allowed to act on both vascular beds. Measurements of changes in bronchial vascular resistance have nearly always included the bronchopulmonary anastomoses. Because of this factor, the results may differ from those for the tracheal vasculature. However, little or nothing is known of the pharmacology of bronchopulmonary anastomoses as distinct from the main bronchial blood vessels.

The methods of studying the lower airways vasculature are diverse (see Chap. 4). The selection of a particular method may influence a pharmacological result, certainly quantitatively and possibly even qualitatively. The two methods most used in recent years have been the measurement of bronchial blood flow by an appropriate flow probe placed around the main bronchial artery, and perfusion of a tracheal artery, either with a constant-flow pump while measuring pressure or by the animal's own blood pressure while measuring flow. For surgical reasons, dogs, sheep, and pigs have been used for most studies, although smaller animals have occasionally been used. It is worth emphasizing and regreting that no good methods exist for studying the lower airways vascular pharmacology in humans. Indeed, almost the *only* method is laser Doppler flowmetry; this method shows some promise, but we must wait to see if that promise is fulfilled (Corfield et al., 1991b).

A final general consideration is the means of administering pharmacological agents. They can be directly administered into the arterial inflow to the tracheal or bronchial vascular bed, and this has the advantage that small doses are used. The natural way for many inflammatory mediators to reach vascular smooth muscle is through the interstitium, however, and this route presents different features compared with the intravascular. The latter may more directly involve endothelially derived factors, which can have a profound effect on vascular smooth muscle. With the same methods of assessing airways vascular resistance, drugs can be administered intravenously to reach the airway vasculature. However, this method has the disadvantage that the drugs may have systemic effects that can interact with the airways vascular bed via general hemodynamic responses or via reflexes.

It is clear that there are many different models and methods for studying the pharmacology of the airway vasculature. In general the published results are consistent qualitatively, as is described in the following sections. The quantitative aspects of airways vascular pharmacology are less well worked out, however; in particular, the precise relevance of individual pharmacological experiments on animals to the mechanisms of control of the human airways vasculature is very difficult to assess.

II. Neurotransmitters and the Tracheobronchial Circulation

A. Parasympathetic Cholinergic Mechanisms

Nerve Section and Stimulation

The role of the parasympathetic cholinergic nervous system in the control of tracheobronchial blood flow is still unclear. Horisberger and Rodbard (1960) found that total bronchial blood flow decreases after bilateral vagotomy, suggesting a significant resting parasympathetic dilator tone. However, other investigators have not seen any change in bronchial blood flow when the vagi are sectioned (De Letona et al., 1961; Jindal et al., 1985). Tracheal vascular resistance in dogs is significantly increased when the cervical vagi are cut (Salonen et al., 1988) and decreased when the superior laryngeal nerves are cut (Laitinen et al., 1987b); both nerves supply the cervical trachea. The effects of nerve section on local tracheobronchial blood flow are difficult to interpret because this intervention can cause profound changes in systemic arterial blood pressure. In addition the nerves are mixed, containing not only parasympathetic fibers but also sensory and possibly sympathetic motor fibers. Therefore such experiments do not clearly establish whether there is tonic activity in parasympathetic motor fibers to the tracheobronchial vasculature, but in a negative sense they may suggest that any such tone is not a dominant influence.

Stimulation of the distal cut (motor) end of the vagus nerve increases bronchial blood flow in dogs (Murao, 1965), cats (Martling et al., 1985), and pigs (Matran et al., 1989b). Similarly, stimulation of the motor superior laryngeal nerve increases blood flow in the superior laryngeal artery supplying the upper trachea and larynx of pigs (Matran et al., 1989b) and reduces tracheal perfusion pressure, indicating vasodilation, when the superior laryngeal artery of dogs is perfused at constant flow (Fig. 1) (Laitinen et al., 1987b). The increased bronchial blood flow in cats (Martling et al., 1987) and pigs (Matran et al., 1989b) on motor vagal nerve stimulation is not affected by pretreatment with atropine, suggesting that these responses are entirely noncholinergic (see later). In contrast, vasodilation of the tracheal vasculature in dogs (Laitinen et al., 1987b) and the increased blood flow in the pig superior laryngeal artery on stimulation of the motor superior laryngeal nerve (Matran et al., 1989b) are substantially reduced by atropine, suggesting, at least in part, a cholinergic mechanism (Figs. 1 and 2). The difference in results could depend on species,

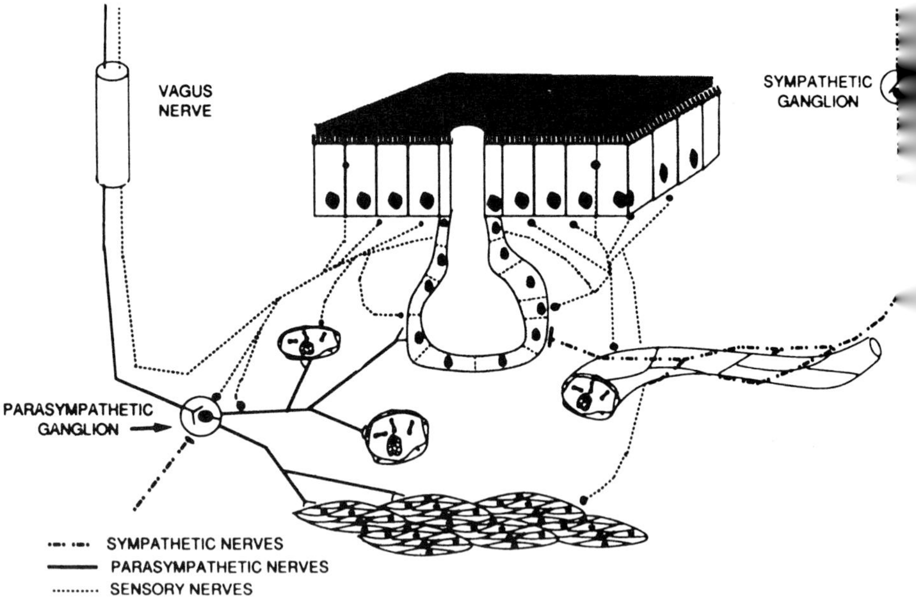

Figure 1 Nervous control of the tracheobronchial circulation.

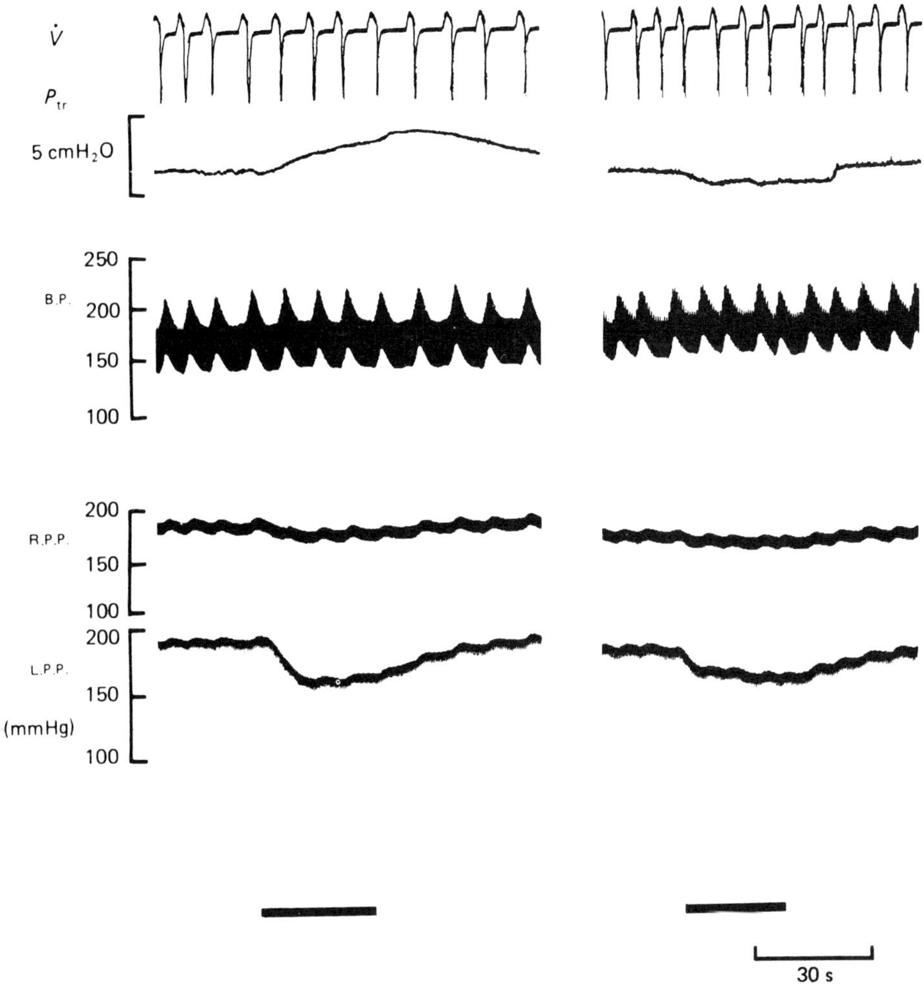

Figure 2 Electrical stimulation (5 V, 1 ms, 10 Hz) of the peripheral end of the cut left superior laryngeal nerve in a spontaneously breathing dog before (left) and after (right) administration of atropine (1 mg/kg IV). From above down, V̇, airflow; Ptr, tracheal pressure; B.P., blood pressure; R.P.P., right and L.P.P., left perfusion pressures. Before atropine, stimulation causes falls in both perfusion pressures, greater on the ipsilateral side, an increase in tracheal pressure, and no change in blood pressure. After atropine the falls in perfusion pressure are smaller, and there is a decrease in tracheal pressure. (From Laitinen et al., 1987b).

on methods, or on experimental conditions, such as anesthesia. Thus nerve stimulation experiments, like nerve sectioning, are not strongly definitive but suggest that parasympathetic motor nerves cause airway vasodilation by cholinergic and/or noncholinergic (presumably peptidergic) mechanisms (Fig. 3).

Exogenous Agonists

Injections of acetylcholine into the bronchial artery of dogs produce large increases in bronchial blood flow (Bruner and Schmidt, 1947; Aramendia et al., 1962; Cudkowitz, 1968). Similar injections of methacholine (a stable analog of acetylcholine) in dogs (De Letona et al., 1961) and sheep (Parsons et al., 1985; Link et al., 1985) also increases flow. Similarly, aerosolized muscarinic agonists increase bronchial blood flow in dogs (Bruner and Schmidt,

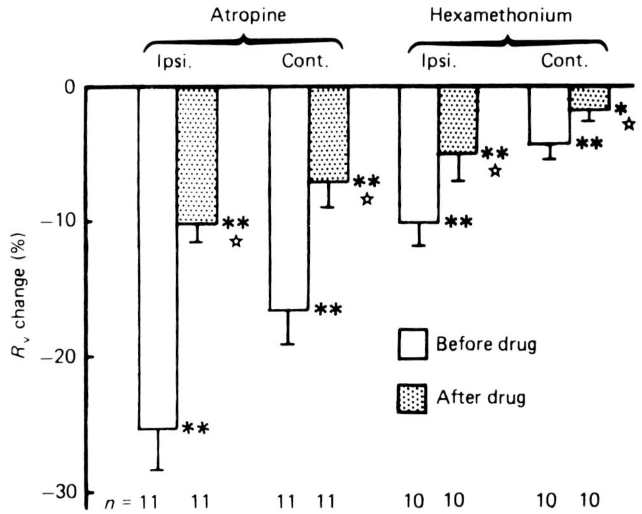

Figure 3 Changes in tracheal vascular resistance R_V in anesthetized dogs. Electrical stimulation (10V, 1 ms, 10 Hz) of the peripheral end of one superior laryngeal nerve, both being cut, causes vasodilatation on both sides (open columns), the larger effect being ipsilateral. After giving atropine (0.5–1.0 mg/kg IV) the responses are about halved (stippled columns, left). After giving the ganglionic blocking agent hexamethonium (0.5 mg/kg IV) in addition to atropine, the responses are again reduced but there is a residual vasodilatation (stippled columns, right), presumably due to sensory nerve stimulation. Ipsi., ipsilateral; Cont., contralateral. $*P < 0.05$; $**P < 0.01$ for change compared with zero effect. ☆ $P < 0.05$ for response after drug compared to response before drug. (From Laitinen et al., 1987b.)

1947; Lakshminarayanan et al., 1985) and sheep (Parsons et al., 1985). The tracheal circulation also responds to exogenous muscarinic agonists. Close arterial injection of acetylcholine into the dog tracheal circulation produces dose-dependent increases in tracheal blood flow (Himori and Taira, 1976). In addition, methacholine induces dose-dependent decreases in tracheal vascular pressure in dogs (Fig. 4) (Laitinen et al., 1987a) and sheep (Webber et al., 1989) when the tracheal circulation is perfused at constant flow. In contrast, methacholine fails to elicit any change in tracheal mucosal blood flow in sheep when administered as an aerosol, even when flow is first reduced by vasopressin (Barker et al., 1988); however, this negative result may be due to weak penetration of the drug through the thick tracheal mucosa to the vasculature.

The increase in bronchial blood flow in dogs with aerosolized methacholine (Lakshminarayanan et al., 1985) and the increased tracheal blood flow with intra-arterial acetylcholine (Himori and Taira, 1976) are significantly attentuated by atropine, suggesting they are mediated by stimulation of muscarinic receptors. It is not clear whether the agonists act directly on muscarinic receptors on the vascular smooth muscle to elicit relaxation or whether recep-

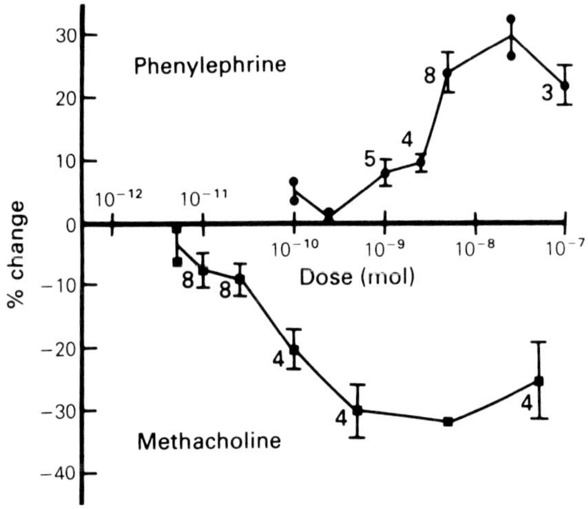

Figure 4 Dose-response curves for methacholine (■) and phenylephrine (●) showing dose (moles, abscissa scale) given by close-arterial injection against the percentage change in tracheal vascular resistance (ordinate scale) in dogs. Methacholine decreased vascular resistance, whereas phenylephrine increased it. Vasodilatation is downward. N values are shown against mean points, and the vertical lines are SEM. (From Laitinen et al., 1987a.)

tor stimulation leads to the release of endothelium-derived relaxing factor(s) (EDRF) as occurs in other vascular beds (Furchgott and Vanhoutte, 1989). Methacholine-induced increases in tracheal blood flow in sheep are abolished by pretreatment with oxyhemoglobin, which prevents the dilator action of EDRF (Fig. 5) (Corfield et al., 1991a). These last results suggest that, at least in the tracheal circulation, methacholine increases blood flow by stimulating muscarinic receptors to release EDRF.

It is also possible that the effects of muscarinic agonists on the tracheobronchial vasculature are secondary to the bronchoconstriction they produce (Lakshminarayanan et al., 1985). This seems unlikely, however, since other agonists (e.g., salbutamol) that do not contract airway smooth muscle can produce a potent vasodilation of the airway vasculature and agents that change smooth muscle tone do not always have a converse effect on vascular resistance (e.g., vasocative intestinal polypeptide, VIP).

Thus it is clear that exogenous application of muscarinic agonists potently dilates the tracheobronchial vasculature. It is still uncertain, however, whether the cholinergic parasympathetic nervous system plays a major role in the physiological regulation of airway blood flow.

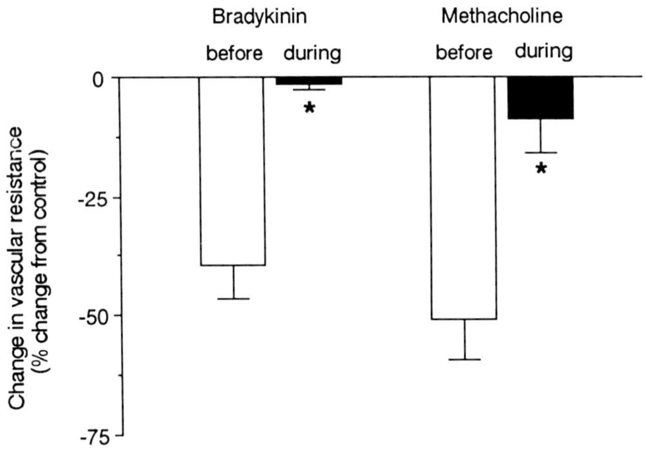

Figure 5 Effects of a local arterial infusion of oxyhemoglobin on the vasodilations produced by bradykinin and methacholine in anesthetized sheep. Open columns represent the response before and filled columns after oxyhemoglobin. The results are the means of four determinations, with the SEM shown by the vertical lines. *Significantly less than control value ($P < 0.05$, Wilcoxon signed-rank one-tailed test). (From Corfield et al., 1991a.)

B. Sympathetic Adrenergic Mechanisms

Nerve Stimulation

Physiological and pharmacological studies suggest that the main nervous control of the tracheobronchial circulation is by the sympathetic system. Stimulation of sympathetic nerves to the bronchial vasculature of dogs produces a potent vasoconstriction (De Letona et al., 1961; Aviado, 1963; Murao, 1965). Stimulation of sympathetic nerves to the tracheal vasculature of the dog when perfused at constant flow increases perfusion pressure, indicating vasoconstriction (Sahin et al., 1987).

Exogenous Agonists

Exogenous application of agonists with actions on α- and β-adrenoceptors has potent effects on the tracheobronchial vasculature. Close-arterial injections or infusions of epinephrine or norepinephrine into dog (Bruner and Schmidt, 1947; Himori and Taira, 1976; Lung et al., 1976) and sheep (Charan et al., 1985; Link et al., 1985; Parsons et al., 1985) bronchial arteries markedly reduce bronchial blood flow. The reduced bronchial blood flow produced by epinephrine in the dog (Himori and Taira, 1976) is blocked by phentolamine, suggesting it is mediated by α-receptors. Similarly, the relatively specific α-adrenoceptor agonist phenylephrine reduces bronchial blood flow in the sheep when administered as an aerosol (Barker et al., 1988); this response is also blocked by phentolamine. Phenylephrine also increases perfusion pressure in the dog when the tracheal circulation is perfused at constant flow, indicating vasoconstriction (Fig. 4) (Laitinen et al., 1987a).

Clearly, agonists that act on α-adrenoceptors are powerful constrictors in the tracheobronchial circulation, and it seems likely that the reduction in bronchial blood flow on sympathetic nerve stimulation is mediated by α-receptors. β-Receptors are present on bronchial arteries in large numbers, however (Carstairs et al., 1984). These receptors may respond to mediators released from sympathetic nerves or to circulating catecholamines. Exogenously applied β-adrenoceptor agonists certainly have potent effects on the bronchial vasculature. Closed-arterial injection of isoproterenol into dog (Lung et al., 1976; Himori and Taira, 1976) and sheep (Parsons et al., 1985; Barker et al., 1988) bronchial circulations produces a large increase in bronchial blood flow. These effects are blocked by propranolol, suggesting they are mediated by β-adrenoceptors. Furthermore, salbutamol, a more specific β_2-agonist, reduces tracheal perfusion pressure, indicating vasodilation in both the dog (Laitinen et al., 1987a) and sheep (Webber et al., 1989).

C. Nonadrenergic, Noncholinergic Mechanisms

There is now considerable evidence from anatomic and histological studies that both the parasympathetic and sympathetic nervous systems to the airways, including to the airway vasculature, release transmitters that are nonadrenergic and noncholinergic (NANC) in nature. The transmitters of these NANC systems are thought to be neuropeptides. Vasoactive intestinal polypeptide and peptide histidine isoleucine (PHI; peptide histidine methionine, PHM, in the human) probably coexist with acetylcholine in parasympathetic motor nerves to the airway vasculature (Lundberg et al., 1984). Similarly, neuropeptide Y (NPY) probably coexists with norepinephrine in sympathetic motor nerves (Lundberg et al., 1987). In addition, there is a third type of nerve in the airway, the sensory (including C fiber) nerves, which also innervate the vasculature. The transmitters of these sensory nerves include the peptides substance P (SP), neurokinin A (NKA), neurokinin B (NKB), and calcitonin gene-related peptide (CGRP) (Hua et al., 1985b). All these neuropeptides, except NKB in some species, have been identified by immunohistochemical methods and shown to be localized to nerves in the airway mucosa of humans and many experimental animals, often concentrated around blood vessels (Uddman and Sundler, 1986, 1987; Karlsson and Persson, 1990). It should be noted that the absence of histological identification of a neuropeptide at a vascular site does not necessarily mean it has no action on the blood vessel, since it may be released from other sites and diffuse to the blood vessels. Results from physiological and pharmacological studies (nerve stimulation or exogenous application of peptides) however suggest that the neuropeptides may play an important role in the control of the tracheobronchial vasculature.

Nerve Stimulation

Parasympathetic Nerves

Stimulation of the parasympathetic nervous supply (superior laryngeal nerve) to the tracheal vasculature of cat, pig, and dog causes vasodilation. In the pig and dog this is partially blocked by atropine (Figs. 1 and 2), indicating that a component is due to the release of acetylcholine (see earlier). The residual vasodilation is also partially blocked by hexamethonium (Fig. 2) or other ganglionic blocking agents, however, indicating the release of a parasympathetic motor neuropeptide, such as VIP or PHI (Laitinen et al., 1987a; Matran et al., 1989b). In the cat, the tracheal vasodilation is entirely noncholinergic (Martling et al., 1985).

With regard to the bronchial vasculature, parasympathetic stimulation causes vasodilation in the pig and cat (see earlier). This vasodilation is not affected by atropine, however, suggesting it is noncholinergic, and is also unaffected by hexamethonium, suggesting it is not mediated by the release of a parasympathetic motor neuropeptide (Martling et al., 1985; Matran et al., 1989b). It is likely that these particular responses are mediated almost entirely by the release of sensory neuropeptides (see later).

Sympathetic Nerves

There seem to have been no studies on the effect of stimulation of sympathetic nerves with release of sympathetic neuropeptides on the tracheal or bronchial vasculature, probably because of difficulties in the surgical approach to the sympathetic supply to this tissue. Early experiments establish that these nerves are vasoconstrictive, with evidence that the transmitter is norepinephrine, (see earlier), but the possible involvement of NPY was not tested (Daly and Hebb, 1966) because its role elsewhere had not been identified at that time.

Neurogenic Inflammation

There has been much research in recent years on the effect of sensory neuropeptides on the tracheobronchial vasculature. Much of this is in relation to extravasation of protein into the interstitial space, that is, neurogenic inflammation and edema, discussed in detail elsewhere (McDonald, 1987; Persson and Erjefalt, 1988; Karlsson and Persson, 1990). Extensive studies by Persson and his colleagues show that this extravasation occurs mainly from the postcapillary venules and that the liquid and protein may flow into the airway lumen (Persson and Erjefelt, 1986). The main methods of study are (1) antidromic stimulation of nerves to the airways in the presence of ganglionic blocking agents to prevent the release of motor transmitters, and often in the presence of anticholinergic and antiadrenergic agents as well; (2) stimulation of sensory nerves to release their neuropeptides by such agents as capsaicin, by such mediators as bradykinin and histamine, and by such irritants as cigarette smoke, ammonia, and ether; and (3) testing the responses to the same stimuli when sensory, presumed C fiber nerves have been made to degenerate by large doses of capsaicin. In general, the results of all three methods lead to the same conclusion, that activation of sensory receptors in the airway mucosa causes local release of neurotransmitters (including SP, NKA, NKB, and CGRP), which among other actions produce vasodilation. At the same time, stimulation of these nerves when intact sets up reflexes that are usually vasodilating to the airway mucosa but may involve far larger parts of the respiratory tract than the local area where the stimulus is applied.

As indicated earlier, antidromic stimulation of parasympathetic nerves, such as the vagus and superior laryngeal nerves, causes vasodilation and extravasation of protein in the presence of atropine and of ganglionic blocking agents, suggesting that the response is due to the release of sensory neuropeptides (Persson and Erjefalt, 1986, 1988; McDonald, 1987; Lundberg et al., 1990). This view is supported by the fact that (1) the extravasation is prevented by large doses of capsaicin that deplete sensory nerves of their neuropeptides, and (2) the responses are mimicked by application of sensory neuropeptides. Such results have been obtained mainly in the rat and guinea pig, species especially susceptible to neurogenic edema and inflammation. Similar experiments on the bronchial circulation of the cat and pig suggest that this vasodilation due to sensory neuropeptides is the dominant neural mechanism, with appreciable components of control due to parasympathetic or sympathetic motor neuropeptides (Martling et al., 1985, 1988; Matran et al., 1989b). Application of small doses of capsaicin, cigarette smoke, and inflammatory mediators to the tracheobronchial mucosa of rats and guinea pigs causes neurogenic edema. In the dog and pig there is usually mucosal vasodilation with no evidence of edema. The release of sensory neuropeptides is thought to mediate these responses.

Exogenous Application of Neuropeptides

VIP, PHI, and PHM all increase tracheal blood flow, as do the sensory neuropeptides, (Fig. 6) (Laitinen et al., 1987a, d; Salonen et al., 1988; Matran et al., 1989a). The relative order of potency is NKA > VIP > CGRP > SP > PHI in the dog, and in the pig VIP is 10 times more active than PHI. NPY decreases blood flow in the dog (Fig. 7) (Salonen et al., 1988). In dog trachea the vasodilation with SP and VIP is not associated with an appreciable increase in mucosal thickness (Laitinen et al., 1986). Under these particular conditions and with these doses of neuropeptides the dominant effect seems to be an increase in blood flow rather than interstitial fluid volume. Bombesin, found in airway epithelium, also constricts the tracheal vasculature, but galanin, found in motor and sensory nerves, has no effect (Salonen et al., 1988).

There have been fewer studies on the effect of neuropeptides on the bronchial vessels, but McCormack et al. (1989) tested them on the isolated dog bronchial artery. The order of potency was SP > NKA > CGRP > NKB. It is not clear why the order of potency is different for the tracheal vasculature in vivo compared with the bronchial vasculature in vitro, both for the dog. There may be a true difference between the vascular tissues, or there may be some methodological reason. It is interesting that, for the dog bronchial artery in vitro, NPY, a powerful constrictor of the tracheal vasculature in vivo (Salonen et al., 1988), has no consistent effect.

With the bronchial circulation in vivo, SP, CGRP, and VIP all cause vasodilation (Martling et al., 1988), although the last is less active at this site than in the trachea, at least for the pig. The action of NKA on this preparation does not seem to have been studied.

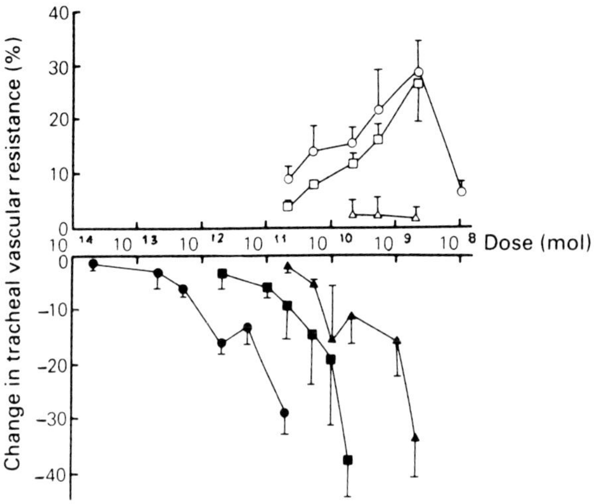

Figure 6 Dose-response curves showing the effects of the neuropeptides on tracheal vascular resistance in dogs. Five to six doses of each neuropeptide (only three doses of galanin) were injected into the arterial catheters supplying the tracheal vascular bed: (○) bombesin, (□) neuropeptide Y, (△) galanin, (●) neurokinin A, (■) calcitonin gene-related peptide, and (▲) peptide histidine isoleucine. The values presented are mean percentage changes from control values in three to four separate dogs; vertical lines indicate SEM. (From Salonen et al., 1988.)

III. Nonneural Mediators and the Tracheobronchial Circulation

A. Histamine

Histamine is probably the best characterized of all nonneural mediators of inflammation in the airways (Table 1). It is formed by the decarboxylation of histidine and stored in preformed cytoplasmic granules of mast cells and basophils in close connection with proteoglycans; these are mainly heparin in mast cells and chrondroitin 4-sulfate in basophils. Histamine is released from mast cells or basophils by an active secretory process in response to a number of stimuli, including cold air or allergen challenge (Freidman and Kaliner, 1987). When released, histamine exerts its effects in the airways by interacting with specific receptors on target cells. Histamine is a potent constrictor of human tracheal and bronchial smooth muscle in vitro (Schild et al., 1951; Finney et al., 1985) and contracts airway smooth muscle from other species both in vitro and in vivo (Castillo and Debeer, 1947; Drazen and Austen, 1974). The contractile effect of histamine on airway smooth muscle is mediated through H_1-

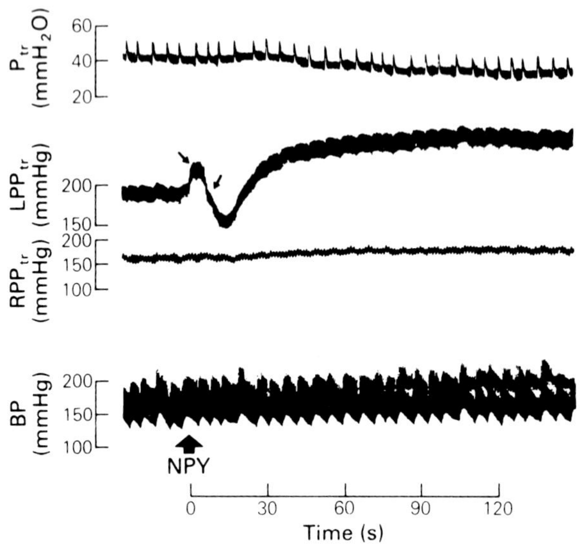

Figure 7 Tracheal vascular response to neuropeptide Y (NPY, 2 nmol) injected into the arterial catheter supplying the left side of the tracheal vascular bed of a dog. A long-lasting increase in left arterial perfusion pressure (LPPtr) is seen after two transient artifacts (small arrows); the initial increase in perfusion pressure is due to injection, and the subsequent decrease is caused by lowered viscosity of the blood due to the saline. There are also a small increase in right arterial perfusion pressure (RPPtr) and a decrease in intratracheal pressure (Ptr; not seen in two other dogs) but no change in systemic arterial blood pressure (BP). (From Salonen et al., 1988.)

receptor activation (Schild et al., 1951). There is some evidence from animal studies that histamine can also stimulate H_2-receptors to induce bronchodilation (Chand and Eyre, 1975), but the relevance of this action in the human is unclear. Histamine also increases microvascular permeability in the airways via H_1-receptors (Brigham and Owen, 1975), stimulates mucus secretion probably by activation of H_2-receptors (Webber and Widdicombe, 1987; Shelhamer et al., 1980), and vasoconstricts the pulmonary circulation (H_1-receptors) (Tucker et al., 1975). A third type of histamine receptor (H_3) was identified by radioligand binding studies in the brain (Arrang et al., 1987). Stimulation of this receptor inhibits cholinergic neurotransmission in the airways (Barnes and Ichinose, 1989).

For the sheep tracheal vasculature perfused at constant flow, we found that histamine has a complex action (Webber et al., 1988). In 40% of sheep, close-arterial injections of histamine produces a short-lasting vasoconstriction that is dose dependent (Fig. 8a). In the remaining 60% of sheep histamine has

Table 1 Effects of Nonneural Mediators on the Tracheobronchial Circulation

Mediator	Species	Vascular Response	Receptor
Histamine	Sheep	Dilation, constriction	H_1
		Dilation	H_2
	Dog	Dilation	?
Serotonin	Sheep	Dilation	$5HT_1$
	Sheep	Constriction	$5HT_2$
Prostaglandins			
PGE_2	Dog	Dilation	?
$PGF_{2\alpha}$	Dog	Dilation	?
PGI_2	Dog	Dilation	?
Leukotrienes			
LTC_4	Sheep	Constriction	?
LTD_4	Sheep	Constriction	?
LTE_4	Sheep	Constriction	?
PAF	Dog	Dilation	?
	Sheep	Dilation	?
Bradykinin	Sheep	Dilation	B_2

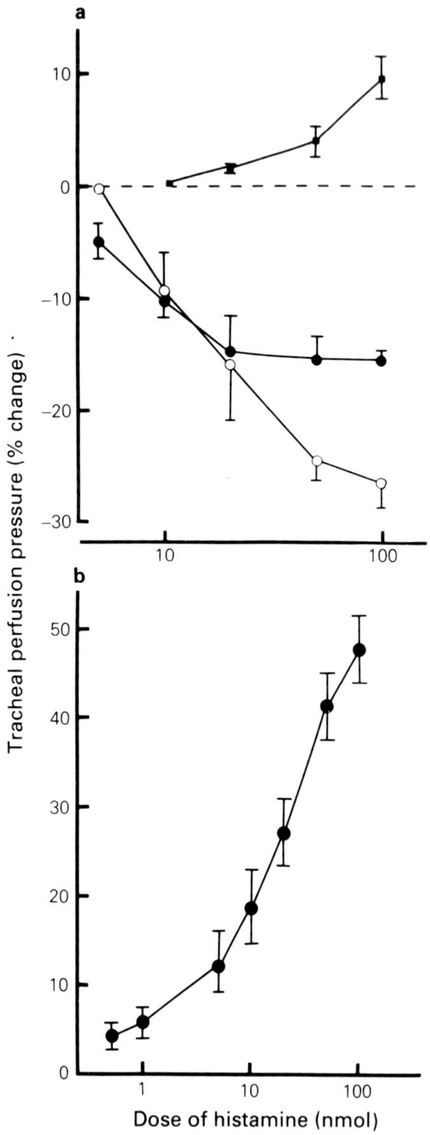

Figure 8 Dose-response curves for (a) the triphasic effect of closed-arterial injections of histamine on tracheal vascular resistance in sheep: (●) early dilatation (maximum at 20 s); (■) constriction (50–60 s); and (○) late dilatation (3–5 min). (b) The constrictor effect of histamine on tracheal vascular resistance. Points are the means of three to four determinations, and the vertical lines represent SEM. (From Webber et al., 1988.)

a triphasic effect, an initial vasodilation followed by a vasoconstriction and then a further long-lasting vasodilation. All phases of this response are dose dependent (Fig. 8b). The long-lasting vasodilation is blocked by bilateral cervical vagotomy, but the mechanism of this effect is not known. The short-lasting initial vasodilation and the vasoconstriction are both unaffected by the H_2-receptor antagonist cimetidine but are blocked by mepyramine, suggesting H_1-receptor–mediated effects (Fig. 9). Although H_2-receptors do not seem to be involved in the responses of sheep tracheal vasculature to histamine, direct stimulation of H_2-receptors with the specific H_2-receptor agonist dimaprit produces a tracheal vasodilation (Webber et al., 1988). Histamine has a less complex action on dog tracheal vasculature, producing only short-lasting vasodilations that are dose-dependent (Laitinen et al., 1987a); the receptors mediating this effect are not known.

Histamine has a simpler action on sheep and pig bronchial circulations than on sheep tracheal circulation. An increase in bronchial blood flow is

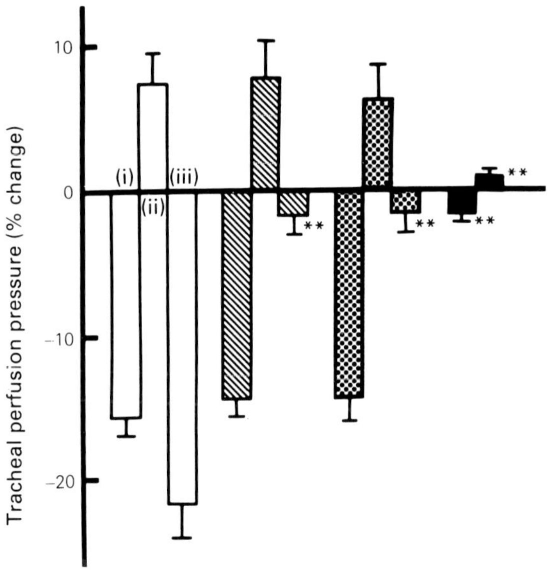

Figure 9 Effect of vagotomy (hatched columns), cimetidine (250 mg, IV, stippled columns), and mepyramine (50 mg IV, solid columns) on (i) early dilatation, (ii) constriction, and (iii) late dilatation induced by closed-arterial injections of histamine into the tracheal circulation of sheep. The results are the means of 5–11 determinations, with SEM shown by vertical lines. **Highly significantly different ($P < 0.01$) from control value (open columns) by Student's paired *t*-test. (From Webber et al., 1988.)

observed when histamine is injected intravenously in the sheep (Parsons et al., 1989) or pig (Matran et al., 1989a), when it is injected directly into the sheep bronchial artery (De Letona et al., 1961; Link et al., 1985), or when it is administered by aerosol inhalation to sheep (Long et al., 1985b). The method of measuring bronchial blood flow also makes no difference to the response observed with histamine. Thus an increase in flow in sheep is seen with histamine when flow is measured using an electromagnetic flow probe (Baier et al., 1985; Long et al., 1985b), video dilution technique (Link et al., 1985), or laser Doppler flowmetry (Parsons et al., 1989).

Unlike the actions of histamine on the tracheal circulation of sheep that are mediated by H_1-receptors, the increase in sheep bronchial blood flow with aerosolized histamine measured using an electromagnetic flow probe (Long et al., 1985b) is not affected by H_1-receptors antagonists. These responses are blocked by H_2-receptor antagonists, suggesting H_2-receptor–mediated effects. In contrast, the increased bronchial blood flow observed with intravenous histamine and measured using the laser Doppler technique is blocked by an H_1-receptor antagonist and is not affected by H_2-antagonists (Parsons et al., 1989). Clearly, the receptors mediating the action of histamine on the tracheobronchial vasculature depend on the part of the vasculature being studied, the method used to study the vasculature, and the route of administration of histamine.

The effect of H_3-receptor stimulation on the control of the tracheobronchial vasculture by parasympathetic nerve stimulation has not been investigated, so it is not known if histamine released in airway inflammation can modify cholinergic-induced vasodilation by acting on H_3-receptors on the parasympathetic cholinergic ganglia. However, the limited effectiveness of antihistaminic drugs in the treatment of clinical asthma suggests that histamine-induced mucosal thickening due to hyperemia and edema is probably not the major cause of airway narrowing in this condition (Lewiston et al., 1982).

B. Serotonin

Serotonin (5-hydroxytryptamine, 5HT) is formed by the decarboxylation of dietary tryptophan and is stored in secretory granules. In rodents serotonin is present in mast cell granules, but this is not the case in larger animals, such as dogs, sheep, or humans (Parrott and West, 1957). 5HT in human airways is principally localized to epithelial neuroendocrine cells and the dense secretory granules of platelets (Sirek and Sirek, 1970). Recently the role of platelets in inflammatory airway diseases, such as asthma, has been reappraised with the identification of a platelet activating factor (PAF; see later). The bronchoconstriction, mucosal edema, and hyperemia produced by PAF may be due to the release of 5HT from platelets (Morley et al., 1984).

Exogenously applied 5HT has a potent bronchoconstrictive effect in several species, including guinea pig, cat, rat, dog, sheep, and monkey (Table 1) (Brocklehurst, 1975; Simonsson and Svedmyr, 1981; Selig et al., 1988). Its effects on human airway caliber are variable: constriction (Panzini, 1962), no effect (Cushley et al., 1986), and dilation (Raffestin et al., 1985) have all been reported. 5HT also causes microvascular leakage into guinea pig airways (Saria et al., 1983) and is a powerful vasoconstrictor of the pulmonary circulation (Raffestin et al., 1985; Selig et al., 1988).

At least three types of receptor mediate the actions of 5HT, and there are probably subdivisions of these receptors. $5HT_1$-receptors are inhibitory or excitatory, whereas $5HT_2$-receptors are always excitatory and usually mediate smooth muscle contraction. $5HT_3$-receptors are present on nerves and stimulate neurotransmitter release from certain peripheral nerves (Richardson and Engel, 1986). The bronchoconstriction produced by 5HT is mediated either by $5HT_1$-receptors (Webber et al., 1990) or $5HT_2$-receptors (Selig et al., 1988).

The first report of the effect of 5HT on the bronchial circulation was by Horisberger and Rodbard (1960). They isolated and perfused a segment of aorta in dogs that contained the main bronchial artery branches. Blood flow through this segment was measured with a rotameter. Injections of 5HT (1 μg/kg) into the aorta increased bronchial artery blood flow up to three times. In contrast, De Letona et al. (1961), using the same method as Horisberger and Rodbard, found that 5HT has a variable effect on dog bronchial blood flow. In three dogs an increase in flow was seen, whereas in the other five dogs a decrease was observed. Despite these early reports, until recently there was no systematic examination of the effects of 5HT on the tracheobronchial circulation.

We examined the effect of 5HT on the perfused tracheal circulation of sheep. Like histamine, 5HT has a complex action on tracheal blood flow (Webber et al., 1990). In 55% of sheep 5HT dose dependently constricts the tracheal vasculature (Fig. 10a). In the remaining 45% of sheep a rapid vasoconstriction is followed by a more prolonged vasodilation (Fig. 10b). The vasodilator effect of 5HT on sheep tracheal vasculature is interesting since only constrictor responses to 5HT have been observed in the pulmonary circulation. However, some systemic vessels relax on addition of 5HT in vitro (Stewart et al., 1987) and in vivo (Chu and Cobb, 1987). The 5HT-induced vasoconstrictions are blocked by ketanserin ($5HT_2$-receptor antagonist), suggesting they were mediated by $5HT_2$-receptors (Fig. 11). The vasodilation is not affected by ketanserin but is blocked by methysergide (combined $5HT_1$ and $5HT_2$-receptor antagonist), indicating a $5HT_1$-receptor effect (Fig. 11). The

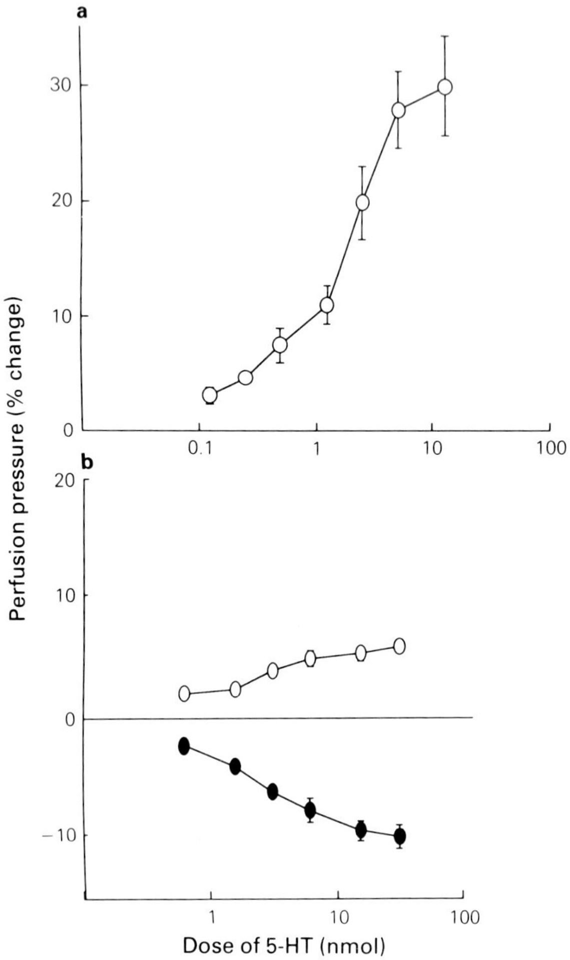

Figure 10 Dose-response curves for (a) the constrictor only effect of serotonin (5HT) on the tracheal vasculature of anesthetized sheep (maximum at 30–40 s), and (b) the biphasic effect of 5HT on the tracheal vasculature: (○) early constriction (maximum at 20–30 s); and (●) later dilatation (2.5–3 min). Points are means of four to eight determinations, and the vertical lines represent SEM. (From Webber et al., 1990.)

5HT-induced relaxation of rabbit coronary arteries occurs by $5HT_1$-receptor–mediated release of an endothelium-derived relaxing factor (Stewart et al., 1987). This possibility cannot be ruled out for the $5HT_1$-induced vasodilation of the tracheal vasculature but has not yet been examined. The selective

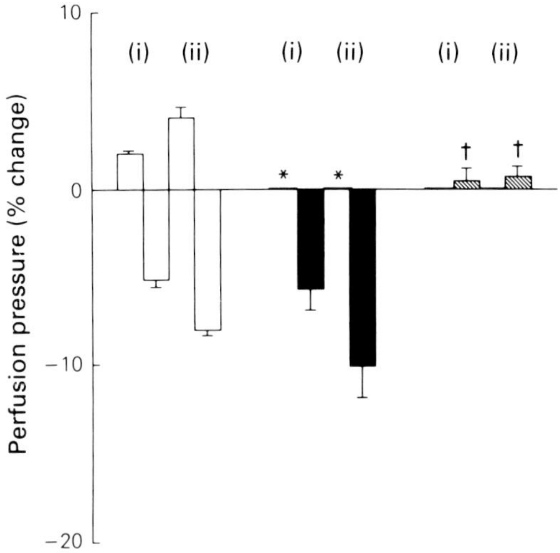

Figure 11 Effect of the $5HT_2$-antagonist ketanserin (0.5 mg/kg IV; solid columns) and ketanserin plus the $5HT_1$-antagonist methysergide (1 mg/kg IV; hatched columns) on the early vasoconstriction and later dilatation produced by (i) control low and (ii) control high doses of 5HT. Open columns, response without antagonists. The results are the means of four to six determinations, with SEM shown by vertical lines. *Significantly different ($P < 0.05$) from control value (open column) and †significantly different from value in the presence of ketanserin alone (solid column) by Student's paired *t*-test. (From Webber et al., 1990.)

$5HT_3$-receptor agonist 2-methyl-5HT has no significant effect on the tracheal vasculature, suggesting a lack of involvement of $5HT_3$-receptors in this tissue (Webber et al., 1989).

The effects of 5HT on the dog tracheal vasculature, the bronchial circulation in general, and the receptors mediating these effects remain to be investigated.

C. Bradykinin

Bradykinin is generated from kininogens in plasma by the action of kininogenase enzymes, which are produced by the liver (plasma kallikrein) or other tissues (tissue kallikrein). In addition, human lung mast cells and basophils produce another kininogenase distinct from kallikreins (Proud et al., 1983). At least two receptors mediate the actions of bradykinin and related kinins. These receptors are classified on the basis of agonist potency ratios. Thus, B_1-

receptors are selectively activated by lys-bradykinin and des-Arg-bradykinin, whereas B_2-receptors are more potently stimulated by bradykinin itself (Regoli and Barabe, 1980).

Bradykinin is a powerful bronchoconstrictor agent in vivo in guinea pigs (Collier and Shorley, 1960) and asthmatic humans (Simonsson et al., 1973; Newball et al., 1975; Fuller et al., 1987), but not in healthy individuals (Simonsson et al., 1973). Bradykinin has little effect on airway smooth muscle in vitro (Fuller et al., 1987), suggesting that the in vivo bronchoconstrictive action may be indirect. The bronchoconstriction in guinea pigs is blocked by cyclooxygenase inhibitors, suggesting the involvement of prostaglandins or thromboxane (Collier and Shorley, 1960). In contrast, the bronchoconstriction in asthmatic humans is resistant to aspirin but is partially blocked by anticholinergic agents, such as atropine, suggesting a vagal reflex mechanism (Fuller et al., 1987). Bradykinin also causes microvascular leakage in guinea pig airways (Dijk et al., 1988; Saria et al., 1983) and is a potent stimulant of ion transport across canine tracheal epithelium (Leikauf et al., 1985). This latter effect is blocked by indomethacin. Furthermore, bradykinin releases PGE_2 from canine tracheal epithelium (Leikauf et al., 1985).

Bradykinin and lys-bradykinin strongly increase tracheal blood flow in the sheep when measured using an electromagnetic flow probe (Table 1) (Corfield et al., 1991a). Bradykinin is slightly more potent than lys-bradykinin, suggesting that the vasodilation is mediated by stimulation of B_2-receptors (Fig. 12). The vasodilations produced by bradykinin and lys-bradykinin are extremely long-lasting (>10 min), indicating that, like the in vivo bronchoconstriction in guinea pigs and the increased tracheal ion transport in the dog, they occur by an indirect mechanism. Unlike the bronchoconstriction and increased ion transport, however, the tracheal vasodilations produced by the kinins are not blocked by indomethacin, indicating that this effect is not mediated by kinin-induced release of prostaglandins or thromboxane. The increased tracheal blood flow with the kinins is prevented by prior perfusion of the tracheal vasculature with hemoglobin (which inactivates preformed EDRF; Fig. 5). It therefore seems that the kinins stimulate B_2-receptors to release EDRF, which dilates the tracheal blood vessels and produces an increase in tracheal blood flow.

Bradykinin is also a potent vasodilator of the dog tracheal circulation when perfused at constant flow (Laitinen et al., 1987a) and of the pig tracheal circulation when measured with a transonic blood flowmeter (Matran et al., 1989a). The action of the kinins on the bronchial circulation has been little studied, although bradykinin increases pig bronchial blood flow (Matran et al., 1989a). The receptors mediating the effects of bradykinin and the mechanism of action of bradykinin on dog and pig tracheal blood flow and bronchial blood flow in general have not been investigated.

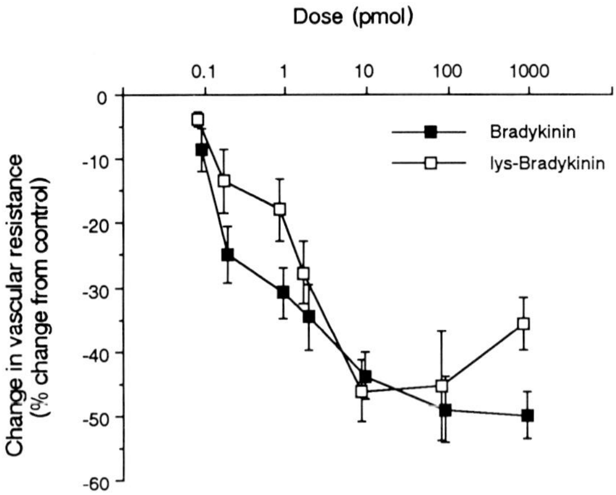

Figure 12 Dose-response curves showing the effects of bradykinin and lys-bradykinin on tracheal vascular resistance in anesthetized sheep. Points are means of four to eight determinations; the vertical lines represent SEM. (From Corfield et al., 1990b.)

D. Cyclooxygenase and Lipoxygenase Products

Arachidonic acid is the precursor for prostaglandins, thromboxanes, leukotrienes and several hydroxyacids. It is formed by the action of phospholipase A_2 on cell membrane phospholipids (Barnes et al., 1988). The synthesis of arachidonic acid is the rate-limiting step that determines the amount of substrate available for prostaglandin and leukotriene synthesis (Lands and Samuelsson, 1968).

Arachidonic acid is oxidized by cyclooxgenase to form PGG_2, which is then reduced to PGH_2, which is unstable and gives rise to $PGF_{2\alpha}$, PGE_2, and PGD_2. Other enzymatic pathways of PGG_2 and PGH_2 lead to the formation of thromboxane A_2 (TXA_2) and prostacyclin (PGI_2). Lipoxygenation of arachidonic acid initiates the formation of leukotrienes and hydroeicosatetraenoic acids (HETE). The initial compounds generated from arachidonic acid by lipoxygenase are hydroperoxyeicosatetraenoic acids (HPETE), which can be reduced by peroxidases to HETE or catalyzed by 5-lipoxygenase to form LTA_4. LTA_4 is unstable and is hydrolyzed to LTB_4 or oxygenated with glutathione to LTC_4 . LTC_4 can be converted to LTD_4, which can be further metabolized to LTE_4 (Parker et al., 1980).

In the airways, cyclooxygenase and lipoxygenase products can be released from almost any cell, including mast cells, basophils, neutrophils, macrophages, eosinophils, and endothelial and epithelial cells. When released, these compounds have potent effects on the airways. The prostanoids PGD_2,

PGF_2, and TXA_2 all contract airway smooth muscle in vitro (Gardner and Collier; 1980; Black et al., 1986) and in vivo (Wasserman and Griffin, 1976), as do LTC_4 and LTD_4 (Dahlen et al., 1980; Barnes et al., 1984). In contrast, PGE_1 relaxes airway smooth muscle in vitro (Adaikan and Karim, 1979) and PGE_1 and $PGF_{2\alpha}$ are bronchodilators in vivo (Kawakami et al., 1973).

PGD_2, PGF_2, LTC_4, and LTD_4 all increase the output of mucus glycoprotein from human airways (Marom et al., 1981; 1982), whereas PGE_2 has an inhibitory effect (Marom et al., 1981. The effects of cyclooxygenase products on airways vascular permeability have not been systematically studied. LTC_4, LTD_4, and LTE_4 all potently increase microvascular permeability in the airways of guinea pigs (Hua et al., 1985a).

PGE_1, $PGF_{2\alpha}$, and PGD_2 are all powerful vasodilators of the dog tracheal circulation when injected closed-arterially (Fig. 13 and Table 1) (Laitinen et al., 1987 a, c). Inhaled $PGF_{2\alpha}$ also increases bronchial blood flow in the dog (Lakshminarayan et al., 1985). PGI_2 increases bronchial blood flow in dogs when given as an infusion into the pulmonary artery (Deffebach et al., 1986), although its effect on the tracheal circulation is unknown. Similarly, although thromboxane A_2 is a potent vasoconstrictor of the pulmonary circulation, its effect on tracheobronchial blood flow has not been examined.

Leukotrienes C_4 and D_4 decrease bronchial blood flow in the sheep (Long et al., 1986), and leukotriene C_4 is a vasoconstrictor of the sheep tracheal circulation when injected closed-arterially (Table 1) (Webber et al., 1989). The effects of leukotrienes B_4 and E_4 on tracheobronchial blood flow have not been examined.

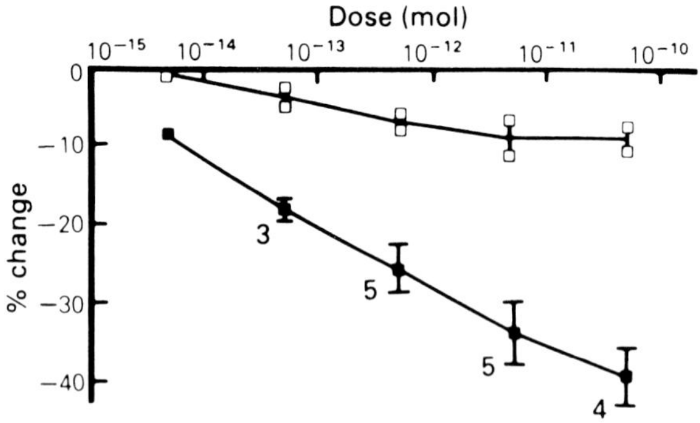

Figure 13 Dose-response curves for PGE_1 showing decreases in vascular resistance (ordinate scale) against dose (abscissa scale) in dogs: (■) ipsilateral side into which drug was injected; (□) contralateral side. Points are the means of the values shown, with SEM as vertical lines. (From Laitinen et al., 1987a.)

E. Platelet Activating Factor

Platelet activating factor is released from a number of inflammatory cells in the airways. When released it exerts its effects via specific membrane receptors on target cells (Braquet and Godfroid, 1986). PAF is a potent inducer of bronchoconstriction in vivo in experimental animals (Table 1) and humans (Cuss et al., 1986; Morley et al., 1984); this effect seems to depend on the presence of circulating platelets (Vargaftig et al., 1980). PAF does not contract airway smooth muscle in vitro (Schellenberg, 1987) but is a powerful inducer of microvascular leakage in the airways (Evans et al., 1987) and has a weak stimulatory effect on tracheal submucosal gland secretion (Lang et al., 1987). Perhaps the most important property of PAF, and the reason it is thought to be such an important mediator in inflammatory airway diseases, is its ability to produce a nonselective and long-lasting increase in bronchial hyperresponsiveness in experimental animals and humans (Cuss et al., 1986). Many of the effects of PAF in the airways, including hyperresponsiveness, are probably due to its potent chemotactic action on other inflammatory cells, such as eosinophils and platelets, and to its ability to produce a secondary release of other inflammatory mediators, such as 5HT, prostaglandins, leukotrienes, bradykinin, and oxygen radicals, from these cells (Barnes et al., 1988). Despite the importance of PAF in inflammatory airway disease and although PAF has been shown to be a weak vasodilator in the dog tracheal vasculature (Laitinen et al., 1987a) and to increase tracheal blood flow in the sheep (Corfield, Webber, and Widdicombe, unpublished observations), its actions on the tracheobronchial circulation in general have not been investigated in detail.

F. Other Mediators

Other mediators, such as adenosine, complement fragments, and oxygen radicals, are released in the airways particularly when there is inflammation, and they may be important regulators of airway blood flow both in health and in inflammatory airway disease. The oxygen radical H_2O_2 relaxes pulmonary vascular smooth muscle in vitro (Greenberg et al., 1986), and both H_2O_2 (Del Maestro et al., 1981) and the complement fragments (Dias da Silva and Lepow, 1967) are strong stimulants of microvascular leakage. Although adenosine was reported to lower tracheal blood pressure (Johnson and McNee, 1985), the direct action of these mediators on tracheal and bronchial blood flow has not been fully examined. Blood-borne hormones may also affect the tracheobronchial vasculature. Epinephrine is a powerful vasoconstrictor (see earlier), as is exogenous vasopressin (Barker et al., 1988; Wanner et al., 1990). Whether these hormones are active endogenously is not known.

IV. Allergen Challenge

In susceptible individuals inhalation of a specific antigen results in an immediate bronchoconstriction (early response) that peaks at 10 min and recovers by 60–90 min. This constriction is sometimes followed by more prolonged increases in airflow resistance (late response) that begin 6–12 h after antigen inhalation. This later response is associated with the development of inflammation in the airways and hyperresponsiveness of airway tissues.

The tracheobronchial circulation may play an important role in the response of the airways to allergen challenge in several ways. It may be involved in edema formation during the inflammatory phase of the allergen response, and it may regulate the penetration and clearance of inflammatory mediators released after antigen challenge. The inhalation of antigen certainly has effects on the human airway vasculature because the mucosa is often red, indicating hyperemia.

A. Allergen and the Tracheobronchial Circulation

Many sheep are spontaneously sensitive to *Ascaris suum* antigen, and we have used the model of the sheep perfused trachea to investigate the effects of local closed-arterial injections of ascaris on the tracheal circulation (Webber et al., 1989). Airway and vascular smooth muscle sometimes lose sensitivity to chemical mediators released during aging. It was not known, however, if aging affects airway responses to allergen challenge. The tracheal vascular effects of allergen were therefore investigated in two groups of sheep, the first group 1 year old and the second group 5 years old. The sheep were shown to be sensitive to the antigen by a skin test. Close-arterial injection of ascaris in young sheep produces a rapid vasodilation that persists for 5–10 min. The vasodilation depends on the dose of antigen injected (Fig. 14). In contrast, in the older sheep ascaris produces a vasoconstriction that has a time course similar to that of vasodilation in young sheep and is also dose dependent (Fig. 14).

The effects of allergen challenge on bronchial blood flow have been studied in sheep and pigs that are spontaneously sensitive to ascaris. The ascaris delivered as an aerosol produces a rapid increase in blood flow in sheep (Long et al., 1988) and pigs (Alving et al., 1988), which lasts for up to 1 h. In sheep, this is followed by a second increase in bronchial blood flow 5 h after challenge that persists for several hours (Long et al., 1985a). The rapid increases in bronchial blood flow in the sheep and pig are consistent with the vasodilation observed with antigen in the tracheal circulation of young sheep but are at variance with the vasoconstriction seen in the older sheep.

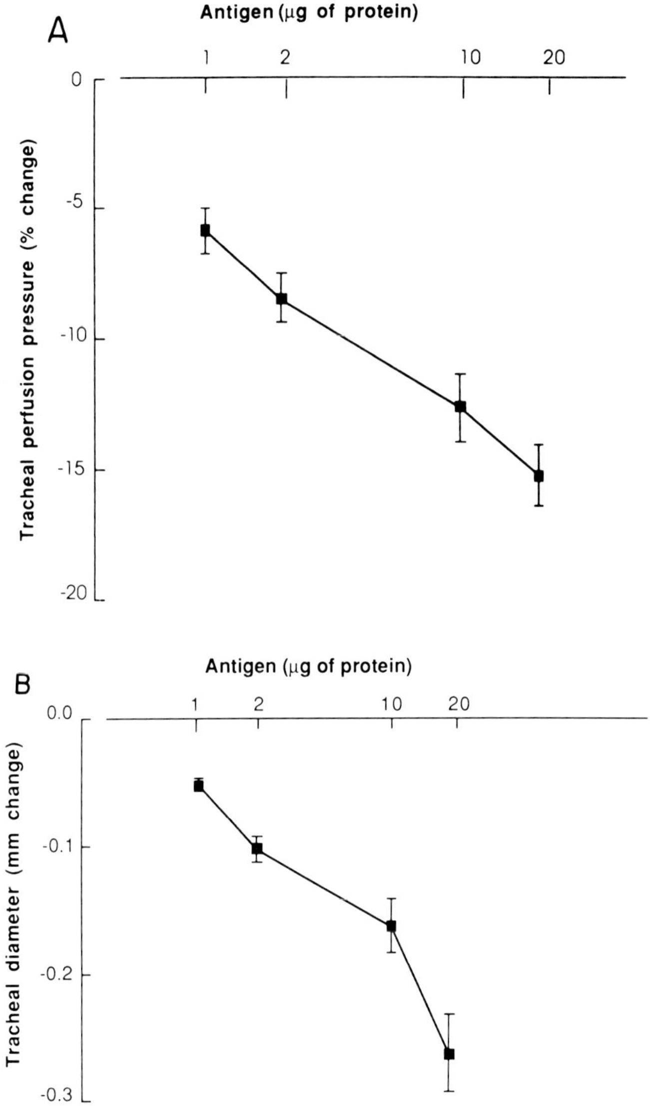

Figure 14 Dose-response curves showing the effect of close-arterial injections of *Ascaris* antigen on (A) tracheal perfusion pressure and (B) tracheal diameter in young sheep. Doses of antigen are given in micrograms of protein. Three or four different doses of antigen were given once to each sheep. The values shown are mean percentage changes from control values obtained in 8–12 sheep. Vertical lines represent SEM. (From Webber et al., 1989.)

B. Mechanisms of Allergen-Induced Effects on the Tracheobronchial Vasculature

The vasodilation of the tracheal circulation in young sheep and the vasoconstriction in older sheep are not affected by the H_1-receptor antagonist mepyramine or the H_2-receptor antagonist cimetidine, suggesting they are not mediated by antigen-induced release of histamine from mast cells in the airways (Fig. 15). Similarly, antihistamines have only a very weak antagonist effect on the immediate increase in sheep bronchial blood flow produced by ascaris (Long et al., 1988). The tracheal vasodilation in young sheep and the vasoconstriction in older sheep are both attenuated by the cyclooxygenase inhibitor indomethacin and further reduced by the leukotriene receptor antagonist FPL55712 (Fig. 15). Similarly, both the immediate- and late-phase increases in sheep bronchial blood flow with aerosolized ascaris are reduced by

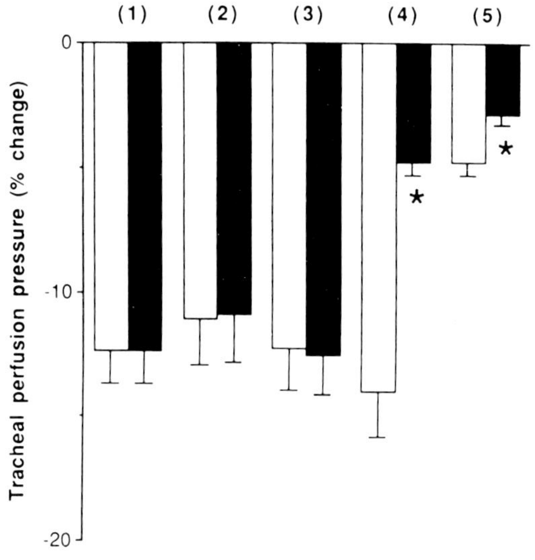

Figure 15 Effect of (1) vagotomy, (2) vagotomy and cimetidine (10 mg/kg IV), (3) vagotomy, cimetidine, and mepyramine (2 mg/kg IV), (4) indomethacin (5 mg/kg IV), and (5) indomethacin and FPL55712 (2 mg/kg IV) on the change in perfusion pressure produced by *Ascaris* in young sheep. Open bars, control responses to *Ascaris* obtained before each of five interventions; filled bars, responses to *Ascaris* after each intervention. Vagotomy, cimetidine, and mepyramine were tested in eight sheep and indomethacin and FPL55712 in four different sheep. The control before FPL55712 is low because the response to antigen was already attentuated by indomethacin. The bars represent means of four to eight determinations, with the vertical lines indicating SEM. *Significantly ($P < 0.05$) different from control value by Student's paired t-test.

indomethacin (Long et al., 1985a). Thus, tracheobronchial blood flow changes produced by allergen challenge in the sheep seem to be mediated by the release of a mixture of cyclooxygenase products and leukotrienes. $PGF_{2\alpha}$, PGI_2, and PGE_1 are all possible mediators of the increased tracheal blood flow in young sheep and the increased bronchial blood flow in response to antigen since they are all vasodilators of the tracheal and bronchial circulations when applied exogenously (Lakshminarayanan et al., 1985; Deffebach et al., 1986; Laitinen et al., 1987a). The vasoconstriction of the tracheal circulation in older sheep cannot be mediated by the dilating prostaglandins but could be mediated by thromboxane A_2, which is a vasoconstrictor in the pulmonary circulation, or by leukotrienes C_4 or D_4, both of which are vasoconstrictors in the sheep tracheal circulation (Webber et al., 1989) and reduce bronchial blood flow in the sheep (Long et al., 1986). The difference in response of the tracheal vasculature of young and older sheep to antigen challenge is probably due to a different combination of mediators being released in the two groups of sheep, with vasodilators dominant in young sheep and vasoconstrictors in older sheep.

In contrast to sheep, the increase in bronchial blood flow observed with ascaris in pigs is almost abolished by pretreatment with capsaicin (Alving et al., 1988). Since capsaicin depletes sensory nerves of such neuropeptides as SP, NKA, and CGRP, the antigen-induced increase in bronchial blood flow in the pig is probably due to the release of these peptides. The effect of capsaicin on the tracheobronchial vascular response to antigen in sheep has not been examined.

V. Mucosal Thickness Changes

Since the tracheobronchial circulation comprises a complex and dense system of vessels and is known to occupy up to 20% of the tissue volume (Hill et al., 1988), it is possible that large changes in blood volume may have a considerable effect on airway caliber. In addition, if there is edema formation and plasma exudation into the airway lumen, these will compound any effects of increased blood flow on resistance. Using a microprocessor-controlled surface probe, we developed a method that gives a direct measurement of changes in tracheal mucosal thickness in vivo and allows simultaneous measurement of blood flow or vascular resistance.

In dogs, the changes in mucosal thickness produced by a series of vasoactive drugs were over a range of 150μm, or about 20% of the tissue volume (Table 2) (Laitinen et al., 1986). Vasodilator drugs increased thickness and phenylephrine, a vasoconstrictor, decreased thickness. It was thought that the changes in thickness produced were not sufficiently large to alter appreciably airflow resistance in the trachea, but if similar changes occur in smaller

Table 2 Effects of Vasoactive Drugs on Tracheal Mucosal Thickness (MTtr) in Dogs and Sheep[a]

	Sheep		Dog	
Agonist	Dose (nmol)	ΔMTtr (μM)	Dose (nmol)	ΔMTtr (μM)
Phenylephrine	100	−104 ±18	50–400	−24 ±3
Methacholine	50	154 ±47	15–100	46 ±6
Bradykinin	0.01	308 ±121	0.1–20	119 ±25
Albuterol	85	45 ±10	5–500	34 ±14
Histamine	55	153 ±31	30–300	62 ±20

[a] In sheep the results for one dose are given, whereas in dogs the results from different doses have been pooled. Values are means ±SEM (Standard error of the mean).

airways they may be important. The time course of the mucosal thickness responses in dogs are similar to those for changes in vascular resistance, suggesting they are due predominantly to changes in blood volume. The experiments in dogs were performed with the vasculature perfused with blood at constant flow. This method of perfusion may underestimate the magnitude of the possible changes in mucosal thickness. Also, the tracheal vasculature of dogs lacks the large venous capacitance vessels (sinuses), which are profuse in rabbits and sheep and also present in humans (Hill et al., 1988). We therefore examined the effects of the same vasoactive drugs on the tracheal mucosal thickness of sheep with the vasculature perfused at systemic arterial pressure. The changes in mucosal thickness produced in the sheep are qualitatively the same as in dogs. Equivalent doses of vasoactive drugs produce considerably larger effects, however (Table 2). The maximum increases in mucosal thickness increase airways resistance by about 10% in the normal trachea and by substantially more if similar changes are produced in smaller or narrowed airways. In sheep, unlike dogs, the maximum changes in mucosal thickness occur substantially later (up to 120 s) than the changes in blood flow, particularly with the vasodilating drugs (Corfield et al., 1991c). This suggests that in sheep the changes in mucosal thickness may not only be due to changes in tracheal blood volume but may also reflect the effects of tissue edema and mucus secretion.

VI. Removal of Inhaled Drugs and Allergens

The pharmacology of the airway vasculature includes not only pharmacological actions on the blood vessels but the effects of changes in blood flow on the uptake, distribution, and removal of drugs and mediators from the airway wall. This aspect of pharmacology is potentially important because it influences the life of active mediators in the mucosa and also the distributions and activities of aerosolized agents used to treat or test airways diseases. There are few studies on this subject, however.

A clear clue to the importance of airway blood flow in affecting mediator concentration was seen in the study of Kelly et al. (1986). They showed that the peripheral airway bronchoconstriction seen in dogs with inhalation of a histamine aerosol is prolonged when bronchial blood flow is decreased. Csete et al. (1989; see also Wanner et al., 1990) varied tracheal blood flow in the sheep with vasoactive drugs and measured the effects of antigen challenge on tracheal smooth muscle tone; vasodilation decreases the smooth muscle response to antigen and vasoconstriction prolongs it. Thus airway blood flow plays an important role in the strength and duration of mediator actions on airway smooth muscle.

Using the perfused sheep tracheal vascular preparation, we changed blood flow by drugs or directly by controlling a perfusion pump and measured ^{99m}technetium-labeled diethylenetriamine penta-acetic acid (DTPA) uptake from the lumen into venous drainage (Corfield et al., 1989, 1990a). Surprisingly, when blood flow is increased DTPA uptake is less, and vice versa when blood flow is decreasd (Corfield et al., 1989, 1990a), and this was true for in blood flow induced both by vasoactive drugs and by altering perfusion flow rate. The explanation for these paradoxical results is uncertain, but increases in blood flow increase microvascular pressure and result in more interstitial fluid and a greater interstitial barrier to diffusion to DTPA. Another possibility is that changes in blood flow could alter the release of such endothelial agents as EDRF and endothelins, which in turn may affect epithelial permeability. In vitro PAF increases epithelial permeability, but the drugs that alter DTPA uptake in sheep trachea in vivo have little or no effect (Hanafi et al., 1990). Thus the barrier to drug uptake and action depends on epithelium, interstitium, and vasculature, and changes in mucosal blood flow affect drug uptake and mediator actions. In view of the potential clinical importance of the subject, more investigations are clearly needed.

VII. Conclusions

Virtually all the neurotransmitters and inflammatory and immunological mediators can be shown to affect lower airways vasculature in pharmacological experiments. This is not surprising because experiments are usually designed to increase the dose or concentration of the agent until it becomes effective. What is less clear is whether these agents exert a pathophysiological role on the airway vasculature in health and disease. It seems reasonably certain that the main functional neurotransmitters in healthy airways are in the sympathetic nerves, namely norepinephrine and NPY. The vasculature responds strongly to parasympathetic transmitters, such as acetylcholine and VIP, but the importance of these under natural conditions has not been established. With regard to the sensory neuropeptides, these are all active on the airways vascular bed in experimental condition, and their release in vivo presumably underlies the axon reflex vasodilatation seen in asthma and airways inflammation. The sensory neuropeptides are coreleased, and the exact combination that is effective in life has not been established. A major problem in studying their importance is the absence of specific antagonists. Most inflammatory and immunological mediators cause vasodilation. For many of these we have specific antagonists, and it should be possible to determine their importance in airway disease. There are no good ways to measure lower airways blood flow in humans, however, although laser Doppler flowmetry shows some promise. To take an example of our ignorance, in the mucosal hyperemia seen in a condition like asthma, we have no idea of the relative importance of the various neurogenic and inflammatory mediators that may be acting on the blood vessels to dilate them. Nor can we say to what extent a change in sympathetic constrictor tone contributes to the total vascular response. The extensive pharmacological studies of the tracheobronchial vasculature described here must be relevant to the control of the airways circulation in human health and disease, but definitive studies are almost entirely lacking.

References

Adaikan, P. G. and Karim, S. M.M. (1979). Effects of some prostaglandin analogues on guinea-pig and human respiratory tract. *Prostaglandins* **18**:787–791.

Alving, K., Matran, P., Lacroix, J.-S. and Lundberg, J. M. (1988). Allergen challenge induces vasodilation in pig bronchial circulation via capsaicin-sensitive mechanism. *Acta Physiol. Scand.* **134**:571–572.

Aramendia, P., Martnex, L., De Letona, J., and Aviado, D. M. (1962). Responses of the bronchial veins in a heart-lung-bronchial preparation. *Circ. Res.* **10**:3–10.

Arrang, J. M., Garbarg, M., Lancelot, J.-C., Leconte, J.-M., Pollard, H., Robba, M., Schunak, W., and Schwartz, J.-C. (1987). Highly potent and selective ligands for histamine H_3-receptors. *Nature* **327**:117–123.

Aviado, D. M. (1963). Pharmacology of the bronchial circulation. *First International Pharmacology Meeting.* Edited by B. Uvnas. London, Pergamon Press, pp. 125–149.

Baier, H., Long, W. M., and Wanner, A. (1985). Bronchial circulation in asthma. *Respiration* **48**:199–205.

Barker, J. A., Chediak, A. D., Baier, H. J., and Wanner, A. (1988). Tracheal mucosal blood flow responses to autonomic agonists. *J. Appl. Physiol.* **65**:829–834.

Barnes, N. C., Piper, P. J., and Costello, J. F. (1984). Comparative effects of inhaled leukotriene C_4, leukotriene D_4 and histamine in normal human subjects. *Thorax* **39**: 500–504.

Barnes, P. J., and Ichinose, M. (1989). H_3-receptors in airways. *Trends Pharmacol. Sci.* **10**:264.

Barnes, P. J., Fan Chung, K., and Page, C. P. (1988). Inflammatory mediators and asthma. *Pharmacol. Rev.* **40**:49–84.

Black, J. L., Armour, C. L., Vincenc, K. S., and Johnson, P. R. A. (1986). A comparison of the contractile activity of PGD_2 and $PGF_{2\alpha}$ in human isolated bronchus. *Prostaglandins* **32**: 25–31.

Braquet, P., and Godfroid, J. J. (1986). Platelet-activating factor (PAF-acether) specific binding sites. 2. Design of specific antagonists. *Trends Pharmacol. Sci.* **7**:397–403.

Brigham, K. L., and Owen, P. J. (1975). Increased sheep lung vascular permeability caused by histamine. *Circ. Res.* **148**:647–666.

Brocklehurst, W. F. (1975) Pharmacological mediators of hypersensitivity reactions. In *Clinical Aspects of Immunology*, 3rd ed. Edited by P. G. H. Gell and R. A. Coombs. Oxford, Blackwell Scientific, pp. 360–381.

Bruner, H. D., and Schmidt, C. F. (1947). Blood flow in the bronchial artery of the anesthetised dog. *Am. J. Physiol.* **148**:648–666.

Carstairs, J. R., Nimmo, A. J., and Barnes, P. J. (1984). Autoradiographic localisation of beta-adrenoreceptors in human lung. *Eur. J. Pharmacol.* **103**:189–190.

Castillo, J. C. and Debeer, E. J. (1947). The tracheal chain. 1. A preparation for the study of antispasmodics with particular reference to the bronchodilator drugs. *J. Pharmacol. Exp. Ther.* **90**:104–119.

Chand, N., and Eyre, P. (1975). Classification and biological distribution of histamine receptor subtypes. *Agents Actions* **5**:277–295.

Charan, N. B., Turk, G. M., and Ripley, R. (1985). Measurement of bronchial blood flow and bronchovascular resistance in sheep. *J. Appl. Physiol.* **59**:305–308.

Chu, A., and Cobb, F. R. (1987). Vasoactive effects of serotonin on proximal coronary arteries in awake dogs. *Circ. Res.* **61**:81–87.

Collier, H. O. J., and Shorley, P. G. (1960). Analgesic antipyretic drugs as antogonists of bradykinin. *Br. J. Pharmacol.* **15**:601–610.

Corfield, D. R., Hanafi, Z., Webber, S. E., and Widdicombe, J. G. (1989). Clearance of ^{99m}Tc-DTPA from the tracheal lumen in anaesthetised sheep. *J. Physiol. (Lond.)* **415**:85P.

Corfield, D. R., Hanafi, Z., Webber, S. E., and Widdicombe, J. G. (1990). Tracheal clearance of ^{99m}Tc-DTPA at controlled arterial perfusion flow rates in anaesthetised sheep. *J. Physiol. (Lond.)* **423**:20P.

Corfield, D. R., Webber, S. E., Hanafi, Z., and Widdicombe, J. G. (1991a). The actions of bradykinin and lys-bradykinin on tracheal blood flow and smooth muscle in anaesthetised sheep. *Pulm. Pharmacol.* **4**:85–90.

Corfield, D. R., Deffebach, M. E., Erjefalt, I., Salonen, R. O., Webber, S. E., and Widdicombe, J. G. (1991b). Laser Doppler measurement of tracheal mucosal blood flow: Comparison with tracheal arterial flow in dogs and sheep. *J. Appl. Physiol.* **70**:274–281.

Corfield, D. R., Hanafi, Z., Webber, S. E., and Widdicombe, J. G. (1991c). Changes in tracheal mucosal thickness and blood flow in sheep. *J. Appl. Physiol.* In Press.

Csete, M. E., Chediak, A. D., and Wanner, A. (1989). Mucosal blood flow influences the duration of allergic airway smooth muscle contraction in the trachea. *Am. Rev. Respir. Dis.* **139**:A228.

Cudkowitz, L. (1968). The pharmacology of the normal bronchial circulation. In *The Human Bronchial Circulation in Health and Disease*. Edited by

L. Cudkowitz. Baltimore: Williams & Wilkins, pp. 84–104.

Cushley, M. J., Wee, L. H., and Holgate, S. T. (1986). The effect of inhaled 5-hydroxytryptamine (5HT, serotonin) on airway calibre in man. *Br. J. Clin. Pharmacol.* **22**:487–490.

Cuss, F. M., Dixon, C. M. S., and Barnes, P. J. (1986). Effects of inhaled platelet activating factor on pulmonary function and bronchial responsiveness in man. *Lancet* **2**:189–192.

Dahlen, S.-E, Heqvist, P., Hammerstorm, B., and Samuelsson, B. (1980). Leukotrienes are potent constrictors of human bronchi. *Nature* **288**:484–486.

Daly, M. de B., and Hebb, C. (1966). *Pulmonary and Bronchial Vascular Systems.* London, Edward Arnold.

Deffebach, M., Agostoni, P., Lakshminarayan, S., and Butler, J. (1986). Prostacyclin (PGI_2) increases bronchial blood flow in the dog. *Am. Rev. Respir. Dis.* **133**:162.

De Letona, J. M.L., De La Mata, R. C., and Aviado, D. M. (1961). Local and reflex effects of bronchial artery injection of drugs. *J. Pharmacol. Exp. Ther.* **133**:295–303.

Del Maestro, R. F., Bjork, J., and Arfors, K. E. (1981). Increase in microvascular permeability induced by enzymatically generated free-radicals. In vivo study. *Microvasc. Res.* **22**: 239–254.

Dias da Silva, W., and Lepow, I. H. (1967). Complement as a mediator of inflammation. II. Biological properties of anaphylotoxin prepared with purified components of human complement. *J. Exp. Med.* **125**:921–946.

Dijk, S., Rogers, D. F., and Barnes, P. J. (1988). Bradykinin-induced microvascular leakage in guinea-pig airways: Involvement of platelet activating factor. *Clin. Sci.* **74**:29P.

Drazen, J. M., and Austen, K. F. (1974). Effects of intravenous administration of slow-reacting substances of anaphylaxis, histamine, bradykinin and prostaglandin $F_{2\alpha}$ on pulmonary mechanics in the guinea pig. *J. Clin. Invest.* **53**:1679–1688.

Evans, T. W., Chung, K. F., Rogers, D. F., and Barnes, P. J. (1987). Effect of platelet activating factor on airway vascular permeability: Possible mechanisms. *J. Appl. Physiol.* **63**:479–484.

Finney, M. J. B., Karssan, J.-A., and Persson, C. G. A. (1985). Effects of bronchoconstrictors and bronchodilators on a novel human small airway preparation. *Br. J. Pharmacol.* **85**:29–36.

Freidman, M. M., and Kaliner, M. A. (1987). Human mast cells and asthma. *Am. Rev. Respir. Dis.* **135**:1157–1164.

Fuller, R. W., Dixon, C. M. S., Cuss, F. M. C., and Barnes, P. J. (1987). Bradykinin-induced bronchoconstriction in man: Mode of action. *Am. Rev. Respir. Dis.* **135**:176–180.

Furchgott, R. F., and Vanhoutte, P. M. (1989). Endothelium-derived relaxing

and contracting factors. *FASEB J.* **3**:2007–2018.
Gardiner, P. J., and Collier, H. O. J. (1980). Specific receptors for prostaglandins in airways. *Prostaglandins* **19**:819–841.
Greenberg, B., Rhoden, K. J., and Barnes, P. J. (1986). Activated oxygen molecules generated by electrical stimulation affect vascular smooth muscle. *J. Mol. Cell. Cardiol.* **18**:975–981.
Hanafi, Z., Corfield, D. R., Webber, S. E., and Widdicombe, J. G. (1990). PAF-induced changes in epithelial permeability of the ferret trachea in vitro. *J. Appl. Physiol.* In Press.
Hill, P. Goulding, D., Webber, S. E., and Widdicombe, J. G. (1989). Blood sinuses in the submucosa of the large airways of the sheep. *J. Anat.* **162**:235–247).
Himori, N., and Taira, N. (1976). A method for recording smooth muscle and vascular responses of the blood-perfused dog trachea in situ. *Br. J. Pharmacol.* **56**:293–299.
Horisberger, B., and Rodbard, S. (1960). Direct measurement of bronchial artery flow. *Circ. Res.* **8**:1149–1156.
Hua, X. Y., Dahlen, S. E., Lundberg, J. M., Hammerstrom, S., and Hedqvist, P. (1985a). Leukotrienes C_4 and E_4 cause widespread and extensive plasma extravasation in the guinea-pig. *Naunyn Schmeidebergs Arch. Pharmacol.* **330**:136–141.
Hua, X. Y., Theodorsson-Norheim, E., Brodin, E., Lundberg, J. M., and Hokfelt, T. (1985b). Multiple tachykinins (neurokinin A, neuropeptide K and substance P) in capsaicin-sensitive sensory neurons in the guinea-pig. *Regul. Pept.* **13**:1–19.
Jindal, S. K., Lakshminarayanan, S., Kirk, W., and Butler, J. (1985). Effect of cervical vagotomy on anastomotic bronchial blood flow after pulmonary artery obstruction in dogs. *Indian J. Med. Res.* **91**:83–85.
Johnson, H. G., and McNee, M. L. (1985). Adenosine-induced secretion in the canine trachea: Modification by methylxanthines and adenosine derivatives. *Br. J. Pharmacol.* **86**:63–67.
Karlsson, J. -A., and Persson, C. G. A. (1990). Novel autonomic neurotransmitters and control of the airways. *Pharmacol. Ther.* In Press.
Kawakami, Y., Uchiyama, K., Irie, T., and Murao, M. (1973). Evaluation of aerosols of prostaglandins E_1 and E_2 as bronchodilators. *Eur. J. Clin. Pharmacol.* **6**:127–132.
Kelly, L., Kolbe, J., Mitzner, W., Spannhake, E. W., Bromberger-Barnea, B., and Menkes, H. (1986). Bronchial blood flow affects recovery from constriction in dog lung periphery. *J. Appl. Physiol.* **60**:1954–1959.
Laitinen, L. A., Robinson, N. P., Laitinen, A., and Widdicombe, J. G. (1986). Relationship between tracheal mucosal thickness and vascular resistance in dogs. *J. Appl. Physiol.* **61**:2186–2193.

Laitinen, L. A., Laitinen, M. A., and Widdicombe, J. G. (1987a). Dose-related effects of pharmacological mediators on tracheal vascular resistance in dogs. *Br. J. Pharmacol.* **92**:703–709.

Laitinen, L. A., Laitinen, A., and Widdicombe, J. G. (1987b). Parasympathetic control of tracheal vascular resistance in the dog. *J. Physiol. (Lond.)* **385**:135–146.

Laitinen, L. A., Laitinen, A., and Widdicombe, J. G. (1987c). Effects of inflammatory and other mediators on airway vascular beds. *Am. Rev. Respir. Dis.* **135**:567–570.

Laitinen, L. A., Laitinen, A., Salonen, R. O., and Widdicombe, J. G. (1987d). Vascular actions of airway neuropeptides. *Am. Rev. Respir. Dis.* **136**:S59–S64.

Lakshminarayanan, S., Jindal, S. K., Kirk, W., and Butler, J. (1985). Increases in bronchial blood flow following bronchoconstriction with methacholine and prostaglandin $F_{2\alpha}$ in dogs. *Chest* **87**:183s–184s.

Lands, W. M., and Samuelsson, B. (1968). Phospholipid precursor of prostaglandins. *Biochim. Biophys. Acta.* **164**:426–430.

Lang, M., Hansen, D., and Hahn, H. L. (1987). Effect of the PAF antagonist CV-3988 on PAF-induced changes in mucus secretion and in respiratory and circulatory variables in ferret. PAF, platelet and asthma. *Agents Actions* 21 (Suppl.):245–251.

Leikauf, G. D., Ueki, I. F., Nadel, J. A., and Widdicombe, J. H. (1985). Bradykinin stimulates chloride secretion and prostaglandin E_2 release by canine tracheal epithelium. *Am. J. Physiol.* **248**:F48–F55.

Lewiston, N. J., Johnson, S., and Sloan, E. (1982). Effect of anithistamine on pulmonary function of children with asthma. *J. Pediatr.* **101**:458–460.

Link, D. P., Parsons, G. H., Lantz, B. M. T., Gunther, R. A., Green, J. F., and Cross, C. E. (1985). Measurement of bronchial blood flow in the sheep by video dilution technique. *Thorax* **40**:143–149.

Long, W. M., Yerger, L. D., Codias, E. K., Pfeffer, M., Sprung, C. L., Wanner, A., and Abraham, W. M. (1985a). Early and late antigen-induced changes in bronchial artery blood flow and bronchomotor tone in allergic sheep. *Fed. Proc.* **44**:1756.

Long, W. M., Sprung, C. L., El Fawal, H., Yerger, L. D., Eyre, P., Abraham, W. M., and Wanner, A. (1985b). Effects of histamine on bronchial artery blood flow and bronchomotor tone. *J. Appl. Physiol.* **59**:254–261.

Long, W. M., Yerger, L. D., Sprung, C. L., Wanner, A., and Abraham, W. M. (1986). Differential effects of lipoxygenase and cycloxgenase products on antigen-induced late phase increases on bronchomotor tone and bronchial artery blood flow. *Am. Rev. Respir. Dir.* **133**:175.

Long, W. M., Yerger, L. D., Martinez, H., Codias, E., Sprung, C. L., Abraham, W. M., and Wanner, A. (1988). Modification of bronchial blood flow during allergic airway responses. *J. Appl. Physiol.* **65**:272–282.

Lundberg, J. M., Fahrenkrug, J., Hokfelt, T., Martling, C.-R., Larsson, O., Tatemoto, K., and Anggard, A. (1984). Co-existence of peptide HI (PHI) and VIP in nerves regulating blood flow and bronchial smooth muscle tone in various mammals including man. *Cell Tissue Res.* **235**:251–261.

Lundberg, J. M., Lundbland, L., Martling, C.-R., Saria, A., Stjarne, P., and Anggard, A. (1987). Co-existence of multiple peptides and classical transmitters in airway neurons: Functional and pathophysiologic aspects. *Am. Rev. Respir. Dis.* **136**:S16–S22.

Lundberg, J. M., Alving, K., Lacroix, J.-S., and Matran, R. (1990). Local and central reflex mechanisms in neural control of microcirculation in airway mucosa. *Eur. Respir. J.* **3**:(suppl. 1). **2**:624S–629S.

Lung, M. A., Wang, J. C. C., and Cheng, K. K. (1976). Bronchial circulation: An autoperfusion method for assessing its vasomotor activity and the study of alpha adrenoceptors in the bronchial artery. *Life Sci.* **19**:577–580.

Marom, Z., Shelhamer, J. H., and Kaliner, M. (1981). The effects of arachidonic acid, monohydroxyeicosatatraenone acid and prostaglandins on the release of mucus glycoproteins from human airways in vitro. *J. Clin. Invest.* **671**:695–1703.

Marom, Z., Shelhamer, J. H., Bach, M. K., Morten, D. R., and Kaliner, M. (1982). Slow-reacting substances LTC_4 and D_4 increase the release of mucus from human airways in vitro. *Am. Rev. Respir. Dis.* **126**:449–451.

Martling, C. R., Anggard, A., and Lundberg, J. M. (1985). Non-cholinergic vasodilation in the tracheobronchial tree of the cat induced by vagal nerve stimulation. *Acta Physiol. Scand.* **125**:343–346.

Martling, C. R., Gazelius, B., and Lundberg, J. M. (1987). Nervous control of tracheal blood flow in the cat measured by the laser doppler technique. *Acta. Physiol. Scand.* **125**:343–346.

Martling, C. R., Matran, R., Alving, K., Lacroix, J.-S., and Lundberg, J. M. (1988). Vagal vasodilatory mechanisms in the bronchial circulation preferentially involve capsaicin-sensitive nerves. *Neurosci. Lett.* **96**:306–311.

Matran, R., Alving, K., Martling, C. R., Lacroix, J.-S., and Lundberg, J. M. (1989a). Effects of neuropeptides and capsaicin on tracheobronchial blood flow in the pig. *Acta Physiol. Scand.* **135**:335–342.

Matran, R., Alving, K., Martling, C. R., Lacroix, J.-S., and Lundberg, J. M. (1989b). Vagally mediated vasodilation by motor and sensory nerves in the tracheal and bronchial circulation of the pig. *Acta Physiol. Scand.* **135**:29–35.

McCormack, D. G., Salonen, R. O., and Barnes, P. J. (1989). Effect of sensory neuropeptides on canine bronchial and pulmonary vessels in-vitro. *Life Sci.* **45**:2405–2412.

McDonald, D. M. (1987). Neurogenic inflammation in the respiratory tract: Actions of sensory nerve mediators on blood vessels and epithelium of the airway mucosa. *Am. Rev. Respir. Dis.* **136**:S65–S71.

Morley, J., Page, C. P., and Sanja, S. (1984). The platelet in asthma. *Lancet* **2**:1142–1144.

Murao, H. (1965). Nervous regulation of the bronchial vascular system. *Jpn. Circ. J.* **29**:855–865.

Newball, H. M., Keiser, H. R., and Pisario, J. J. (1975). Bradykinin and human airways. *Respir. Physiol.* **24**:139–146.

Panzini, R. (1962). 5-Hydroxytryptamine (serotonin) in human (bronchial) asthma. *Ann. Allergy* **20**:721–732.

Parker, C. W., Falkenhein, S. F., and Huber, M. M. (1980). Sequential conversion of the glutathionyl side chain of slow reacting substance (SRS) to cysteinyl-glycine and cysteine with A23187. *Prostaglandins* **20**:863–866.

Parrott, J. R., and West, G. B. (1957). 5-Hydroxytryptamine and tissue mast cells. *J. Physiol.* (*Lond.*) **137**:169–193.

Parsons, G. H ., Kramer, G. C., Link, D. P., Lantz, B. M. T., Gunther, R. A., Green, J. F., and Cross, C. E. (1985). Studies of reactivity and distribution of bronchial blood flow in sheep. *Chest* **87**:180s–182s.

Parsons, G. H., Villablanca, S., and Howard, R. (1989). Histamine increases bronchial blood flow (Doppler) in conscious sheep via H_1-receptor stimulation. *Am. Rev. Respir. Dis.* **139**:65P.

Persson, C. G. A., and Erjefalt, I. (1986). Inflammatory leakage of macromolecules from the vascular compartment into the tracheal luman. *Acta Physiol. Scand.* **126**:615–616.

Persson, C. G. A., and Erjefalt, I. (1988). Non-neural and neural regulation of plasma exudation in airways. In *The Airways. Neural Control in Health and Disease.* Edited by M. A. Kaliner and P. J. Barnes. Marcel Dekker, New York, pp. 523–550.

Proud, D., Togias, A., Naclerio, R., Gush, S. A., Norman, P. S., and Lichtenstein, L. M. (1983). Kinins are generated in vivo following nasal airway challenge of allergic individuals with allergen. *J. Clin. Invest.* **72**:1678–1685.

Raffestin, B., Cerina, J., Boullet, C., Labat, C., Benveniste, J., and Brulik, C. (1985). Response and sensitivity of isolated human pulmonary muscle preparations to pharmacological agents. *J. Pharmacol. Exp. Ther.* **264**:186–194.

Regoli, D., and Barabe, J. (1980). Pharmacology of bradykinin and related kinins. *Pharmacol. Rev.* **32**:1–46.

Richardson, B. P., and Engel, G. (1986). The pharmacology and function of $5HT_3$-receptors. *Trends Neurol. Sci.* **2**:424–428.

Salonen, R. O., Webber, S. E., and Widdicombe, J. G. (1988). Effects of neuropeptides and capsaicin on the canine tracheal vasculature in vivo. *Br. J. Pharmacol.* **95**:1262–1270.

Sahin, G., Webber, S. E., and Widdicombe, J. G. (1987). Nervous control of tracheal vascular resistance. *Clin. Respir. Physiol.* **23**:384S.

Saria, A., Lundberg, J. M., Skofitsch, G., and Leubeck, F. (1983). Vascular protein leakage in various tissues induced by substance P, capsaicin, bradykinin, serotonin, histamine and by antigen challenge. *Naunyn Schmeidebergs Arch. Pharmacol.* **324**:212–218.

Schellenberg, R. R. (1987). Airway responses to platelet-activating factor. *Am. Rev. Respir. Dis.* **136**:S28–S31.

Schild, H. O., Hawkins, D. F., Mongar, J. L., and Herxheimer, H. (1951). Reactions of isolated asthmatic lung and bronchial tissue to a specific antigen. Histamine release and muscular contraction. *Lancet* **2**:376–382.

Selig, W. M., Bloomquist, M. A., Cohen, M. L., and Fleish, J. H. (1988). Serotonin-induced pulmonary responses—the perfused guinea-pig lung; evidence for 5HT receptor-mediated pulmonary vascular and airway smooth muscle constriction. *Pulm. Pharmacol.* **1**:93–99.

Shelhamer, J., Marom, Z., and Kaliner, M. (1980). Immunologic and neuropharmacologic stimulation of mucous glycoprotein release from human airways in vitro. *J. Clin. Invest.* **66**:1400–1408.

Simonsson, B. G., and Svedmyer, N. (1981). Bronchoconstrictor drugs. In *Respiratory Pharmacology.* Edited by J. G. Widdicombe. Oxford, Pergamon Press, pp. 577–582.

Simonsson, B. G., Skoogh, B.-E., Bergh, N. P., Anderson, R., and Smedmyr, N. (1973). In vivo and in vitro effect of bradykinin on bronchial motor tone in normal subjects and in patients with airway obstruction. *Respiration* **30**:378–388.

Sirek, A., and Sirek, O. V. (1970). Serotonin. A review. *Can. Med. Assoc. J.* **102**:846–849.

Stewart, D. J., Holtz, J., Pohl, V., and Bansenge, E. (1987). Balance between endothelium-mediated dilating and direct constricting actions of serotonin on resistance vessels in the isolated rabbit heart. *Eur. J. Pharmacol.* **143**:131–134.

Tucker, A., Wier, E. K., Reeves, J. T., and Groover, R. F. (1975). Histamine H_1- and H_2-receptors in pulmonary and systemic vasculature of the dog. *Am. J. Physiol.* **229**:1008–1013.

Uddman, R., and Sundler, F. (1986). Innervation of the upper airways. In *Clinics in Chest Medicine,* Vol. 7, *The Upper Airways.* Edited by J. H. Widdicombe. W. B. Saunders, Philadelphia.

Uddman, R., and Sundler, F. (1987). Neuropeptides in the airways: A review.

Am. Rev. Respir. Dis. **136**:53–58.

Vargaftig, B. B., Lefort, J., Chignard, M., and Benveniste, J. (1980). Platelet activating factor induces a platelet dependent bronchoconstriction unrelated to the formation of prostaglandin derivatives. *Eur. J. Pharmacol.* **65**:185–192.

Wanner, M. D., Chediak, A. D., and Csete, M. D. (1990). Airway mucosal blood flow: Response to autonomic and inflammatory stimuli. *Eur. Respir. J.* **3**: (Suppl. 12), 618S–623S.

Wasserman, M. A., and Griffin, R. L. (1976). In vivo and in vitro bronchoconstrictor responses to prostaglandin $F_{2\alpha}$, cyclic endoperoxide analogues and thromboxane B_2. In *Lung Cells in Disease*. Edited by A. Bouhuys. North Holland, Amsterdam, pp. 309–312.

Webber, S. E., and Widdicombe, J. G. (1987). The actions of methacholine, phenylephrine, salbutamol and histamine on mucus secretion from the ferret in vitro trachea. *Agents Actions* **22**:82–85.

Webber, S. E., Salonen, R. O., and Widdicombe, J. G. (1988). H_1- and H_2-receptor characterisation in the tracheal circulation of sheep. *Br. J. Pharmacol.* **95**:551–561.

Webber, S. E., Salonen, R. O., and Widdicombe, J. G. (1989). Effects of antigen on tracheal circulation and smooth muscle in sheep of different ages. *J. Appl. Physiol.* **67**:1256–1264.

Webber, S. E., Salonen, R. O., and Widdicombe, J. G. (1990). Receptors mediating the effects of 5-hydroxytryptamine on the tracheal vasculature and smooth muscle of sheep. *Br. J. Pharmacol.* **99**:21–26.

9

Respiratory Air Conditioning and the Bronchial Circulation

JULIAN SOLWAY

University of Chicago
Chicago, Illinois

I. Introduction

One of the physiological duties of the pulmonary airway is to warm and humidify inspired air: by the time ambient gas reaches the alveoli, it is fully water saturated at body temperature. Although in the human the process of warming and humidifying inspired air ordinarily goes unnoticed, having little influence on whole-body thermoregulation (Phelipeau et al., 1982) or pulmonary function (O'Cain et al., 1980), there are two circumstances in which heat and water loss through the respiratory tree *can* lead to trouble. First, deep-sea divers breathing gas mixtures, made dense by compression to several atmospheres of pressure, can lose large amounts of heat to exhaled gas, making underwater hypothermia a hazard (Hayes et al., 1982). Second, subjects with exercise-induced asthma sometimes experience an asthma attack after they breathe cool or dry air, especially at high minute ventilation (as during exercise or voluntary hyperventilation) (Aitken and Marini, 1985; Anderson et al., 1982, 1985; Chen and Horton, 1977; Deal et al., 1979a–c, 1980; Higenbottam et al., 1983; Zeballos et al., 1978). It is this association between repiratory heat or water loss and bronchoconstriction in exercise-induced asthma that has kindled substantial recent interest in respiratory air conditioning.

Much of the heat and water vapor added to inspired air comes from the mucosa of pulmonary airways. This chapter examines key factors that determine the magnitude and distribution of airway heat and water losses and how the bronchial circulation and its physiological responses to these airway thermal exchanges may help to resist mucosal cooling and dessication. Several important aspects of the delicate balance of factors that promote or resist airway cooling and drying remain unknown. Because respiratory air conditioning seems so important in precipitating bronchoconstriction in exercise-induced asthma, parallels are drawn between the physiology of air conditioning and the severity of bronchoconstriction to examine possible events leading to bronchoconstriction in exercise-induced asthma.

This chapter is organized in three sections. The first reviews the heat and mass transfer principles underlying respiratory heat and water exchange and describes theoretical predictions based on these principles, and the second examines experimental tests of these theoretical predictions. In this section, particular attention is given to how the bronchial circulation modulates the mucosal effects of respiratory air conditioning. The third section explores the converse issue, how airway heat and water losses affect the bronchial circulation.

II. Principles of Respiratory Heat and Water Exchange

A. Historical Background

Before the nineteenth century, it was widely held that ambient air reached the alveoli without much alteration (Inglestedt, 1956). The notion that inspired air was conditioned by warming and humidification in the nose was first proposed by Magendie in 1829, but Goodale's observation (1896) that air exhaled from the nose is cooler than body temperature led to our current recognition of the nose as a heat exchanger. In this construct, cool inspired air removes heat and water from the nasal mucosa during inspiration, cooling the mucosal surface (Webb, 1951). During exhalation, warm humid air from the alveoli loses some of its heat (and thus its water content as a result of condensation) to the cooler nasal mucosa. In some species, like the kangaroo rat, this mechanism for heat and water conservation is dramatically effective (Cole, 1982); in a resting human breathing temperate air, about one-third of the energy required for inspired air conditioning is recovered from exhaled air (Cole, 1982).

Although the nose and, to a lesser extent, the mouth are remarkably effective, they do not fully condition inspired air under all conditions (Cole, 1954; Inglestedt, 1956). Inglestedt (1956) found that when subjects breathed cold air through the mouth and nose, their inspiratory subglottic temperatures fell as low as 24.3°C, with expiratory subglottic temperatures recorded as low as 35.4°C. These data, obtained during resting ventilation, clearly demonstrated that the pulmonary airways also participate in the conditioning of inspired air and, like the nose, may act as a heat exchanger by recovering heat and water during exhalation; exhalation of air at a temperature below body temperature demonstrates the latter function. The ability of pulmonary airways to condition inspired air was not unexpected: a decade earlier Moritz and Weisiger (1945) demonstrated that dog lower airways could warm frigid air blown directly into the trachea. The extent to which unconditioned air penetrates into the lung was still unclear, however.

Over the two decades since Inglestedt's studies little further insight was gained, until Deal et al. (1979b) demonstrated a stimulus-response relationship between total respiratory heat and water exchange during exercise and the ensuring bronchoconstriction seen in subjects with exercise-induced asthma. They, and others (Anderson et al., 1982; Chen and Horton, 1977; Chen et al., 1979; Higenbottam et al., 1983; Sheppard et al., 1983; Zeballos et al., 1978), proposed that respiratory heat and/or water loss may serve as the bronchoconstrictive stimulus. An initial explanation (Enright et al., 1980) was that neural reflex mechanisms triggered by oropharyngeal heat and water loss may result in the observed bronchoconstriction. Neither afferent (Fanta et al., 1980) nor efferent (Griffin et al., 1982; Sheppard et al., 1983) blockade of this potential reflex completely abolished the lower airways response, however. Thus, if heat or water exchange were indeed the bronchoconstrictive stimulus, then the site of that exchange must be within the pulmonary airways themselves. After gathering indirect evidence that pulmonary heat exchange might be substantial (Deal et al., 1979a), McFadden et al. (1982) used a bronchoscopically positioned thermocouple to detect inspiratory airstream temperatures as low as 27°C in a sixth-generation airway within the right lower lobe during rapid hyperventilation of frigid air by normal subjects. Under these conditions, unconditioned air penetrated substantially farther into the pulmonary airways than had been appreciated previously. This finding supported the notion that heat and/or water loss from the pulmonary airways could be an initiating stimulus for exercise-induced asthma.

B. Theoretical Considerations

The following examination of the physical principles underlying respiratory heat and water exchange is adapted from a recent computational model of this phenomenon by Ingenito and colleagues (1984; 1986). What emerges from this analysis is that the airway wall may lose heat and water to the airstream, tending to cool and dry the airway mucosa. The net effect of these losses upon mucosal temperature and hydration, however, depends upon how effectively heat and water are replenished to the mucosa by physiological replenishing sources. The detailed analysis follows.

During ventilation, heat and water vapor may be exchanged between the airstream and the airway mucosa. A careful accounting of these fluxes must include energy balance within the airstream and within the airway mucosa and must also allow for conservation of the mass of water vapor exchanged.

First, consider the balance of energy in air contained within any small length Δx of the airways, positioned at location x along the airways (Fig. 1). By conservation of energy, the time rate of change in energy of the contents of that "control volume" (dE/dt) must at any instant equal the sum of the energy fluxes into and out of the control volume. *Two* factors contribute to the total energy that must be conserved: (1) thermal energy of the gas within the control volume; and (2) the latent heat due to vaporization of water "stored" within humid gas. The total energy balance equation for the control volume in Fig. 1 can be written as

$$\frac{dE}{dt} = \dot{m}_{air}[H_{air}(x + \Delta x) - H_{air}(x)] + \dot{q} + \dot{m}_{H_2O}h_{fg} \tag{1}$$

where $\dot{m}_{air}$ is the mass flow rate through the control volume, H_{air} is the standard enthalpy of the air-water vapor mixture, $\dot{q}$ is the heat flow from airway mucosa to luminal gas, $\dot{m}_{H_2O}$ is the mass flow of water vapor from mucosa to airstream within the control volume, and h_{fg} is the heat of vaporization of water. Each of the terms in Eq. (1) can be expressed in terms of a number of physical constants and only three independent variables: airstream temperature $[T_{air}(x, t)]$, mucosal surface temperature $[T_{wall}(x, t)]$, and airstream absolute water content [Wair(x, t)]:

$$\frac{dE}{dt} = \frac{M_{air}dH_{air}}{dt} \tag{2}$$

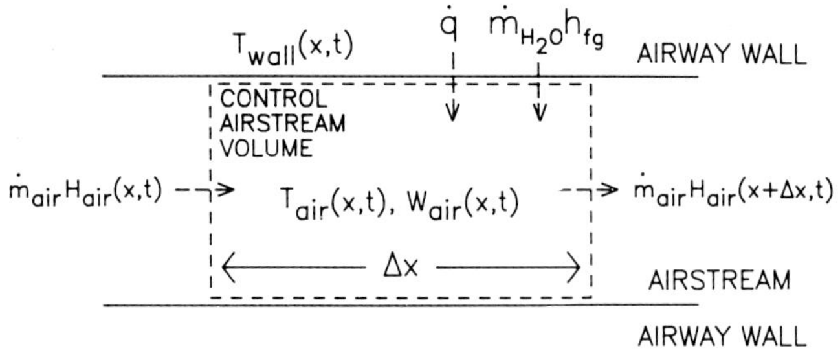

Figure 1 Control volume for analysis of airstream energy balance. (Adapted from Ingenito et al., 1986, with permission from the *Journal of Applied Physiology*.)

where M_{air} is the mass contained within the control volume.

$$M_{air} = A(x)\Delta x \rho_{air} \tag{3}$$

where A(x) is the total airway cross-sectional area at the locus of the control volume (i.e., at x) and ρ_{air} is the density of the air-water vapor mixture.

$$\frac{dH_{air}}{dt} = \frac{(Cp_{air} + W_{air}(x, t)Cp_{H_2O})\delta T_{air}(x, t)}{\delta t} + \frac{(h_{fg} + T_{air}(x, t)Cp_{H_2O})\delta W_{air}(x, t)}{\delta t} \tag{4}$$

where Cp_{air} and Cp_{H_2O} are the specific heat capacities of air and water, respectively. Similarly, the first term on the right side of Eq. (1) can be expanded as

$$\dot{m}_{air}[H_{air}(x + \Delta x) - H_{air}(x)] = -\rho_{air}\dot{V}_{air}\Delta x \left[\frac{(Cp_{air} + W_{air}(x, t)Cp_{H_2O})\delta T_{air}(x, t)}{\delta x} + \frac{(h_{fg} + T_{air}(x, t)Cp_{H_2O})\delta W_{air}(x, t)}{\delta x}\right] \tag{5}$$

where $\dot{V}_{air}$ is the volume flow of air through the control volume. Principles of heat and mass transfer (Rohsenow and Choi, 1961) can be used to estimate the energy transferred from the airway mucosa to the control volume gas as follows:

$$\dot{q} = P(x)\Delta x\, h(x)(T_{wall}(x, t) - T_{air}(x, t)) \tag{6}$$

where P(x) is the total airway perimeter at locus x and h(x) is the local gas-wall heat transfer coefficient. It should be noted that h(x) itself depends upon local airflow regime and velocity, airway geometry, and gas physical properties. Finally, the energy exchange due to water vapor transfer from wall to gas is found as

$$\dot{m}_{H_2O}h_{fg} = h_{fg}P(x)\Delta x\, h_D(x)(W_{wall}(x, t) - W_{air}(x, t)) \tag{7}$$

where $h_D(x)$ is the gas-wall *mass* transfer coefficient for water, which is proportional to the gas-wall *heat* transfer coefficient h(x) according to the Chilton-Colburn heat-mass transfer analogy (Rohsenow and Choi, 1961). $W_{wall}(x, t)$ is the water content of saturated gas at the wall temperature and is therefore a function of $T_{wall}(x, t)$. Thus, the energy balance equation [Eq. (1)] for the gas contained within the control volume includes several parameters that are known or may be estimated (such as airway geometry, heat and mass transfer coefficients, heat capacity of air, and heat of vaporization of water), but only three independent variables—airstream temperature, airway mucosal temperature, and airstream water content. By considering the airways as longitudinally divided into many tiny contiguous control volumes with shared boundaries, one can express the airstream energy balance as a single nonlinear, first-order partial differential equation in these three variables, each a function of time and longitudinal airway position. Two more equations in these three variables are needed for solution of this problem; these are derived by considering energy conservation in the mucosa and water vapor mass balance, as summarized below.

A similar control volume approach can be used to derive an energy balance equation for the airway mucosa, as illustrated in Fig. 2. Here, four energy fluxes must be considered: (1) heat conduction from mucosal tissue in the control volume to axially contiguous tissues (i.e., mucosa in adjacent control volumes) ($\dot{q}_{contig}$); (2) radial heat conduction from heat-replenishing sources, such as the underlying capillary bed, into the control volume of mucosa ($\dot{q}_{replen}$); (3) conductive heat transfer from the mucosa to the adjacent airsteam ($\dot{q}$); and (4) the energy provided by the mucosa for evaporation of water into the airstream ($\dot{m}_{H_2O}h_{fg}$). The sum of these four fluxes determines the net change of energy within the mucosal control volume and is reflected in a change in wall temperature (T_{wall}). The first flux, heat transfer by axial conduction to or from adjacent mucosal tissues, is much smaller than the other fluxes and can be neglected for simplicity (Ingenito, 1984; Ingenito et al., 1986). The third and fourth fluxes are identical to those that entered the airstream, as discussed in our consideration of airstream energy balance. Therefore, only the second flux, heat conduction from heat-replenishing sources to the airway wall, remains to be examined.

Both Ingenito et al. (1986) and Hanna and Scherer (1986a, b) assumed that the principal heat-replenishing source for the pulmonary airway walls is the bronchial capillary network that invests the submucosa (Charan et al., 1984; Deffebach et al., 1987; Murata et al., 1986). To the extent that this assumption is correct (experimental tests of this assumption are reviewed

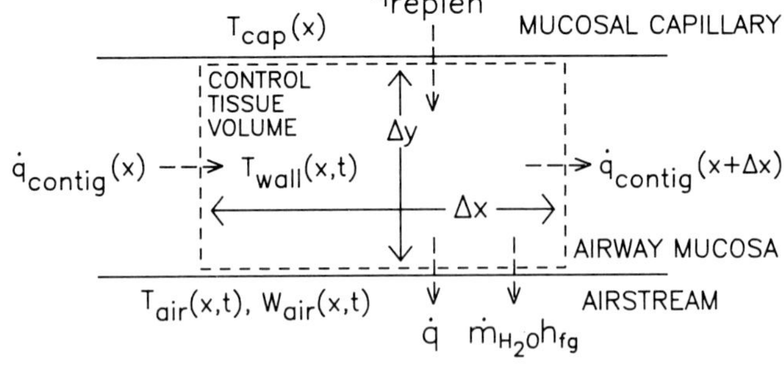

Figure 2 Control volume for analysis of airway mucosal tissue energy balance. (Adapted from Ingenito et al., 1986, with permission from the *Journal of Applied Physiology.*)

later), capillary blood temperature dramatically influences heat replenishment to the airway wall, and thereby its temperature, $T_{wall}(x, t)$. If Δy is the distance from the capillary bed to the mucosal control volume, then the replenishing heat flow from this souce to the mucosa is

$$\dot{q}_{replen} = \frac{k_{tis}(T_{cap}(x) - T_{wall}(x,t))\, P(x)\Delta x}{\Delta y} \tag{8}$$

where k_{tis} is the thermal conductivity of the tissue and $T_{cap}(x)$ is the capillary blood temperature. The net mucosal energy balance equation, including the three important fluxes, is

$$\frac{\rho_{tis} Cp_{tis} \delta T_{wall}(x, t)}{\delta t} = \frac{k_{tis}(T_{cap}(x) - T_{wall}(x, t))}{\Delta y^2}$$
$$- \frac{h(x)(T_{wall}(x,t) - T_{air}(x,t))}{\Delta y} + h_D(x)\rho_{air} h_{fg}(W_{wall}(x,t) - W_{air}(x,t)) \tag{9}$$

where ρ_{tis} is the wall tissue density and Cp_{tis} is mucosal specific heat capacity.

The last balance is that of water vapor mass in the airstream. Here, the change in mass of water vapor within the airstream control volume (Fig. 1) is determined by the fluxes of water vapor into the control volume (by convection through its upstream boundary or evaporation from the airway wall) and out of the control volume (i.e., convection of water vapor out through the downstream boundary of the control volume). Using the symbols just defined, the mass balance is

$$\frac{\rho_{air} A(x) \delta W_{air}(x, t)}{\delta t} = \frac{-\rho_{air} \dot{V}_{air} \delta W_{air}(x, t)}{\delta x}$$
$$+ P(x) h_D(W_{wall}(x, t) - W_{air}(x, t)) \tag{10}$$

These three conservation equations in three variables can be solved simultaneously (with the aid of a large computer) to provide insight into the physiology of respiratory heat and water transfers and how important physiological parameters—minute ventilation, inspired gas conditions, and mucosal blood temperature—determine the magnitude and distribution of these thermal exchanges. Following are some of the predictions made by Ingenito's model and by a similar construct put forth by Hanna and Scherer (1986a, b). First, however, a brief aside is presented to familiarize the reader with the notions of global and local respiratory heat and water exchanges.

C. Global Versus Local Respiratory Heat and Water Exchanges

When, in the 1970s, several investigators recognized that the physical qualities (temperature and humidity) of inspired air were closely related to the severity of bronchoconstriction that followed exercise in subjects with exercise-induced asthma, they sought to identify a stimulus-response relationship between the physical consequences of breathing cool or dry air (i.e., heat and/or water loss through the respiratory tree to the environment) and the physiological consequences that ensued (i.e., bronchoconstriction). To do so, it was necessary to quantify the physical stimulus; thus, the notion of "respiratory heat loss" (RHL) was born. This is the *global* rate of heat loss (including both conductive and evaporative components) from the entire respiratory tree, and is calculated as

$$RHL = \dot{V}_E[\rho_{air}Cp_{air}(T_{exp} - T_{insp}) + h_{fg}(W_{exp} - W_{insp})] \tag{11}$$

where $\dot{V}_E$ is minute ventilation and T_{exp}, T_{insp}, W_{exp}, and W_{insp} are airstream temperature and absolute water content measured (at the airway opening) during expiration or inspiration, respectively. The first term in the bracketed quantity on the right side of the equation reflects conductive heat loss and is (under most circumstances of breathing cool, dry air) quantitatively far smaller than the second term in that quantity, which represents heat loss due to evaporation. When investigators found that the severity of bronchoconstriction induced by cool, dry air breathing did follow a stimulus-response relationship with global RHL (Chen and Horton, 1977; Chen et al., 1979; Deal et al., 1979a–c, 1980; Zeballos et al., 1978), they inferred that airway *cooling* (due to the heat loss) represents the key initial step in the pathogenesis of an asthma attack (Gilbert et al., 1987, 1988; McFadden, 1983). However, since evaporative heat loss dominates RHL, and evaporative heat loss simply reflects respiratory water loss [RWL, Eq. (12)],

$$RWL = \dot{V}_E(W_{exp} - W_{insp}) \tag{12}$$

it was also true that the severity of hyperpnea-induced bronchoconstriction also followed a stimulus-response relationship with global respiratory water loss, suggesting that airway *drying* may be the key bronchoconstrictor stimulus. There has ensued a "heated exchange" about which consequence of the physical stimulus is more important (Aitken and Marini, 1985; Anderson et al., 1982, 1985; Chen et al., 1979; Eschenbacher and Sheppard, 1985; Gilbert et al., 1987, 1988; Higenbottam et al., 1983; Ingenito et al., 1988; McFadden, 1983; McFadden and Ingram, 1986; Zawadski et al., 1988) in precipitating asthma. This is an important question, but the focus of this chapter remains on how respiratory air conditioning and the bronchial circulation interact.

The global RHL or RWL, measured in these clinical studies, reflects the sum of all the local mucosal heat and water losses or recoveries that occur throughout the respiratory tree. As such, these global measurements can hide profound axial heterogeneity in local mucosal heat and water exchanges. Since local mucosal temperature and hydration depend upon local heat and water vapor exchanges with the airstream and local heat and water replenishment, it is important to partition global repiratory heat and water losses along the length of the respiratory path to reveal this heterogeneity. A conceptually simple approach can be applied in both theoretical and experimental studies. Values of RHL and RWL can be calculated from inspiratory and expiratory airstream temperatures and water contents obtained at sites *within* the airways, for example in the airstream at the glottis or at the main carina. In such cases, these RHL and RWL values would not represent *global* heat and water losses but would account only for heat and water losses from airways *distal* to the airstream observation site (Ray et al., 1989c). Note that the *difference* between such "cumulative" RHL and RWL values obtained at two different airstream sites would reflect *local* mucosal heat or water losses from the airways bounded by the two observation sites. Thus, measurement (or theoretical prediction) of local temperature and water vapor fluctuations at various sites along the airways allows inference about local heat and water losses from airways at various depths into the lung (Ingenito et al., 1986; Ray et al., 1989c).

D. Computational Model Predictions

Effects of Breathing Pattern and Inspired Gas Conditions

As noted earlier, the severity of the bronchoconstriction that occurs after asthmatic subjects breathe cold or dry air is related to the rate of respiratory heat and/or water loss during dry air breathing. Breathing conditions that lead to greater respiratory heat and/or water loss precipitate more severe airway obstruction (Aitken and Marini, 1985; Anderson et al., 1982; Chen and Horton, 1977; Deal et al., 1979c; Higenbottam et al., 1983; Zeballos et al., 1978). Two primary factors tend to increase total respiratory heat or water exchange: (1) decreasing inspired air temperature and/or humidity, and (2) increasing minute ventilation. Clinical studies of exercise-induced asthma have exploited this to generate stimulus-response relationships between the magnitude of respiratory heat and/or water loss and the severity of airflow obstruction by subjecting asthmatic subjects to periods of hyperventilation using various inspired air conditions or various minute ventilations. Either of these approaches can increase respiratory heat or water loss, but do they lead to similar intraairway thermal conditions?

Actually, they do not. Figures 3 and 4 illustrate predicted longitudinal profiles of airstream temperature at the end of inspiration under a variety of mouth-breathing circumstances (Ingenito et al., 1986). Figure 3 shows the effects of decreasing inspired air temperature and water content while keeping minute ventilation fixed at 15 L/min. When room temperature or cool air is breathed, the inspired gas is warmed and humidified primarily in the orophar-

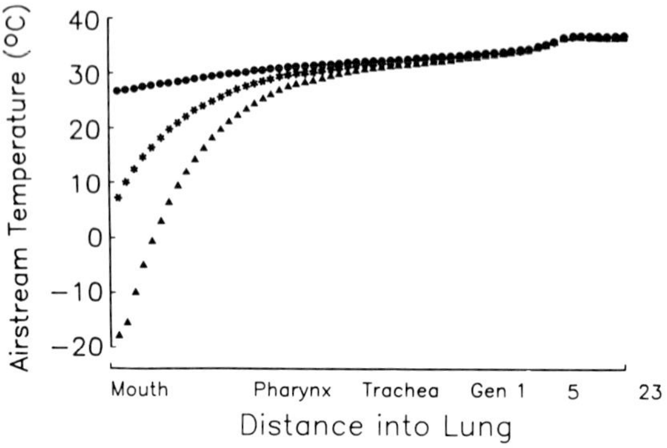

Figure 3 Predicted end-inspiratory airstream temperature versus airway location profiles for three inspired gas conditions: (triangles) inspired gas temperature −17.8°C, humidity 0.42 mgH_2O/L; (stars) inspired gas temperature 7.22°C, humidity 3.00 mgH_2O/L; (circles) inspired gas temperature 26.7°C, humidity 11.84 mgH_2O/L. Minute ventilation is constant at 15 L/min. (Adapted from Ingenito et al., 1986, with permission from the *Journal of Applied Physiology.*)

ynx, so that little penetration of cool, dry air occurs beyond the trachea. When frigid, very dry air is breathed, it too warms quickly within the oropharynx. From the point of view of the deeper airways (e.g., the bronchi beyond the main carina), there is relatively little difference whether the inspired gas is warm or cold! Thus, the principal effect of lowering inspired gas temperature and humidity is to increase proximal heat and water losses without changing the relative longitudinal distribution of those thermal exchanges.

In contrast, increasing minute ventilation (with fixed inspired gas temperature and humidity) alters the longitudinal pattern of heat and water loss along the airways. As shown in Fig. 4, increasing the minute ventilation of room air from 15 to 30 to 60 L/min increases the penetration depth of still cool and dry (relative to alveolar) air considerably. As this unconditioned air reaches farther into the lung, it acquires heat and water from these deeper airways, so that they too now participate in respiratory heat and water exchange, along with the more proximal respiratory mucosal surfaces. Clearly, increasing minute ventilation alters the relative distribution of airway heat and water losses, shifting these losses from the most proximal central airways toward the more distal central airways (Hanna and Scherer, 1986a; Ingenito et al., 1986). Indeed, Ingenito calculated that while breathing room air, doubling minute ventilation from 15 to 30 L/min raises total respiratory heat loss from the trachea plus main and lobar bronchi 2.6-fold but disproportionately raises energy loss from the bronchi beyond generation 2 by over 5.6 times. Thus, the princi-

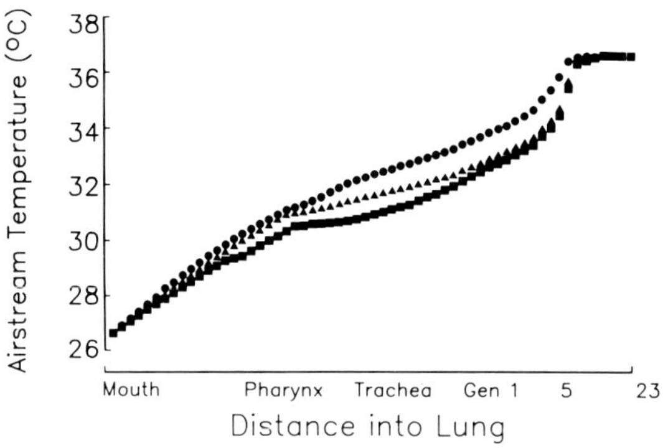

Figure 4 Predicted end-inspiratory airstream temperature versus airway location profiles for three minute ventilations: (circles) 15 L/min; (triangles) 30 L/min; (squares) 60 L/min. Inspired gas temperature is 26.7°C with 40% relative humidity for all cases. (Adapted from Ingenito et al., 1986, with permission from the *Journal of Applied Physiology.*)

pal effect of increasing minute ventilation is to place, somewhat selectively, an increased thermal burden of mucosal heat and water losses upon the more distal central airways.

Why is there a difference between lowering inspired air temperature or humidity and increasing minute ventilation? The answer lies primarily in Eqs. (6) and (7). The rates of heat or water vapor transfer between the airway mucosa and the airstream depend largely upon the gas-wall heat transfer coefficient or gas-wall mass transfer coefficient (which scales along with the heat transfer coefficient). When minute ventilation is raised, the airstream velocity increases and results in more effective heat transfer between the airstream and the airway wall; that is, the heat transfer coefficient increases with velocity. In the central airways (Ray et al., 1986; Solway et al., 1985), as in fully developed turbulent flow in rigid pipes (Rohsenow and Choi, 1961), the gas-wall heat transfer coefficient increases with velocity only to the 0.8 power. The total amount of heat transferred to the airstream, for a heat transfer *rate*, decreases linearly as exposure time to the airway decreases. When minute ventilation is raised, airstream velocity increases and the heat transfer rate increases, but not quite as much as the gas-wall exposure time decreases. The net result is that during inspiration, less heat (and water vapor, for the same reasons) is transferred from the wall to the luminal gas and "unconditioned" air penetrates farther into the airway tree. When inspired gas temperature or humidity is lowered, the gradient driving thermal heat flow or water vapor evaporation into the airstream is increased proportionally to the reduction in inspired gas temperature or humidity [Eqs. (6) and (7)]. Thus, the rates at which heat and water are added to the inspirate are fully proportional to the severity of its increased coolness or dryness, and the relative distribution of local airway heat and water losses remains roughly constant.

Importance of Heat-Replenishing Sources

A key determinant of heat and water transfers between the luminal gas and the airway mucosa is the temperature of the airway wall [Eqs. (6) and (7)]. In turn, mucosal (wall) temperature depends ultimately upon a balance of energy lost to the airstream and heat restored to the tissue from heat-replenishing sources, such as the bronchial circulation. Consider, hypothetically, that heat-replenishing sources for the airway wall were remarkably effective, providing all the heat lost to the airstream. Then, airway wall temperature would remain at body temperature, never cooling despite conductive and evaporative heat losses. Clearly this cannot be the case, for ample evidence indicates that the central airways cool below body temperature, allowing recovery of heat and water vapor by the wall during exhalation (Cole, 1954; Ferrus et al., 1980; Inglestedt, 1956; Solway et al., 1985; Webb, 1951; Zawadski et al., 1988). Thus, heat-replenishing sources available to the airway mucosa, at least in the most proximal airways, are not "infinitely" effective.

The authors of both computational models of respiratory heat and water exchange (Hanna and Scherer, 1986a; Ingenito et al., 1986) approached this problem as follows. Because the mucosal blood flow is finite (and perhaps relatively small), the total rate of heat delivery to the region of any control volume of tissue may be small. As such, heat transfer from the mucosal blood to the mucosal tissue could constitute a considerable fraction of the total heat stored within the inflowing circulation. With substantial heat loss, especially in the most proximal airways, the blood perfusing the mucosa is expected to cool considerably. [Indeed, upper airway venous blood cooled in this way may play an important role in cooling the brain (Cabanac, 1986).] In the steady state, one could calculate the precise blood temperature if local mucosal blood flow and tissue-capillary distances were known, assuming that no sources other than mucosal circulation provided appreciable heat replenishment (Hanna and Scherer, 1986a, b). In fact, mucosal blood flow, at each airway locus, is not known throughout the respiratory tree. Therefore, to simulate the cooling of capillary blood that would occur during ambient, cool, or dry air breathing, the authors assumed a temperature distribution for capillary blood that increased from 27°C (Ingenito et al., 1986) or 32°C (Hanna and Scherer, 1986a) at the airway opening to body temperature at the level of the midtrachea. In doing so, they "lumped" all potential heat-replenishing sources into a single "as if" source whose apparent effectiveness is determined according to Eq. (9).

Hanna and Scherer (1986a) examined the sensitivity of their heat and water transfer predictions to changes in the effectiveness of heat-replenishing sources within the most proximal airways (implemented by changing the assumed capillary blood temperature axial distribution). Figure 5 shows their results, expressed as local net (cycle averaged) mucosal water loss versus distance into the respiratory tree. Increasing the effectiveness of proximal airway heat-replenishing sources (dashed lines) raised water loss from the pharynx and spared local water loss from airways beyond the trachea by raising the temperature of the pharyngeal wall. Under the "control" heat-replenishing conditions (solid lines), the proximal pharynx actually underwent net water gain as a result of condensative recovery of humid exhalate passing over the cooled pharynx. Conversely, upon extending the zone of submaximal heat replenishment deeper into the lung (dotted lines), Hanna's model predicts that in exchange for slightly further penetration of unconditioned air into the lung (and, thus, heat or water loss from yet deeper airways), there is considerable

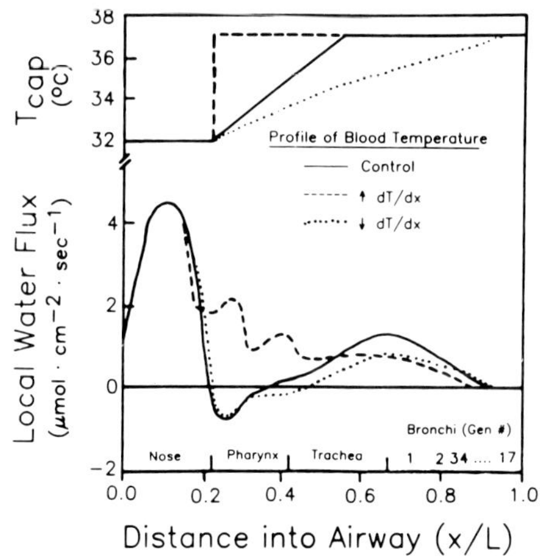

Figure 5 Predicted local water flux from airway wall to airstream versus distance into the lung for three profiles of capillary blood temperature: x/L, local distance into the lung as a fraction of the distance from airway opening to alveoli; T_{cap}, capillary blood temperature; dT/dx, rate of change of T_{cap} with distance into the lung. (Adapted from Hanna and Scherer, 1986a, with permission from the *Journal of Applied Physiology.*)

sparing of water loss from the more proximal airways. This stems from greater mucosal cooling in the trachea and bronchi, which both impairs humidification of inspired gas and improves mucosal recovery of heat and water vapor during exhalation.

This profound sensitivity of regional mucosal heat and water loss to the effectiveness of local mucosal heat-replenishing sources underscores the importance of this aspect of the physiology of heat and water exchange. Experimental tests of these theoretical predictions are presented subsequently, with particular attention given to the nature and effectiveness of heat- and water-replenishing sources that oppose the mucosal dehydration and cooling attending respiratory heat and water exchange.

III. Experimental Evaluations of Regional Airway Heat and Water Exchange

A. Studies in Human Subjects

Intraairway Thermal Profiles

McFadden has led the principal effort to partition repiratory heat and water losses along the respiratory tree of normal and asthmatic human subjects. Using a multiple-thermistor probe positioned bronchoscopically within the airways, his group recorded airstream temperature fluctuations at several sites along the airways of six normal volunteers, from the glottis to the right lower lobe subsegmental bronchi (McFadden et al., 1985). Figure 6 illustrates their results, obtained during breathing of frigid, dry air. Inspiratory and expiratory temperature extremes are plotted against distance into the lung, with the positions of several anatomic landmarks designated along the top of each panel. At the lowest minute ventilation (15 L/min), both inspiratory and expiratory temperatures rose with distance into the lung. As minute ventilation of frigid air was increased, inspiratory and expiratory airstream temperatures fell, although both temperature extremes showed progressive increase with distance into the lung. These patterns support the notion that cold inspired air acquires heat and humidity from the airway walls as it traverses the respiratory tree and that warm, humid exhalate loses some of its heat and water vapor as it passes over the proximal airway mucosa cooled during inspiration. These data also confirm the prediction that increasing minute ventilation recruits more distal airways into the air-conditioning process by allowing further penetration of incompletely warmed and humidified gas into the lung.

These measurements do not allow precise quantitation of local airway heat and water transfers because the thermistors embedded within the polyvinyl catheter probe did not respond rapidly to changes in airstream tempera-

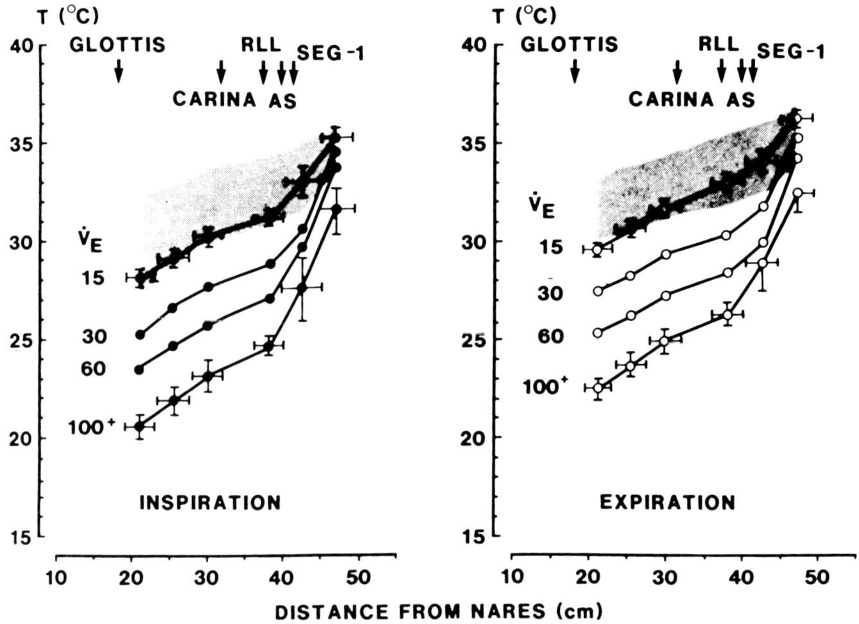

Figure 6 Inspiratory and expiratory airstream temperature extremes versus distance into the lung. Longitudinal airstream temperature profiles were collected during frigid air hyperpnea at several minute ventilations (V_E) as shown in L/min. The shaded region shows the range of values obtained during room air hyperpnea. Anatomic landmarks are as shown; RLL, right lower lobe orifice; AS, RLL anterior segment orifice; SEG^{-1}, RLL AS subsegmental orifice. (From McFadden et al., 1985, with permission from the *Journal of Applied Physiology*.)

ture fluctuation (McFadden et al., 1985). As such, it is likely that the actual intraairway temperature fluctuations exceeded those recorded in these and subsequent experiments (Gilbert et al., 1987, 1988; McFadden and Pichurko, 1985) using similar instrumentation. A reduction in measured temperature fluctuations would lead to underestimation of local heat losses, and of local water losses, if airstream temperatures were used to estimate airstream water vapor content by assuming full water saturation. Hence, estimates of changes in mucosal hydration based on these measurements may have minimized potentially larger water losses (Gilbert et al., 1987, 1988).

Despite these possible limitations upon the precise quantification of local heat and water transfers, this approach has proved extremely useful in addressing several questions regarding the physiology and pathophysiology of respiratory heat and water exchange in normal and asthmatic subjects. It is well established that hyperpnea of frigid air, induced either by exercise or by voluntary isocapnic hyperventilation, can elicit bronchoconstriction in asthmatic subjects (McFadden, 1983; McFadden and Ingram, 1986) and that extremely rapid frigid gas hyperpnea can induce bronchoconstriction in normal subjects as well (O'Cain et al., 1980). These observations raise two interesting questions: (1) are intraairway thermal events similar when exercise or voluntary hyperventilation is used to increase minute ventilation? (2) Do normal and asthmatic subjects exhibit similar respiratory processing of frigid inspired air as it traverses the airways?

To address the first question, McFadden and Pichurko (1985) recorded axial airstream temperature fluctuation profiles in seven normal subjects as they exercised while breathing frigid air. As minute ventilation rose progressively through the 5 min exercise period, local inspiratory temperatures fell throughout the airways, in much the same pattern as that seen in Fig. 6. After 30 min rest, each subject performed isocapnic voluntary hyperventilation of frigid air, his or her breathing pattern adjusted [with a biofeedback "target balloon" (Deal et al., 1979c) and metronome] so that minute ventilation and breathing frequency increased through the hyperpnea period in a fashion identical to the breathing pattern observed during exercise. Inspiratory airstream temperatures throughout the central airways to segmental bronchi were similar during exercise and voluntary hyperpnea, indicating that similar intraairway thermal events occur, independent of the mode of elevation of minute ventilation. A subsequent study by Gilbert and colleagues (1988) found similar results in asthmatic subjects. One interpretation of these data (McFadden and Pichurko, 1985) has been that the pulmonary circulation has little physiological role in replenishing heat to the airways, because increasing its blood flow greatly during exercise (compared with no increase during voluntary hyperpnea) did not affect airstream temperature modification by the airways. However, an alternative view is that the pulmonary circulation, even at rest, represents so vast a heat reservoir that its blood temperature remains constant despite heat lost to the airways. Although increasing cardiac output with exercise would further increase the pulmonary circulation heat reservoir, this would have no significant impact upon pulmonary arterial blood cooling: In neither case would blood temperature within the pulmonary circulation fall significantly below body core temperature. Evidence that supports this view is cited subsequently.

Is the difference in sensitivity between asthmatic and normal airways to dry gas hyperpnea attributable to differences in intraairway thermal processing? To test this second question, Gilbert's group (1987) again used a multiple thermistor intraairway probe to compare airstream temperature profiles in 10 asthmatic subjects and 10 age- and gender-matched normal volunteers during 4 min of cycle ergometry while breathing frigid air. Minute ventilation rose through the exercise period and gradually fell toward baseline thereafter, with no significant differences in minute ventilation between normal or asthmatic subject groups. Although axial temperature profiles were also similar *during* exercise (and again resembled the patterns shown in Fig. 6), upon ceasing exercise the asthmatic subjects' airstreams rewarmed more quickly than did airstream temperatures in the normal control subjects. The authors suggested that if the bronchial blood flow had slowed during hyperpnea because of mucosal cooling (McFadden and Ingram, 1986), then the more rapid rewarming in asthmatic subjects may reflect improved heat replenishment to the airway wall by a more rapid and overexuberant mucosal blood reflow in these subjects compared with normal individuals. Additional studies of the effects of airway heat and water loss upon the bronchial circulation are examined later.

Estimation of Airway Wall Temperature

To date, there has been no direct assessment of the changes in airway mucosal temperature that accompany cold or dry air hyperpnea in human subjects. Nonetheless, indirect evidence of airway mucosal cooling has long been available. Studies by Webb (1951), Inglestedt (1956), Cole (1954), and others (Ferrus et al., 1980; Solway et al., 1985; Zawadski et al., 1988) demonstrated that air is exhaled below body temperature, especially during cold air breathing. Since alveolar air is now uniformly held to exist at body core temperature, the finding of relatively cool expirate confirms that warm alveolar gas must have traversed airways whose temperature is lower than core temperature.

Solway and colleagues (1985) recently explored the influence of breathing pattern upon airway mucosal cooling with a new, noninvasive technique, the single-breath temperature washout (SBTW) curve. Analogous to its nitrogen counterpart, the SBTW curve is a plot of exhaled gas temperature versus exhaled volume, inscribed during a constant flow rate exhalation following a vital capacity inspiration of frigid gas. They compared SBTW curves obtained after "preconditioning" the airways with cold gas breathed at various minute ventilations or with varying inspiration-expiration duration (I/E) ratio. Typical SBTW curves, obtained after quiet breathing (Fig. 7a) or airway preconditioning by cold air hyperventilation at 40 (Fig. 7c) or 80 (Fig. 7b) L/min, are shown in Fig. 7. Exhaled gas temperature rises within the initial 200 ml expirate to a plateau value, which is maintained through the remainder of exhalation. As evident in Fig. 7d, increasing minute ventilation during preconditioning resulted in lower exhaled gas temperature at every exhaled volume,

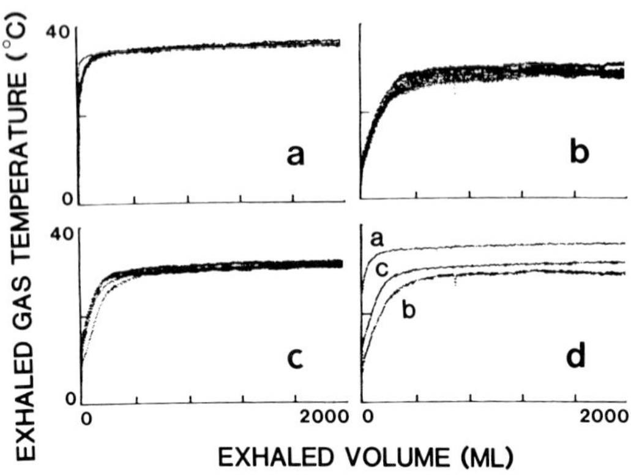

Figure 7 Single-breath temperature washout curves obtained in a single subject. (a, b, and c) Multiple repetitions obtained in a single subject after airway preconditioning by breathing: (a) frigid or room air quietly; (b) frigid air at 80 L/min; (c) frigid air at 40 L/min. (d) Averaged curves obtained from data in a, b, and c. (From Solway et al, 1985, with permission from the *American Review of Respiratory Disease* and the authors).

suggesting that increasing minute ventilation caused greater airway mucosal cooling. Further, gas temperatures within the initial expirate were lower than directly measured end-inspiratory airstream temperatures at corresponding locations within the airways, confirming that appreciable cooling occurred upon exhalation. Since the expiratory plateau temperature reflects the summed heat losses from alveolar gas (because warm, humid exhalate traverses airways of various temperatures), it cannot reveal the axial distribution of mucosal temperatures. Although a novel reanalysis (Solway et al., 1986a) of the temperature rise within the initial expirate has provided insight into the distribution of heat transfer coefficients within human lungs (Ray et al., 1986), inference of airway wall temperature from SBTW curves remains to be achieved. Solway also used SBTW curves to identify one way to modify airway cooling despite breathing at constant minute ventilation. When normal subjects breathed with high I/E ratio (long inspiration and brief exhalation), SBTW plateau temperatures were 1.5 ±0.4°C colder than when hyperpnea was performed using a small I/E ratio. Thus, it appears that breathing with small I/E ratio reduced airway wall cooling, perhaps by allowing farther penetration of cold inspired gas into the lung, thus distributing a fixed thermal burden over more airways (perhaps to deeper airways that are better able to resist cooling, as we discuss subsequently). Most recently, Zawadski and his colleagues (1988) adopted the SBTW curve to prove that mucosal cooling also accompanies hyperpnea of hot, dry gas.

Invasive estimation of airway mucosal temperature in humans has been performed in two approaches. First, Deal et al., (1979a) measured retrotracheal esophageal temperature in exercising normal and asthmatic subjects breathing frigid air and recorded an average 3.3°C (asthmatic) to 4.0°C (normal) fall at peak exercise. No decrease in retrocardiac esophageal temperature occurred, indicating that local cooling of the tracheal wall occurred. Similar results have been confirmed by studies from Anderson's group (1985). Note that the fall in esophageal temperature represents the minimum decrease in adjacent tracheal temperature, so that the latter may have been considerably colder than the retrotracheal esophagus. Second, Ingenito devised a scheme by which, using McFadden's thermistor probe, airway wall temperatures along the airways could be estimated from the rate of rise in airstream temperature during an inspiratory breath hold performed during cold air hyperpnea (Ingenito et al., 1987). The analysis is based on the assumption that, in the absence of airflow (i.e., the breath hold), airstream temperature decays exponentially toward the temperature of the adjacent airway wall. Tests of this method by direct wall temperature measurement in canine airways and in the human pharynx supported the validity of these experiments. Figure 8 shows the longitudinal profiles of airway wall temperatures estimated using this approach. Estimated wall temperatures increased with distance into the lung and fell by over 5°C upon increasing minute ventilation of frigid air from 30 to 80 L/min. Of particular note is that wall temperatures below 32°C were calculated for generation 5 airways during rapid cold air hyperpnea. Direct measurement of airway mucosal temperature to confirm these intriguing indirect estimates would be of considerable interest.

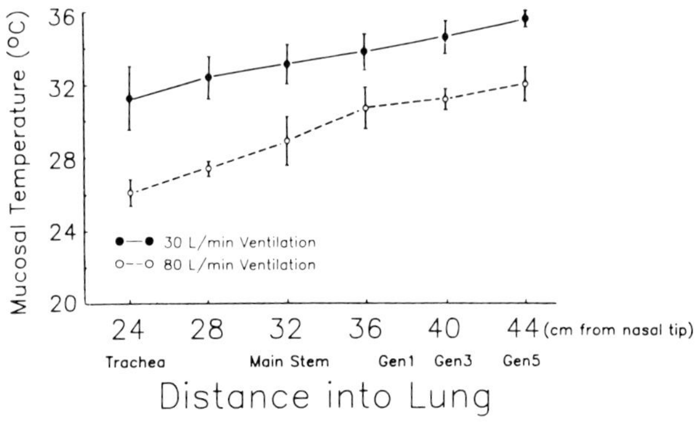

Figure 8 Axial profiles of estimated airway wall temperature versus airway location obtained from measurements made while hyperventilating frigid air at 30 or 80 L/min as shown. (Adapted from Ingenito et al., 1987 with permission from the *Journal of Applied Physiology*.)

B. Studies in Animals

Sites and Magnitudes of Local Respiratory Heat and Water Exchanges

To circumvent potential limitations of prior instrumentation and to evaluate airstream humidity fluctuations directly, Ray et al. (1989c) used rapidly responding temperature (40 ms response time) and humidity (110 ms response time) probes to record longitudinal profiles of canine airstream temperature and humidity fluctuations, as well as airway wall temperature, from the airway opening to 6 cm beyond the main carina. From these primary measurements, local respiratory heat and water losses were calculated according to the analysis presented earlier, and these local thermal exchanges could then be related to their effects on local airway mucosal temperature. To assess the influence of breathing pattern and inspired gas temperature, these authors obtained axial profiles in six endotracheally intubated dogs during mechanically imposed ventilation using three breathing patterns: low minute ventilation of 4.8–5.1 L/min, achieved with low tidal volume (200 ml) and high frequency (about 24 breaths/min), or with high tidal volume (600 ml) and low frequency (approximately 8 breaths/min); or high minute ventilation (14.2–15.8 L/min, using 600 ml tidal volumes at about 24 breaths/min) while breathing either frigid or body temperature dry inspired gas. The tidal volume-frequency combination chosen to effect low minute ventilation had no effect upon local thermal exchanges or on airway mucosal temperature. These data are therefore grouped together to facilitate focus on the influences of minute ventilation and inspired gas temperature.

Figure 9 shows the longitudinal airstream temperature and water vapor content fluctuation profiles observed during these studies. The upper left panel presents airstream temperature plotted as a function of intraairway location. Both inspiratory (lower traces) and expiratory (upper traces) temperature extremes are shown for each of the two minute ventilations as indicated. At low minute ventilation, cold inspired gas progressively warmed as it penetrated farther into the lung, approaching but not reaching body temperature, even by 6 cm beyond the main carina. Note that raising minute ventilation promoted further penetration of cool air into the lung, exposing more of the bronchi to relatively cool air. This finding is consonant with theoretical predictions (Hanna and Scherer, 1986a; Ingenito et al., 1986) and previous observations in human subjects (McFadden et al., 1982, 1985). In contrast to the gradual rise of inspired gas temperature with distance into the lung, however, exhaled gas temperature remained fairly constant as it passed from the alveoli toward the airway opening, until it reached the most proximal airways and the endotracheal tube. Thus, there was little conductive "recovery" of heat on exhalation in the bronchi beyond the main carina, although recovery

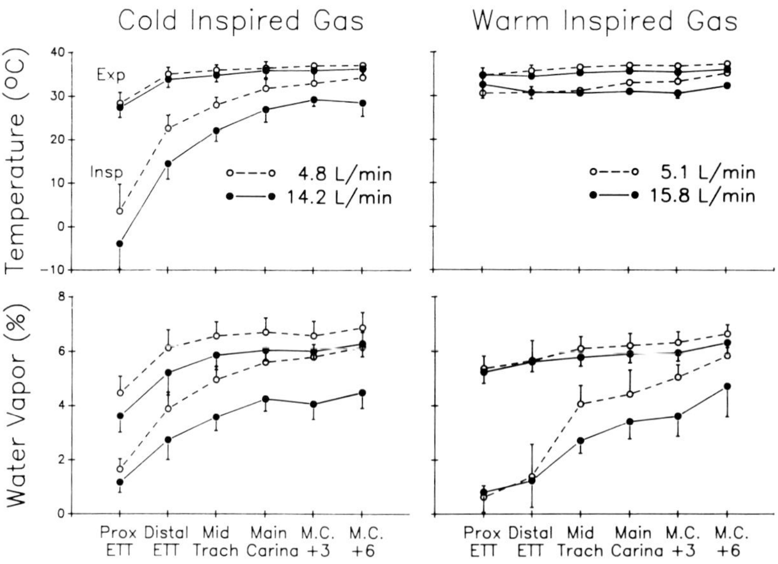

Figure 9 Longitudinal profiles of end-expiratory (Exp) and end-inspiratory (Insp) airstream temperature and humidity obtained during hyperpnea in endotracheally intubated dogs for cold or warm dry inspired gas at either of two minute ventilations, as shown. Airway locations are Prox ETT, proximal end of the endotracheal tube; Distal ETT, distal end of the endotracheal tube; Mid Trach, midtrachea; M.C. + 3, 3 cm distal to the main carina within the lower lobe; M.C. + 6, 6 cm distal to the main carina. (Adapted from Ray et al., 1989c, with permission from the *Journal of Applied Physiology*.)

occurred in the trachea and endotracheal tube. As discussed later, this pattern occurs because canine airways beyond the main carina remain rather warm, with mucosal cooling occurring only in the more proximal airways. Yet, airstream cooling during exhalation was apparent throughout central human airways in the studies of McFadden and colleagues (Gilbert et al., 1987, 1988; McFadden and Pichurko, 1985; McFadden et al., 1985). Whether this difference reflects species variation in air-conditioning dynamics, the greater minute ventilations used in human studies, or differences in measurement technique remains uncertain.

Absolute airstream water vapor fluctuations are plotted in the lower left panel of Fig. 9 using the same format as for temperature fluctuations. The y axis is now absolute humidity, with water vapor expressed as a percentage of total gas molecules. In this scale, full saturation at body temperature corresponds to about 6.2%. The key features of these profiles are that dry cold inspired gas gradually increases its absolute water content with penetration into the lung over the same distance scale as temperature (indeed, full saturation was present throughout the airways and endotracheal tube during cold air breathing), and as with temperature, increasing minute ventilation promotes further penetration of incompletely humidified gas into the lung. Again, most of the water recovery from exhaled gas took place in the most proximal airways.

Breathing warm dry air reduced airstream temperature fluctuations (upper right panel, Fig. 9), but (especially during hyperpnea) inspired gas actually cooled with penetration into the airways, reflecting passage over proximal airway walls cooled by evaporation. As shown in the lower right panel, warm dry inspired gas, like cold gas, progressively increased in water content as it traversed the respiratory tree, and again, increasing minute ventilation promoted further penetration of relatively dry inspirate.

Ray used these primary data to partition total pulmonary heat and water losses between the trachea and the bronchi distal to the main carina (Ray et al., 1989c). Figure 10 shows local total respiratory heat losses from the trachea and from the bronchi during ventilation with cold or warm dry inspired air. Within each bar, the shaded portion represents the conductive, or temperature gradient, component of total local heat loss, and the clear portion represents the evaporative component of total local heat loss. Increasing minute ventilation raised local total heat loss from the trachea about 2½ times during cold air breathing. Raising minute ventilation caused a much greater four to five

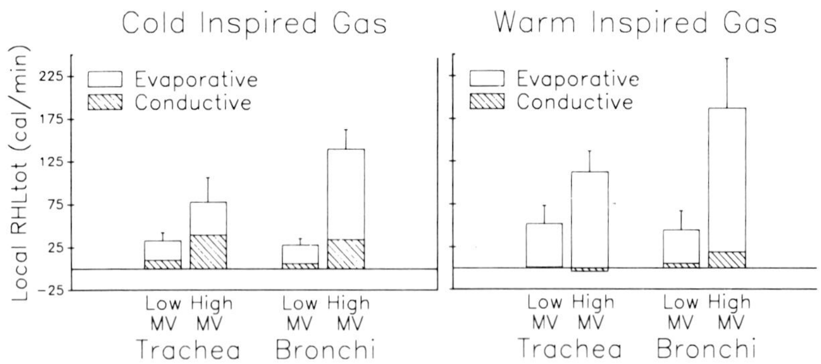

Figure 10 Local total respiratory heat loss (RHLtot) from the trachea or bronchi during hyperpnea of cold or warm dry inspired gas at the low or high minute ventilations (MV) shown in Fig. 9. (Adapted from Ray et al., 1989c, with permission from the *Journal of Applied Physiology*.)

fold rise in heat loss from the bronchi distal to the main carina, however, shifting the *principal* site of pulmonary heat loss distally from the trachea to the first few bronchial generations beyond the main carina. Similar results were obtained during warm dry air breathing, with the central bronchi again suffering a disproportionate increase in local heat loss compared with the trachea. These findings correspond closely with the theoretical predictions of Ingenito et al. (1986) detailed earlier. With these relatively greater increases in heat loss from the bronchi beyond the main carina, one might have expected to find more substantial cooling of the bronchi than of the trachea with increased minute ventilation.

This is not what Ray and his colleagues (1989c) found, however. Figure 11 shows longitudinal profiles of canine airway mucosal temperature during the various breathing conditions. Airway wall temperature increased with distance into the lung in the proximal airways, almost reaching body core temperature by 6 cm beyond the carina. A most interesting result was the effect of increasing minute ventilation. In the midtrachea, tripling the minute ventilation of cold dry air caused the mucosal temperature to fall by 3.3°C. In marked contrast, only a small, nonsignificant change in bronchial wall temperatures accompanied the increase in minute ventilation. During warm dry air breathing, increasing the minute ventilation by three-fold precipitated a 4°C fall in midtracheal temperature but again had little influence upon bronchial wall temperatures. Thus, increasing the minute ventilation of either cold or warm dry

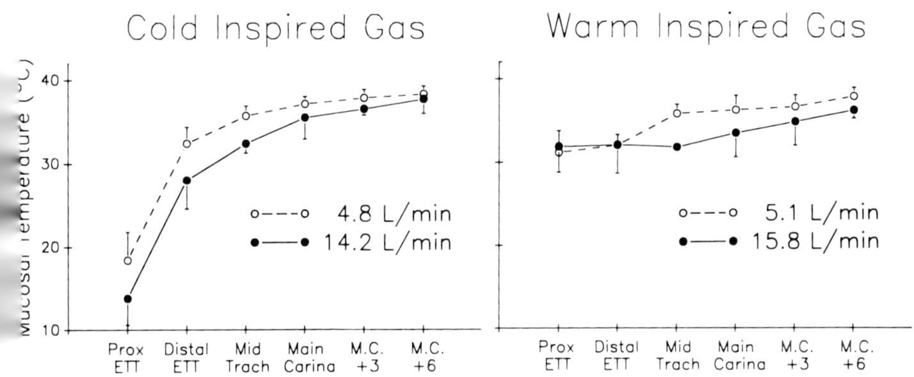

Figure 11 Longitudinal profiles of airway mucosal temperature obtained during hyperpnea in endotracheally intubated dogs for cold or warm dry inspired gas at either of two minute ventilations, as shown. Airway locations are as designated in Fig. 9. (Adapted from Ray et al., 1989c, with permission from the *Journal of Applied Physiology*.)

air cools the canine trachea but does not substantially cool the bronchi beyond the main carina. Recall that increasing minute ventilation resulted in substantially greater bronchial heat loss than tracheal heat loss. Apparently, the bronchi were better able to resist cooling than was the trachea. The role of local heat replenishing sources is considered in the light of this result.

In their studies relating respiratory heat and water loss to airway blood flow, Baile and her associates also measured airstream (Baile et al., 1985, 1986, 1987b) and tracheal wall (Baile et al., 1987a) temperatures during mechanical ventilation of tracheostomized dogs. Time-averaged mean airstream temperatures (Baile et al., 1985) fell as low as 21.7°C in the trachea during rapid hyperpnea of frigid air (about 24 L/min) and rose progressively with distance into the lung. Mean tracheal wall temperature (Baile et al., 1987a) fell during both frigid and warm dry gas rapid hyperpnea, although the fall was more marked during cold air breathing than during warm air breathing (tracheal wall temperature 26.2 ±4.9 versus 32.0 ±3.4°C for cold or warm dry inspired air, respectively). Such a difference in tracheal temperature was not apparent in the studies reported by Ray et al. (1989c) and may stem from the presence in the experiments of Ray et al. of an endotracheal tube that clearly participated in warming and humidification of inspired gas (Fig. 9).

Airway Wall Heat-Replenishing Sources

The tracheal and bronchial circulations invest the airway submucosa and adventitia (Charan et al., 1984; Deffebach et al., 1987; Dunnill, 1960; Hill et al., 1989; Murata et al., 1986) with prominent venular plexuses that are ideally positioned to supply heat to the airway wall. However, the magnitude of the blood flow to the airways is small, often less than 1% of the cardiac output (Deffebach et al., 1987), so that the total amount of heat brought to the airway wall by the airway circulation may also be small. To test whether the tracheal and bronchial circulation could indeed supply all the heat necessary for respiratory heat exchange, Baile et al. (1985) used radioactive microspheres to measure airway systemic blood flow during warm humid or cold dry gas hyperpnea in dogs while measuring respiratory heat loss and mean tracheal airstream temperature. They estimated the maximum possible heat delivery (HD) from the airway circulation to the airway wall by assuming that blood entered the airway wall at body temperature (T_b) but left at mean tracheal airstream temperature (T_{tr}):

$$HD = \dot{Q}[(T_b - T_{tr})HC_{blood}] \quad (13)$$

where $\dot{Q}$ is airway blood flow and HC_{blood} is the heat capacity of blood. They found that even though tracheal and bronchial blood flow increased from 4.5 ±0.7 ml/min during warm air hyperventilation to 7.1 ±1.0 ml/min during cold air hyperpnea, the maximum estimate of heat delivered to the airways through the bronchial circulation fell far below the measured respiratory heat loss: During cold air hyperpnea, RHL [as measured in Eq. (11)] was 0.60 ±0.16 kcal/min but HD was only 0.15 ±0.07 kcal/min. Because these measurements were made 25 min into the hyperventilation period, and reflected a thermal steady state, clearly some other heat-replenishing source must have supplied the rest of the heat being lost from the mucosa to the airstream.

Solway and his associates (1986b) investigated the nature of airway heat-replenishing sources by comparing the effectiveness of the pulmonary and bronchial circulations in keeping the airways warm. They measured airstream temperature fluctuations at 7–13 cm beyond the main carina in the lower lobes of intubated, mechanically hyperventilated dogs and compared the changes in airstream temperature attending temporary occlusion of one lower lobe pulmonary artery (LLPA) or of the major sources of the canine bronchial circulation. Figure 12 shows an example of the intraairway temperature fluctuations they measured in the right and left lower lobes of an intubated dog during hyperventilation of cold air. At the point indicated by the left-hand arrow, they inflated a Swan-Ganz catheter balloon in the left lower lobe pulmonary artery, obstructing pulmonary blood flow to the left lower lobe. Airstream temperatures fell in the left lower lobe but not in the right lower lobe, demonstrating that the left pulmonary artery was acting as an important local airway heat source. Upon deflating the balloon to restore blood flow (at the point indicated by the right-hand arrow), airstream temperatures quickly rose, reflecting rapid rewarming of the airway wall. On average, occlusion of the lower lobe pul-

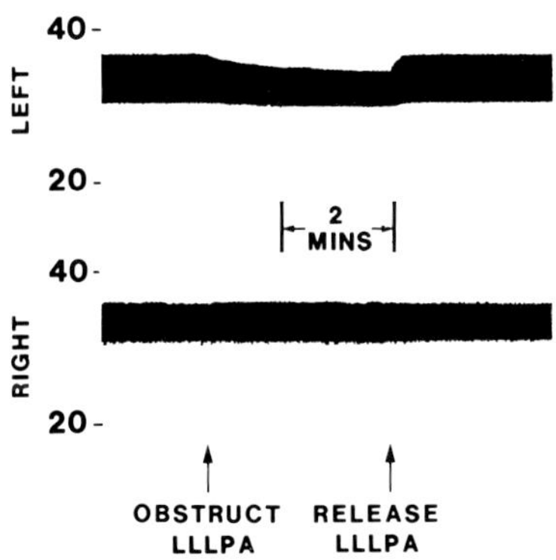

Figure 12 Airstream temperature fluctuations recorded in the left or right lower lobe of an endotracheally intubated dog subjected to mechanical hyperventilation of frigid air. LLLPA, left lower lobe pulmonary artery. (From Solway et al., 1986b.)

monary arteries for 3 min lowered end-expiratory and end-inspiratory airstream temperatures by 2.8 ±0.2 and 1.1 ±0.2°C, respectively, during hyperpnea with room temperature dry gas and by 3.5 ±0.5 and 1.8 ±0.2°C, respectively, during hyperpnea with frigid gas. To explore how heat gets from the pulmonary artery to the airways, Solway measured blood temperature in the pulmonary artery (PA) just beyond the obstructing balloon (Fig. 13). After inflating the balloon, both airstream and blood temperatures fell together, suggesting that heat transfer occurs by lateral conduction from the pulmonary artery to the adjacent airway within the bronchovascular bundle, an interesting feature of the functional anatomy of the lung. In marked contrast to the prominent fall in airsteam temperature attending pulmonary arterial occlusion, temporary interruption of the bronchial circulation had no effect on airstream temperature within the lung, even in the presence of pulmonary arterial occlusion.

Recently, Barman et al. (1988) discovered another way that the pulmonary circulation may act as an important airway wall heat-replenishing source for the bronchi beyond the main carina: direct perfusion of the main and lower bronchi. Although in these microsphere studies the pulmonary circulation contributed little to tracheal blood flow, it apparently supplied as much as 50% of the total blood flow to the main bronchi, and preliminary

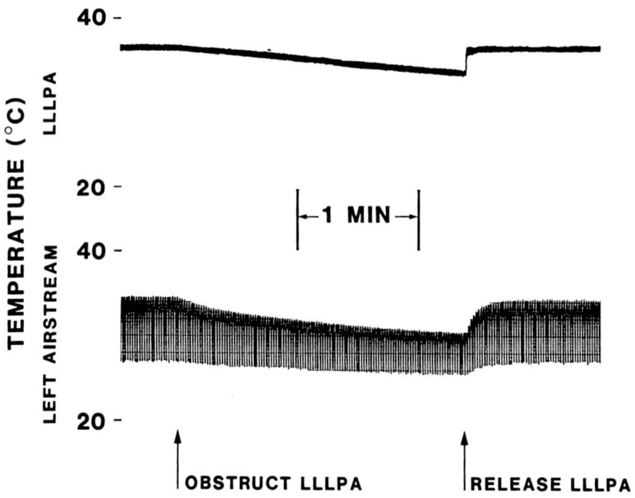

Figure 13 Simultaneous recordings of left lower lobe airstream temperature and left lower lobe pulmonary arterial blood temperature (measured at a site distal to an obstructing balloon) obtained during mechanical hyperventilation of an endotracheally intubated dog using frigid inspired gas. LLLPA, left lower lobe pulmonary artery. (From Solway et al., 1986b.)

studies suggested that blood flow to the lower airways is even more markedly contributed by the pulmonary circulation. Latent heat in blood supplied by this route would certainly increase total heat delivery above that estimated from measurements of bronchial blood flow alone (Baile et al., 1985) and could provide an additional explanation for Solway's observation (Solway et al., 1986b) that the pulmonary circulation is a more important heat source for the lower lobe airways than the bronchial systemic circulation during conditions of elevated respiratory heat loss. Potential changes in the pulmonary circulatory perfusion of the lower airways during hyperpnea remain to be studied.

Recall that upon increasing the minute ventilation of dry gas, Ray et al. (1989c) found that the canine bronchi suffered a disproportional increase in local heat and water losses. Despite their greater thermal burden with increased minute ventilation, however, the bronchi remained warm whereas the trachea cooled significantly. A likely explanation for their greater resistance to mucosal cooling is that the bronchi possess an effective heat source for replenishing energy lost to the airstream, one not available to the trachea: the pulmonary circulation. Thus, the pulmonary circulation, but *not* the systemic bronchial circulation (Baile et al., 1985; Solway et al., 1986b), acts as an important heat-replenishing source and enables the canine bronchi to resist cooling despite large local heat losses. The trachea lacks this effective heat source, and so its temperature is more susceptible to even modest elevations in local heat loss. These results demonstrate that the net change in airway wall temperature with a change in minute ventilation reflects a balance between increased losses and the ability to replace those losses.

Airway Wall Water-Replenishing Sources

The bronchial circulation seems to play only a small role in opposing airway wall cooling, at least in dogs (Baile et al., 1985; Solway et al., 1986b) if not humans (Gilbert et al., 1987). What role does it play in resisting airway desiccation due to respiratory water loss? It is clear that considerable water loss can occur from the pulmonary airways. For example, Ray et al. (1989c) measured canine pulmonary water losses of 0.5 ml/min during warm, dry gas hyperpnea at 15.8 L/min, with over 60% contributed by the bronchi beyond the main carina. In tracheostomized dogs, Baile et al. (1987a) found even higher water losses (0.9 ml/min) during warm, dry gas hyperpnea at 30 L/min. Does this represent substantial water loss? Although the precise extent of the water compartment that provides humidity for conditioning of inspired air is unknown, one possibility is readily examined. Let us assume, as did Gilbert et al. (1987), that the airway fluid lining depth is uniform along the airways at 10 μ and that airways from the trachea through 0.5 mm bronchioles participate in humidifying inspired air, probably an overly inclusive estimate (Baile et al., 1985;

Hanna and Scherer, 1986a, b; Ingenito et al., 1986). Using Horsfield and Cumming's (1976) canine airway morphometric model and assuming a tracheal length of 24 cm, the surface water compartment comprises only 2.3 ml. If this is the true size of the water compartment from which respiratory water loss occurs, then even the lower measured water loss of 0.5 ml/min constitutes a compartmental turnover of over 20%/min!

With such appreciable water loss relative to the available compartment size, it is clear that water replenishment must play a key role in opposing mucosal desiccation, or that substantial mucosal dehydration occurs, or that each is true to some extent. Experimental evidence suggests that mucosal water loss *can* lead to mucosal dehydration and surface secretion hyperosmolarity. Both Man et al. (1979) and Boucher and colleagues (1981) analyzed surface secretions from the trachea of spontaneously breathing dogs. In each study, tracheal surface secretions were hyperosmolal (about 330 mOsm/L) compared with plasma during nasal breathing of ambient room air. Warming and humidification of the inspired gas to "alveolar conditions" reduced tracheal secretion tonicity to about 305 mOsm/L, only 3% higher than plasma osmolality (Man et al., 1979). In addition, changing from nasal breathing to oral breathing of ambient air caused a significant increase in tracheal secretion osmolarity to 380–410 mOsm/L (Boucher et al., 1981; Man et al., 1979), an effect seen within 10 min of instituting mouth breathing. Thus, interventions that undoubtedly decreased or increased tracheal water loss, respectively, caused concomitant decreases or increases in tracheal secretion tonicity. These studies led both groups of investigators to conclude that local respiratory water loss plays an important role in determining the composition of surface secretions. By inference, it seems that local water-replenishing sources must not be completely effective in opposing the mucosal effects of local respiratory water losses.

Even stronger evidence of this notion comes from the work of van Oostdam et al. (1986). As shown graphically in Fig. 14, when guinea pigs spontaneously breathed room-temperature dry air through a tracheostomy for 1 h, substantial desiccation of the airway wall was evident, with contraction of the loose connective tissue and of the epithelium apparently the most prominent effects of local water loss. In a similar study, Barbet et al. (1988) demonstrated tracheal but not bronchial epithelial denudation, ciliary loss, subepithelial vascular congestion, and inflammatory cellular infiltration after tracheostomized guinea pigs breathed warm, dry air for 1 h. These epithelial changes were much less marked or were absent in control animals that received a tracheostomy but breathed fully humidified air.

Together, these studies (Barbet et al., 1988; Boucher et al., 1981; Man et al., 1979; van Oostdam et al., 1986) demonstrate that the water-replenishing

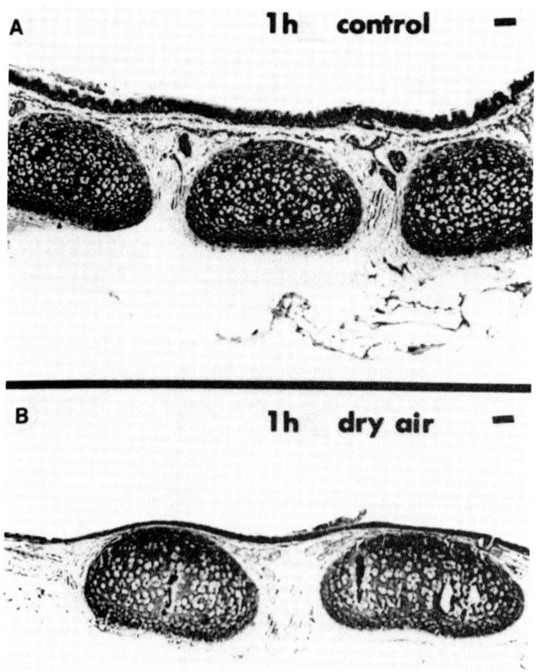

Figure 14 Representative histological sections of guinea pig trachea breathing humidified gas quietly through the nose (A) or breathing dry air through a tracheostomy (B). The scale shown is 100 μ in length. Note the profound loss of contraction of epithelium and submucosal tissue due to dehydration after dry air breathing. (From van Oostdam et al., 1986, with permission from the *Journal of Applied Physiology*.)

sources available to the tracheal mucosa can be overwhelmed, even during resting ventilation, and especially if the normal upper airway humidification mechanism (Cole, 1982) is bypassed. Although a double-indicator dilution method for local mucosal water estimation was developed recently (Baier et al., 1986; Wanner et al., 1988), application of this technique to ascertain axial profiles of local mucosal hydration during hyperpnea has not yet been reported.

What are the water-replenishing sources for tracheal and bronchial water loss? Although this question has not been studied experimentally, it seems likely that here the systemic circulation to the airways plays a key role. In contrast to its role in heat delivery, the tracheobronchial circulation carries a considerable volume of fluid to the airways relative to the volume of water lost. For example, estimates of systemic blood flow to the airways of dogs range from about 12 to 65 ml/min, or up to 3.9% of the cardiac output (Deffebach et al., 1987), under resting conditions. Even if one takes Baile's (1987a) higher value for pulmonary water loss of 0.9 ml/min, complete replacement of mucosal water from the plasma within the airway systemic circulation would concentrate this blood by less than 8%, assuming the minimum value of airway blood flow. If, as Barman's (1988) recent evidence suggests, the pulmonary circulation also perfuses the bronchi, then it, too, could act as a water-replenishing source for these lower airways. Furthermore, the volume of blood in mucosal venous sinuses found in some species—rabbits (Hughes, 1965), sheep (Hill et al. 1989), and probably humans (Hill et al., 1989), but not dogs (Laitinen et al., 1987)—might act as an additional reservoir for airway hydration, at least during non–steady-state conditions. Yet the airway circulation, well positioned to influence mucosal hydration and more than adequate in its total potential water supply to the airway, still seems to be a suboptimal water-replenishing source; that is, mucosal drying still occurs (Barbet et al., 1988; Boucher et al., 1981; Man et al., 1979; van Oostdam et al., 1986). A likely explanation is that the ratio of local airway water loss to local airway blood flow may vary considerably along the airways (Deffebach et al., 1989). Clearly, airway water losses are axially distributed along the airways, with more proximal airways suffering greater losses than more distal airways (Hanna and Scherer, 1986a; Ingenito et al., 1986; Ray et al., 1989c). If airway blood flow is *evenly* distributed along the airway tree, then local proximal water losses would be relatively high and the apparent adequacy of total airway blood flow for total airway water loss may not hold true for the proximal airways. Another possible explanation is that the permeability-limited rate of transudation of intravascular fluid to the bronchial wall interstitium may be slow relative to the rate of local water loss, resulting in airway drying even when the volume of local water-replenishing sources available is more than adequate.

IV. Effects of Respiratory Heat and Water Losses on the Bronchial Circulation

The previous sections reviewed the details of local respiratory heat and water transfers and how the tracheal and bronchial circulations modulate the effects of those thermal exchanges upon local mucosal temperature and hydration. This section examines how respiratory heat and water exchanges influence the bronchial circulation. The respiratory air-conditioning process is now known to affect the airway systemic circulation in two ways. First, it appears to cause bronchial arterial vasodilation; second, it results in bronchovascular hyperpermeability.

A. Effects on Airway Blood Flow

McFadden (1983) noticed blanching of the tracheobronchial mucosa when normal subjects hyperventilated frigid air, suggesting that human bronchial vessels may constrict when subjected to tissue cooling (McFadden and Ingram, 1986), further lowering airway temperature and thus improving water conservation (by reducing evaporation during inhalation and enhancing water recovery on exhalation). It is interesting, in this regard, that lowering bronchial blood flow promotes bronchoconstriction during cold dry gas hyperpnea in sheep (Wagner et al., 1986) and prolongs the recovery from histamine-induced peripheral bronchoconstriction in dog lungs (Kelly et al., 1986). The potential role of a fall in airway blood flow in hyperpnea-induced bronchoconstriction in human asthmatic subjects remains unknown. A more rapid rise in intraairway airstream temperature following cessation of exercise while breathing frigid air, evident in asthmatic compared with normal subjects, suggested to Gilbert and colleagues (1987) that restoration of bronchial blood flow (and consequent tissue rewarming) occurred faster in asthmatic subjects and that this difference in vascular response may be integral to the generation of airflow obstruction following exercise. However, in a recent preliminary study, Baile et al. (1989) used laser Doppler flowmetry (Godden et al., 1988a; Martling et al., 1987) to track changes in tracheal blood flow as normal volunteers hyperventilated cold dry or warm humid air. Although considerable variability was evident among subjects, airway mucosal blood flow was maintained or possibly increased during hyperpnea with either gas, and no posthyperpnea hyperemia was evident. This result contrasts with McFadden's bronchoscopic observations (1983), and so the precise influence of respiratory heat and water losses on tracheobronchial blood flow rate in human subjects remains uncertain.

Results from studies in animals, though, are more conclusive. Using radioactive microspheres (Baile et al., 1982), Baile and her colleagues (1985) demonstrated that 30 min of frigid air hyperpnea increased tracheal and bronchial systemic blood flow from 0.22 $\pm$0.01% of the cardiac output (measured after 30 min of warm humid air hyperpnea) to 0.37 $\pm$0.05% of the cardiac output. Airway blood flow returned to baseline after another 30 min hyperventilating air at body conditions. Parsons et al. (1989) found similar results in sheep. Microsphere-derived estimates of tracheal and bronchial blood flow during rapid warm dry gas hyperpnea were increased at least twofold over values found during warm humid gas hyperpnea, although airway blood flow did not increase during warm dry air breathing at lower minute ventilation. Thus, the magnitude of minute ventilation during dry gas hyperpnea partially determined the magnitude of the airway blood flow response. In a different approach, Salonen et al. (1988a) measured the perfusion pressure during constant-flow pump perfusion as an index of canine tracheal artery caliber. After 10 min exposure to warm humid air, blowing cold dry air through the isolated tracheal segment caused sustained vasodilation, and subsequent return to warm humid air insufflation resulted in even further vasodilation rather than a return to baseline vascular tone, as Baile's results had suggested (Baile et al., 1985). These results support Gilbert's speculation (1987) that the more rapid airway rewarming they observed in asthmatic compared with normal human subjects may reflect more prominent posthyperpnea airway hyperemia in asthma. Conceivably, the vascular engorgement that may ensue plays a role in the generation of post-hyperpnea airflow obstruction in asthma, although this potential mechanism remains to be tested directly.

Both cooling and drying of the airway wall result from hyperventilation of dry gas. To identify whether cooling or drying was the more important physical stimulus in eliciting the observed increase in airway blood flow, Baile et al. (1985) measured tracheobronchial blood flow following 30 min periods of hyperventilation with warm humid, warm dry, or cold dry air and compared these values with changes in tracheal tissue temperature measured directly (Baile et al., 1987a). They found that although cold dry gas increased tracheobronchial blood flow by about 80% compared with warm humid gas hyperpnea, warm dry gas hyperpnea raised airway blood flow even more (about 2.6 times), despite significantly less tracheal cooling [6°C fall in tracheal tissue temperature (warm dry) versus 11°C fall (cold dry)]. The fractional increases in airway blood flow upon changing from warm humid to dry gas ventilation correlated well with respiratory water loss during both cold dry and warm dry gas hyperpnea. Together, these results suggest that airway drying may be the key stimulus that influences tracheobronchial blood flow during dry gas hyperpnea. However, when Deffebach et al. (1989) superfused the lumen of an isolated tracheal segment with fluids of varying temperature or tonicity, they found tracheal arterial vasodilation of about the same magnitude when either cold isotonic or warm hypertonic superfusate was applied (warm isotonic solution was the control condition). This study suggests that both cooling and increasing surface osmolarity [as probably occurs during dry gas breathing (Boucher et al., 1981; Man et al., 1979)] modulate airway vascular tone. Godden et al. (1988b) found no change in canine airway perfusion following inhalation of hypertonic saline. Surface osmolarity was not measured directly in Godden's study, and it remains possible that a smaller change in osmolarity with aerosol inhalation may have occurred and this could explain the apparent contradiction. Finally, Agostoni et al. (1987) has demonstrated that anastomotic airway blood flow is affected by the temperature of the airways, which he altered by perfusing the pulmonary circulation with blood at a controlled temperature. In this study, bronchial blood flow was maximum when pulmonary blood temperature was 36°C and fell at temperatures above or below this value. Thus, the precise nature of the physical stimulus (cooling, drying, or both) that elicits hyperpnea-induced bronchovascular dilatation remains to be clarified.

The mechanism by which airway cooling or drying leads to bronchovascular vasodilation also remains unknown, although considerable insight has been gained. Baile et al. (1986) showed that neither α nor β-adrenergic blockade affected the bronchovascular blood flow response to cold or warm dry gas hyperventilation. These authors also found that bilateral vagotomy had no effect on this response, although cold air-induced vasodilation was enhanced by atropine in Salonen's study (1988b). In all, these data suggest that hyperpnea-induced changes in blood flow are not mediated by vagal or adrenergic reflexes. Furthermore, hyperpnea-induced changes in pulmonary airway blood flow do not seem to be related to thermoregulation (Baile et al., 1987b). In dogs panting in response to raised body temperature, significant increases in tracheal muscosal blood flow were found only in tracheostomized animals breathing warm dry air; no such changes were observed in nontracheostomized animals breathing through the nose and mouth or in tracheostomized animals breathing warm humid air. This pattern of tracheal mucosal blood flow response stands in marked contrast to changes observed in nasal and lingual blood flow, which increased during hyperthermia independently of the humidity of inspired air breathed and independently of whether the upper airway was bypassed with a tracheostomy. Thus, it seems that the effects of airway heat and water loss upon the airway wall per se determine the local increase in tracheal mucosal blood flow during dry gas hyperpnea.

In another study, the Vancouver group demonstrated that lidocaine topically applied to the tracheal mucosa substantially attentuates the local increase in blood flow caused by warm dry air hyperpnea (Baile et al., 1990). Because autonomic efferent blockade does not blunt the increase in airway blood flow, this effect of lidocaine is probably not due to suppression of afferent activity in a classic autonomic reflex arc. Rather, it may be that lidocaine suppresses a sensory neuronal axon reflex that leads to neuropeptide release ("neurogenic inflammation") under these conditions (Barnes, 1986). Several experimental results support this view. First, it is well established that several neuropeptides, including substance P and calcitonin gene-related peptide (CGRP), can vasodilate the bronchial circulation (Barnes, 1987a, b; Laitinen et al., 1987a; McCormack et al., 1989; Salonen, et al., 1988b). Second, lidocaine can inhibit neuropeptide release in response to known stimulants of the axon reflex (Karlsson and Persson, 1984), as demonstrated by its ability to block the tracheal vascular hyperpermeability caused by capsaicin superfusion (Persson et al., 1986). Finally, and most intriguing, both Chapman and Danko (1985) and

Ray et al. (1988b) recently demonstrated that room-temperature dry gas hyperpnea elicits bronchoconstriction in tracheostomized guinea pigs, and Ray (1989b) has further demonstrated that tachykinin release from airway sensory nerves mediates this response. Thus, it is certainly plausible that mucosal heat or water loss leads to neuropeptide release, which then modulates mucosal blood flow. Potentially confounding this notion, though, is Salonen's (1988b) finding that the vasodilating effect of cold gas exposure was not prevented by acute capsaicin desensitization or by local anesthesia.

It is also conceivable that mucosal water loss leads to inflammatory mediator secretion from mast cells (Eggleston et al., 1987; Kay, 1987; Lee et al., 1982, 1984; Nagakura et al., 1983) or other secretory cells (Ingenito et al., 1990). Several studies from Lichtenstein's group (Togias et al., 1985, 1986) document the appearance of mediators in nasal secretions after nasal breathing of cold, dry air, and clinical studies have sometimes (Lee et al., 1982, 1984; Nagakura et al., 1983), although not uniformly (Deal et al., 1980), found evidence for secretory cell mediator release during exercise-induced bronchoconstriction in human subjects with atopic asthma. Recently, Ingenito and his colleagues (1990) found elevations in eicosanoid mediators in bronchoalveolar lavage fluid obtained at the peak of hyperpnea-induced bronchoconstriction in guinea pigs. Since a variety of secretory cell mediators, including prostaglandins, histamine, and platelet activating factor, have all been shown to dilate bronchial vessels (Baier et al., 1985; Laitinen et al., 1986, 1987b, 1987c; Long et al., 1985, 1988), it is conceivable that these agents participate in the vasodilation of dry gas hyperpnea as well.

B. Effects on Airway Vascular Permeability

The tracheobronchial vasculature becomes hyperpermeable when exposed to a variety of inflammatory mediator substances, including neuropeptides (Barnes, 1987a, 1987b; Laitinen et al., 1987a; McDonald, 1987), histamine, platelet activating factor, and leukotrienes (Baier et al., 1986; Evans et al., 1987; Fick et al., 1987; Laitinen et al., 1987b; Persson, 1987, 1988; Pietra and Magno, 1978; Woodward et al., 1983). As noted earlier, several of these agents may be released during or after dry gas hyperpnea, raising the question of whether bronchovascular hyperpermeability results from dry gas hyperpnea. Ray et al. (1988a) addressed this question in their guinea pig model of hyperpnea-induced bronchoconstriction (Chapman and Danko, 1985; Ray et al., 1988b). Just before hyperpnea, they treated each animal with intravenous monastral blue, an intravascular dye suspension whose large particles extravasate from bronchial vessels only when postcapillary venules become hyperpermeable (McDonald, 1987). Dry gas hyperpnea for 5 min provoked bronchoconstriction and also caused monastral blue staining of the trachea and central airways up to 4 cm beyond the main carina (about generation 4), but humid gas hyperpnea caused neither bronchoconstriction (Ray et al., 1988b) nor airway mucosal staining. Thus, bronchovascular hyperpermeability is elicited by dry gas hyperpnea in guinea pigs. Garland et al. (1991) addressed the mechanism of this response by quantifying Evans blue-labeled albumin extravasation along the central airways. Tachykinin depletion by capsaicin pretreatment ablated the bronchoconstrictor response to dry gas hyperpnea and prevented hyperpnea-induced albumin extravasation in the intrapulmonary airways but did not suppress hyperpnea-induced microvascular hyperpermeability in the trachea or main bronchi. Thus, it seems likely that different mechanisms leading to this response dominate in different airway regions. Perhaps this axial variation reflects the distributed nature of airway heat and water losses cited earlier.

Dry gas hyperpnea elicits bronchovascular hyperpermeability in other species as well. Ferrets exhibit airway vascular leak (evident in monastral blue staining of airways) after dry but not humid gas hyperpnea (Ray et al., 1989a). It is unknown whether dogs develop bronchovascular permeability changes following dry gas hyperpnea, but Deffebach et al. (1989) recently showed that warm or cold hypertonic solutions superfusing an isolated canine tracheal segment increased the flux of intravenously administered albumin into the superfusate, compared with warm isotonic control solution. No such increase was evident following cold isotonic solution exposure, suggesting that increased airway mucosal tonicity was the key stimulus provoking vascular leak in these studies.

C. Localization of Hyperpnea-Induced Airway Responses

As observed earlier, the influence of dry gas hyperpnea upon airway wall temperature and hydration varies substantially along the length of the airways, with mucosal cooling and drying often more marked in the most proximal airways than in the more distal central bronchi. When such heterogenous stimuli are applied to the airways, are the bronchial and bronchovascular responses uniform, or are they also heterogeneous, with local airway responses determined by local mucosal stimuli? Three recent studies address this question, each focused on one of the three hyperpnea-induced airway responses: bronchoconstriction, increased airway blood flow, and bronchovascular hyperpermeability. First, Ray et al. (1990) obtained tantalum bronchograms in guinea pigs before and during dry gas hyperpnea-induced bronchoconstriction. At relatively low minute ventilation, only the proximal central bronchi narrowed. As minute ventilation was raised [and the resultant bronchoconstriction worsened (Ray et al., 1988b)], these proximal airways narrowed progressively, but constriction also appeared in more distal central airways that did not narrow at lower minute ventilation. This pattern was markedly different from methacholine- or capsaicin-induced bronchoconstriction, in which both proximal and more distal central airways narrowed in concert. Prior work established that increasing minute ventilation during dry gas hyperpnea raises proximal airway heat and water losses but also disproportionately enhances heat and water losses from more distal bronchi (Ray et al., 1989c). As such, Ray's tantalum bronchography data suggest that local bronchoconstriction occurs in response to a locally applied airway thermal stimulus.

Next, Baile et al. (1987b) identified that a similar principle applies to the increase in tracheal blood flow caused by warm dry air hyperpnea in tracheostomized dogs. Tracheal blood flow increased substantially when dogs panted warm dry air through a tracheostomy. However, simultaneously measured blood flow to tracheal tissue above the tracheostomy (i.e., not directly exposed to the cooling and drying stimulus) remained constant at control values. Thus, local mucosal drying appears to determine the local mucosal vasodilator response.

Finally, Ray and his colleagues (1989a) have recently reported that bronchovascular hyperpermeability occurs in tracheostomized ferrets subjected to room temperature dry gas hyperpnea. As in guinea pigs, this response is ablated by humidification of inspired air. The ferret's long trachea allowed these investigators to deliver dry gas to a limited segment of proximal trachea while ventilating the remaining lung with humidified air. In all animals studied, bronchovascular hyperpermeability (identified by monastral blue extravasation) occurred in the airway segment directly subjected to the cooling and drying stimulus. Of 10 animals, 2 also exhibited faint staining in airways beyond the limited zone of direct stimulation. If these preliminary observations are confirmed in further studies, they suggest that an additional mechanism acts to extend the bronchovascular response to distant, nonstimulated airways. Conceivably, antidromic transmission along sensory axons within the airways may represent the mechanism of extension, though this possibility remains speculative at present.

V. Summary

Dry air hyperpnea leads to considerable heat and water losses from the conducting pulmonary airways. This respiratory air-conditioning process is not uniform along the respiratory tree. Rather, local heat and water losses are axially distributed, and the distribution depends upon minute ventilation. During quiet breathing, only the most proximal central airways participate in the heating and humidification of inspired air. During hyperpnea, however, the zone of respiratory air conditioning extends farther into the lung, so that deeper airways also lose heat and water to inspired air. These local thermal transfers tend to cool and dry the airways in which they occur, but their net effects upon local airway temperature and hydration are modulated by heat and water replacement from local circulatory replenishing sources; these also vary along the airways. Heat is brought to the trachea primarily through its systemic circulation, but the bronchi have two heat sources: the systemic bronchial circulation and the pulmonary circulation. Since its blood flow rate is relatively small, the systemic tracheobronchial circulation replaces little of the heat lost to inspired air. Rather, the pulmonary circulation plays the principal role in opposing bronchial cooling, transferring heat to the airway by lateral conduction and perhaps by direct perfusion. Nonetheless, the tracheobronchial systemic circulation may be important in minimizing the airway dehydration that would otherwise accompany respiratory water loss. The airway circulation thus modulates the net airway effects of respiratory air conditioning, but it also responds to airway heat and water flux in two important ways. Dry gas hyperpnea dilates the tracheobronchial vasculature and also increases bronchovascular permeability to macromolecules. Although the mechanisms by which these vascular changes occur are not fully known, each appears primarily as a local response to local airway heat and water flux. Perhaps these hyperpnea-induced bronchovascular responses act to minimize the cooling and drying promoted by dry gas breathing, by enhancing the rates of heat and water replenishment to those airways suffering the greatest thermal burdens. Thus, the respiratory air-conditioning process and the tracheobronchial circulation share bidirectional interactions. Further evaluation of these interactions may promote our understanding of the normal role of the airway vessels in human physiology and may disclose derangements that could contribute to the pathogenesis of hyperpnea-induced bronchoconstriction in subjects with exercise-induced asthma.

Acknowledgments

Supported by NHLBI Grants HL02205 and HL41009, and by the Whitaker Foundation.

References

Agostoni, P., Deffebach, M. E., Kirk, W., and Brengelmann, G. L., (1987). Temperature dependence of intraparenchymal bronchial blood flow. *Respir. Physiol.* **68**:259–267.

Aitken, M.L., and Marini, J. J. (1985). Effect of heat delivery and extraction on airway conductance in normal and in asthmatic subjects. *Am. Rev. Respir. Dis.* **131**:357–361.

Anderson, S. D., Schoeffel, R. E., Follet, R., Perry, C. P., Daviskas, E., and Kendall, M. (1982). Sensitivity to heat and water loss at rest and during exercise in asthmatic patients. *Eur. J. Respir. Dis.* **63**:459–471.

Anderson, S. D., Schoeffel, R. E., Black, J. L., and Daviskas, E. (1985). Airway cooling as the stimulus to exercise-induced asthma—a re-evaluation. *Eur. J. Respir. Dis.* **66**:1–11.

Baier, H., Yerger, L., Moas, R., and Wanner, A. (1985). Vascular and airway effects of endogenous cycloxygenase products during lung inflation. *J. Appl. Physiol.* **59**(3):884–889.

Baier, H., Moas, R., Yerger, L., and Wanner, A. (1986). In vivo estimation of tracheal wall water: Effects of histamine and carbachol. *J. Appl. Physiol.* **60**(5):1680–1685.

Baile, E. M., Nelems, J. M. B., Schulzer, M., and Pare, P. D. (1982). Measurement of regional bronchial arterial blood flow and bronchovascular resistance in dogs. *J. Appl. Physiol.* **53**(4):1044–1049.

Baile, E. M., Dahlby, R. W., Wiggs, B. R., and Pare, P. D. (1985) Role of tracheal and bronchial circulation in respiratory heat exchange. *J. Appl. Physiol.* **58**(1):217–222.

Baile, E. M., Osborne, S., and Pare, P. D. (1986). Effect of autonomic blockade on tracheobronchial blood flow. *J. Appl. Physiol.* **62**(2):520–525.

Baile, E. M., Dahlby, R. W., Wiggs, B. R., Parsons, G. H., and Pare, P. D. (1987a). Effect of cold and warm dry air hyperventilation on canine airway blood flow. *J. Appl. Physiol.* **62**(2):526–532.

Baile, E. M., Guillemi, S., and Pare, P. D. (1987b). Tracheobronchial and upper airway blood flow in dogs during thermally inducing panting. *J. Appl. Physiol.* **63**(6):2240–2246.

Baile, E. M., Godden, D. J., and Pare, P. D. (1989). Effect of cold dry and warm humid air hyperventilation on tracheal wall blood flow in humans. *Am. Rev. Respir. Dis.* **139**(4, Part 2):A63.

Baile, E. M., Godden, D. J., and Pare, P. D. (1990). Mechanism for increase in trachebronchial blood flow induced by hyperventilation of dry air in dogs. *J. Appl. Physiol.* **68**(1):105–112.

Barbet, J. P., Chauveau, M., Labbe, S., and Lockhart, A. (1988). Breathing dry air causes acute epithelial damage and inflammation of the guinea pig trachea. *J. Appl. Physiol.* **64**(5):1851–1857.

Barman, S. A., Ardell, A. L., Parker, J. C., Perry, M. L., and Taylor, A. E. (1988). Pulmonary and systemic blood flow contributions to upper airways in canine lung. *Am. J. Physiol.* **225**(24):H1130–1135.

Barnes, P. J. (1986). Neural control of human airways in health and disease.

Am. Rev. Respir. Dis. **134**(6):1289–1314.

Barnes, P. J. (1987a). Neuropeptides in human airways: Function and clinical implications. *Am. Rev. Respir. Dir.* **136**(6, Part 2):S77–S83.

Barnes, P. J. (1987b). Regulatory peptides in the respiratory system. *Experientia* **43**(7):832–839.

Boucher, R. C., Stutts, M. J., Bromberg, P. A., and Gatzy, J. T. (1981). Regional differences in airway surface liquid composition. *J. Appl. Physiol.* **50**(3):613–620.

Cabanac, M. (1986). Keeping a cool head. *News Physiol. Sci.* **1**:41–44.

Chapman, R. W., and Danko, G. (1985). Hyperventilation-induced bronchoconstriction in guinea pigs. *Int. Arch. Allergy Appl. Immunol.* **78**:190–196.

Charan, N. B., Turk, G. M., and Dhand, R. (1984). Gross and subgross anatomy of the bronchial circulation in sheep. *J. Appl. Physiol.* **57**:658–664.

Chen, W. Y., and Horton, D. J. (1977). Heat and water loss from the airways and exercise-induced asthma. *Respiration* **34**:305–313.

Chen, W. Y., Weiser, P. C., and Chai, H. (1979). Airway cooling: Stimulus for exercise-induced asthma. *Scand. J. Respir. Dis.* **60**:144–150.

Cole, P. (1954). Respiratory mucosal vascular responses, air conditioning and thermoregulation. *J. Laryngol. Otol.* **68**:613–622.

Cole, P. (1982). Modification of inspired air. In *The Nose: Upper Airway Physiology and the Atmospheric Environment,* pp. 351–375. Edited by D. F. Proctor and I. Andersen. Amsterdam, Elsevier Biomedical Press (Chap. 14).

Deal, E. C., McFadden, Jr., E. R., Ingram, Jr. R. H., and Jaeger, J. J. (1979a). Esophageal temperature during exercise in asthmatic and nonasthmatic subjects. *J. Appl. Physiol.* **46**(3): 484–490.

Deal, E. C., McFadden, Jr., E. R., Ingram, Jr. R. H., and Jaeger, J. J. (1979b). Hyperpnea and heat flux: Initial reaction sequence in exercise-induced asthma. *J. Appl. Physiol.* **46**(3):476–483.

Deal, E. C., McFadden, Jr., E. R., Ingram, Jr., R. H. Strauss, R. H., and Jaeger, J. J. (1979c). Role of respiratory heat exchange in production of exercise-induced asthma. *J. Appl. Physiol.* **46**(3):467–475.

Deal, E. C., Wasserman, S. I., Soter, N. A., Ingram, Jr., R. H., and McFadden, Jr., E. R. (1980). Evaluation of role played by mediators of immediate hypersensitivity in exercise-induced asthma. *J. Clin. Invest.* **65**:659–665.

Deffebach, M. E., Charan, N. B., Lakshminarayan, S., and Butler, J. (1987). The bronchial circulation: Small, but vital attribute of the lung. *Am. Rev. Respir. Dis.* **135**:463–481.

Deffebach, M. E., Salonen, R. O., Webber, S. E., and Widdicombe, J. G. (1989). Cold and hyperosmolar fluids in canine trachea: Vascular and smooth muscle tone and albumin flux. *J. Appl. Physiol.* **66**:1309–1315.

Dunnill, M. S. (1960). The pathology of asthma, with special reference to changes in the bronchial mucosa. *J. Clin. Pathol.* **13**:27–33.

Eggleston, P. A., Kagey-Sobotka, A., and Lichtenstein, L. M. (1987). A comparison of the osmotic activation of basophils and human lung mast cells. *Am. Rev. Respir. Dis.* **135**:1043–1048.

Enright, P. L., McNally, J. F., and Souhrada, J. F. (1980). Effect of lidocaine on the ventilatory and airway responses to exercise in asthmatics. *Am. Rev. Respir. Dis.* **122**:823–828.

Eschenbacher, W. L., and Sheppard, D. (1985). Respiratory heat loss is not the sole stimulus for bronchoconstriction induced by isocapnic hyperpnea with dry air. *Am. Rev. Respir. Dis.* **131**:894–901.

Evans, T. W., Chung, K. F., Rogers, D. F., and Barnes, P. J. (1987). Effect of platelet-activating factor on airway vascular permeability: possible mechanisms. *J. Appl. Physiol.* **63**(2):479–484.

Fanta, C. H., Ingram, Jr., R. H., and McFadden, Jr., E. R. (1980). A reassessment of the effects of oropharyngeal anesthesia in exercise-induced asthma. *Am. Rev. Respir. Dis.* **122**:381–386.

Ferrus, L., Guenard, H., Vardon, G., and Varene, P. (1980). Respiratory water loss. *Resp. Physiol.* **39**:367–381.

Fick, Jr., R. B., Metzger, W. J., Richerson, H. B., Zavala, D. C., Moseley, P. L., Schoderbek, W. E. and Hunninghake, G. W. (1987). Increased bronchovascular permeability after allergen exposure in sensitive asthmatics. *J. Appl. Physiol.* **63**(3):1147–1155.

Garland, A., Ray, D. W., Doerschuk, C. M., Alger, L., Eappen, S., Hernandez, C., Jackson, M., and Solway, J. (1991). The role of tachykinins in hyperpnea-induced bronchovascular hyperpermeability in guinea pigs. *J. Appl. Physiol.* **70**(1):27–35.

Gilbert, I. A., Fouke, J. M., and McFadden, Jr., E. R. (1987). Heat and water flux in the intrathoracic airways and exercise-induced asthma. *J. Appl. Physiol.* **63**(4):1681–1691.

Gilbert, I. A., Fouke, J. M., and McFadden, Jr., E. R. (1988). Intra-airway thermodynamics during exercise and hyperventilation in asthmatics. *J. Appl. Physiol.* **64**(5):2167–2174.

Godden, D. J., Okazawa, M., Baile, E. M., and Pare, P. D. (1988a). Measurement of tracheal and bronchial mucosal blood flow in dogs using laser doppler velocimetry (abstract). *Am. Rev. Respir. Dis.* **137**(4, Part 2):370A.

Godden, D. J., Okazawa, M., Pare, P. D., and Baile, E. M. (1988b). Hypertonic aerosol inhalation does not alter central airway blood flow in dogs. *J. Appl. Physiol.* **65**(5):1990–1994.

Goodale, J. L. (1896). An experimental study of the respiratory function of the nose. *Boston Med. Surg. J.* **135**:457.

Griffin, M. P., Fung, K. F., Ingram, Jr., R. H., McFadden, Jr., E. R., and MacDonald, N. (1982). Dose-response effects of atropine on thermal stimulus response relationships in asthma. *J. Appl. Physiol.* **53**(6):1576–1582.

Hanna, L. M., and Scherer, P. W. (1986a). Regional control of local airway heat and water vapor losses. *J. Appl. Physiol.* **61**(2):624–632.

Hanna, L. M., and Scherer, P. W. (1986b). A theoretical model of localized heat and water vapor transport in the human respiratory tract. *J. Biomech. Eng.* **108**(1):19–27.

Hayes, P. A., Padbury, E. H., Florio, J. T., and Fyfield, T. P. (1982). Respiratory heat transfer in cold water and during rewarming. *J. Biomech. Eng.* **104**(1):45–49.

Higenbottam, T., Stokes, T., Jamieson, S., and Hill, L. (1983). A comparison of exercise, hyperventilation with cold air and warm air, and the inhalation of "fog" in the provocation of asthma. *Eur. J. Respir. Dis.* **64**:421–423.

Hill, P., Goulding, D., Webber, S. E., and Widdicombe, J. G. (1989). Blood sinuses in the submucosa of the large airways of the sheep. *J. Anat.* **162**:235–247.

Horsfield, K., and Cumming, G. (1976). Morphology of the bronchial tree in the dog. *Respir. Physiol.* **26**:173–182.

Hughes, T. (1965). Microcirculation of the tracheo-bronchial tree. *Nature* **206**:425–426.

Ingelstedt, S. (1956). Studies on the conditioning of air in the respiratory tract. *Acta Otolaryngol. (Stockh.) (Suppl.)* **131**:1–180.

Igenito, E. P. (1984). *Respiratory Fluid Mechanisms and Heat Transfer.* Ph. D. Thesis. Cambridge, MA; Massachusetts Institute of Technology.

Ingenito, E. P., Solway, J., McFadden, Jr., E. R., Pichurko, B. M., Cravalho, E. G., and Drazen, J. M., (1986). Finite differences analysis of respiratory heat transfer. *J. Appl. Physiol.* **61**(6):2252–2259.

Ingenito, E. P., Solway, J., McFadden, Jr., E. R., Pichurko, B., Bowman, H. F., Michaels, D., and Drazen, J. M. (1987). Indirect assessment of mucosal surface temperature in airways: theory and tests. *J. Appl. Physiol.* **63**(5):2075–2083.

Ingenito, E. P., Solway, J., Lombardo, A., Drazen, J. M., and Pichurko, B.

(1988). Dissociation of temperature-gradient and evaporative heat loss during cold gas hyperventilation in cold-induced asthma. *Am. Rev. Respir. Dis.* **138**:540–546.

Ingenito, E. P., Pliss, L. B., Ingram, Jr., R. H., and Pichurko, B. M. (1990). Bronchoalvelar lavage cell and mediator responses to hyperpnea-induced bronchoconstriction in the guinea pig. *Am. Rev. Respir. Dis.* **141**:1162–1166.

Karlsson, J. A., and Persson, C. G. A. (1984). Local anesthetics selectively inhibit non-cholinergic neural contractions in guinea pig airways. *Acta Physiol. Scand.* **210**:469–471.

Kay, A. B. (1987). Provoked asthma and mast cells. *Am. Rev. Respir. Dis.* **135**:1200–1203.

Kelly, L., Kolbe, J., Mitzner, W., Spannhake, E. W., Bromberger-Barnea, B., and Menkes, H. (1986). Bronchial blood flow affects recovery from constriction in dog lung periphery. *J. Appl. Physiol.* **60**(6):1954–1959.

Laitinen, A., Laitinen, L. A., Moss, R., and Widdicombe, J. G. (1987). The organization and structure of tracheal and bronchial blood vessels in the dog. *J. Physiol. (Lond.)* **382**:10P.

Laitinen, L. A., Robinson, N. P., Laitinen A., and Widdicombe, J. G. (1986). Relationship between tracheal mucosal thickness and vascular resistance in dogs. *J. Appl. Physiol.* **61**(6):2186–2193.

Laitinen, L. A., Laitinen, A., Salonen, R. O., and Widdicombe, J. G. (1987a). Vascular actions of airway neuropeptides. *Am. Rev. Respir. Dis.* **136**(6, Part 2):S59–S64.

Laitinen, L. A., Laitinen, A., and Widdicombe, J. (1987b). Effects of inflammatory and other mediators on airway vascular beds. *Am. Rev. Respir. Dis.* **135**(6, Part 2):S67–S70.

Laitinen, L. A., Laitinen, M. A., and Widdicombe, J. G. (1987c). Dose-related effects of pharmacological mediators on tracheal vascular resistance in dogs. *Br. J. Pharmacol.* **92**(4):703–709.

Laitinen, L. A., Laitinen, M. V. A., and Widdicombe, J. G. (1987d). Parasympathetic nervous control of tracheal vascular resistance in the dog. *J. Physiol. (Lond.)* **385**:135–146.

Lee, T. H., Nagy, L., Nagakura, T., Walport, M. J., and Kay, A. B. (1982). Identification and partial characterization of an exercise-induced neutrophil chemotactic factor in bronchial asthma. *J. Clin. Invest.* **69**:889–899.

Lee, T. H., Nagakura, T., Cromwell, O., Brown, M. J., Causon, R., and Kay, A. B. (1984). Neutrophil chemotactic activity and histamine in atopic and nonatopic subjects after exercise-induced asthma. *Am. Rev. Respir. Dis.* **129**:409–412.

Long, W. M., Sprung, C. L., Fawal, H. E., Yerger, L. D., Eyre, P., Abraham, W. M., and Wanner, A. (1985). Effects of histamine on bronchial artery blood flow and bronchomotor tone. *J. Appl. Physiol.* **59**(1):254–261.

Long, W. M., Yerger, L. D., Martinez, H., Codias, E., Sprung, C. L., Abraham, W. M., and Wanner, A. (1988). Modification of bronchial blood flow during allergic airway responses. *J. Appl. Physiol.* **65**(1):272–282.

Magendie (1829) in Hetderks, D. R. (1927). Observations on reaction of normal nasal mucous membrane. *Am. J. Med. Sci.* **174**:231.

Man, S. F. P., Adams, III, G. K., and Proctor, D. F. (1979). Effects of temperature, relative humidity, and mode of breathing on canine airway secretions. *J. Appl. Physiol.* **46**(2):205–210.

Martling, C. R., Gazelius, B., and Lundberg, J. M. (1987). Nervous control of tracheal blood flow in the cat measured by the laser Doppler technique. *Acta Physiol. Scand.* **130**(3):409–417.

McCormack, D. G., Salonen, R. O., and Barnes, P. J. (1989). Effect of sensory neuropeptides on canine bronchial and pulmonary vessels in vitro. *Life Sci.* **45**(25):2405–2412.

McDonald, D. M. (1987). Neurogenic inflammation in the respiratory tract: Actions of sensory nerve mediators on blood vessels and epithelium of the airway mucosa. *Am. Rev. Respir. Dis.* **136**:S65–S72.

McFadden, E. R., Jr. (1983). Respiratory heat and water exchange: Physiological and clinical implications. *J. Appl. Physiol.* **54**(2):331–336.

McFadden, E. R., Jr., and Ingram, R. H. Jr., (1986). Thermal factors in respiratory mechanics. In *Handbook of Physiology.* Section 3. *The Respiratory System.* Volume III. *Mechanics of Breathing,* Part 2. pp. 703–709. Edited by A. P. Fishman, P. T. Macklem, and J. Mead. Baltimore, Williams & Wilkins, (Chap. 39).

McFadden, E. R., Jr., and Pichurko, B. M. (1985). Intraairway thermal profiles during exercise and hyperventilation in normal man. *J. Clin. Invest.* **76**(3):1007–1010.

McFadden, E. R., Jr., Denison, D. M., Waller, J. R., Assoufi, B., Peacock, A., and Sopwith, T. (1982). Direct recordings of the temperatures in the tracheobronchial tree in normal man. *J. Clin. Invest.* **69**:700–705.

McFadden, E. R., Jr., Pichurko, B. M., Bowman, H. F., Ingenito, E., Burns, S., Dowling, N., and Solway, J., (1985). Thermal mapping of the airways in humans. *J. Appl. Physiol.* **58**(2):564–570.

Moritz, A. R., and Weisiger, J. R. (1945). Effects of cold air on air passages and lungs. *Arch. Intern. Med.* **75**:233–240.

Murata, K., Itoh, H., Todo, G., Itoh, T., Kanaoka, M., Furuta, M., and Torizuke, K. (1986). Bronchial venous plexus and its communication with pulmonary circulation. *Invest. Radiol.* **21**(1):24–30.

Nagakura, T., Lee, T. H., Assoufi, B. K., Newman-Taylor, A. J., Denison, D. M., and Kay, A. B. (1983). Neutrophil chemotactic factor in exercise- and hyperventilation-induced asthma. *Am. Rev. Respir. Dis.* **128**:294–296.

O'Cain, C. F., Dowling, N. B., Slutsky, A. S., Hensley, M. J., Strohl, K. P., McFadden, Jr., E. R., and Ingram, Jr. R. H. (1980). Airway effects of respiratory heat loss in normal subjects. *J. Appl. Physiol.* **49**(5):875–880.

Parsons, G. H., Pare, P. D., White, D. A., and Baile, E. M. (1989). Airway blood flow response to eucapnic dry air hyperventilation in sheep. *J. Appl. Physiol.* **66**:1443–1447.

Persson, C. G. A. (1987). Leakage of macromolecules from the tracheobronchial microcirculation. *Am. Rev. Respir. Dis.* **135**(6, Part 2):S71–S75.

Persson, C. G. A. (1988). Plasma exudation and asthma. *Lung* **166**:1–23.

Persson, C. G. A., Erjefalt, I., and Andersson, P. (1986). Leakage of macromolecules from guinea pig tracheobronchial microcirculation. Effects of allergen, leukotrienes, tachykinins, and anti-asthma drugs. *Acta Physiol. Scand.* **127**:95–106.

Phelipeau, D., Ferrus, L., and Varene, P. (1982). Les echanges thermiques respiratoires chez l'homme en fonction de la temperature de gas inspire. *J. Physiol. (Paris)* **78**(2):163–169.

Pietra, G. G., and Magno, M. (1978). Pharmacological factors influencing permeability of the bronchial microcirculation. *Fed. Proc.* **37**(11):2466–2470.

Ray, D. W., Crawford, G., Strek, M., Ingenito, E., and Solway, J. (1986). Non-invasive determination of intrapulmonary heat exchange (abstract). *Physiologist* **29**(4):146.

Ray, D. W., Doerschuk, C. M., Jackson, M., Hernandez, C., Eappen, S., Leff, A. R., and Solway, J. (1988a). Bronchial vascular hyperpermeability accompanies hyperpnea-induced bronchoconstriction (HIB) in guinea pigs (abstract). *Physiologist* **31**(4):A65.

Ray, D. W., Hernandez, C., Munoz, N., Leff, A. R., and Solway, J. (1988b). Bronchoconstriction elicited by isocapnic hyperpnea in guinea pigs. *J. Appl. Physiol.* **65**(2):934–939.

Ray, D. W., Alger, L., Hernandez, C., Eappen, S., Leff, A. R., and Solway, J. (1989a). Local mucosal cooling/drying causes local bronchovascular hyperpermeability in ferrets (abstract). *Am. Rev. Respir. Dis.* **139**(4, Part 2):A233.

Ray, D. W., Hernandez, C., Leff, A. R., Drazen, J. M., and Solway, J. (1989b). Tachykinins mediate bronchoconstriction elicited by isocapnic hypernea in guinea pigs. *J. Appl. Physiol.* **66**:1108–1112.

Ray, D. W., Ingenito, E. P., Strek, M., Schumacker, P. T., and Solway, J. (1989c). Longitudinal distribution of canine respiratory heat and water exchanges. *J. Appl. Physiol.* **66**:2788–2798.

Ray, D. W., Eappen, S., Hernandez, C., Jackson, M., Alger, L., Leff, A. R., and Solway, J. (1990). Distribution of airway narrowing during hyperpnea-induced bronchoconstriction in guinea pigs. *J. Appl. Physiol.* **69**(4):1323–1329.

Rohsenow, W. M., and Choi, H. Y. (1961). *Heat, Mass, and Momentum Transfer.* Englewood Cliffs, NJ: Prentice Hall.

Salonen, R. O., Deffebach, M. E., and Widdicombe, J. G. (1988a). Cold dry air-induced smooth muscle and vascular responses in the trachea of the anesthetized dog. *J. Physiol. (Lond.)* **407**:35P.

Salonen, R. O., Webber, S. E., and Widdicombe, J. G. (1988b). Effect of neuropeptides and capsaicin on the canine tracheal vasculature in vivo. *Br. J. Pharmacol.* **95**(4):1262–1270.

Sheppard, D., Epstein, J., Hotzman, M. J., Nadel, J. A., and Boushey, H. A. (1983). Effect of route of atropine delivery on bronchospasm from cold air and methacholine. *J. Appl. Physiol.* **54**(1):130–133.

Solway, J., Picurko, B. M., Ingenito, E. P., McFadden, Jr., E. R., Fanta, C. H., Ingram, Jr., R. H., and Drazen, J. M. (1985). Breathing pattern affects airway wall temperature during cold air hyperpnea in humans. *Am. Rev. Respir. Dis.* **132**:853–857.

Solway, J., Ray, D. W., Crawford, G., Strek, M., and Ingenito, E. (1986a). Non-invasive estimation of intra-airway heat transfers (abstract) *Physiologist* **29**(4):145.

Solway, J., Leff, A. R., Dreshaj, I., Munoz, N. M., Ingenito, E. P., Michaels, D., Ingram, Jr., R. H., and Drazen, J. M. (1986b). Circulatory heat sources for canine respiratory heat exchange. *J. Clin. Invest.* **78**:1015–1019.

Togias, A. G., Naclerio, R. M., Proud, D., Fish, J. E., Adkinson, Jr., N. F., Kagey-Sobotka, A., Norman, P. S., and Lichtenstein, L. M. (1985). Nasal challenge with cold, dry air results in release of inflammatory mediators: Possible mast cell involvement. *J. Clin. Invest.* **76**:1375–1381.

Togias, A. G., Naclerio, R. M., Peters, S. P., Nimmagadda, I., Proud, D., Kagey-Sobotka, A., Adkinson, Jr., N. F., Norman, P. S., and Lichtenstein, L. M. (1986). Local generation of sulfidopeptide leukotrienes upon nasal provocation with cold, dry air. *Am. Rev. Respir. Dis.* **133**:1133–1137.

van Oostdam, J. C., Walker, D. C., Knudson, K., Dirks, P., Dahlby, R. W., and Hogg, J. C. (1986). Effect of breathing dry air on structure and function of airways. *J. Appl. Physiol.* **61**(1):312–317.

Wagner, E. M., Mitzner, W. A., and Bleecker, E. R. (1986). Role of the bronchial circulation in cold air induced bronchospasm (abstract). *Am. Rev. Respir. Dis.* **133**(4, Part 2):A174.

Wanner, A., Barker, J. A., Long, W. M., Mariassy, A. T., and Chediak, A. D. (1988). Measurement of airway mucosal perfusion and water volume with an inert soluble gas. *J. Appl. Physiol.* **65**(1):264–271.

Webb, P. (1951). Air temperatures in respiratory tracts of resting subjects in cold. *J. Appl. Physiol.* **4**:378–382.

Woodward, D. F., Weichman, B. M., Gill, C. A., and Wasserman, M. A. (1983). The effect of synthetic leukotrienes on tracheal microvascular permeability. *Prostaglandins* **25**(1):131–142.

Zawadski, D. K., Lenner, K. A., and McFadden, Jr., E. R. (1988). Comparison of intraairway temperatures in normal and asthmatic subjects after hyperpnea with hot, cold, and ambient air. *Am. Rev. Respir. Dis.* **138**:1553–1558.

Zeballos, R. J., Shturman-Ellstein, R., McNally, Jr., J. F., Hirsch, J. E., and Souhrada, J. F. (1978). The role of hyperventilation in exercise-induced bronchoconstriction. *Am. Rev. Respir. Dis.* **118**:877–884.

10

Regulation of Respiratory Heat and Water Loss by Lung Circulation

MARK E. DEFFEBACH

University of Washington
School of Medicine
Seattle, Washington

PIERGIUSEPPE AGOSTONI

Cardiology Institute
University of Milan
Milan, Italy

I. Introduction

Heat in the form of warm, moist exhaled air is continuously lost from the airways of all air-breathing animals. This is, in part, a consequence of the transfer of heat and water into the inspired air so that it is properly conditioned before reaching the alveolar and gas-exchanging surfaces. These heat losses can be viewed as an unavoidable and perhaps unfortunate consequence of a conditioning process, or they can be looked at as an opportunity to transfer heat from the organism into the environment. Many species, including several of the species currently used to study the airway circulation, rely on respiratory heat loss as a primary mechanism of thermoregulation. The purpose of this review is to examine some of the ways the airway circulation participates in thermal regulation. These processes involve the circulation of both the upper and lower airways as well as the pulmonary circulation.

II. Mechanisms

A. Countercurrent Heat Exchange

The basic physical principle that underlies much of respiratory thermoregulation is that of countercurrent heat exchange. Schmidt-Nielsen and colleagues have applied this principle to the study of a variety of biological systems, including regulation of respiratory heat losses (Jackson and Schmidt-Nielsen, 1964; Schmidt-Nielsen et al., 1970b; Schmidt-Nielsen, 1981). The simplest form of countercurrent heat exchange is that between fluids that are spatially separated and flowing in opposite directions (Fig. 1). In the respiratory tract a very similar form of heat exchange occurs, but rather than two fluids that are spatially separated, there is temporal separation of a single fluid, air, in a single tube (Fig. 2). During inspiration cooler air passes over warm moist airway surfaces, with cooling of the mucosa and warming of the air. As the air is warmed the relative humidity decreases and water evaporates off the mucosal surface. Thus, there are two components to mucosal cooling: convection and evaporation. Of these two, evaporation accounts for the bulk of the heat loss from the mucosal surface. The inhaled air is fully saturated and warmed to body temperature before exhalation begins. As this heat- and water-laden air passes over the previously cooled airway surface, heat is transferred back to the mucosa. Heat conservation occurs as a result of the cooling of the exhaled air. Heat recovery would be complete if three criteria were met: (1) all exchange was convective, (2) there was no heat exchange with the airway surface (such as from the circulation) other than the countercurrent heat exchange with the airstream, and (3) at each point on the airway, heat exchange reaches equilibrium. In life none of these criteria are met, although there is considerable conservation of respiratory heat. As a result of counter current heat exchange, recovery of up to 70% of the heat required for the conditioning of

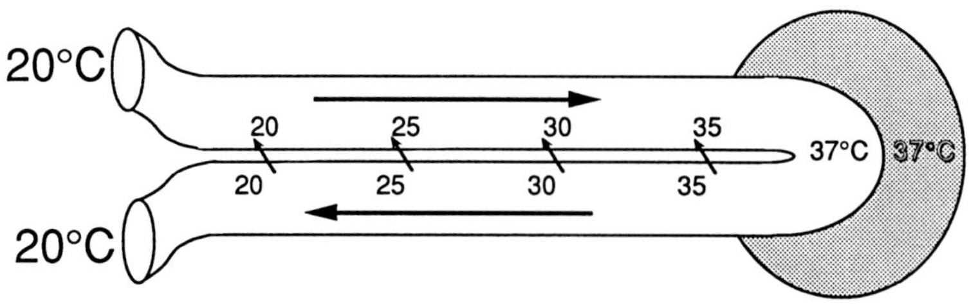

Figure 1 Countercurrent heat exchange between two fluids with spatial separation and flow in opposite directions. A biological example of a very similar kind of heat exchange occurs in extremities between arteries and veins.

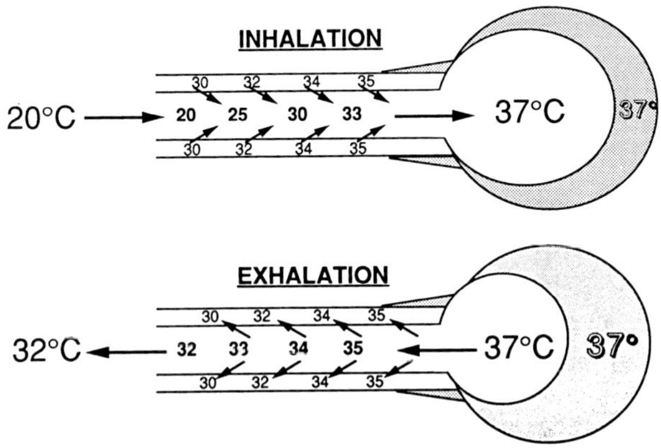

Figure 2 Countercurrent heat exchange as it occurs in the respiratory tract. Rather than spatial separation, there is temporal separation, with heat transferred to the airway mucosa during inspiration and recovered during exhalation. The shaded area represents the pulmonary blood volume. This form of countercurrent heat exchange is most efficient when no additional heat is supplied to the surface.

the inspired air can occur (Folkow and Blix, 1987). With rare exceptions, the exhaled air is 100% humidified. Because the water content of saturated air (a function of air temperature) is lower at a lower temperature, substantial water recovery occurs as well.

Regulation

Respiratory heat loss can be regulated in three ways. One mechanism is for inhalation and exhalation to occur over different surfaces, as can occur through the oral and nasal portions of the upper airway. Another involves regulation of airway surface temperature. As shown in Fig. 2, if the airway surface remains cool, maximal heat recovery occurs during exhalation. This is why an endotracheal tube can be very effective at recovering exhaled heat and water (Ray, et al., 1989). To the extent that this cooling is prevented, the gradient for heat recovery during exhalation is lost and heat escapes to the environment (Fig. 3). Last, and perhaps most potent, is a change in total minute ventilation. Changing the pattern of ventilation for a given minute ventilation has a small effect on the total amount of heat loss and a large effect on the site of heat losses along the repiratory tract (Solway et al., 1985).

Role of the Circulation

It is in these last two methods (regulation of airway temperature and ventilation) of regulating respiratory heat losses that the lung and airway circulations

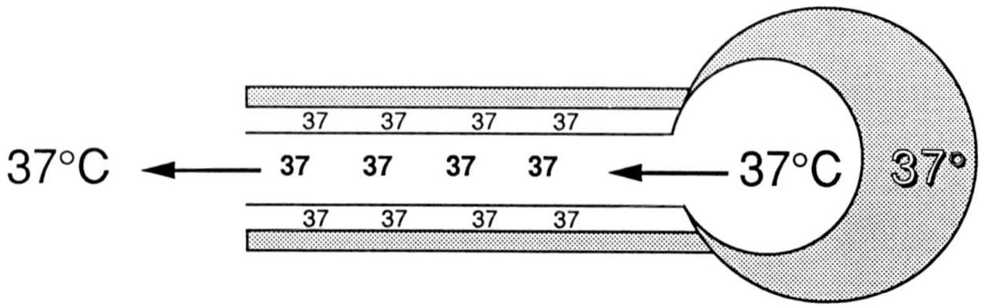

Figure 3 Countercurrent heat exchange is eliminated by keeping the mucosal surface warm. The shaded area along the airway represents increased airway blood flow, and the air escaping to the environment remains at the same temperature and water content as alveolar air.

play an important role. When conservation of heat and water is required and the mucosa is passively cooled during inspiration, vasoconstriction prevents rewarming. This is seen particularly in small animals (less than 1 kg), which, because of their high body surface area to heat production ratio, are able to dissipate all excess heat by surface convection (Taylor, 1977). In rats, for example, nasal mucosal and exhaled air temperatures remain low even during exercise (Raab and Schmidt-Nielsen, 1972). Airway surface cooling by evaporation can be so great that exhaled air can be as much as 6°C below inspired air temperature (Jackson and Schmidt-Nielsen, 1964). Anesthesia, which prevents nasal vasoconstriction, results in an increase in the exhaled air temperature (Raab and Schmidt-Nielsen, 1972). Thermoregulation-related nasal vasoconstricting responses are seen in the human as well. Burgess and Whitelaw (1984) found that nasal airflow resistance decreases during tidal breathing of cold air, suggesting that vasoconstriction occurred. In addition, selective cooling of the skin causes a reflex-mediated decrease in nasal mucosa temperature (Speisman, 1936). Similar responses are seen in seals, which forego all food and water during three months of breeding. Heat, and therefore water, conservation may be so great as to allow metabolic water production to exceed respiratory water losses, although on occasion the vasoconstricting responses may be compromised to prevent freezing of the nose (Folkow and Blix, 1987; Huntley et al., 1984).

Vascular responses also promote respiratory heat losses by a vasodilation that causes warming of the mucosal surface. In dogs, the first response to a heat load, even before panting begins, is vasodilation of the infraorbital and sphenopalatine nasal vessels (Pleshka et al., 1979). Nasal and lingual blood flow also increase during elevations in body temperature, even when the upper airway is completely bypassed (Baile et al., 1987). This illustrates that these responses are part of an overall systemic thermoregulation, not a response to local heat and water losses. Similarly, in the human, selective warming of the skin increases nasal mucosal temperature (Speisman, 1936).

Structural Adaptations

The vascular responses just described occur in the upper airway, primarily in the nose and tongue. Several upper airway structural adaptations are correlated with the efficient use of thc airways for thermal regulation (Langman et al., 1979; Schmidt-Nielsen, 1981). A large surface area with close approximation of mucosal surfaces and turbulent airflow favors heat transfer between the mucosal surfaces and the airstream. This type of structure can improve countercurrent heat recovery or promote heat loss from the surface. It is through vascular responses that the upper airway can be transformed from an efficient heat radiator to a heat conservation device. The human, in contrast, has a small nasal mucosal surface and a limited ability to conserve respiratory heat and water.

Another structural adaptation present in many species, including the human, is a large number of arteriovenous (AV) anastomoses in the nose and tongue. These contribute to very large changes in surface blood flow that are independent of local metabolic needs. In the dog, AV shunting can account for 60% of nasal blood flow. Blood flow through the shunts is controlled by the release of vasoconstriction (Krönert and Pleschka, 1976).

An even more specialized structural arrangement allows airway cooling to contribute to selective brain cooling (Fig. 4). (Baker, 1972, 1982; Blumberg and Moltz, 1988; Cabanac, 1986; Johnsen and Folkow, 1988). Blood that is cooled during its passage through the nose is directed to the base of the brain. In the carotid rete, heat exchange with the carotid blood cools the arterial blood on its way to the brain. Because the brain is the most temperature-sensitive structure, even a small amount of cooling can result in a significant selective advantage, especially in animals adapted for endurance exercise. The gazelle, for example, demonstrates the most efficient brain cooling, with brain temperature as much as 3.2°C below that of the central blood (Cabanac, 1986). Brain cooling during exercise occurs in several other species and has even been shown in the copulating rat (Blumberg and Moltz, 1988).

B. Lower Airways Heat Exchange

In contrast to the upper airways, there are few structural adaptations for thermoregulation in the airways below the larynx. After accounting for body size, the mucosal surface area and blood flow of the large airways is fairly constant throughout many different animal species (Deffebach et al., 1987). AV anastomoses have not been demonstrated in the lower airways, where vascular

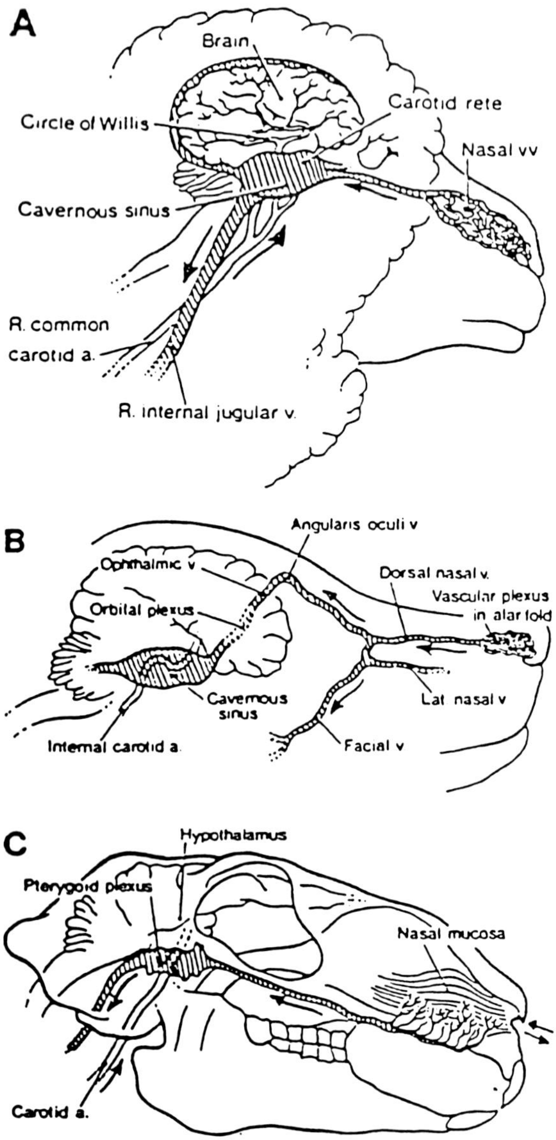

Figure 4 Specialized vascular arrangement for brain cooling: (A) sheep; (B) dog; and (C) rabbit; v, vein; a, artery. Blood is cooled in the nasal mucosa and then directed to the base of the brain, where it cools the carotid blood. (Cabanac, 1986.)

responses are not part of overall thermoregulation but rather due to local heat and, probably, water losses. In the dog, for example, tracheal blood flow increases only when the upper airway is bypassed by a tracheostomy and the trachea exposed to poorly conditioned air (Baile et al., 1987). This is in clear contrast to the tongue, where elevation in body temperature causes blood flow to rise (Fig. 5). In the human, cold and dry air ventilation results in substantial cooling of the trachea, with surface temperatures as low as 27°C deep within the lung (McFadden et al., 1982). In the trachea, dry air ventilation, cooling, and hypertonic fluid exposure all result in vasodilation (Deffebach et al., 1989). The intrapulmonary airways, however, are much more resistant to cooling (Ray et al., 1989). This resistance is because of the surrounding pulmonary circulation. In this region of the lung, it is likely that the pulmonary circulation

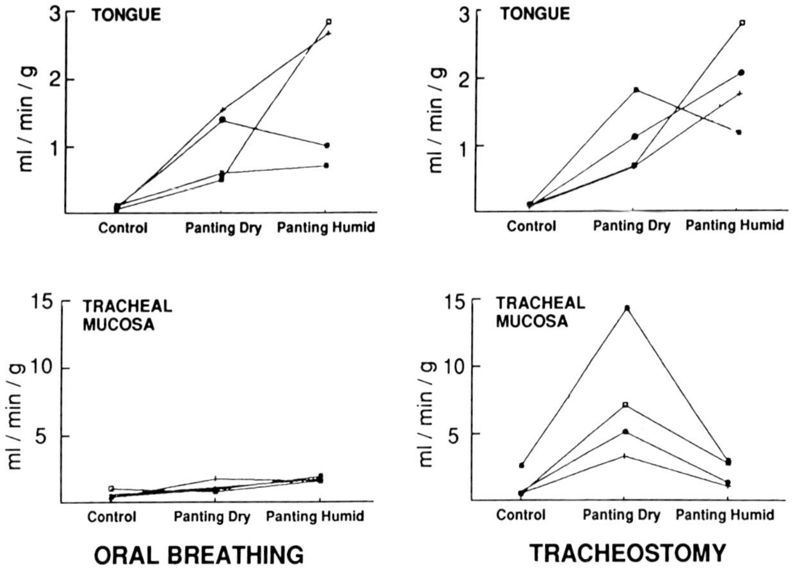

Figure 5 Blood flow responses in the tongue and tracheal mucosa during panting induced by raising body temperature in the dog. On the left the upper airway was intact and ventilation was through the mouth and nose. On the right the upper airway was bypassed and ventilation was through a tracheostomy. Each symbol represents an individual dog. Blood flow in the tongue is related to overall thermoregulation and was increased whether there was airflow across the tongue or not. Tracheal blood flow increased only when the tracheal surface was exposed to cold, dry air. (Baile et al., 1987.)

supplies the heat to prevent cooling of the mucosal surface, and the bronchial circulation supplies water to prevent desiccation. The pulmonary blood flow represents an almost unlimited supply of heat (the entire cardiac output), and the amount of water required is sufficiently small to represent only a fraction of the bronchial blood flow (Deffebach et al., 1989). This arrangement prevents any heat transferred into the airstream from the intrapulmonary airways from being recovered within the lung during exhalation (see Fig. 3). The surface area in the trachea and extrapulmonary bronchi is too small for signficant amounts of heat recovery to occur.

Heat transfer from the mucosa to the airstream occurs in the intrapulmonary airways in both humans and dogs. The factors that determine whether heat exchange occurs in this region are total minute ventilation and the size of the tidal volume (Ray et al., 1989; Solway et al., 1985). Thus, the lower airways can be recruited for respiratory thermoregulation, primarily through alterations in ventilation, not through changes in blood flow.

III. Integration of Heat Exchange

A. Panting

Panting is the most familiar mechanism for increasing respiratory heat loss. It is not a single response but rather a series of responses, each resulting in greater amounts of respiratory heat loss. It has some advantages over sweating as a thermoregulatory mechanism (Taylor, 1977). First, a link between respiratory heat loss and breathing already exists as heat production and ventilation are both increased during exercise. Second, because the skin is not used for dissipation of heat, skin blood flow can remain low and skin temperature can approach ambient temperature. This greatly reduces simultaneous heat gain from a hot environment, and the salt losses that occur with sweating are minimized as well. In addition, the cooling of the respiratory mucosal surfaces can be utilized for brain cooling. The additional work due to the increased ventilation does not add significantly to heat production. Panting can occur at the natural resonant frequency of the respiratory system (approximately 300 breaths/min in dogs), which results in very little increase in the work of breathing (Crawford, 1962).

The earliest response to heat load in the dog is vasodilation of nasal blood vessels, even before panting begins (Pleshka et al., 1979). As excess heat production increases, there is an abrupt increase in respiratory rate to over 300 breaths/min. There is also a dramatic fall in tidal volume; from 215 to 30 ml, for instance, in a 15 kg dog (Hales and Bligh, 1969). This results in an increase in total ventilation without a change in alveolar ventilation. If the rapid, shallow breathing were to and fro across the same surface, countercurrent heat recovery would remain, although it would be less efficient because mucosal vasodilation would limit cooling of the surface (see Fig. 3). If the flow of air were over different surfaces during inhalation and exhalation, however, this problem would be solved. This is what occurs during shallow thermal panting in dogs (Fig. 6) (Schmidt-Nielsen et al., 1970a). Air enters through the nose and is exhaled through the mouth so that exhaled air leaves at

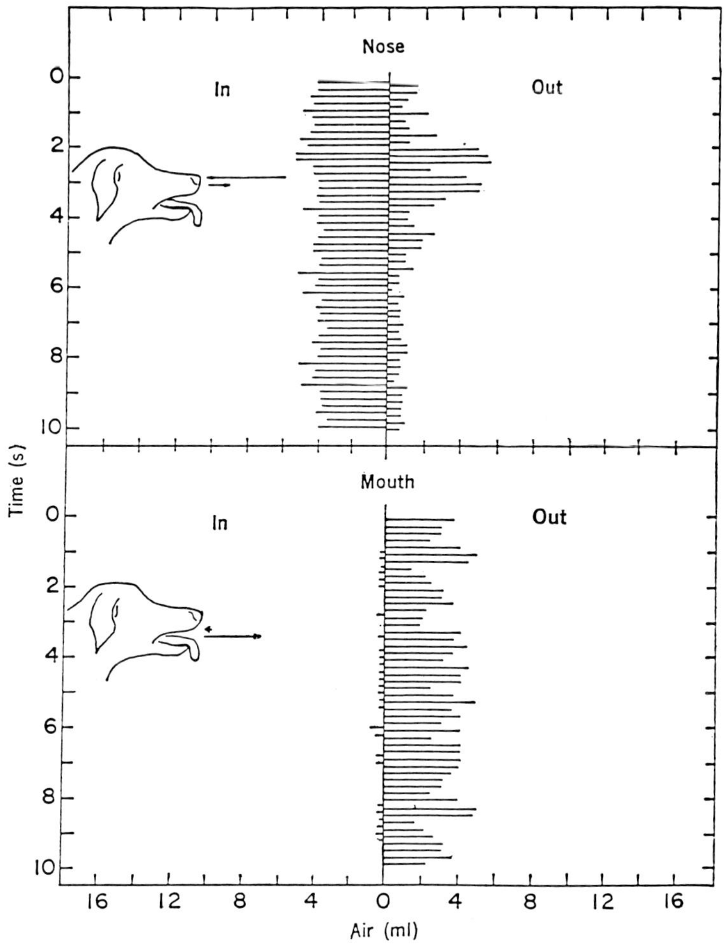

Figure 6 Respiratory pattern during early panting in the dog. Inflow of air is through the nose, with the outflow through the mouth. This results in unidirectional airflow over two different mucosal surfaces and eliminates countercurrent heat recovery. Note that the respiratory frequency during panting is ≈5 Hz. (Schmidt-Nielsen et al., 1970a.)

nearly the same temperature and water content as the alveolar air. If the dog is forced to pant through the mouth, exhaled temperature falls to 29°C. The nasal mucosal surface is an important site of water transfer into the airstream, with the lateral nasal gland supplying hypotonic fluid to the surface (Blatt et al., 1972). This fluid accounts for only about one-third of the total fluid lost during exhalation. The increase in nasal blood flow is limited (Baile et al., 1987; Hales and Dampney, 1975; Pleshka et al., 1979), suggesting that other regions of the respiratory tract must be important sites of heat transfer into the inspired air. Lingual blood flow is actually decreased during the early stages of panting (Kindermann and Pleschka, 1973). This, coupled with the fact that there is unidirectional flow of fully saturated, body-temperature air over the surface (Schmidt-Nielsen et al., 1970a), suggests that the tongue is not a major site of heat loss during the changes of early panting.

As heat stress continues, the pattern of ventilation again changes, from nasal in and oral out to strictly oral breathing (Fig. 7) (Schmidt-Nielsen et al., 1970a). Respiratory frequency decreases, and tidal volume increases with a

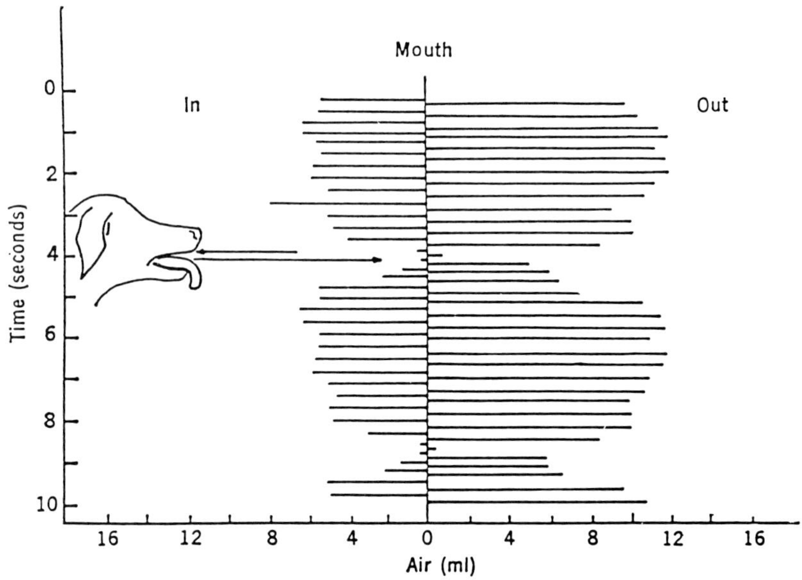

Figure 7 Respiratory pattern during deep thermal panting in the dog. Frequency is decreased, tidal volume increased, and all airflow is through the mouth. (Schmidt-Nielsen et al., 1970a.)

large increase in the total alveolar ventilation (Hales and Bligh, 1969). Without an increase in CO_2 production, a marked respiratory alkalosis develops. This pattern of breathing results in a shift of the primary sites of respiratory heat dissipation from the upper airway to the smaller airways of the lung and allows poorly conditioned air to penetrate the intrapulmonary airways (Ray et al., 1989). At this point, lingual blood flow increases greatly, primarily through AV anastomoses (Kindermann and Pleschka, 1973; Krönert and Pleschka, 1976), and the tongue is extended out of the mouth. Fluid for evaporation from the tongue is supplied by the salivary glands (Blatt et al., 1972; Taylor, 1977). A significant amount of heat is lost from the tongue, probably during both inhalation and exhalation.

B. Panting and Nonpanting Comparison

It is interesting to compare respiratory heat exchange in a panting animal with that of other species, including the human. Although the primary thermoregulatory mechanism in the human is sweating and changes in skin blood flow, substantial respiratory heat and water losses can be regulated. The nasal vasoconstricting and vasodilatory reflexes seen with skin cooling and warming are examples of systemic reflexes that can regulate respiratory heat losses (Speisman, 1936). During nasal breathing with cold air in the human, the ventilatory response to inspired CO_2 is decreased (Burgess and Whitelaw, 1984), suggesting that a reduction in ventilation could be another mechanism for conserving respiratory heat and water. More recently, Diesel et al. (1990) found in calves that reductions in inspired air or ambient temperature changed the pattern of ventilation, changing the ventilatory equivalent (V_{O_2}/V_e) and resulting in hypoxia and hypercarbia. This substantially reduced the fraction of metabolic heat production lost through the respiratory tract (Diesel et al., 1990). In primates, spinal cord and hypothalamic heating results in an abrupt increase in ventilation (Chai and Lin, 1972; Elizondo, 1977), confirming that manipulation of respiratory heat losses can be part of an overall thermoregulatory response.

If analogies between thermoregulation in dogs and human can be made, then dog tongue and human skin probably have a similar function. Both provide surfaces for evaporation of fluid secreted onto the surface by specialized glands; both are richly supplied by a vasculature containing AV anastomoses; and the blood flow and fluid secretion of both are controlled by central thermoregulatory mechanisms. The utilization of the lower airways is similar in both species, as is the structure of the lower airways. In both humans and dogs, recruitment of the lower airways is determined by the pattern of ventilation, and when excess heat production is great, the pattern of ventilation in both becomes that of oral breathing with large tidal volumes.

C. The Camel

The camel is faced with four major problems related to thermoregulation. Access to water is limited and very episodic; it exercises in an extremely hot and dry environment; it cannot escape to a less hostile environment, such as a burrow; and because it is a large animal, it is dependent on evaporation for dissipation of excess heat. This results in very conflicting goals: water conservation and dissipation of excess heat. Because of these challenges, respiratory heat losses may be more closely regulated in the camel than in any other species.

In a series of studies by Schmidt-Nielsen and colleagues, a remarkable pattern emerges (Langman et al., 1978; Schmidt-Nielsen et al., 1957, 1967, 1981a; Schmidt-Nielsen 1964; Schroter et al., 1987). The most important thermoregulatory strategy is heat storage during the day and dissipation at night. This is accomplished by several mechanisms. During the day, there is nasal vasodilation and heat losses are primarily through respiratory evaporation, with the exhaled air fully saturated and at body temperature. The vasodilation also contributes to brain cooling. Respiratory heat losses are limited, and body temperature increases up to 6°C during the day. Over many days, as the animal becomes more dehydrated, daytime respiratory heat losses decrease and the daily rise in body temperature increases. As dehydration progresses further, there may be vasoconstriction during the day, which although limiting respiratory water loss, also limits brain cooling. At night, the gradient for radiant heat losses from the skin is much greater and the heat stored during the day can be gradually dissipated by nonevaporative mechanisms. At night, therefore, water conservation mechanisms are in full force. These include nasal vasoconstriction, leading to lowering of exhaled air temperature. In addition, the relative humidity of the exhaled air is decreased to 75%, probably by hygroscopic (water-absorbing) secretions on the nasal mucosa (Schmidt-Nielsen et al., 1981b). Despite all these manipulations, the camel can lose 30% of its body weight during water deprivation but is able to replace the entire amount in a single drinking session.

IV. Airway Circulation Responses to Temperature

Thus far, we have discussed how the airway circulation can control heat and water losses from the animal and regulate body temperature. The reverse situation, that is, how changes in body or tissue temperature can influence circulatory responses, is also of interest in both the pulmonary and bronchial circulations.

Selective cooling of blood perfusing the lung increases pulmonary arterial pressure, probably by increasing blood viscosity (Pennington et al., 1971). Specific pulmonary vascular responses can be temperature sensitive, with diminution of both hypoxia- and ATP-induced vasoconstriction at 27°C as compared with body temperature (Haavik-Nilsen and Hauge, 1968).

The temperature of the pulmonary blood also influences bronchial blood flow in the same region of the lung. Agostoni et al. controlled the pulmonary perfusion temperature in open-chested dogs while measuring the total and anastomotic bronchial blood flow to the perfused lobe (Agostoni et al., 1987a). Systemic temperature did not vary. The bronchial blood flow was temperature dependent, showing a maximal blood flow at 36°C, 2°C below body temperature (Fig. 8). Because there were no changes in pulmonary perfusion pressure and the change in flow occurred with both raising and lowering of the perfusion temperature, this is not an effect of blood viscosity. The temperature dependence of the lobar bronchial blood flow may explain some of the variability in reported values for bronchial blood flow.

An imporant aspect of the temperature dependence of bronchial blood flow is illustrated in studies on the role of the bronchial circulation in pul-

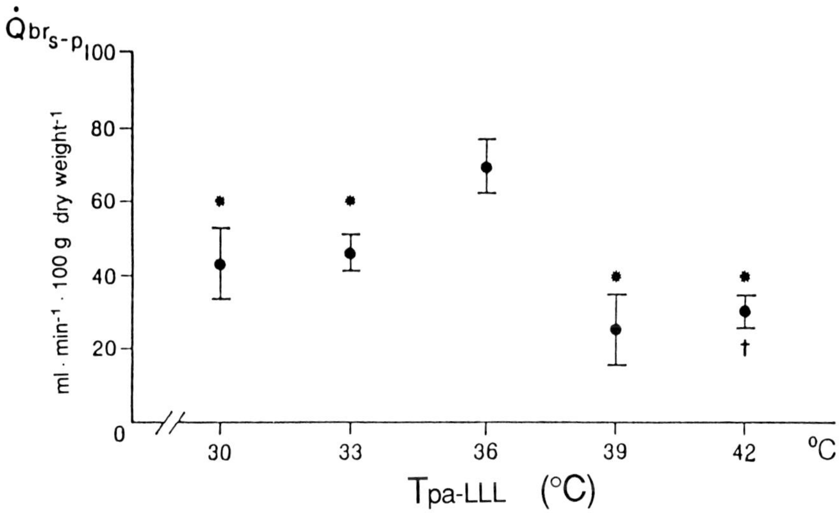

Figure 8 Relationship between lobar systemic-to-pulmonary anastomotic bronchial blood flow Q̇br(s-p) and temperature in the lung (pulmonary vein) when lobar temperature was altered by adjusting the temperature of the pulmonary artery blood perfusing the lobe Tpa-LLL. Q̇br(s-p) decreases at lobar temperatures above and below 36°C. *$P < 0.005$ compared to 36°C ($n = 7$ †except where $n = 6$). (Agostoni et al., 1987a.)

monary vascular obstruction. Early studies did not demonstrate any alteration of bronchial blood flow for 4 h following pulmonary artery ligation in dogs (Williams and Towbin, 1955). These studies were in animals with a limited thoracotomy. Similarly, in closed-chested animals, Malik and Tracy (1980) did not see any acute changes in bronchial blood flow following pulmonary microembolism. Jindal et al. (1984), also in dogs, examined the responses of left lower lobe systemic to pulmonary anastomotic bronchial blood flow in open-chested animals. In contrast to earlier studies, they found an acute increase in bronchial blood flow following interruption of pulmonary perfusion. A major difference in the studies of Jindal et al. and the other cited studies is that the studies of Jindal et al. were performed in open-chested animals without temperature controls, such as warming of the perfusing blood. A very similar study performed with both environmental and blood temperatures carefully controlled showed that during interruption of pulmonary perfusion there was actually a slight reduction in anastomotic lobar bronchial blood flow, due to a reduction in lobar temperature, when the perfusion of warmed pulmonary blood was stopped (Agostoni et al., 1987b). In the same study, if the lobe was perfused with room-temperature blood and then flow was stopped without external control of temperature, as was done in the studies of Jindal et al., there was an increase in total and anastomotic bronchial blood flow. These results suggested that the lobe was continuously cooled during perfusion with pulmonary blood at room temperature. When this flow was interrupted, the influx of body-temperature bronchial blood, now making up the entire perfusion to the lobe rather than a fraction, warmed the lung. Because of the temperature dependence of lobar bronchial blood flow (Agostoni et al., 1987a), as lobar temperature increased so did the bronchial blood flow. The relationship between pulmonary vein temperature (a reflection of the lung parenchymal temperature) and bronchial blood flow is the same whether the temperature is varied by controlling lobar perfusing blood temperature or allowing the temperature to change in an uncontrolled manner during interruption of pulmonary blood flow (Fig. 8 and 9). Thus, it is important to carefully control experimental temperature when studying the airway circulation. As described here, tracheal blood flow is also dependent on local temperature (Baile et al., 1987; Deffebach et al., 1989).

V. Conclusion

This review has focused on the interaction of the lungs, circulation, and thermoregulation. The systemic circulation of the upper and lower airways, as well as the pulmonary circulation, participates in various aspects of

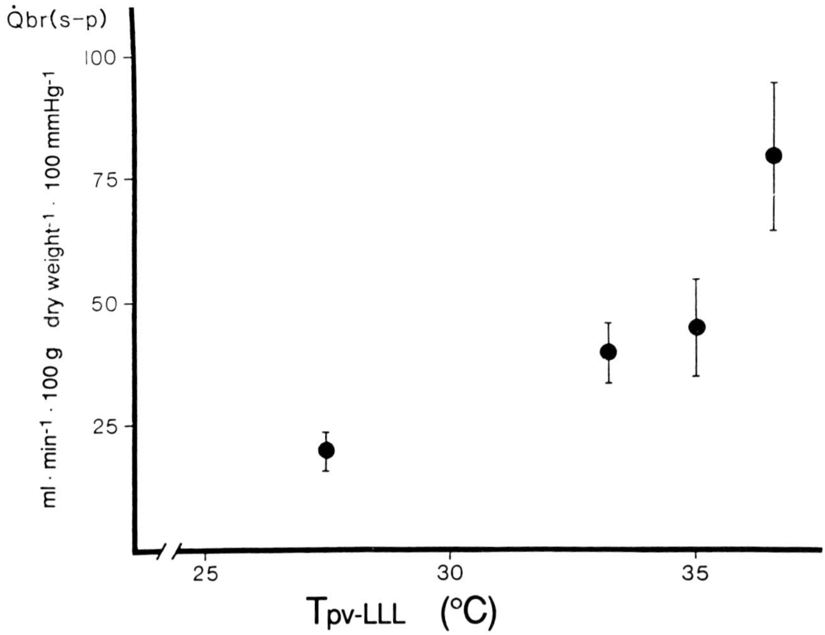

Figure 9 Relationship of lobar systemic to pulmonary anastomotic bronchial blood flow $\dot{Q}$br(s-p) and left lower lobe pulmonary venous blood temperature Tpv-LLL when lobar temperature was altered because of interruption of pulmonary perfusion. In these experiments, unlike those shown in Fig. 8, the temperature of the perfusing pulmonary artery blood was not controlled and was at room temperature. The systemic blood remained at body temperature, and with interruption of pulmonary blood flow, the inflow of bronchial blood warmed the lung. (Adapted from Agostoni et al., 1987b.)

thermoregulation. The upper airways are of primary importance in determining the amount of heat lost from the respiratory tract, and this highly regulated process is accomplished by varying the blood perfusion to the airway surfaces. Although more developed in them, these processes are not confined to panting animals. The lower airways can also be recruited for thermoregulation. This is determined primarily by the amount and pattern of ventilation and is likely to be the same in panting and nonpanting animals. Last, the tracheal and bronchial blood flow is very dependent on local temperature, and these effects should be carefully considered in the study of the physiological responses of the lung circulations.

References

Agostoni, P., Deffebach, M. E., Kirk, W., and Brengelmann, G. L. (1987a). Temperature dependence on intraparenchymal bronchial blood flow. *Respir. Physiol.* **68**:259-267.

Agostoni, P. G., Deffebach, M. E., Kirk, W., and Butler, J. (1987b). Temperature alters bronchial blood flo\' response to pulmonary artery obstruction. *J. Appl. Physiol.* **62**:1907–1911.

Baile, E. M., Guillemi, S., and Paré, P. D. (1987). Tracheobronchial and upper airway blood flow in dogs during thermally induced panting. *J. Appl. Physiol.* **63**:2240–2246.

Baker, M. A. (1972). Influence of the carotid rete on brain temperature in cats exposed to hot environments. *J. Physiol. (Lond.)* **220**:711–728.

Baker, M. A. (1982). Brain cooling in endotherms in heat and exercise. *Anna. Rev. Physiol.* **44**:85–96.

Blatt, C. M., Taylor, C. R., and Habal, M. B. (1972). Thermal panting in dogs: The lateral nasal gland, a source of water for evaporative cooling. *Science* **177**:804–806.

Blumberg, M. S., and Moltz, H. (1988). How the nose cools the brain during copulation in the male rat. *Physiol. Behav.* **43**:173–176.

Burgess, K., and Whitelaw, W. (1984). Reducing ventilatory response to carbon dioxide by breathing cold air. *Am. Rev. Respir. Dis.* **129**:687–690.

Cabanac, M. (1986). Keeping a cool head. *News Physiol. Sci.* **1**:41–44.

Chai, C. Y., and Lin, M. T. (1972). Effects of heating and cooling the spinal cord and medulla oblongata on the thermoregulation in monkeys. *J. Physiol. (Lond.)* **225**:297–308.

Crawford, E. C. (1962). Mechanical aspects of panting. *J. Appl. Physiol.* **17**:249–251.

Deffebach, M. E., Charan, N. B., Lakshminarayan, S., and Butler, J. (1987). The bronchial circulation: Small, but vial attribute of the lung. *Am. Rev. Respir. Dis.* **135**:463–481.

Deffebach, M. E., Salonen, R. O., Webber, S. E., and Widdicombe, J. G. (1989). Cold and hyperosmolar fluids in the in situ canine trachea: Vascular and smooth muscle tone. *J. Appl. Physiol.* **66**:1606–1609.

Diesel, D. E., Tucker, A., and Robertshaw, D. (1990). Cold-induced changes in breathing pattern as a strategy to reduce respiratory heat loss. *J. Appl. Physiol.* **69**:1946–1952.

Elizondo, R. (1977). Temperature regulation in primates. *Int. Rev. Physiol. Environ. Physiol. II* **15**:71–118.

Folkow, L., and Blix, A. (1987). Nasal heat and water exchange in gray seals. *Am. J. Physiol.* **253**:R883–R889.

Haavik-Nilsen, K., and Hauge, A. (1968). Effects of temperature changes on the pressor response to acute alveolar hypoxia in isolated rat lungs. *Acta Physiol. Scand.* **73**:111–120.

Hales, J. R. S., and Bligh, J. (1969). Respiratory responses of the conscious dog to severe heat stress. *Experientia* **25**:818–819.

Hales, J. R. S., and Dampney, R. A. L. (1975). The redistribution of cardiac output in the dog during heat stress. *J. Therm. Biol.* **1**:29–34.

Huntley, A., Costa, D., and Rubin, R. (1984). The contribution of nasal countercurrent heat exchange to water balance in the northern elephant seal, *Mirounga angustirostris. J. Exp. Biol.* **113**:447–454.

Jackson, D., and Schmidt-Nielsen, K. (1964). Countercurrent heat exchange in the respiratory passages. *Proc. Natl. Acad. Sci.* **51**:1192–1197.

Jindal, S. K., Lakshminarayan, S., Kirk, W., and Butler, J. (1984). Acute increase in anastomotic bronchial blood flow after pulmonary artery obstruction. *J. Appl. Physiol.* **57**:524–528.

Johnsen, H. K., and Folkow, L. P. (1988). Vascular control of brain cooling in reindeer. *Am. J. Physiol.* **254**:R730–739.

Kindermann, W., and Pleschka, K. (1973). Local blood flow and metabolism of the tongue before and during panting. *Pflugers Arch.* **340**:251–262.

Krönert, H., and Pleschka, K. (1976). Distribution of lingual blood flow in the panting dog. *Pflugers Arch.* **365**:R8.

Langman, V. A., Maloiy, G. M., Schmidt-Nielsen, K., and Schroter, R. C. (1978). Respiratory water and heat loss in camels subjected to dehydration. *J. Physiol. (Lond.)* **278**:35P.

Langman, V. A., Maloiy, G. M., Schmidt-Nielsen, K., and Schroter, R. C. (1979). Nasal heat exchange in the giraffe and other large mammals. *Respir. Physiol.* **37**:325–333.

Malik, A. B., and Tracy, S. E. (1980). Bronchovascular adjustments after pulmonary embolism. *J. Appl. Physiol.* **49**:476–481.

McFadden, E. R., Denison, D. M., Waller, J. F., Assoufi, B., Peacock, A., and Sopwith, T. (1982). Direct recordings of the temperatures in the tracheobronchial tree in normal man. *J. Clin. Invest.* **69**:700–705.

Pennington, D., Hyman, A., and Woolverton, W. (1971). Pulmonary vascular responses to selective lung cooling in intact dogs. *Proc. Soc. Exp. Biol. Med.* **137**:1375–1380.

Pleshka, K., Kühn, P., and Nagai, M. (1979). Differential vasomotor adjustments in the evaporative tissues of the tongue and nose in the dog under heat load. *Pflugers Arch.* **382**:255–262.

Raab, J. L., and Schmidt-Nielsen, K. (1972). Effect of running on water balance of the kangaroo rat. *Am. J. Physiol.* **222**:1230–1235.

Ray, D., Ingenito, E., Strek, M., Schumacker, P., and Solway, J. (1989).

Longitudinal distribution of canine respiratory heat and water exchanges. *J. Appl. Physiol.* 61(6):2252–2259.

Schmidt-Nielsen, K. (1964). *Desert Animals.* New York: Oxford University Press.

Schmidt-Nielsen, K. (1981). Countercurrent systems in animals. *Sci. Am.* **244**:118–128.

Schmidt-Nielsen, K., Schmidt-Nielsen, B., Jarnum, S. A., and Houpt, T. R. (1957). Body temperature of the camel and its relation to water economy. *Am. J. Physiol.* **188**:103–112.

Schmidt-Nielsen, K., Crawford, E. C., Jr., Newsome, A. E., Rawson, K. S., and Hammel, H. T. (1967). Metabolic rate of camels: Effect of body temperature and dehydration. *Am. J. Physiol.* **212**:341–346.

Schmidt-Nielsen, K., Bretz, W. L., and Taylor, C. R. (1970a). Panting in dogs: Unidirectional air flow over evaporative surfaces. *Science* **169**:1102–1124.

Schmidt-Nielsen, K., Hainsworth, F. R., and Murrish, D. E. (1970b). Countercurrent heat exchange in the respiratory passages: Effect on water and heat balance. *Respir. Physiol.* **9**:263–276.

Schmidt-Nielsen, K., Crawford, E. C., and Hammel, H. T. (1981a). Respiratory water loss in camels. *Proc. R. Soc. Lond.* [*Biol.*] **211**:291–303.

Schmidt-Nielsen, K., Schroter, R. C., and Shkolnik, A. (1981b). Desaturation of exhaled air in camels. *Proc. R. Soc. Lond.* [*Biol.*] **211**:305–319.

Schroter, R. C., Robertshaw, D., Baker, M. A., Shoemaker, V. H., Holmes, R., and Schmidt-Nielsen, K. (1987). Respiration in heat stressed camels. *Respir. Physiol.* **70**:97–112.

Solway, J., Pichurko, B. M., Ingenito, E. P., McFadden, E. R., Fanto, C. H., Ingram, R. H., and Drazen, J. M. (1985). Breathing pattern affects airway wall temperature during cold air hyperpnea in humans. *Am. Rev. Respir. Dis.* **132**:853–857.

Speisman, I. G. (1936). Vasomotor responses of the mucosa of the upper respiratory tract to thermal stimuli. *Am. J. Physiol.* **115**:181–187.

Taylor, C. (1977). Exercise and environmental heat loads: Different mechanisms for solving different problems? *Int. Rev. Physiol.* **15**:119–146.

Williams, M. H., and Towbin, E. J. (1955). Magnitude and time of development of the collateral circulation to the lung after occlusion of the left pulmonary artery. *Circ. Res.* **3**:422–424.

Part V

FUNCTION

11

Nutrition and Ischemic Injury of the Lung

JOHN BUTLER

University of Washington School of Medicine
Seattle, Washington

I. Introduction

This chapter examines current concepts of the role of the bronchial circulation in the preservation of the lung after a loss of pulmonary artery blood flow. It also considers other mechanisms that provide blood flow to prevent nutritional deprivation under these conditions. Methods for preserving lung tissues that do not depend on blood perfusion are discussed, and finally, I look at our woefully inadequate knowledge about healing after ischemic injury and the factors that lead to hypertrophy of the bronchial circulation.

Ischemia is defined as a loss of blood flow. In the lung, unlike other organs, ischemia does not necessarily result in hypoxia because the lung is ventilated. As in other organs, however, ischemia does lead to a lack of the chemical substrates necessary for cell function and an inability to clear certain metabolites. The lung has come to be regarded as an extraordinarily tough organ in its ability to withstand ischemia caused by obstruction of the pulmonary artery. The famous pathologist Virchow was struck by this in the middle of the last century (Virchow, 1856). An obvious reason is the presence of the bronchial circulation, which gives the lung, like the liver, a double blood supply. A more important explanation is that the lung is ventilated and thus is unique in its continued exposure to an oxygen environment. All parts of the lung are within a very short distance (0.3 mm) of the gas in the airspaces (Weber and Visscher, 1969). Thus, blood flow may not be necessary to prevent the hypoxia that in other organs, like the heart and the brain, is usually considered the most important factor in causing ischemic damage. Nor is blood flow necessary in preventing metabolic tissue acidosis, another factor implicated in worsening ischemic damage, since the most important metabolite, CO_2, can be ventilated away from the lungs.

Maintenance of the nutrition of lung tissues is of clinical importance as well as basic physiological interest. Whether the stoppage of the pulmonary circulation leads to necrotic changes, such as those found in infarcts, survivable damage manifested by edema, hemorrhage, and atelectasis, or simply minor inflammatory reactions, must depend on the sensitivity of the tissues to ischemia and the mechanisms available to prevent nutritional deprivation. Clinically, the problem of pulmonary embolism affects over 500,000 people a year in the United States, the great majority surviving the temporary ischemia of the lung (Moser, 1990). The survival of lung tissues without pulmonary blood flow when heart and lung bypass techniques are used in surgery or in medicine is of obvious clinical importance. The exciting, newly invigorated science of lung transplantation is focusing attention on two aspects of lung ischemia: (1) the need to preserve lung tissues isolated from donors, and (2) the need to prevent ischemic lesions of the airways after transplantation on which only the pulmonary circulation can be reanastomosed (see Chap. 23).

This review focuses on the human lung. Of necessity, however, many of the ideas discussed come from studies of the lungs of other species. Since their anatomy is different and their physiological reactions may be, this must be borne in mind in interpreting the relevance of the data to the human situation.

II. Functional Anatomy

All the tissues of the lung can be nourished by blood from two circulations, the pulmonary and the bronchial, and the lung also has its ventilatory safeguard against oxygen deprivation when the airways are patent. It now appears that the blood flowing in from either systemic arterial (bronchial) or systemic venous (pulmonary arterial) sources is capable of perfusing a component of the vessels of the other's vasculature within the lungs. This is because of the widespread anastomoses between the pulmonary and bronchial vascular beds that occur around the airways, beneath the pleura, and perhaps at other sites. It also appears that, even if both these arterial inputs are reduced or cut off upstream, the alveolar tissues can still be perfused by reverse flow up the pulmonary veins from the left atrium (Butler et al., 1989).

The vessels of the pulmonary vasculature are adapted for gas exchange, for the filtering out of particles (thus protecting the coronary, cerebral, or other systemic vascular beds), and for the processing of chemicals, such as neuropeptides and vasoactive peptides in the circulating blood. Less well appreciated is that the pulmonary circulation is normally the sole blood supply for the very active endothelial and epithelial tissues and the other constituents of the alveolar walls. These form almost all the lung substance and are spread over a very wide area. It is also possible that the pulmonary arterial input constitutes a proportion of the normal nutritional supply to the bronchi, particularly the smaller airways (see Chap. 6) (Barman et al., 1988).

The predominant function of the bronchial circulation is, under normal conditions, to nourish the nonalveolar lung tissues, particularly, of course, the bronchi. Inflow comes from several systemic arteries (Fig. 1 and Chap. 2).

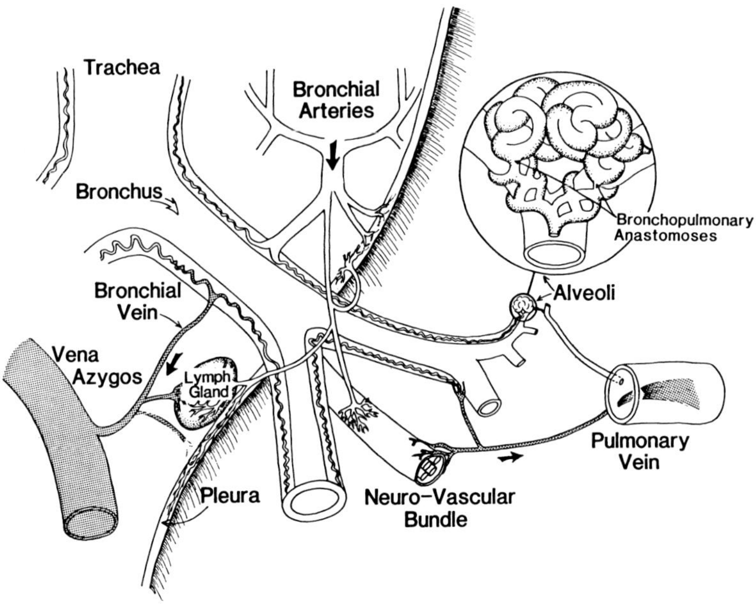

Figure 1 The bronchial circulation. Multiple bronchial arteries supply the extrapulmonary airways and pleura, from which the drainage is into the right heart, and more extensive intrapulmonary airways and other structures, from which the drainage is into the pulmonary vasculature. These bronchopulmonary anastomoses and the vasa vasorum of the pulmonary arteries can supply systemic blood to regions with restricted pulmonary artery inflow.

The upper trachea has a separate systemic arterial inflow, but this is from the laryngeal and thyroid vessels and is not considered part of the bronchial circulation since it is outside the chest (see Chap. 8). The lower trachea and the large, first-division extrapulmonary bronchi within the chest are perfused by the bronchial blood flow. The venous blood from these intrathoracic but extrapulmonary bronchial vessels drains mostly through the vena azygos into the vena cavae and the right heart. Bronchial flow to the intrapulmonary airways, the pleural vessels, the intrapulmonary vasculature, lymphatics, and lymph glands drains into the pulmonary vessels and so to the left atrium. These drainage routes to the right and left atria are linked through the rich complex of bronchial vessels in the airways, so if one pathway is impeded, outflow can still occur through the other. There are three anatomic routes from which blood flow may reach an alveolar region suffering a loss of pulmonary arterial inflow: surrounding pulmonary microvessels, bronchial-to-pulmonary anastomoses, and pulmonary veins (Fig. 2). It is likely that sufficient blood to prevent damage in the potentially ischemic region is usually available from the surrounding pulmonary microvessels (Fig. 2A) (Karsner and Ash, 1912). The pulmonary capillaries form a network from side to side and top to bottom of the lungs. Where the region abuts a lung surface, however, and particularly where it occupies a restricted edge at the anterior or posterior tip of a lobe, there are few normally perfused adjacent vessels to sustain it. It is in these regions that infarction is more common clinically and experimentally (Fig. 2B) (Karsner and Ash, 1912). After a pulmonary embolism due to a large blood clot, thrombolysis fragments the clot so it is washed onward and smaller lumps obstruct the peripheral vessels. A larger region at risk in this way could cause the inflow from surrounding pulmonary microvessels to be inadequate. However, the bronchial blood flow can perfuse the pulmonary vessels that are compromised, via the vasa vasorum of the pulmonary artery and arterial and capillary anastomoses (Fig. 2D). This is only a trickle at first. In fact, experimental studies have shown a fall in the bronchial blood flow immediately after widespread pulmonary vascular obstruction (Kowalski et al., 1990). This is unexpected and unexplained because a fall in pulmonary vascular pressure such as occurs after pulmonary artery obstruction leads to an increase in the driving pressure between the systemic and pulmonary vessels and should encourage an increase in bronchial blood flow.

Reverse pulmonary venous flow could help to sustain the potentially ischemic tissues in the period soon after the loss of pulmonary artery inflow. Reflux flow from the left atrium up the pulmonary veins to the alveolar tissues is an intriguing but previously little considered alternative source of nutrients for the alveolar cells when there is no inflow from the pulmonary artery. In this situation reverse pulmonary venous flow could wash into the compromised parts of the lungs through the pulmonary microvenular network until the bron-

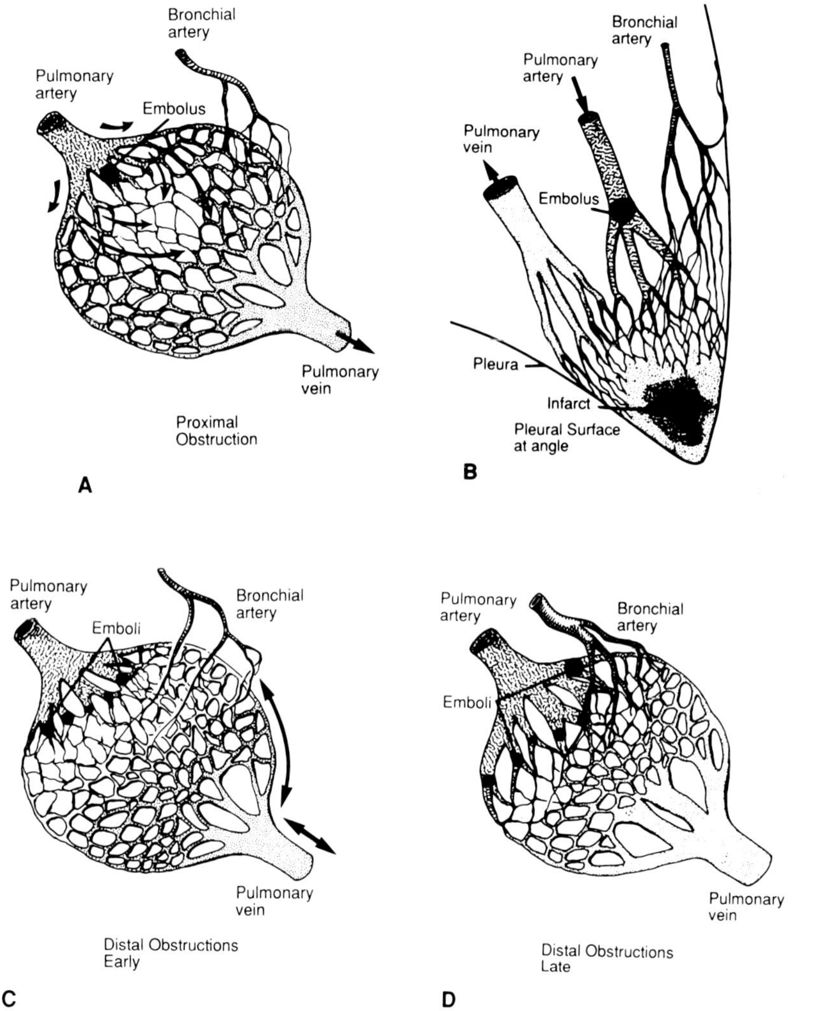

Figure 2 Vascular responses to ischemia. (A) A single small obstruction compromises a localized alveolar region that can be perfused from the surrounding pulmonary microvessels. (B) Where the potentially ischemic region abuts pleural surfaces there are no surrounding pulmonary microvessels and the anatomy compromises reverse pulmonary venous flow. Infarction could occur before bronchopulmonary anastomotic flow increases. (C) When a larger region is compromised, reverse pulmonary venous flow can supply blood for the period before bronchopulmonary anastomotic flow increases. (D) Hours or days after obstruction of the pulmonay artery flow to a large region, the bronchopulmonary anastomotic flow increases sufficiently to prevent ischemic damage and eventually restore function.

chial blood flow increased (Fig. 2C). A longer period of substrate supply from reverse pulmonary venous flow may occur if the bronchial as well as the pulmonary circulation is compromised. Zahn (1897) and Karsner and Ash (1912) demonstrated the probable mechanism of reverse pulmonary venous flow in pulmonary arterial obstruction. By strapping the chest of rabbits (Zahn) or filling one hemithorax of dogs with oil (Karsner and Ash), they reduced the lung volume changes that are now thought to cause the alveolar vessels to expel blood into the veins on inflation and aspirate it on deflation (Fig. 3). They showed that this, like tying the veins, led to infarction when the pulmonary and bronchial blood supply was interrupted.

Over the few days after pulmonary artery obstruction, the bronchial flow increases markedly as a result of vasodilation (Fig. 2D) (Mathes et al., 1932) and then more gradually because of the subsequent hypertrophy of the bronchial vascular bed with the formation of new vessels (Weibel, 1960). Eventually, when the left or right pulmonary artery or a main branch is obstructed, the amount of the bronchial flow that enters the pulmonary vasculature can be large enough to restore some alveolar gas exchange (Liebow, 1962). This exchange is mainly CO_2 excretion, but O_2 uptake can occur if the systemic bronchial blood is hypoxemic.

Only recently recognized is the opposite of this response: the ability of the pulmonary circulation to perfuse the bronchial vessels and nourish the air-

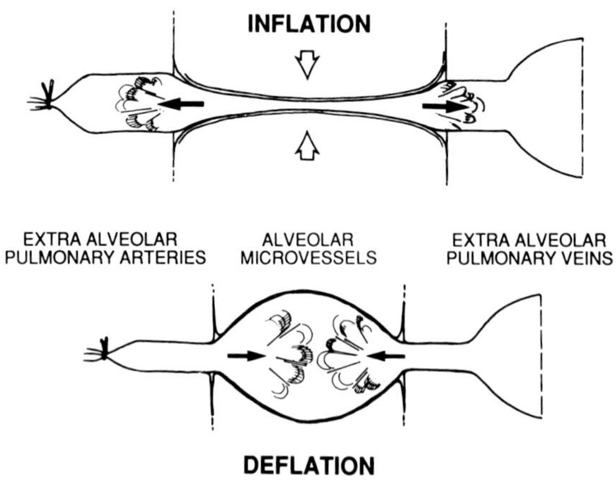

Figure 3 Mechanism driving reverse pulmonary venous flow. Lung inflation (top) squeezes blood from the pulmonary capillaries back to the pulmonary veins, and then deflation (bottom) draws it back.

ways when the bronchial input is compromised (Barman et al., 1988). Such a lack of bronchial arterial flow could occur in atherosclerotic systemic vascular disease, in traumatic separation of the airways, and after lung transplant operations. In these conditions, the adjacent and torrential pulmonary circulation immediately begins to flow into the bronchial vasculature. The high pressure systemic arterial inflow rapidly redevelops, however, because previously unperfused bronchial vessels open up and existing systemic vessels in other lung regions and from other sources in the mediastinum enlarge and spread.

It is unlikely that systemic venous blood from the azygos system could reflux up the bronchial veins to nourish the bronchi, like the pulmonary venous blood reverses up to the alveoli, because the impetus of the pulmonary capillary volume changes with breathing is not provided by the bronchial vasculature. Also, the valves in the veins of the azygos system would stop reverse flow.

In the very unusual event that pulmonary arterial, bronchial arterial, and pulmonary venous reverse flows are obstructed, pulmonary infarction always occurs (Veith et al., 1971). Ventilation alone is not sufficient to prevent injury in this situation.

III. Tissue Susceptibility

Normally the alveolar wall tissues seem most susceptible to lack of substrates. In the warm, *in situ* lungs of rats, lack of both perfusion with chemical nutrients and of ventilation to provide oxygen resulted in alveolar cell dysfunction, causing surfactant deficiency within 5 min; and alveolar septal necrosis followed (Amthor, 1973). The type I epithelial cells were most susceptible. In contrast, the smooth muscle in the bronchial walls was able to survive after such a deprivation for about 5 h. The bronchial mucosa was intermediate, with survival when deprived of both chemical nutrients and oxygen for about 30 min. Ventilation alone or perfusion alone approximately doubled the survival time.

The nutritional demands of the lung tissues are larger in smaller animals because their metabolic rates are higher. Thus, the demands of each unit of tissue of the lungs of rats are more than those of dogs or humans. The lung tissues of small animals, such as the rat, cannot tolerate periods of substrate deficiency for as long as can those of larger animals (Amthor, 1973). Nutritional demands are also high in periods of growth and development, so developing organisms are more susceptible to the lack of substrates than adults. Demands are high for the rapidly growing tissues in neoplasms and when the temperature and metabolic activity is increased in inflammation. The metabolic O_2 demand of a solid, unventilated lung consolidated with leukocytes in pneumonia is higher than can be supplied by a pulmonary arterial flow that has been reduced because of hypoxic vasoconstriction, so blood perfusing such regions, instead of being oxygenated, actually loses oxygen (Light, 1988).

Demands for particular functional substrates may arise when there are specific tissue activities. For instance the metabolic burst of the airway leukocytes, the outpouring of airway secretions from goblet cells, or the replenishment of the chemicals in the submucosal glands when these have been secreted must increase the local demands for nutrients. Presumably these are distributed by the bronchial circulation. The increase in bronchial blood flow necessary for such changes could result from local regulation or be part of a more generalized response.

Nutritional demands are relatively lower in the lungs of large animals. They are reduced in hypometabolic states, such as hypothyroidism. They are low when the lungs are atrophic in the elderly or as a result of diseases, such as α 1-antitrypsin emphysema. It is likely that a lack of substrates would be tolerated longer in these situations. Similarly, the depression of metabolism that takes place in hypothermia prolongs the period that isolated tissues may be preserved. This is used extensively in storing lungs for transplant surgery. In fact, the period the lung can be preserved when kept cool after a single pulmonary artery flushing with a cold electrolyte solution has been reported to range up to 48 h (Hoyer et al., 1980).

IV. Metabolism

The lung as a whole depends on oxygen. When this is restricted, anaerobic glycolysis of glucose provides for its metabolism. Despite the size of the lungs, their metabolism, reflected as O_2 consumption (about 0.05 ml/min/g dry weight), is only about 1% of the total oxygen uptake of the animal and appears to be related to lung weight. On this basis it is less than one-sixth that of the working muscle of the heart (Weber and Visscher, 1969). The metabolic rate of the alveolar tissues is comparable to that of intestines, salivary glands, or resting muscle (Fisher et al., 1974). About 80% of the available oxygen is used by the cellular mitochondria that reside most profusely in the alveolar type II and the endothelial cells. There are rather few mitochondria in the type I alveolar cells. The alveolar cells' mitochondria have an oxygen consumption of 40–50 μmol/min/g mitochondrial protein. This is about half the demand of the mitochondria of liver hepatocytes. This low level may be artifactual, however, as a result of the greater trauma required in obtaining mitochondria from the lung than from the liver because there is more fibrous tissue in the lung (Fisher et al., 1974).

A. Hypoxia

The lung is relatively insensitive to hypoxia alone, as in atelectasis or bronchial obstruction (Pattle, 1956; Fisher et al., 1972). In the isolated warm, unventilated, but perfused rat lung intermediate oxidative metabolites (lactate/pyruvate ratios, ATP, and ATP/ADP ratios) are not altered until alveolar Po_2 falls to less than 1 mmHg (Fisher and Dodie, 1981). Pig lungs similarly treated and subjected to 1/4 h of anoxia experience a reduction in ATP by only about one-third. If they are perfused with oxygenated blood, ATP levels remain stable within 10% for more than 4 h. There is recovery during a subsequent 1/2 h of normoxia (Hall et al., 1988). To damage by anoxia most of the pulmonary endothelial cells from the rat in a culture takes almost an hour (Ratych et al., 1987).

The tissues of the airways are even more resistant to hypoxia alone at body temperature. It is known from organ culture studies that the cilia of the bronchial epithelium continue beating for 30 min of nitrogen ventilation and that the ability of the bronchial smooth muscle to contract continues but diminishes at low oxygen tensions. The bronchial mucosa glandular secretions cease after exposure to agents that block metabolic oxygen uptake, however.

B. Substrate Deficiency

Unlike its resistance to hypoxia, the lung is quite sensitive to substrate deficiency. Only 1/4 h of ischemia causes a profound (90%) drop in ATP and in pH (7.5→6.4) in warm, isolated pig lungs. In the warm, nonventilated rabbit lung, the small initial amount of glucose drops 50% in the 1/2 h after perfusion is stopped, and after 2 h, ATP falls by 80% (Von Wichert, 1972). Under these conditions, about one-third of the glucose goes to lactic acid: this anaerobiasis starts when the hilum is clamped despite the presence of trapped blood and gas in the lungs. Lactic acid levels can exceed 100 mgm per 100 ml tissue, failing to increase further only when the glucose runs out after about 2 h. This lactic acid accumulation evidently does not depress metabolism (Weber and Visscher, 1969). The remaining two-thirds of the glucose normally goes to form fats (surfactants) and other end products. Surfactant levels only fall after a day or more of substrate deficiency.

Of particular importance to transplantation is that hypothermia (4°C) preserves ATP in nonperfused, degassed rabbit lungs, at about two-thirds the initial ratio (in relation to inorganic phosphate) for at least 2 h: control (warm) lungs show a drop of nearly 90% (Fig. 4). However, warm lungs with ATP reduced by 90% can recover to normal levels on reperfusion, particularly if leukocyte-depleted blood is used. The importance of leukocytes in the reaction to anoxic or ischemic damage is discussed later.

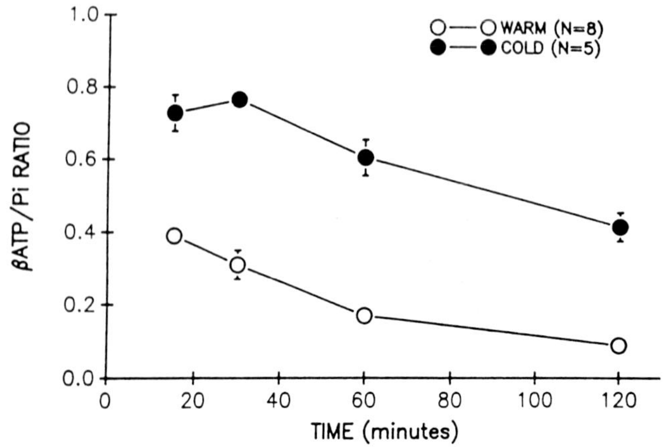

Figure 4 ATP ratios in hypothermia. Measurements were made by [31]p nuclear magnetic resonance in excised, degassed, bloodless rabbit lungs kept warm (36°C) or cold (4°C). Cooling preserved a much higher energy state = βATP/P_i. (adenosine triphosphate/inorganic phosphate). (From Hall et al., 1988.)

C. Cell Functional Requirements

The substrates required by each group of cells are different and differ with changes in their function at different times, in their maturation from fetal to adult life, and in their environment.

The type I alveolar epithelial cell is thinly spread, with an important barrier function. Since its other abilities, if any, are unknown, it is not possible to say if it requires specific substrates. The alveolar type II cells are usually concerned with making surfactant from fatty acid residues already in the alveoli or provided by the blood. At other times, however, when repairing the alveolar surface, their main function is to reproduce themselves and form type I epithelial cells. Again, in some circumstances, they are capable of transporting ions and fluid out of the alveoli, a feature shown well when the amniotic fluid is absorbed into the circulation after air breathing commences at birth.

The type II epithelial cell requires energy and a variety of substrates for its different abilities. The high rate of aerobic glycolysis found in type II cells may be partly responsible for the brisk lactate generation by the lung.

Vascular endothelial cells make up the largest proportion of the alveolar tissues. It is likely that they require specific substrates since they are very active in locally reacting to blood flow changes, producing anticoagulant factors and vasoactive amines and locally degrading them (Petty and Pearson, 1989). They are also involved in regulating the levels of many chemicals, such as bradykinin and angiotensin, that have general systemic functions in the body. Endothelial cells can also show some reticuloendothelial function by taking up particles as they pass through the lungs in the bloodstream.

It is interesting that pulmonary arterial endothelial cells, normally exposed to $Po_2 \sim 40$ torr differ from aortic endothelial cells normally exposed to $Po_2 \sim 100$ torr in showing more pyruvate kinase and phosphofructokinase activity. This agrees with the results of cell culture studies showing that hypoxia favors glycolytic enzyme activity whereas normoxia favors the oxidative phosphorylation enzymes (Cummiskey et al., 1981). The ability of O_2 to modify the activity of rate-limiting bioenergetic enzymes could be a mechanism for ensuring the maintenance of ATP stores.

The other main cell in the alveolus, the alveolar macrophage, appears to move freely and be very active in defending the lung against inhaled particles and organisms. It is presumed to be nourished by alveolar fluids and by oxygen from its gaseous environment. The macrophage has been shown to depend on the availability of oxygen for its dramatic "metabolic burst" when it engages in phagocytosis (Oren et al., 1963).

The airway wall muscle, the airway mucosa, and its associated glands are nourished by the diminutive bronchial blood flow. Although the flow is very small, the bronchial vascular bed is quite extensive, particularly in the mucosa, where there is a superficial and a deep venous capillary plexus and, in some animals, lacunae of blood spread widely through the membrane. It is now much better appreciated that the resistance of the airways to hypoxic and ischemic damage is because this rich vasculature can be perfused by the pulmonary as well as the bronchial blood flow.

V. Injuries Caused by Ischemia

Ischemic damage is mediated by at least three mechanisms (Fig. 5). First, the lack of O_2 and other substrates can cause cellular dysfunction. Many cells at the periphery of an ischemic region are only slightly affected and capable of rapid recovery. Although cell function is abnormal, there may be no visible changes. In the absence of perfusion, such injuries as are present are localized and dry: with perfusion the more vulnerable vessels may leak (Fig. 5B) (Bishop et al., 1989). Since these lesions are due to the ischemia, not the inflammatory response to it, they are not reversed by specific free oxygen radical scavengers (catalase and superoxide dismutase) or by inhibitors of the reactions that generate oxygen radicals (allopurinol and dimethylsulfoxide).

Second, if more severe ischemia causes a critical fall in energy levels, an intracellular "self-destruct" mechanism, discussed later, can come into play (Fig. 5C). Although the presence of lysozomes in cells has been appreciated

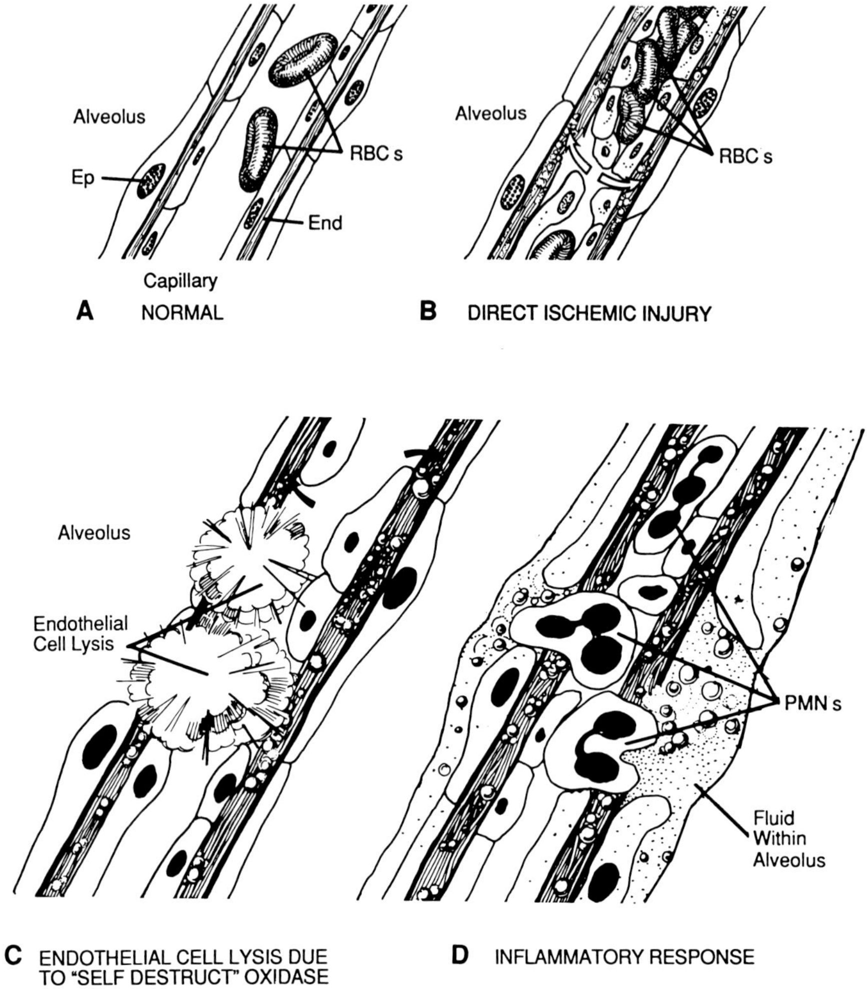

Figure 5 Histological phases of ischemic damage. (A) A normal capillary: RBC, red blood cell; Ep, epithelium of alveolar lining (types 1 and 2); End, endothelium of microvessel. (B) Direct ischemic injury damages the endothelium, allowing fluid to leak out. Red blood cells agglomerate, stopping flow. (C) More severe injury to the cells, particularly those of the endothelium, causes damage (low-energy state) from which they cannot recover. The self-destruct mechanism causes them to lyse so that the capillary wall is breached. (D) After the ischemic injury the inflammatory response via the pulmonary and bronchial blood flow causes leukocyte accumulation and exudation. The leukocytes block further pulmonary capillary flow and lyse the damaged cells. Exudates containing protein and cells fill the alveoli.

for a long time, the possibility of the release of powerful oxygen radicals has caused considerable controversy. Paradoxically, the correction of hypoxia by reperfusion seems to be capable of completing the biochemical cycle leading to cellular disintegration. The initial injury is thought to be in the endothelial cell (Bulkley, 1987). When there is blood in the vessels, the damage caused by these and other cytolytic mechanisms, when added to that directly due to the ischemia, allows leakage of fluid and spreading edema. In contrast to the direct effects of ischemia, it seems that some of these cytolytic mechanisms can be modified by inhibitors of xanthine oxidase and scavengers of oxygen radicals (McCord, 1985).

Third, there is the inflammatory reaction of the body, stimulated by ischemic cell injury, that takes some time to develop (Fig. 5D). Leukocytes accumulate and themselves release oxygen radicals. Exudates develop as the inflammation makes the vessels more permeable. This is neutrophil mediated because neutrophil depletion appears to ameliorate it (Bishop et al., 1989b; Ide et al., 1990). In the heart, the overall 'reperfusion injury" and the attendant "no reflow" phenomenon are not seen in the absence of granulocytes (Engler et al., 1986). No reflow is the failure to reperfuse some of the ischemic regions immediately after removing the arterial obstruction. The blockers of this reaction, steroidal and nonsteroidal antiinflammatory compounds, are quite different from those modifying the earlier stages of the ischemic damage.

A transplanted lung must be subjected to these three biochemical abnormalities, because although cooled, it has not been perfused for a considerable time before being reperfused by the transplant recipient. Thus, the temporary loss of function, called "reimplantation injury," usually seen for 1 or 2 days after lung transplant surgery (Veith et al., 1971), can be attributed to the transient abnormalities of slight, recoverable ischemic injury and probably some irreversible damage generating the toxic oxygen radicals as well. The lung is more evidently susceptible to these problems than other organs because its edema is easily seen on x-ray.

In summary, hypoxia or nonhypoxic ischemia injures the cell to a small extent, from which it can recover, or to a critical extent that may lead to its disintegration and death. This cell lysis could be a necessary step in healing, since irreparably damaged cells must be scoured out by the imflammatory process (particularly leukocytic phagocytosis) before new tissues can be laid down to replace them (Metchnikov, 1891).

A. The Self-Cytolytic Mechanism

Although the following discussion is based on ideas that have, like the inflammatory reaction, generated much heat, it is included because an appreciation of the framework of the response is necessary in our consideration of the effects of ischemia. This is an exciting focus of research in cell biology at the moment, so the ideas about it are changing rapidly.

The cell appears to contain its own cytolytic mechanism that is triggered when its energy charge drops below a certain level. It is postulated that this self-destruction is caused by oxygen-derived free radicals, similar to those released when leukocytes liquefy tissues, radicals that have tremendous toxic potential. Thus far this has been better documented in organs other than the lung. Normally, antioxidants in the tissues and the blood protect other cells from destruction by these free radicals (Bulkley, 1987).

The main source of oxygen radicals in cells is thought to be from the action of an enzyme, xanthine oxidase, on intracellular xanthine. In healthy cells xanthine dehydrogenase accounts for almost all the xanthine activity. When the cell is injured by ischemia it is postulated that there is a redistribution of calcium ions that converts the dehydrogenase to the oxidase by a proteolytic attack. The energy depletion starting the redistribution of calcium ions simultaneously changes ATP to AMP and eventually to hypoxanthine, which together with xanthine is the oxidizable purine substrate for xanthine oxidase. In the presence of molecular O_2 (in short supply until reperfusion), the toxic oxygen radicals are produced. The conversion of xanthine dehydrogenase to xanthine oxidase seems to be slower in the lung than in other organs (Engerson et al., 1987).

B. Detection of Injury

Investigators have studied the effects caused by deprivation of oxygen and blood nutrients in several ways. In the past only histological criteria could be used. Now biochemical analyses of specific cellular functions (Hall et al., 1988) and of the general cellular effects of lack of substrates (Fisher and Dodia, 1981) are also being applied. These approaches have been used for the brain and the heart for some time, but sampling difficulties, the ability of oxygen to reach the tissues via the airways, and their multiple vascular sources of perfusion have impeded their application to the lungs. The only certain way of excluding blood nutrients from the lung tissues is by excising the lungs and flushing the pulmonary vasculature with an inert solution. Unfortunately, active compounds, including the lower molecular weight ADP and AMP, are washed out with this flushing. Ironically, washing out the pulmonary vessels with an electrolyte solution, although in this case a very cold one, is the technique used in preparing excised lungs for transplantation.

The severity of the ischemic damage due to preserving the lung outside the body is usually assessed from abnormalities seen after reimplantation. The rise in pulmonary artery pressure has been reported as the best indicator of the extent of the injury (Pegg et al., 1982). It probably reflects vasospasm caused by local falls in alveolar oxygen, obstruction due to ischemic and inflammatory vascular injury, and the blockage of microvessels by granulocytes. Others have championed either the drop in arterial P_{O_2} (rise in AaP_{O_2} difference), the impairment of O_2 uptake, or the fall in diffusing capacity as indicators of injury. Still others rely on the indications of edema: increase in lung weight (not a feasible measurement in vivo), the decrease in compliance, or the change in density on X-ray. Increases in protein and cells in the fluid from broncho-alveolar lavage (BAL) have been considered to reflect the re-implantation edema phase.

We can now look at the effects of depriving the lung of ventilation and perfusion in the light of the preceding analysis. The discussion is arranged in two sections. The first section deals with the consequences of hypoxia and ischemia at body temperature and details animal studies that could mimic clinical conditions. The second section deals with the survival of lungs for transplantation that have been cooled before being stored. It draws on the burgeoning experience of transplant centers around the world.

C. Damage Due to Substrate Deprivation at Body Temperature

No Ventilation with No Perfusion

These conditions are met when all perfusion and ventilation are interrupted. Clinically this could follow trauma but is more likely to occur in a region of sepsis when all the vessels and airways are involved. It is relevant to the unusual situation of lung excision and preservation for transplant without cooling.

In a very interesting study in 1973, Amthor clamped, at the hilum, the upper lobe of the right lung of anesthetized rats, preventing both ventilation and perfusion. He closed the chest for periods of 5 or 10 min or an hour or more; after which he removed the clamp so both ventilation and perfusion could resume and then sacrificed the rats after hours or days. Changes consistent with cellular damage and leakage from the vasculature were present after clamping for only 5 min before ventilation and perfusion were restored. The lobe became atelectatic after 1 or 2 days. This was attributed to loss of surfactant. Lymphatics were dilated around the bronchovascular bundles. The alveolar walls were edematous and the alveoli filled with exudates. These were initially watery but became more exudative after reperfusion. After clamping for 10 min, the alveolar septa were necrotic and all the other changes were exaggerated. Emphysema, caused by necrosis of alveolar walls, often followed reinflation. After clamping for 1 h, the bronchial mucosa was also damaged, but the bronchial muscle survived 5 h of ischemia and hypoxia. Inexplicably, unless some systemic flow reached the pleura, there was always a narrow sub-pleural zone that remained intact around the lung.

In rabbit lungs, similarly clamped at the hilum but then excised and stored at body temperature before being quick frozen, Von Wichert found that aerobic metabolism soon gave way to anaerobic, with the generation of lactic acid (Von Wichert, 1972). Only half the glucose remained after 1/2 h (the lung has no glycogen stores), and all the glucose was used up in 2 h. Since there was insufficient energy generation, the ATP fell rapidly. ADP-to-AMP catabolism was slow, but after 1 h these nucleotides still constituted a considerable energy-providing system that could reestablish ATP levels rather quickly after reperfusion (see Fig. 4). The large amount of surfactant-associated phospholipids was not noticeably altered after 3 h. However, atelectasis with abnormalities of surfactant takes 1–2 days to appear after reperfusion in rats (Amthor, 1973).

Because the blood and gas remain in the lungs after hilar clamping and since blood makes up about two-thirds of the weight of the lungs, only 10–20% of their weight is made up of fully metabolically active lung tissue. This and the presence of glucose in the trapped blood confuses the interpretation of these studies as reflections of the time course of deprivations of the lung tissue alone. On the other hand, the studies (although carried out in animals) could be relevant to a clinical setting.

In blood-free excised lungs the fall in the ATP, the ADP, and the ATP/ADP ratio, together with the increase in lactate and the reduction in glucose measured in random biopsies of rapidly frozen tissues gives an overall reflection of the effect of hypoxia and ischemia on the lung tissues only (Bassett et al., 1975). Fisher et al. (1972) studied the effects of hypoxia in isolated, warmed, electrolyte-perfused rat and hamster lungs ventilated with nitrogen or given cyanide as a metabolic blocker. CO_2 concentrations rose continuously. Serotonin uptake by the endothelial cells, thought to be linked to active sodium transport, was impaired to the extent that only about half the normal amount was cleared on each circulatory cycle. Lung surfactant synthesis was decreased. There is some uncertainty in these observations, however, because the time between the sacrifice of the animal and the setting up of the excised, perfused lung preparation is unknown.

The longest period that airway, pulmonary, and bronchial artery occlusion could be tolerated by the warm dog lung without subsequent impairment of pulmonary function due to edema was 30 min (Blades 1954). Although the pulmonary veins were open, there was no ventilation to cause reverse venous flow. Apparently this period can be increased to 2–3 h if the warm lung is held inflated while ischemic (Veith et al., 1971). Obstruction of one lung's airway, pulmonary artery, pulmonary veins, and bronchial vascular supplies caused lung pallor and atelectasis in open-chested dogs with the lung maintained at body temperature (Connaughton et al., 1962). After 2–6 h the clamps were removed and the *in situ* lungs reperfused and reventilated. Most of the dogs with lungs that were ischemic and nonventilated for 6 h died. Most of those clamped for 4 h or less lived.

No Ventilation with Perfusion

To meet these conditions there is vascular perfusion by the normal routes but no oxygenation from ventilation. This occurs clinically in atelectasis or pnenumonia. The amount of pulmonary arterial perfusion is usually reduced by hypoxic vasoconstriction.

At body temperature, atelectic dog lungs perfused with oxygenated blood *in situ* maintained bioenergetic levels of ATP, ADP, and ATP/ADP ratios for 5 h. They developed ultrastructural changes before biochemical (ATP and lactic acid) alterations (Modry et al., 1977). The effects of the interruption of ventilation alone were worse when pulmonary arterial hypoxemia was added. Since these *in situ* lungs were still perfused with oxygen-containing systemic bronchial arterial blood, presumably the hypoxic stress was not total. This experiment indicates that perfusion of the lung with oxygenated blood protects it against serious injury when it is not ventilated, as in clincial bronchial obstruction and atelectasis.

Ventilation with Partial Ischemia

These conditions are met when ventilation is maintained but either bronchial or pulmonary artery occlusion is produced and pulmonary venous reflux is possible. Clinically, bronchial artery obstruction occurs at lung transplantation and pulmonary artery obstruction after pulmonary embolism.

Bronchial artery occlusion in animals seldom causes any demonstrable lesions. It is likely that a single upstream obstruction does not stop distal bronchial capillary flow because of the network of bronchial and pulmonary anastomoses (Ricketts and Carrington, 1965). In the human, however, the lack of all systemic (bronchial) arterial flow despite the restoration of pulmonary flow after lung transplantation has heretofore been the main cause of death (see Chap. 23). The airway anastomosis failed to heal or became necrotic, leading to dehiscence.

In other animals, bronchial tissue can be made necrotic by ischemia if the small vessels themselves are occluded by the injection of tissue glue (Ricketts and Carrington, 1965), latex (Ellis et al., 1951), or small glass beads (Boushy et al., 1969). Further, ischemic damage is apparent if both bronchial and regional pulmonary arteries are ligated (Hughes et al., 1954). In animals, the pulmonary arterial flow seems able to perfuse the bronchial vasculature when the bronchial arterial flow has been selectively interrupted, so the ischemic damage after human lung transplantation could be due to differences in the extent of bronchopulmonary anastomoses at the site where the airway is rejoined (Trummer and Berg, 1968).

Experimental temporary unilateral pulmonary artery occlusion is analogous to massive main branch pulmonary embolization in the human. Some ischemic changes always occur because there can be no inflow from surrounding pulmonary microvessels when a whole lung or lobe is involved. There is considerable variation in the response between species. In the rabbit and dog, when pulmonary artery occlusion was sustained for several hours in a ventilated lung *in situ*, the pulmonary vasculature became abnormally leaky, as judged by studies of permeability (Bishop et al, 1989). ATP remained normal until ventilation was stopped, however, when it decreased dramatically. When the pulmonary venous reverse flow was also stopped, histological changes were present in less than 1 h despite an uninterrupted bronchial blood flow and the adequate oxygenation assured by continued ventilation (Modry et al., 1977). On pulmonary arterial reperfusion, the severity of the damage becomes evident because it causes ipsilateral and, to some extent, bilateral pulmonary edema., Flow is reduced, and the distribution of perfusion is patchy. This can be so marked as to merit description as a "no reflow" phenomenon. Obviously, a failure of reperfusion of the lung or notable regions of a lung that has sustained ischemic damage is a serious defect, potentially exacerbating the injury.

What is the cause of the "no reflow" phenomenon? One explanation is that ischemia increases the permeability of the pulmonary vessels (Bishop et al., 1989a) so that they leak fluid. This causes high local intravascular red cell concentrations that can plug the vessels and stop flow (Amthor, 1973). Another is that granulocytes can obstruct the microvessels in the alveoli. The granulocyte is large enough to block the alveolar microvessel, but normally it is soon swept away because it is soft and able to streamline its shape (Lien et al., 1989). However, the cell that has been activated by ischemia is apparently harder and more apt to adhere to the endothelium, acting as a cork (Schmid-Schonbein, 1988). Only a few leukocytes are required to stop flow through a considerable part of the capillary network (Lien et al., 1989). As the period of ischemia lengthens, the vessels become more permeable and there is endothelial and alveolar cell damage, together with alveolar exudation and hemorrhage on reperfusion. An inflammatory response marked by fever, leukocytosis, and inflammatory cell infiltrates in the ischemic lung and, to a much lesser extent, the other lung can then occur with frank pulmonary edema. This is the reperfusion injury syndrome that is usually marked by patches of no reflow. Its severity is decreased when the bronchial blood flow at the time of the pulmonary artery occlusion is high, presumably because the ischemic damage is less severe (Kowalski et al., 1990). It is likely that the "implantation" or "reimplantation" syndrome, occurring soon after lung transplantation and lasting for several days, is a similar phenomenon. The "pump lung" pulmonary edema syndrome, now seldom seen, occurred after pulmonary bypass and could also have been associated with reperfusion after temporary ischemia.

Residual lesions after temporary unilateral pulmonary artery occlusion have been documented in dogs and monkeys. The experiments were analogous to massive central pulmonary embolization in the human. In the dogs, there was patchy hemorrhagic atelectasis, worsening over the 7 days of occlusion, with characteristic changes in type II alveolar cell lamellar bodies (thinning of the concentric lamellae). India ink, injected to study the distribution of the bronchial blood flow, was found later in very small amounts in the viable areas but not in the infarcted regions. Most was present subpleurally (Huber and Edmonds, 1967). In the monkeys, the pulmonary artery occlusion was released after periods up to 7 days and the animals were sacrificed after an additional 1–7 days. Decrease in lung volume, local atelectasis, alveolar exudation, and macrophage infiltration of the alveolar walls worsened for 2 days after release of the occlusion (Davis et al., 1952). When the unilateral pulmonary artery occlusion was prolonged for 7 days or more, bronchial epithelial damage was evident. The patchy atelectasis and regions of more severe damage shown by alveolar exudation and hemorrhage were associated with failure of surfactant function in the damaged atelectatic regions (Huber and Edmunds, 1967; Edmunds and Holm, 1969). Other regions appeared comparatively normal. Damaged regions occurred next to normal regions. The lesions were associated with an intitial extrusion of the lamellar bodies from the type II epithelial cells. These cells were subsequently unable to maintain normal lamellar body and surfactant synthesis. Still unexplained is that increasing the CO_2 in the ventilating gas appeared to prevent these injuries (Edmunds and Holm, 1969). Perhaps the increase in bronchial blood flow caused by the hypercarbia (Charan et al., 1986) supplied the required substrates.

Occlusion of a branch of the pulmonary artery does not usually cause ischemic lung damage. Ventilation of the regions served by the obstructed artery is maintained, although a decrease in compliance (surfactant inadequacy) and bronchoconstriction (hypocarbia and hyperoxia of the ventilating gas) tend to reduce it. Perfusion is maintained from surrounding pulmonary vessels or pulmonary venous reflux and bronchial blood flow.

Ventilation with Severe Ischemia

These conditions are met when pulmonary and bronchial perfusion are interrupted but reverse pulmonary venous flow and ventilation are maintained.

Since bronchial blood flow is seldom compromised for long this is rarely a clinical problem, although some degree of the condition is probably often caused by the drop in bronchial blood flow immediately after pulmonary embolism (Kowalski et al., 1990).

In the intact dog, when both pulmonary artery and bronchial blood flow were interrupted, the lung remained viable (Karsner and Ash, 1912). Volume was decreased, and there were focal atelectases and focal alveolar edema with hemorrhages. However, most regions remained almost normal after 10 days of vascular obstruction. Although oxygenation was maintained by ventilation and some regrowth of bronchial vessels was possible in 10 days, similar studies led Shepard et al. (1981) to suggest that there must be an alternate blood supply for alveolar tissue nutrients and that this may by a reflux from the left atrium via the pulmonay veins. DeMoraes and DeCarvalho (1949) had shown previously that labeled left atrial blood could be detected almost immediately in the distal end of a transected lobar pulmonary artery, and Nordenstrom (1954) had shown by angiography that pulmonary venous reflux could occur. Such a mechanism, dependent on the tidal pumping caused by lung volume changes in ventilation, has now been confirmed (Butler et al., 1989).

Ventilation with Complete Ischemia

These conditions are met when pulmonary, bronchial, and pulmonary venous reflux are interrupted but ventilation is maintained. This probably occurs to a greater or lesser extent in clinical shock.

In 1878, Kuttner showed that ligation of the pulmonary veins worsened the ischemic damage caused by pulmonary artery occlusion. This observation was not appreciated until Karsner and Ash (1912) reinvestigated pulmonary infarction 34 years later. They confirmed that lung infarction in the dog was rare after obstruction of both pulmonary and bronchial blood flow but that tying the pulmonary veins as well always caused an infarction.

Under these conditions it is noteworthy that infarcts, characterized by alveolar necrosis and hemorrhage, took about 2 days to become typical macroscopically and on x-ray. This suggests that the energy stores in the tissues are sufficient to protect against ischemic necrosis for a considerable time if they are not depleted as they would be in hemorrhagic shock. Indeed, venous ligation or high venous pressures due to left heart failure must increase the volume of static, nutrient-filled blood in the vessels.

The extreme hypotension and blood volume depletion of hemorrhagic shock reduces the nutrient supply to the lung tissues from all the sources of blood flow, although ventilation and oxygenation are maintained. The subsequent patchy edema has been called "shock lung" and is presumed to be another example of the reperfusion syndrome (Modry and Chu-Jeng, 1979). In dogs bled for periods ranging up to 1 h and then resuscitated, histological changes were present after less than 1 h. Abnormalities were most evident 2 days after resuscitation, improving thereafter. Pulmonary endothelial cells were swollen and disorganized. The alveolar type I cells degenerated, although the type II cells were less affected. There was an alveolar exudate and conspicuous blockage of the vasculature by aggregations of platelets. These changes were more marked after about an hour (100 min), at which time quite gross hemorrhages were present in some regions of the lungs (Connell et al., 1975). Perbeck et al., (1989) found marked heterogeneity of pulmonary flow following reperfusion after 3 h of hemorrhagic shock in rats. This appears to be another manifestation of the "no reflow" syndrome.

Conclusions from Studies of Hypoxia and Substrate Deficiences at Body Temperature

Oxygen and substrate deprivation when the lung is kept at body temperature result in a pattern of histological and biochemical abnormalities that depends on the differences in technique, the species of animal, and the length of the deficiency. As expected, the greatest damage occurs most rapidly when both ventilation and perfusion are stopped, so hypoxia and substrate deficiency develop. The alveolar type I cell appears to be the most sensitive, followed by the other alveolar epithelial and endothelial cells, then the bronchial mucosal cells, the brochial glands and, finally, the bronchial muscle. Anaerobic glycolysis can maintain alveolar tissue energy supplies for only about 2 h. The ATP falls remarkably rapidly (although less quickly than in active organs like the heart) and more profoundly with ischemia than with hypoxia alone.

Interruption of ventilation alone, leading to atelectasis, causes ultrastructural cell damage and lack of surfactant function. The generation of surfactant may require lung distention. Although pulmonary arterial perfusion is reduced by hypoxic vasoconstriction when alveolar oxygen falls, bronchial arterial flow increases (Charan et al., 1986). It is not known if these changes, found in animal studies, occur to the same extent in clinical atelectasis.

When there is no ventilation, substrate deficiency rather than hypoxia causes the gradations of the severity of damage after pulmonary artery occlusion, pulmonary and bronchial artery occlusion, and, worst of all, pulmonary and bronchial artery and pulmonary vein occlusion.

In some studies, ventilation with N_2 seems to have prevented ischemic damage. This finding, the antithesis of that expected from adding hypoxia to lack of perfusion, has led to the suggestion that perhaps too high a concentration of O_2 causes injury when the lung is not perfused (Koyama et al., 1987). Excised, nonperfused lungs very quickly become edematous and show cellular injury histologically when ventilated with O_2. Injury is still present when air is used, however. To explain this it is noted that when there is little or no perfusion, alveolar oxygen can rise from a normal of about 16% to the 21% present in air. This is a relative hyperoxia and could cause oxygen toxicity (Grum, 1989). However, other studies in dogs have failed to confirm that N_2 breathing alters the "reperfusion injury" response to ischemia (Overand et al., 1989). It is unlikely that tissue O_2 during the ischemic period falls so low as to prevent the formation of toxic O_2 radicals for the self-destruct reaction of severely energy depleted cells, although the resupply of O_2 is thought by some to be why reperfusion seems to worsen the ischemic damage. Perhaps the effect of N_2 breathing in preventing hyperoxia and the different but additive injury of O_2 toxicity can reconcile these views.

The importance of species differences in the reaction to ischemia is illustrated by the finding after reestablishing perfusion that, in dogs, unilateral pulmonary artery occlusion for 1 day caused only patchy atelectasis and local loss of surfactant (Huber and Edmunds, 1967), whereas in rabbits the alveolar tissue damage was sufficiently severe and widespread to cause the "reperfusion injury" (Bishop et al., 1989a). The damage after vascular clamping with continued ventilation could be less severe than it otherwise might be because the lung region involved cools, so the metabolic demands of the tissues fall. Preservation of the lung tissues by cooling is considered in the following section.

D. Damage Due to Substrate Deprivation in the Cold

In preventing ischemic damage, the evidence for the efficacy of cooling in reducing metabolic demands is overwhelming. At room temperature, excised, nonventilated dog lungs perfused with electrolyte solutions show both histological and biochemical abnormalities that worsen with time, whereas when cooled these abnormalities are significantly delayed. In preserving lungs for transplantation, the aim is to rapidly reduce their metabolism by cooling to about 10°C. The lungs are flushed with a cold electrolyte solution and then stored in a similar solution without ventilation. Kaneko et al. (1988) found that 4 h was the maximum time that cold dog lungs could be preserved if adequate function were to be present after transplantation under the stress of excision of the other lung.

The rapidity of reduction in lung temperature appears to be more important than the composition of the solution used. For this reason prostacyclin has been used to dilate the pulmonary vasculature and ensure a more rapid and homogeneous distribution of the cold solution. Distending or ventilating the lungs also appears to help preservation, perhaps by ensuring even distribution of the cooling solution. There is evidence that flushing with a solution containing the low potassium and high sodium of extracellular fluid preserves the lung better than a solution with electrolytes like those present in the intracellular fluid. Raising the oncotic pressure with dextran or glucose should help to prevent pulmonary edema, but the results have been equivocal. However, one would think that cold blood from the donor would be best: it should cool almost as rapidly as an electrolyte solution, be less likely to cause osmotic edema, and have the nutrients required in the critical cooling and rewarming periods. Its viscosity may impair uniform perfusion and cooling, however, and infection considerations could make it less desirable. It has been said that there are as many modifications of the cooling solution as there are lung transplant centers.

In transplant studies using the dogs' own lungs, when the pulmonary vasculature was flushed with a cold electrolyte solution and the lung was cooled externally, most of the transplants survived after a 4 h nonventilated ischemic period. However, few survived after an 8 h period (Kaneko et al., 1988). In sharp contrast, Hoyer et al. (1980) claimed that reanastomosed dog lung homografts, preserved in a similar way for periods up to 2 days, showed no gross morphological changes and only slight alterations by electron microscopy. Oxygen uptake was present, the bronchial smooth muscle reacted to acetycholine, and lung scans showed perfusion and ventilation to be satisfactory.

An interesting recent study of the effects of temperature on excised rabbit lungs suggested that temperatures of about 10°C allowed the longest preservation (Wang et al., 1989). What was unexpected was that lower temperatures (to 6°C) were not so beneficial. It was suggested that this was due to the effect of very low temperatures in uncoupling Na, K, and water reaction pathways.

Transplantation offers an opportunity to assess lung healing after the injuries of ischemia and hypoxia. Methods for assessing initial damage, inflammatory response, and healing range from functional studies to careful histological studies after different lengths of time following transplantation (Hoyer et al., 1980; Keschavjee et al., 1989). Resumption of ventilation and perfusion appears to cause the three ischemic reactions discussed earlier (Fig. 2) to become evident as reimplantation or reperfusion injury.

VI. Healing

If the damage is slight, healing of a lung subjected to a temporary unilateral pulmonary artery occlusion (global ischemic stress) can occur in a few days. Davis et al. (1952) found that after relief of 1–7 days of unilateral pulmonary artery occlusion in the monkey, a decrease in lung volume, atelectasis, alveolar exudation, and macrophage infiltration worsened for 2 days and then began to heal, with almost complete recovery after an additional 7 days. The period to normality depended on the severity of the ischemic damage, which worsened with the length of the initial ischemia. If the damage was gross and led to necrotic changes, normality was never restored. This was particularly evident if the basement membranes disappeared so that the scaffolding for the new cells was no longer present (Vracko, 1972). The original tissues were then replaced by fibroblastic scar tissue. Such scarring seems to be greater in mechanical pump organs, such as the lungs and heart, that continually change shape (Vracko and Benditt, 1972).

The healing after local ischemic stress can be studied by following the changes after a pulmonary embolus. A period of inadequate perfusion immediately after the embolic obstruction leads to cellular changes ranging from minor edema to complete infarction. Healing occurs after the inflammatory response subsides (Karsner and Ash, 1912). This can be a complete restoration of the alveolar architecture and cellular distribution if the original ischemia was slight or a gross disruption with fibrosis if infarction occurred (Webb, 1909: McGoldrick et al., 1979). In dogs, Karsner and Ash found that a leukocytic infiltration was beginning to replace the hemorrhagic alveolar exudate and that fibroblasts were proliferating a week after an infarction. After 2 weeks the edema disappeared and fibrosis was considerably more marked; at 3 weeks the entire region was replaced by fibrous tissue except for some residual open airspaces with thick fibrous walls. In human subjects, about half the pulmonary infarctions, defined as radiological opacities, clear completely. The remainder become small linear and pleurally based scars. However, the frequency of residual pulmonary vascular perfusion defects demonstrated by radionuclide scans is rather greater than the scarring (McGoldrick et al., 1979).

VII. Hypertrophy of the Bronchial Circulation After Pulmonary Artery Occlusion

When the pulmonary blood flow is restricted as a result of congenital heart disease, enormous hypertrophy of the bronchial circulation may develop soon after birth. In adults, the size of the bronchial vascular bed may grow manyfold after pulmonary artery occlusion. This response is considered in Chap. 21. It is interesting that the pulmonary circulation cannot form new bridging vessels around a pulmonary arterial obstruction. However, the bronchial circulation can and very soon does form new channels with the potential of conducting flow across the obstruction.

These new vessels are formed remarkably quickly after the obstruction of major pulmonary arteries (Chiles et al., 1990), but it is uncertain if there is a similar response to small vessel occlusions even if these are severe and diffuse (see Chap. 20). Bronchial arterial angioneogenesis starts within a week or 10 days of pulmonary artery occlusion in the rat, and the hypertrophy is considerable after 3 months (Weibel, 1960). New capillaries grow as offshoots from other capillaries or venules. In response to an angiogenic stimulus, endothelial cells begin to extrude from a vessel by lysing the vascular basement membrane with a specific collagenase. The cells move out, perhaps toward the site of the angiogenic stimulus, and proliferate to form a new sprout. As two columns of cells join to form a loop, a channel forms within. Blood starts to flow within the new loop, and soon new branches sprout and join, finally forming a network.

The angiogenic factors affecting the endothelial cells (endothelial growth factors) are able to regulate the way the sprout forms and the rate of its growth. Mast cell heparin, stored in basement membranes, could be the factor stimulating the hyperplasia. The pericytes around the vessel probably suppress endothelial cell division. It appears that they must have physical contact with the endothelial cells to do this. Angiogenin is one human protein that is thought to promote the growth of blood vessels. Others are the fibroblast growth factors (FGF), acid FGF and basic FGF, and the transforming growth factors TGF-α and TGF-β. The latter attracts macrophages that secrete angiogenic materials, probably including tumor necrosis factor TNF-α, which stimulates endothelial cell locomotion but not proliferation. Mast cell heparin enhances the effect of endothelial cell growth factors, for which it has a high binding affinity. Finally, there are angiostatic steroids that circulate as normal products of steroid metabolism. Previously considered inactive, they could be regulators of the normal growth of the microvasculature.

Most of the increase in the bronchial circulation occurs within 3 months after the obstruction of the pulmonary artery. During this period, the pulmonary vascular bed distal to the occlusion undergoes interesting and inexplicable morphological changes like those seen in severe pulmonary hypertension (Shure et al., 1987). This pulmonary vascular remodeling occurs when the bronchial circulation is hypertrophying. If the pulmonary artery occlusion is then removed so that blood flow can resume, reperfusion-associated edema and even hemorrhages develop in a patchy fashion. As in the immediate postobstruction reperfusion injury syndrome, the reperfusion through the damaged pulmonary vasculature is often very poor (see Chap. 20). Regression of the expanded bronchial circulation follows pulmonary reperfusion, and its size reverts to normal provided there is no marked residual limitation of pulmonary flow (Alley et al., 1960).

The augmented bronchial circulation not only perfuses the airways and the other lung structures it normally supplies but, through the anastomoses with the pulmonary circulation, perfuses the pulmonary capillary bed and nourishes the alveolar tissues. These lungs appear normal morphologically, although there may be some shrinkage and an increase in the fibrous tissue in the alveolar walls and septa. They appear to function normally, but the status of the more specialized attributes of lung tissue, such as the hypoxic vasoconstrictive response and endothelial cell function, is unknown.

Many questions remain about the hypertrophy of the bronchial circulation that follows pulmonary artery occlusion. How is it turned on? What determines its extent? Is this related only to the nutritional demands of the tissues, or are the other functions of the lung, such as gas exchange, involved? What is the mechanism of bronchial circulatory regression if and when the pulmonary circulation is restored? This is such an important response clinically and conceptually that every effort should be made to answer these questions.

VIII. Summary and Conclusions

The lung seldom experiences nutritional deficiency despite its energetic and specialized metabolism. Gram for gram, it is more active in lipid metabolism than the liver (Felts, 1964)! It can survive vascular deprivation of oxygen because ventilation is adequate for oxygenation and CO_2 removal from all its tissues. The substrates for the manufacturing processes of the active cells are provided by the pulmonary and, to a very small extent, by the bronchial arterial blood flow. Should the pulmonary blood flow fall, bronchial flow rapidly increases. The cells of all the lung tissues are still sufficiently nourished and the long-term histological result of pulmonary arterial obstruction is but a mild increase in fibrous tissue. In addition to the bronchial flow, the pulmonary venous blood can reflux up to and through the alveoli to the obstructed pulmonary artery. It floods in and out in a tidal fashion with volume changes of breathing. It appears sufficient, in the period soon after pulmonary artery obstruction when bronchial blood flow falls, to provide for the nutrient inflow and the excretion of metabolities. In the long term, the lung suffering a permanent pulmonary artery occlusion can even regain a noteworthy amount of gas exchange because of the striking hyperplasia of the bronchial circulation. The tiny bronchial vasculature, normally carrying less than 1% of the cardiac output, can enlarge to perfuse the pulmonary vascular bed distal to the obstruction with a flow as large as 25% of the cardiac output. This is another fascinating example of the way the organism can adapt to what would appear to be a crippling loss of function of a vital organ.

References

Alley, R. D., Van Mierop, L. H. S., Peck, A. S., Kausel, H. W., and Stranahan, A. (1961). Bronchial arterial collateral circulation. Effect of experimental ligation of the pulmonary artery and subsequent reanastomosis. *Am. Rev. Respir. Dis.* **83**:31–37.

Amthor, M. (1973). Pulmonary changes after temporary ischemia of varying duration. *Bertr. Path. Bd.* **149**:270–279.

Barman, S. A., Ardell, J. A., Parker, J. C., Perry, M. L., and Taylor, A. E., (1988). Pulmonary and systemic blood flow contributions to upper airways in canine lungs. *Am. J. Physiol.* **255**(24):H1130–H1135.

Bassett, D. J. P., Fisher, A. B., and Rabinowitz, J. L. (1975). Effect of hypoxia on incorporation of glucose carbons into lipids by isolated rat lung. *Am. J. Physiol.* **277**:1103–1108.

Bishop, M. J., Albert, R. K., Lamm, W., and Guidotti, S. M. (1989a). Pulmonary ischemia increases vascular permeability even without reperfusion. *Am. Rev. Respir. Dis.* **139**:415A.

Bishop, M. J., Su, M., Chi, E. Y., and Cheney, F. W. (1989b). Neutrophil depletion with hydroxyurea ameliorates lung reperfusion injury. *J. Crit. Care* **4**:176–183.

Boushy, S., Helgason, A., and North, L. (1969). Occlusion of the bronchial arteries by various size glass microspheres. *Clin. Res.* **17**:412.

Bulkley, G. B. (1987). Free radical mediated reperfusion injury: A selective review. *Br. J. Cancer* **55**(Suppl VIII):66–73.

Butler, J., Kowalski, T. F., Willoughby, S., and Lakshminarayan, S. (1989). An alternative nutrient blood supply after pulmonary artery occlusion. *Fed. Proc.* **3**:567A.

Charan, N. B., Lakshminarayan, S., Albert, R. K., Kirk, W., and Butler, J. (1986). Hypoxia and hypercarbia increase bronchial blood flow through bronchopulmonary anastomoses in anesthetized dogs. *Am. Rev. Respir. Dis.* **134**:89–92.

Chiles, C., Newman, G. E., and Blinder, R. A. (1990). A method for evaluating the bronchial circulation. Preliminary observations. *Invest. Radiol.* **25**:52–57.

Connaughton, P. J., Bahuth, J. J., and Lewis, F. J. (1962). Lung ischemia up to 6 hours: Influence of local cooling in situ on subsequent pulmonary function. *Dis. Chest* **41**:404–408.

Connell, R. S., Swank, R. L., and Webb, M. C. (1975). The development of pulmonary ultrastructural lesions during hemorrhagic shock. *J. Trauma* **15**:116–129.

Cummiskey, J. M., Simon, L. M., Theodore, J., Ryan, U. S., and Robin, E. D. (1981). Bioenergetic alterations in cultivated pulmonary artery and aortic endothelial cells exposed to normoxia and hypoxia. *Exp. Lung Res.* **2**:155–163.

Davis, H. A., Gordon, W. B., Hayes, E. W., and Wasley, M. T. (1952). Effects upon the lung of varying periods of temporary occlusion of the pulmonary artery. *Arch. Surg.* **64**:464–474.

Edmunds, L. H., and Holm, J. C. (1969). Effect of inhaled CO_2 on hemorrhagic consolidation due to unilateral pulmonary arterial ligation. *J. Appl. Physiol.* **26**:710–715.

Ellis, F. H., Jr., Grindlay, J. H., and Edwards, J. E. (1951). The bronchial arteries—experimental occlusion. *Surgery* **30**:810–826.

Engerson, T. D., McKelvey, T. G., Rhyme, D. B., Boggio, E. B., Snyder, S. L., and Jones, H. P. (1987). Conversion of xanthine dehydrogenase to oxidase in ischemic rat tissues. *J. Clin. Invest.* **79**:1964.

Engler, R. L., Dahlgren, M. D., Morris, D. D., Peterson, M. A., and Schmid-Schonbein, G. W. (1986). Role of leucocytes in the response to acute myocardial ischemia and reflow in the dog. *Am. J. Physiol.* **251**(20):H314–H322.

Felts, J. M. (1964). Biochemistry of the lung. In *Health Physics* Edited by Vetter, R. Vol. 10. Pergamon Press. p. 973–979.

Fisher, A. B., and Dodia, C. (1981). Lung as a model for evaluation of critical intracellular Po_2 and PCO. *Am. J. Physiol.* **241**:E47–E50.

Fisher, A. B., Hyde, R. W., and Reif, J. S. (1972). Insensitivity of the alveolar septum to local hypoxia. *Am. J. Physiol.* **223**:770–775.

Fisher, A. B., Steinberg, H., and Bassett, B. S. (1974). Energy utilization by the lung. *Am. J. Med.* **57**:437–446.

Grum, C. M. (1989). Ch. 28. Pulmonary ischemic syndrome. In *Clinical Ischemic Syndromes. Mechanisms and Consequences of Tissue Injury.* Edited by G. B. Zelenack, St. Louis, Mosby, pp. 549–564.

Hall, T. S., Buescher, P. C., Borkon, A. M., Reitz, B. A., Michael, J. R., and Baumgartner, W. A. (1988). ^{31}P nuclear magnetic resonance determination of changes in energy state in lung preservation. *Circulation* **78**(Suppl. 111):95–98.

Hoyer, J., Garbe, S., Delpierre, A., Prieur, G., Macquart-Moulin, G., and Noirclerc, M. (1980). Functional evaluation of the transplanted lung after long term preservation. *Respiration* **39**:322–332.

Huber, G. L., and Edmunds, L. H. (1967). Pulmonary artery occlusion: Morphologic studies. *J. Appl. Physiol.* **22**:1002–1011.

Hughes, F. A., Kehne, J. H., and Fox, J. R. (1954). Replantation and transplantation of pulmonary tissue in dogs. *Surgery* **36**:1101–1108.

Ide, H., Ino, T., Hasegawa, T., and Matsumoto, H. (1990). The role of leukocyte depletion by in vivo use of a leucokyte filter in lung preservation after warm ischemia. *Angiology* **41**:318–325.

Kaneko, M., Perrotta, N. J., and Copeland, J. G. (1988). A simple working heart and lung transplant model for assessing preservation methods in the rabbit. *Transplantation* **46**:624–625.

Karsner, H. T., and Ash, J. E. (1912). Studies in infarction. II. Experimental bland infarction of the lung. *J. Med. Res.* **27**:205–224.

Keshavjee, S. H., Yamazaki, F., Cardoso, P. F., McRitchie, D. I., Patterson, G. A., and Cooper, J. D. (1989). A method for safe twelve-hour pulmonary preservation. *J. Thorac. Cardiovasc. Surg.* **98**:529–534.

Kowalski, T. F., Guidotti, S., Deffebach, M., and Kubulis, M. (1990). Bronchial circulation in pulmonary artery occlusion and reperfusion. *J. Appl. Physiol.* **68**:125–129.

Koyama, I., Toung, T. J. K., Rogers, M. C., Gurtner, G. H., and Traytsman, R. J. (1987). O_2 radicals mediate reperfusion lung injury in ischemic, O_2 ventilated canine pulmonary lobe. *J. Appl. Physiol.* **63**:111–115.

Kuttner, C. (1878). Beitrag zur Kenntniss der Kreislaufsverhaltnisse der Saugethierlunge. *Virchows Arch.* (A) **73**:476–523.

Liebow, A. A. (1962). Recent observations on pulmonary collateral circulation. *Med. Thorac.* **19**:417–430.

Lien, D. C., Capen, R. L., Checkley, L. L., Janke, S. J., and Wagner, W. W. (1989). Mode of neutrophil transit in the pulmonary microcirculation. *FASEB J.* **3**:A1161.

Light, R. B. (1988). Intrapulmonary oxygen consumption in experimental pneumococcal pneumonia. *J. Appl. Physiol.* **64**:2490–2495.

Mathes, M. E., Holman, E., and Reichert, F. L. (1932). A study of the bronchial, pulmonary and lymphatic circulations of the lung under various pathological conditions experimentally produced. *J. Thorac. Surg.* **1**:339–362.

McCord, J. M. (1985). Oxygen-derived free radicals in post ischemic tissue injury. *N. Engl. J. Med.* **312**:159–163.

McGoldrick, P. J., Rudd, T. G., Figley, M. M., and Wilhelm, J. P. (1979). What becomes of pulmonary infarcts? *AJR* **133**:1039–1045.

Metchnikov, E. (1891). Lectures on the comparative pathology of inflammation. Lecture 1. (translated from the French by F. A. Starling and E. A. Starling). New York, Dover, 1968, p. 10.

Modry, D. L., and Chu-Jeng, R. (1979). Pulmonary reperfusion syndrome. *Ann. Thorac. Surg.* **27**:206–215.

Modry, D. L., Chin, C. J., and Hinchey, E. J. (1977). The roles of ventilation and perfusion in lung metabolism. *J. Thorac. Cardiovasc. Surg.* **74**:275–285.

De Moraes, R. B., and De Carvalho, S. (1949). Contribuicao para oestudo da fisiologia das comunicacoes arterio-venosas do pulmao. *Gaz. Med. Port.* **2**:553–562.

Moser, K. M., (1990). State of the art. Venous thromboembolism, *Am. Rev. Respir. Dis.* **141**:235–249.

Nordenstrom, B. (1954). Temporary unilateral occlusion of the pulmonary artery: A method of roentgen examination of the pulmonary vessels. *Acta Radiol. Suppl. (Stockh.)* 108.

Oren, R., Farnham, A. E., Salto, K., Milofsky, E., and Karnovsky, M. L. (1963). Metabolic patterns in three types of phagocytosing cells. *J. Cell Biol.* **17**:487-501.

Overand, P. T., Bishop, M. J., Eisenstein, B. L., Chi, E., Menglung, S., and Cheney, F. W. (1989). Lack of alveolar O_2 during lung reperfusion does not decrease edema formulation. *J. Appl. Physiol.* **67**:528–533.

Pattle, R. E. (1956). Failure of local anoxia in rabbit lung to produce or intensify pulmonary odema. *J. Pathol. Bacteriol.* **72**:211.

Pegg, D. E., Jacobsen, I. A., and Halasz, N. A. (1982). Organ preservation: Basic and applied aspects. Lancaster, England, M. I. P. Press, pp. 329–350.

Perbeck, L., Lund, F., and Thulin, L. (1989). Intrathoracic microvascular circulation in hemorrhagically shocked rats. Studies by fluorescence techniques. *Clin. Physiol.* **9**:567–579.

Petty, R. G., and Pearson, J. D. (1989). Endothelium—the axis of vascular health and disease. *J. Coll. Physicians Lond.* **23**:92–102.

Ratych, R. E., Chucknyiska, and Buckley, G. B. (1987). The primary localization of free radical generation after anoxia/reoxygenation in isolated endothelial cells. *Surgery* **102**:122–131.

Ricketts, H. J., and Carrington, C. B. (1968). Experimental bronchial occlusion in sheep. In *Proceedings of the 11th Aspen Emphysema Conference.* Public Health Service Publication No. 1879. Edited by Mitchell, R., Washington, D. C., U. S. Government Printing Office, p. 187–188.

Schmid-Schonbein, (1988). Granulocyte: Friend and foe. *NIPS* **3**:144–147.

Shepard, J. W., Witztum, K. F., Fletcher, J. W., and Dolan, G. F. (1981). Pulmonary venous pathway for substrate delivery to the lung in the absence of arterial blood flow. *Am. Rev. Respir. Dis.* **123**:246A.

Shure, D., Dockweiler, D. W., and Bloor, C. M. (1987). Post obstructive pulmonary arteriopathy does not precede significant bronchial collateral formation in an animal model. *Am. Rev. Respir. Dis.* **135**:514A.

Smirnow, S. A. (1927). Versuche uber einfache und kombinierte Unterbindung der Sungengefasse. *Arch Klin. Chir.* **146**:215–220.

Starkey, T. D., Sakakibara, N., Hagberg, R. C., Tazelaer, H. D., Baldwin, U. C., and Jamieson, S. W. (1986). Successful six-hour cardiopulmonary preservation with simple hypotonic crystalloid flush. *J. Heart Transplant* **5**:291–297.

Trummer, M. J., and Berg, P. (1968). *Lung Transplantation.* Springfield, IL: Charles C. Thomas, pp. 44, 85.

Veith, F. J., Sinha, S. B. P., Graves, J. S., Boley, S. J., and Dougherty, J. C. (1971). Ischemic tolerance of the lung: The effects of ventilation and inflation. *J. Thorac. Cardiovasc. Surg.* **61**:804–809.

Virchow, R. L. (1856). Gesammelte Werke. In *Abhandlungen zur Wissenschlaftlichen Medizin.* Frankfurt, Meidinger, pp. 285–286.

Von Wichert, P. (1972). Studies on the metabolism of ischemic rabbit lungs. *J. Thorac. Cardiovasc. Surg.* **63**:284–291.

Vracko, R. (1972). Significance of basal lamina for regeneration of injured lung. *Virchows Arch (A)* **355**:264–274.

Vracko, R., and Benditt, E. P. (1972). Basal lamina: The scaffold for orderly cell replacement. *J. Cell. Biol.* **55**:406–419.

Wang, L. S., Yoshikawa, K., Migoshi, S., Nakamoto, K., Hsieh, C. M., Yamazaki, F., Cardoso, P. F. G., Shaefers, H. J. G., Brito, J., Kheshavjee, S. H., Patterson, A., and Cooper, J. D. (1989). The effect of ischemic time and temperature on lung preservation in a simple ex vivo rabbit model used for functional assessment. *J. Thorac. Cardiovasc. Surg.* **98**:333–342.

Weber, K. C., and Visscher, M. B. (1969). Metabolism of the isolated canine lung. *Am. J. Physiol.* **217**:1044–1052.

Weibel, E. R. (1960). Early stages in the development of collateral circulation to the lung in the rat. *Circ. Res.* **8**:353–376.

Welch, W. H. (1909). Embolism. Allbut and Rollestous System of Medicine. London Vi, 798.

Zahn, F. W. (1897). Ueber die Folgen des Verschlusses der Lungenarterien und Pfortaderaste durch Embolie. *Verhandl. Gesellsch. Deutsch. Naturforsch. Aerzte* (Braunschweig) **69**:9.

12

The Bronchial and Systemic Circulations in Lung and Pleural Fluid and Protein Balance

MICHAEL A. MATTHAY

University of California, San Francisco
San Francisco, California

I. Introduction

The overall purpose of this chapter is to consider the influence of the systemic and bronchial circulations on fluid and protein balance in the lung and pleural space under selected pathological conditions. The first objective is to evaluate the contribution of the bronchial and systemic circulations to the development of either hydrostatic or increased permeability pulmonary edema. The second objective is to consider the related issue of the pathogenesis of pleural effusions in both hydrostatic and increased permeability pulmonary edema with specific reference to the relative contribution of the pulmonary and bronchial circulations. The third objective is to examine the contribution of the bronchial, pulmonary, and lymphatic circulations to the resolution of pulmonary edema.

Whenever possible, relevant clinical studies are cited to provide pertinent information regarding the possible role of the bronchial circulation in the development or resolution of pulmonary edema or pleural effusions. However, the most specific information regarding the possible role of the bronchial circulation in lung fluid and protein balance depends primarily on a variety of experimental studies that have been designed to identify the relative contribution of the bronchial and pulmonary circulations under experimentally controlled conditions.

II. Role of the Bronchial and Systemic Circulation in the Development of Hydrostatic Pulmonary Edema

The anatomic relationships between the bronchial and pulmonary circulations and drainage pathways that lead to the right or left heart need to be appreciated to understand the results of experimental studies that were designed, in part, to assess the contribution of the bronchial circulation to the development of hydrostatic pulmonary edema. Note that most of the bronchial circulation drains into the left atrium under normal conditions, via the bronchopulmonary anastomoses through either pulmonary capillaries or pulmonary veins. Some of the bronchial circulation drains into the azygos, hemiazygos, or intercostal veins and therefore returns to the right heart (Fig. 1).

There are two mechanisms by which the bronchial circulation itself may contribute to the development of pulmonary edema. First, an elevation in systemic venous pressure could cause bronchial venous hypertension, with increased fluid filtration in the lobar and segmental bronchial veins that eventually drain into the right side of the heart (Fig. 1) (Bruner and Schmidt, 1947). Second, elevation of left atrial and pulmonary venous pressure may cause leakage from the bronchopulmonary anastomoses (Fig. 1). If the pulmonary venous pressure is high enough, then the bronchial venous drainage can reverse from a left to a right atrial outflow, in which case right atrial pressure elevations could also worsen pulmonary edema (Agostoni et al., 1987).

In addition to considering mechanisms by which the bronchial circulation itself could contribute to hydrostatic pulmonary edema, it is also important to mention how elevations of systemic venous pressure could increase edema in the lung by decreasing lung lymphatic drainage from the thoracic duct and the right lymphatic duct into the superior vena caval system. Indeed, one group of investigators reported that an elevation in systemic venous pressure initially caused a reduction in thoracic duct lymph flow (Wegria et al., 1963). However, lymphatic flow restarted after lymphatic pressure increased to levels above the systemic venous pressure. Also, increased lymphatic flows were observed after the release of venous hypertension. Subsequently, another group reported that after experimentally induced right ventricular failure in dogs, the increase in systemic venous pressure resulted in a significant resistance to thoracic duct lymph flow (Cole et al., 1967). Furthermore, the lymph flow could be increased by anastomosis of the thoracic duct to the low-pressure pulmonary veins. None of these studies, however, actually directly

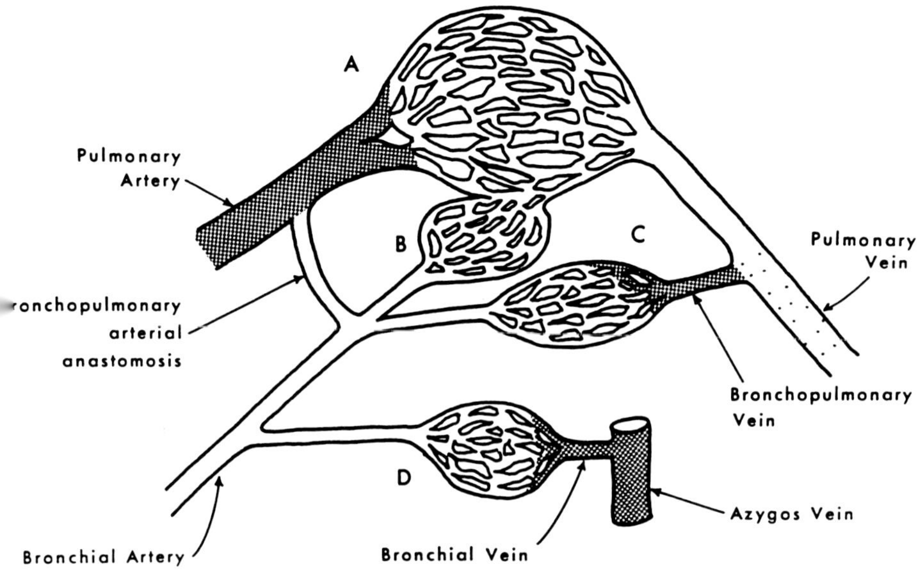

Figure 1 Relationships between the bronchial and pulmonary circulations. The pulmonary artery supplies the pulmonary capillary network (A). A bronchial artery supplies capillary networks B, C, and D. Network B represents the bronchial capillary supply to bronchioles that anastomoses with pulmonary capillaries and drains through pulmonary veins. Network C represents the bronchial capillary supply to most bronchi; these vessels form bronchopulmonary veins that empty into pulmonary veins. Network D represents the bronchial capillary supply to lobar and segmental bronchi; these vessels form true bronchial veins that drain into the axygos, hemiazygos, or intercostal veins. Shaded areas represent blood flow of low O_2 content. (From Murray, 1986.)

measured the accumulation of extravascular lung water in association with systemic venous hypertension. It has been suggested that some patients with right-sided heart failure alone may have increased extravascular lung water clinically (Turino et al., 1968). However, possible coexistent left ventricular failure was not ruled out in this clinical study.

One of the first experiments that was designed to test the role of systemic venous hypertension in the development of hydrostatic pulmonary edema was done in anesthetized dogs (Paré et al., 1981). These investigators evaluated the effects of systemic venous hypertension of 25 cm H_2O with and without left atrial hypertension for 4 h on both the amount of extra-vascular lung water content and the pulmonary function of anesthetized dogs. The results showed that extravascular lung water was not increased in the presence of severe systemic venous hypertension alone compared to control dogs (Fig. 2). Further-

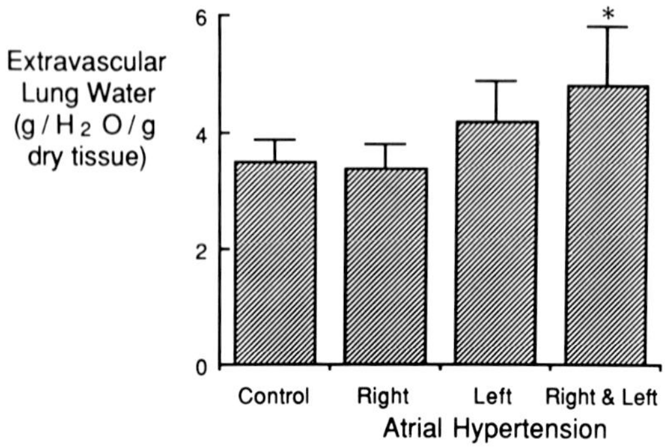

Figure 2 Data (mean ± SD) from experiments in anesthetized dogs on the accumulation of extravascular lung water. When right atrial pressure alone was elevated to 25 cmH_2O, there was no increase in the extravascular lung water. When left atrial pressure was elevated to 16 cmH_2O (control was 8 cmH_2O), these was a modest but insignificant increase in extravascular lung water. However, the combination of both left and right atrial hypertension produces a significant (*) increase in extravascular lung water. (From Paré et al., 1981.)

more, pulmonary function and arterial blood gases were not changed by systemic venous hypertension alone. This experimental observation is supported by a recent clinical study at our institution. Patients with moderate to severe systemic venous hypertension from pulmonary arterial hypertension never had pulmonary edema on the chest radiograph; all the patients had normal left ventricular function and a normal pulmonary arterial wedge pressure (Wiener-Kronish et al., 1987). The explanation for the absence of lung edema with elevation of systemic venous pressure alone may be that the bronchial circulation can drain into the pulmonary circulation if pulmonary venous pressures are not elevated (Charan et al., 1985).

However, the experimental study by Paré et al. (1981) found a small but significant increase in extravascular lung water content when systemic venous hypertension was combined with left atrial hypertension. Right and left atrial pressures were increased by massive volume overload with 100 ml/kg/h of intravenous normal saline for a period of 4 h. In the average 21 kg dog that was studied, this amounted to administration of 8–9 L fluid intravenously over a 4 h time period. In all the volume-loaded dogs, pulmonary arterial wedge pressure doubled from baseline values to approximately 16 cmH_2O. In addition, the plasma protein osmotic pressure fell by more than 50%. In the presence of the volume expansion alone, with a mean left atrial pressure of 16 cmH_2O, the extravascular lung water content increased by 23%. When the volume infusion was coupled with systemic venous hypertension of 25

cmH_2O, the extravascular lung water content increased by 38% over baseline levels (Fig. 2). Quantitatively, the additional increase in extravascular lung water in the presence of systemic venous hypertension was small but statistically significant. Furthermore, arterial oxygen tension tended to be slightly lower in the dogs that had both systemic venous hypertension and volume loading, perhaps indicating more alveolar flooding.

The results of Paré's experimental study in dogs are compatible with an effect of systemic venous hypertension on increased filtration in the bronchial veins in the lung that drain to the right side of the heart, reduced lung lymphatic pumping into the thoracic duct because of the elevated central venous pressures, or reduced reabsorption in the peribronchial edema fluid cuffs because of elevated systemic venous pressure. Another study arrived at a similar conclusion regarding a small additive effect of systemic venous hypertension on the degree of pulmonary edema in the presence of elevated left atrial pressure and lowered plasma protein osmotic pressure (Miller et al., 1978).

Subsequently, another group reported that only blood originating from extrapulmonary bronchi drained into systemic veins (Charan et al., 1984). These investigators argued that an increase in systemic venous hypertension alone would therefore be unlikely to cause increased transvascular fluid flux from intrapulmonary bronchial veins. This observation was further reinforced by a follow-up study in which the direct injection of saline into an isolated bronchial vein did not increase lung lymph flow or change the lung lymph to plasma protein ratio (Charan et al., 1985). However, an increase in pulmonary venous or left atrial pressure could, as mentioned, shift intrapulmonary bronchial venous drainage from the left to the right heart so that elevations in systemic venous pressure would then compound the degree of pulmonary edema (Agostoni et al., 1987).

Finally, a study in sheep reported that elevation of superior vena caval pressure to 20 mmHg over 4 h reduced lung lymph flow, which may account for the additional increase in extravascular lung water when superior vena caval pressure elevation was added to left atrial hypertension (Laine et al., 1986). This study confirmed the findings of Paré et al. in another species and provided some evidence for decreased lung lymph flow as perhaps part of the mechanism. Also, one study in dogs showed that chronic ligation of both the right lymphatic and thoracic ducts in combination with elevated pulmonary vascular pressures increased lung water in dogs (Magno and Szidon, 1976). However, another recent study in perfused open-chested dog lungs concluded that when a lung is already subjected to raised pulmonary vascular pressure sufficient to cause edema, then acute elevation of bronchial systemic venous pressure augments the net rate of outward fluid flux either because of increased filtration or decreased reaborption, but downstream lymphatic pressure elevation does not change the rate of fluid flux (Lakshminarayan, 1991).

It would be more clinically relevant if the experimental studies that have evaluated the effects of both right and left atrial hypertension, or accumulation of extravascular lung water, were carried out for longer time periods. Most of the studies have been acute experiments in anesthetized animals over 4–6 h. It is possible that the small effect of systemic venous hypertension on increasing extravascular lung water would be transient in longer studies in unanesthetized animals if lymphatic flow were allowed to overcome the effect of elevated systemic venous pressures (Wegria et al., 1963).

Clinically, there is good evidence that patients with chronic elevation in left atrial pressure and chronic heart failure have less pulmonary edema radiographically than expected if the same patients had a similar acute elevation in left atrial pressures. For example, in patients with chronic left ventricular failure, the level of pulmonary arterial wedge pressure can be predicted by the radiographic and clinical findings in only a minority of patients. In one study, the roentgenographic findings of pulmonary edema were present in only about 30% of patients with a pulmonary arterial wedge pressure greater than 25 mmHg (Dash et al., 1980). Thus, it is likely that acute elevations in systemic venous pressure have only a transient additive effect on the degree of pulmonary edema from left atrial hypertension. Several possible adaptations may occur in the lymphatic or bronchial circulation. For example, the capacity of the lymphatics may increase sufficiently to pump fluid against the elevated systemic venous pressures. This issue of the chronic adaption of lymphatics and the pulmonary and bronchial circulations to elevated venous pressures deserves further study. With chronic pressure elevations, there may also be a reduction in transvascular leakage because of perivascular fibrosis and a decrease in the interstitial concentration of protein.

Overall, the clinical and experimental evidence indicates that systemic venous hypertension alone is not a cause of hydrostatic pulmonary edema. However, if pulmonary edema has developed because of left atrial hypertension (with or without the contribution of a lowered plasma protein osmotic pressure), then a markedly elevated systemic venous pressure may result in a modest increase in the extravascular lung water.

III. Role of the Bronchial Circulation in the Development of Increased Permeability Pulmonary Edema

Can injury to the bronchial circulation result in sufficient transvascular escape of fluid from the systemic circulation of the lung to result in increased permeability pulmonary edema? The work of Pietra and coworkers (1971, 1974; Pietra and Magno, 1978) is often cited to provide support for the hypothesis that the bronchial circulation may be an important site for fluid leakage in increased permeability pulmonary edema. These investigators reported that colloidal carbon passed through gaps in the bronchial veins into the nearby interstitium in response to infusions of either histamine or endotoxin. More recent studies have suggested that histamine may increase permeability transiently in the pulmonary circulation rather than the bronchial circulation. When histamine was directly injected into the pulmonary circulation, one group of investigators found a marked increased in lung lymph flow that was not reproduced when histamine was directly injected into the left atrium (Nakahara et al., 1979). However, a number of other investigators have shown that histamine and other mediators can increase the permeability of systemic vessels (Maron, 1982; Rippe et al., 1984; Hutchinson et al., 1984). Nevertheless, there are no convincing data in these studies that injury to the bronchial circulation alone causes increased permeability pulmonary edema.

Injury to the bronchial circulation may coexist with injury to the pulmonary circulation in some clinical conditions, however. The best example, perhaps, is acute pneumonitis from aspiration of gastric contents. Injury to the systemic circulation supplying conducting airways may result in exudation of fluid into the extraalveolar interstitial space; injury to the pulmonary circulation in the alveoli could result in accumulation of edema in the distal airspaces, where blood supply primarily originates from the pulmonary circulation. Also, inhalational injuries from smoke or other toxic products could injure the bronchial circulation and result in edema of the lung via direct injury to the conducting airways.

In fact, one group has examined this possibility by studying the effects of smoke inhalation in sheep. These investigators reported the development of pulmonary edema with protein-rich lung lymph flow after smoke inhalation (Bassadre et al., 1988). If 80% of the bronchial circulation was occluded after inhalational injury, then the degree of injury as measured by the increase in lung lymph flow was reduced by 30%.

Also, recent experimental studies have explored the role of the pulmonary and bronchial circulations in delivering neutrophils to the lung in the presence of endotoxin or bacteria. In one study, neutrophil accumulation in the airspaces of the rabbit lung in the presence of *Streptococcus pneumoniae* was dependent on the pulmonary circulation since bronchial flow alone to one lung resulted in minimal neutrophil accumulation in the airspaces (Kowalski et al., 1989). If the same study is done in the presence of an inhalational injury, such as gastric aspiration or smoke inhalation, then the influx of inflammatory cells might depend significantly on the bronchial circulation.

There is some evidence that, in the presence of increased permeability pulmonary edema, elevation in systemic venous pressures may increase the degree of edema. For example, there was a modest increase in extravascular lung water content in sheep after elevation of superior vena caval pressure in the presence of *Escherichia coli* endotoxemia (Allen et al., 1987). In these studies, the investigators reported an increase in the extravascular lung water of 12% above control values with *E. coli* endotoxin alone. In the presence of a systemic venous pressure of 10 cmH_2O, the extravascular lung water increased 33% above baseline values. With a further elevation in systemic venous pressure to 17 cmH_2O, the extravascular lung water increased to 38% above baseline values. The authors were not able to selectively elevate systemic venous pressure alone in this study. In sheep in which the superior vena caval pressure was elevated, pulmonary or left atrial pressure was increased by 3 cmH_2O over baseline values. Although this was a small increase in left atrial pressure, some excellent experimental studies have demonstrated that small increases in left atrial pressure can result in a marked increase in transvascular fluid leak and pulmonary edema in the setting of increased permeability (Ohkuda et al., 1981). However, another recent study reported that elevation of superior vena caval pressure to 11.0 ± 3.1 mmHg increased extravascular lung water after alloxan-induced permeability pulmonary edema in dogs (Ando et al., 1990). One mechanism to account for this effect could be related to the decreased reabsorption of extraalveolar edema fluid by the bronchial circulation that drains to the right heart. Alternatively, an effect on decreasing lymphatic drainage from the lung is possible.

In summary, since the bronchial circulation normally supplies only 1% of the cardiac output to the lung, it seems unlikely that the bronchial circulation plays a major role in the development of increased permeability pulmonary edema when the injury is delivered primarily via the bloodstream, as in sepsis. However, more studies need to be done to identify the contribution of the bronchial circulation to increased permeability pulmonary edema when the injury occurs via the airways, as in gastric aspiration or inhalational injuries, or in the setting of pneumonia that involves the airways as well (i.e., influenza pneumonia). In these circumstances, there may be a significant contribution of the bronchial circulation to the development of pulmonary edema. Also, elevated systemic venous pressures play a small but significant role in reducing the rate of clearance of edema from the lung, thus compounding the extent of pulmonary edema that develops either from increasd pulmonary vascular pressures or an increase in lung vascular permeability.

IV. Contribution of the Systemic and Bronchial Circulations to the Development of Pleural Effusions

Until recently, there was considerable uncertainty regarding the pathogenesis of the transudative pleural effusions associated with congestive heart failure.

One experimental study suggested that right atrial hypertension was the most important factor in the development of pleural effusions in the setting of biventricular heart failure (Mellins et al., 1970). However, the experimental data supporting this theory depended on massive volume-loading studies in dogs with a 50–60% decrease in the plasma protein osmotic pressure. Also, the duration of the study was only 2 h, which may not have allowed enough time for much pulmonary edema to develop. Therefore, the low plasma protein osmotic pressure could have increase filtration across the parietal pleura, causing pleural effusion formation, or the effusions could have formed secondary to elevated systemic venous pressures as well, with increased filtration from the systemic capillaries supplying the parietal pleura.

Subsequently, a prospective clinical study was published that examined the hemodynamic parameters associated with the development of pleural effusions in patients with either left heart failure or biventricular heart failure (mostly chronic), hospitalized in the coronary care unit at our institution (Wiener-Kronish et al., 1985). The investigators measured hemodynamic pressures for 12 h and determined the presence of pleural effusions with ultrasound, a more sensitive technique for detecting pleural effusions than the chest radiograph. A total of 19 patients had pleural effusions, and the mean pulmonary arterial wedge pressure was 24 mmHg in these patients, compared to a mean pulmonary arterial wedge pressure of 17 mmHg ($p < 0.05$) in the 18 patients who did not have pleural effusions (Table 1).

The patients with pleural effusions had more extensive pulmonary edema on their chest radiograph than those who did not have effusions. In addition, the right atrial pressures were not significantly elevated in the patients with pleural effusions versus those without pleural effusions, although the mean right atrial pressure was slightly higher in the patients with pleural effusions. The patients who developed pleural effusions had an elevated pulmonary arterial pressure that correlated with the elevated left atrial pressure. Figure 3 provides a description of how pleural effusions could form in the presence of left atrial hypertension.

In a follow-up study, 29 patients with either primary or secondary pulmonary hypertension but normal left ventricular function were evaluated (Wiener-Kronish et al., 1987). None of the 29 patients had pleural effusions. All the patients had severe pulmonary arterial hypertension, and some of the patients had markedly elevated right atrial pressures, even to levels greater than 20 mmHg. All patients had a normal pulmonary arterial wedge pressure. The data from these two clinical studies provide excellent clinical evidence that right atrial hypertension does not play a major role in the accumulation of pleural effusions in the setting of chronic heart failure.

However, a recent experimental study reported that acute elevation of superior vena caval pressure to very high levels (34–41 cmH_2O) resulted in the accumulation of large, bilateral pleural effusions in unanesthetized sheep

Table 1 Relationship of Right and Left Heart Failure to the Presence of Pleural Effusions[a]

	Right atrial pressure (mmHg)	Pulmonary arterial pressure (mmHg)	Pulmonary arterial wedge pressure (mmHg)	Number of patients with pleural effusions
Right heart failure alone				
Retrospective ($n = 9$)	11 ±7	60 ±22	12 ±3	0
Prospective ($n = 18$)	12 ±2	50 ±5	11 ±1	0
Biventricular heart failure				
Mild ($n = 18$)	10 ±1	31 ±2	17 ±2	0
Severe ($n = 19$)	13 ±2	38 ±2	24 ±1	19

[a] Data shown as mean ± SEM (Standard error of the mean).
Source: Data from Wiener-Kronish and Matthay (1988) and Wiener-Kronish et al. (1985).

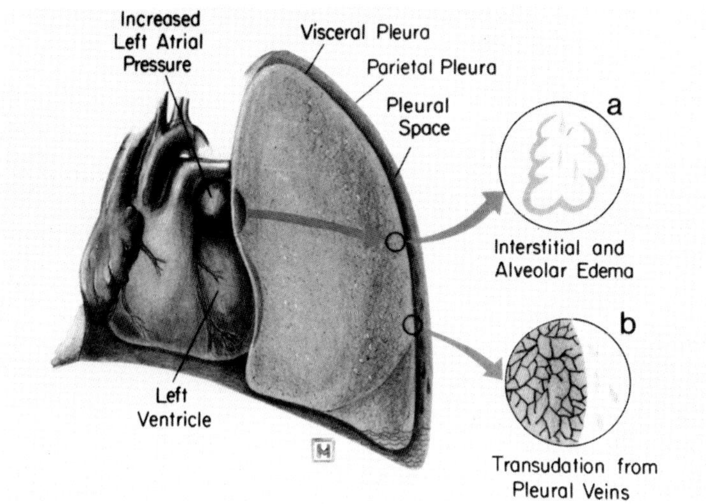

Figure 3 The two possible mechanisms for pleural effusion formation in the setting of left atrial hypertension and pulmonary edema. (a) The pleural liquid is a filtrate of interstitial and alveolar edema. (b) The pleural liquid is formed from the visceral pleural microcirculation because of the increased hydrostatic pressure (left atrial hypertension). (From Wiener-Kronish et al., 1985.)

(Allen et al., 1988). The authors surgically created a carotid artery to internal jugular vein fistula to maintain the markedly elevated superior vena caval pressure; unfortunately there was only one control for the effect of the fistula alone. Nevertheless, in the sheep that did not have a thoracotomy, the pleural protein concentration was low, suggesting that the effusions orginated, at least in part, from increased filtration across the parietal pleural capillaries, although leakage from lymphatics is also a possible explanation. How can we reconcile the data in the human studies with these experimental data? The best explanation may be that the human studies were done in the setting of chronic right atrial hypertension, which allowed time for compensatory mechanisms to develop.

Recent studies from our laboratory have examined the effect of volume loading in sheep on the accumulation of pleural effusions (Broaddus et al., 1990). Broaddus et al found that 100–200 ml pleural liquid formed over 4 h with elevation of pulmonary arterial wedge pressures 20 or 30 cmH_2O above baseline levels. There was a good correlation between the volume of pleural liquid that formed, the increase in extravascular lung water, and the pulmonary arterial wedge pressure; overall, the pleural effusions formed primarily from lung edema crossing the visceral pleura into the pleural space (Table 2).

Table 2 Pleural Effusions in Sheep with Both Sides of the Chest Closed Before and After Volume Loading[a]

Pulmonary arterial wedge pressure elevation (cmH_2O)	Protein concentration			Volume on both pleural sides (ml)
	No.	g per 100 ml	Liquid/plasma	
0[b]	21	1.0 ±0.5	0.15 ±.07	3.7 ±2.9
20	4	1.0 ±0.1	0.27 ±.03[c]	30.8 ±8.8[c]

[a] Data as mean ±SD (standard deviation).

[b] Control data.

[c] $p < 0.05$ compared to controls.

Source: From Broaddus et al. (1990).

Because there was an increase in systemic venous pressure with volume loading, the investigators evaluated the effect of systemic venous pressure elevation to 25 cmH_2O in five additional sheep studies. They also instilled 100 ml autologous plasma diluted to a protein concentration of 1g per 100 ml into one pleural space. Over 4 h, there was a net clearance of 12 ±8 ml despite the elevated systemic venous pressure; the instilled plasma was cleared at a rate of about 0.1 ml/kg/h, which is about half the rate previously reported by this group for the removal of pleural fluid in sheep with normal systemic venous pressure (Broaddus et al., 1988). Thus, the elevated systemic venous pressure did not stop net pleural fluid clearance, but it may have slowed the rate.

Recently, another group reported that left atrial hypertension in sheep, produced with an inflated balloon in the left atrium, resulted in large pleural effusions; there was a good relationship between pleural effusion volume and extravascular lung water (Fig. 4). Systemic venous pressure was not elevated (Allen et al., 1989).

Thus, the pathophysiology of transudative pleural effusions associated with heart failure has some interesting parallels to the pathophysiology of hydrostatic pulmonary edema. Elevated systemic venous pressure alone does not seem to be an adequate mechanism to explain the development of pleural effusions, except perhaps in the acute setting with very high levels. However, systemic venous hypertension may play a small additive role in slowing the clearance of excess pleural liquid that accumulates in the pleural space in the setting of hydrostatic pulmonary edema. Overall, the primary factors contributing to the accumulation of pleural effusions in the setting of congestive heart failure are left atrial hypertension and pulmonary edema.

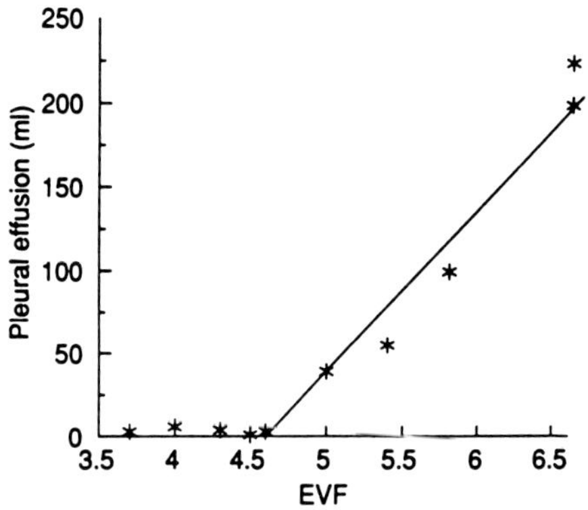

Figure 4 Note the good correlation between pleural effusion volume and extravascular fluid (EVF). (From Allen et al., 1989.)

It should also be mentioned that recent experimental and clinical data from work at our institution indicate that pleural effusions develop in sheep in the setting of acute oleic acid-induced permeability pulmonary edema, probably from movement of edema fluid across the visceral pleura into the pleural space (Wiener-Kronish et al., 1988b). Ultrastructural studies showed no direct injury to the visceral pleura; the studies were carried out over 8 h. During this time period, about 20% of the excess lung water drained into the pleural space. Clinical studies have also confirmed the presence of pleural effusions in patients with increased permeability pulmonary edema (Aberle et al., 1988; Wiener-Kronish and Matthay, 1988a).

V. Resolution of Pulmonary Edema

Before considering the possible routes and mechanisms for clearance of pulmonary edema, it is important to specify the location of the edema fluid to be removed from the lung. If edema fluid is confined to the alveolar interstitial space, then theoretically the fluid can be removed by either the pulmonary circulation or, in the absence of pulmonary blood flow, by the flow of bronchial blood flow through the bronchopulmonary anastomoses in the alveolar capillaries (site 3 in Fig. 5). If the interstitial edema fluid collects in the extra-alveolar interstitial space, as most of it does (Staub, 1974), then there are additional pathways for clearance: the lung lymphatics, the pleural space, peribronchial vessels that drain to the right side of the heart, or drainage into the mediastinum at the hilum. If interstitial edema floods into the airspaces, then some could escape from the lung by the mucociliary escalator. Even though

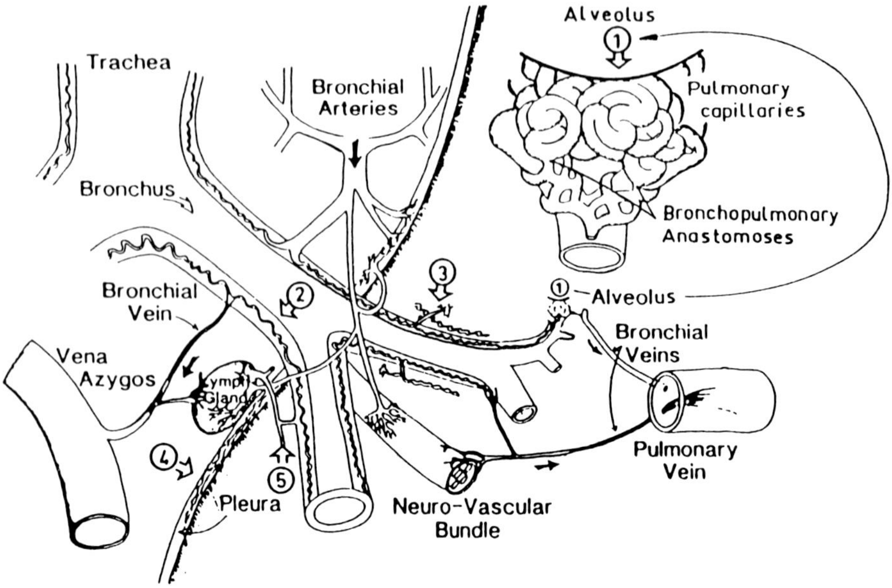

Figure 5 Bronchial circulation. Possible sites of absorption of edema fluid are labeled with numbers and arrows. (1) Alveolar airspace fluid, actively absorbed into the interstitial space and then into the pulmonary circulation by diffusion. (2) Bronchial airspace fluid, actively absorbed into the interstitium and then into the bronchial circulation. (3) Extraalveolar interstitial fluid cuffs, absorbed into the bronchial circulation (peribronchial plexus). (4) Pleural fluid, absorbed into the bronchial circulation (visceral pleural plexus) or into the parietal pleural lmmphatics. (5) Extraalveolar interstitial fluid cuffs, also absorbed into the lung lymphatics. (From Deffebach and Butler, 1989.)

pulmonary edema fluid can be suctioned from the lung by a catheter passed into the distal airways via the endotracheal tube, recent clinical studies indicate that only a small fraction of edema fluid leaves the lung by this route (Matthay et al., 1984; Matthay and Wiener-Kronish, 1990). Therefore, most alveolar edema must be transported across the epithelial barrier into the interstitium for the edema fluid to be removed from the lung by one of the five pathways available for removing interstitial edema fluid.

The first part of this section considers briefly the mechanisms that are important in removing edema fluid from the airspaces to the interstitium. The likely role of the various pathways for clearance of excess liquid and protein from the interstitial space of the lung is then considered.

It is important to emphasize that clearance of edema fluid involves the removal of both the liquid and the protein fractions. Our own studies have demonstrated that removal of edema fluid from the airspaces, experimentally or clinically, involves different mechanisms and pathways for removal of the liquid and the protein fractions of edema fluid (Matthay et al., 1982; 1985; Matthay and Wiener-Kronish, 1990). The primary mechanism driving alveolar liquid clearance is active ion (sodium) transport (Matthay et al., 1982, 1985; Mason et al., 1982; Goodman et al., 1983, Berthiaume et al., 1987).

In our work, the original clue that suggested active ion transport as a critical mechanism for alveolar liquid clearance was the experimental observation that alveolar protein concentration increased to levels well above plasma protein during the clearance of autologous serum from the airspaces of anesthetized sheep (Matthay et al., 1982) and then unanesthetized sheep (Table 3) (Matthay et al., 1985). This observation was subsequently confirmed by studies we completed in other species, including dogs (Berthiaume et al., 1988) and rabbits (Smedira, 1991). We found that 50–75% of the alveolar liquid clearance could be inhibited by amiloride, a sodium channel inhibitor, in sheep and in rabbits. Finally, we recently extended our experimental studies to humans and found that pulmonary edema fluid protein concentration rises to levels well above plasma protein concentration in the resolution of alveolar edema in humans (Matthay and Wiener-Kronish, 1990).

The transport of the protein fraction of edema fluid from the airspaces to the interstitium is the second major issue to be considered in addressing the mechanisms involved in clearance of edema fluid from airspaces of the lung.

Table 3 Alveolar Liquid Clearance in Sheep as Reflected by Progressive Concentration of Protein in the Airspaces of the Lung[a]

	Alveolar protein (g per 100 ml)		
Time (h)	Initial[b]	Final[c]	Lung liquid clearance[d] (% of instilled)
4	6.3 ±0.6	8.4 ±0.6	33.2
12	5.9 ±0.4	10.2 ±1.2	59.2
24	6.4 ±0.6	12.9 ±1.9	75.9

[a] Data shown as mean ±SD.

[b] The protein concentration of the instilled serum (3 ml/kg).

[c] The increase in concentration of protein in the airspaces can be used to estimate the alveolar liquid clearance by a simple proportion calculation since we know the instilled volume and the initial and final alveolar protein concentrations (Berthiaume et al., 1987).

[d] Calculated by the gravimetric method (Matthay et al., 1982).

Our early studies in sheep confirmed that clearance of protein from the airspaces proceeded much more slowly than alveolar liquid clearance (Matthay et al., 1982). Later studies in sheep documented that, after instilling 100 ml serum into the airspaces of one lower lobe in sheep, approximately 75% of the liquid volume was cleared from the lung, whereas only 25% of the protein fraction was removed (Matthay et al., 1985). Finally, a recent study in our laboratory established that removal of protein from the airspaces of unanesthetized sheep over 144 h proceeded at a monoexponential rate: for tracer [^{125}I]-albumin of 1.6%/h and for native protein of 0.9%/h (Berthiaume et al., 1989). Interestingly, alveolar macrophages did not play a major role in the clearance, and most of the [^{125}I]-albumin was recovered as an intact molecule in the plasma or lymph. The exact mechanisms responsible for protein transport across the epithelium are uncertain. Further studies are needed to determine how much of the protein clearance across the epithelium depends on diffusion versus transcytosis.

VI. Role of the Bronchial, Pulmonary, and Lymphatic Circulations in the Clearance of Interstitial Lung Edema

Once the liquid or protein fraction of edema fluid is transported across the epithelium to the interstitium, five pathways are available to remove the excess fluid and protein (Table 4).

For many years, it has been assumed that the lung lymphatic system was the primary route for removal of edema from the lung (Drinker and Hardenbergh, 1947; Courtice and Simmonds, 1949; Staub, 1974). Lung lymphatics are anatomically situated in a favorable location to remove excess liquid and protein that collects or is filtered into the alveolar and juxtaalveolar interstitium. When particles are deposited in the airspaces and cross into the interstitium, they primarily appear within lung lymphatics (Lauweryns and Baert, 1977). Until recently, however, there were virtually no quantitative data con-

Table 4 Five Anatomic Pathways for the Clearance of Pulmonary Edema from the Lung

1. Lung lymphatics
2. Pulmonary circulation
3. Bronchial circulation
4. Pleural space
5. Mediastinal space

cerning the fractional contribution of lung lymphatics to the removal of excess liquid and protein from the lung. Recent experimental studies have now provided valuable new information regarding the quantitative contribution of lung lymphatics to the resolution of pulmonary edema in both adult and newborn animals. In addition, the role of the pulmonary and bronchial circulations has been studied in a variety of these experiments, thus providing some important information on the role of these two circulations in the clearance of excess liquid and protein.

The contribution of the lymphatic circulation to the clearance of edema has been studied in different experimental settings. One group examined the clearance of interstitial pulmonary edema in dogs after saline infusions were given to increase left atrial pressure and to decrease plasma protein osmotic pressure (Gee and Spath, 1980). Lung lymph flow increased markedly; when the infusion was stopped and pulmonary vascular pressures returned to normal, however, lung lymph flow fell to near baseline levels within 1 h (Fig. 6). Morphological examination of the lungs removed at that time showed considerable interstitial pulmonary edema, even though lung lymph flow had returned to nearly normal levels. Thus, these investigators demonstrated that lung lymph flow was primarily sensitive to an elevation in microvascular pressure, not to the quantity of edema fluid present in the interstitium of the lung.

Recent experiments in our laboratory confirmed these findings in anesthetized sheep (Broaddus et al., 1990). Volume loading with saline that was designed to raise left atrial pressure to 20 cmH_2O above baseline levels resulted in a marked increase in lung lymph flow that returned to near baseline lymph flow within 1/2 h after the infusion was stopped and left atrial pressure had declined to normal levels, even though there was extensive interstitial edema. Even in the presence of severe increased permeability edema experimentally produced in sheep, lung lymph accounts for less than 50% of the removal of excess lung liquid after oleic acid-induced lung injury (Weiner-Kronish et al., 1988b).

Our own experimental work in anesthetized, ventilated sheep demonstrated that clearance of excess liquid from the interstitium of the lung does not depend primarily on lung lymphatics. When we instilled either 1.5 ml/kg of Ringer's lactate solution or ultrafiltered serum into the airspaces of one lung, there was no increase in lung lymph flow over a 4 h period, although approximatey 60% of the crystalloid solution and the ultrafiltered serum was removed from the lung during this time (Fig. 7) (Matthay et al., 1982). In addition, other investigators reported that lung lymphatics remove only 10% of the excess fetal lung liquid in lambs at the time of birth (Bland et al., 1982). When we instilled an autologous, isosmolar protein solution into the airspaces of the lung, there was an increase in lung lymph flow that averaged 1–2 ml/h above baseline after 100 ml liquid was instilled in the lung. This increase in

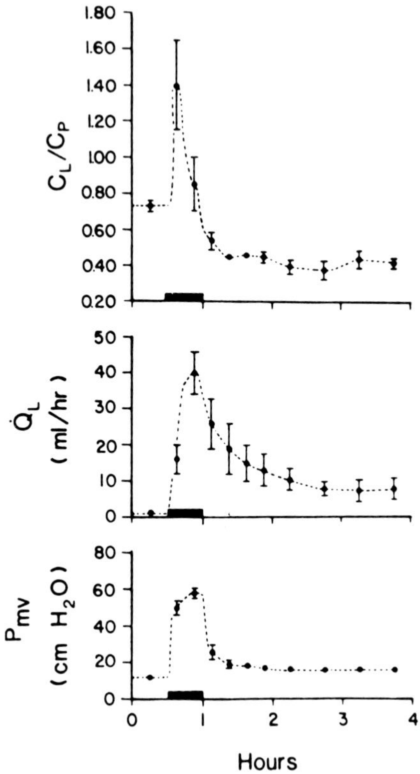

Figure 6 Effect of rapid intravenous fluid infusion on pulmonary microvascular pressure (P_{mv}), right duct lymph flow rate ($\dot{Q}_L$), and the protein concentration ratio in lymph (C_L) and plasma (C_P). The bars indicate the infusion period. Data shown are means ±SEM of measurements in seven dogs. Note that the lung lymph flow declined rapidly to near baseline levels after the fluid infusion was stopped, even though considerable interstitial pulmonary edema was present at that time. (From Gee and Spatts, 1980.)

lymph flow was not simply related to clearance of alveolar liquid, however, since we found that a protein solution causes a sustained increase in lymph flow over a 48 h period in sheep, well after the majority of alveolar liquid has been cleared from the interstitium of the lung (Berthiaume et al., 1989). In this same study, we also found that the lung lymphatics accounted for only 24 ±5% of the clearance of protein ([^{125}I]-albumin tracer) from the lung over a 48 h time period (Table 5).

What about the role of the pleural and mediastinal pathways? Recent experimental data trom our laboratory demonstrated that 20–25% of pul-

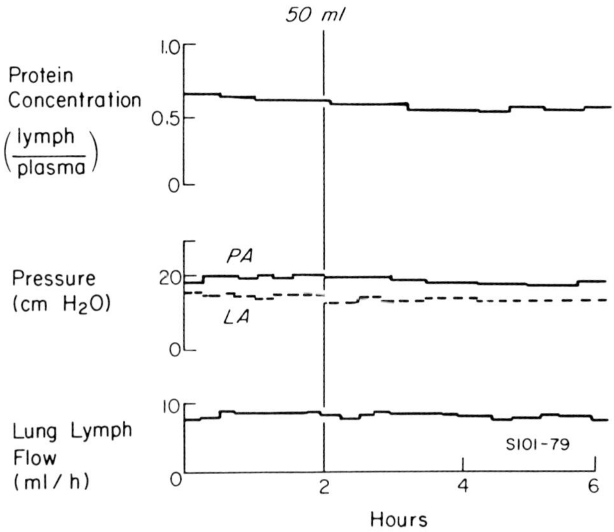

Figure 7 Time course of pulmonary vascular pressure, lung lymph and flow ratio of lymph/plasma protein concentration after 50 ml ultrafiltered serum was instilled into one lower lobe of an anesthetized sheep. During the 4 h time period, 60% of the liquid was removed as shown by gravimetric analysis but there was no increase in lung lymph flow. (From Matthay et al., 1982.)

monary edema fluid drains into the pleural space (Wiener-Kronish and Matthay, 1988; Broaddus et al., 1990). The contribution of the mediastinal pathway has not been well quantified, but there is preliminary evidence indicating that some edema fluid may be cleared from the lung by this route (Jerome et al., 1989).

What is the role of the pulmonary and bronchial circulations in the clearance of interstitial edema fluid? Data from other workers indicated that left atrial hypertension (11 cmH_2O above baseline levels) caused a slowing in the clearance of a crystalloid solution (6 ml/kg) instilled into the airspaces and lungs of newborn lambs compared to control animals with normal pulmonary vascular pressures (Raj and Bland, 1986). Interestingly, this slowdown in clearance was only apparent in the first 2 h; by 6 h, there was no difference in the clearance rate between the lambs with left atrial hypertension and the control animals with normal left atrial pressure (Fig. 8). Histologically, there was accumulation of liquid in the cuffs in the extraalveolar interstitum around peribronchial and perivascular loose connective tissue. It is possible that the catch-up in the liquid clearance of 6 h in the lambs with left atrial hypertension was related to the removal of excess lung liquid by pathways other than the

Table 5 Cumulative Protein Clearance in Lung Lymph[a]

Time (h)	Protein cleared from lung (% instilled)	Protein cleared by lymphatics (% instilled)	Fraction of protein cleared by lymphatics (% cleared)
24	28.5 ±5.2	6.9 ±2.3	24.2
48	38.9 ±9.7	11.5 ±4.3	29.6
96	70.1 ±15.8	14.2	20.3

[a] Data as mean ±SD.
Source: Berthiaume et al., 1989.

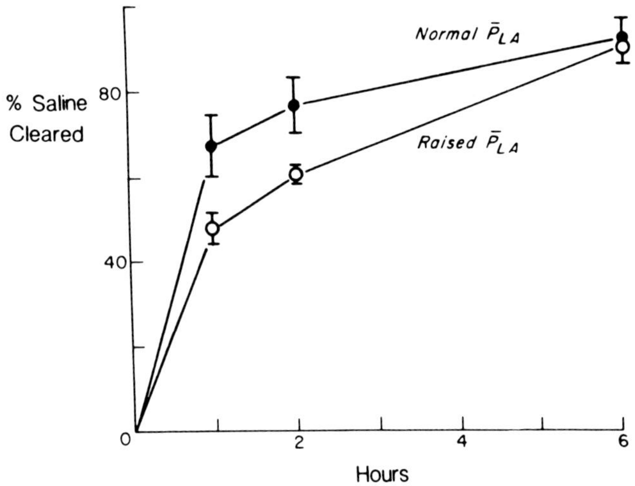

Figure 8 Estimated percentage clearance of the intratracheally instilled saline (6 ml/kg) in 10 lambs with raised left atrial pressure (open circles) and in 9 lambs with normal left atrial pressure (closed circles). Data points represent the mean ±SD. (From Raj and Bland, 1986.)

pulmonary circulation. Some of the liquid may have drained directly into the mediastinum or pleural space, and some may have been cleared into the bronchial veins (site 3 in Fig. 5). Thus, in the presence of left atrial hypertension, with normal central venous pressure, clearance into the bronchial veins may be an alternative route for the clearance of the excess liquid that accumulates in the extraalveolar interstitium.

In our own studies of the resolution of excess alveolar interstitial liquid, changes in pulmonary blood flow have been quantified to determine the influence of pulmonary blood flow on the clearance of excess liquid from the airspaces and interstitium of the lung. After instillation of 100 ml autologous serum into the airspaces of one lower lobe, approximately one-third of the liquid was removed over 4 h (Matthay et al., 1982; Berthiaume et al., 1987). A change in pulmonary blood flow between 20 and 100% of baseline levels did not alter the rate of alveolar and interstitial lung liquid clearance over 4 h in thes studies (Berthiaume et al., 1987).

In a more recent study, we discovered that eliminating pulmonary blood flow altogether does not reduce interstitial liquid clearance in sheep (Jayr and Matthay, 1991). The left pulmonary artery was occluded for 4 or 24 h before instilling 100 ml autologous serum into the left lower lobe. Hemodynamics and lung lymph flow were then measured for 4 h, and the lungs were removed and excess lung water measured gravimetrically. In fact, the residual bronchopulmonary anastomatic flow after pulmonary artery occlusion was 40 ml/min, which was sufficient to maintain normal alveolar epithelial ion transport (alveolar liquid clearance), as well as to remove the excess liquid from the interstitium (Table 6). Lung lymph flow increased and accounted for approximately 35% of the liquid clearance, but the majority of the clearance must have been via the bronchial circulation through bronchopulmonary anastomatic flow (Fig. 5).

These recent experimental data provide excellent evidence for the ability of the bronchial circulation to maintain normal alveolar epithelial function in the absence of pulmonary blood flow. Obviously, there are important implications for the role of the bronchial circulation in pathological conditions in which pulmonary blood flow is markedly reduced or absent. Furthermore, this study demonstrates the capacity of the bronchial circulation to substitute for the pulmonary circulation, at least under the conditions of these experiments.

VII. Summary

An isolated elevation of pressure in the systemic venous system that reduces bronchial systemic venous drainage does not lead to pulmonary edema. However, the presence of an elevated systemic venous pressure in the presence of either hydrostatic or increased permeability edema does increase the degree of

Table 6 Effect of Eliminating Pulmonary Blood Flow (for 4 or 24 h) on Alveolar and Interstitial Liquid Clearance over 4 h in Anesthetized Sheep[a]

Condition	No.	Alveolar protein (g per 100 ml)[b]		Lung liquid[c] cleared (% of instilled)
		Instilled	Final	
Control Sheep	7	6.4 ±0.4	8.4 ±1.1	26.4 ±7.1
PA Occlusion-4h	7	5.9 ±0.5	7.9 ±1.2	27.1 ±3.8
PA OCclusion-24h	3	5.9 ±0.2	7.7 ±0.6	25.6 ±4.6

[a] Data as mean ±SD; PA, pulmonary artery.

[b] Autologous serum (3 ml/kg) was instilled into one lower lobe; then 4 h later a final alveolar protein sample was obtained from the distal airspaces when the lungs were removed. Since the difference between the initial and final alveolar protein concentrations is similar, these data indicate that the quantity of alveolar liquid removed from the airspaces was similar with and without pulmonary blood flow.

[c] The percentage of the 3 ml/kg of serum instilled that was cleared over 4 h was determined by gravimetric methods.

pulmonary edema. The mechanism for this effect is related to decreased reabsorption of edema fluid around airways, increased fluid flux from the lobar and segmental bronchial veins, and/or decreased lymphatic clearance from the lung because of the elevated systemic venous pressures. In the setting of chronic left atrial and systemic venous hypertension, several adaptations may occur that limit the magnitude of the pulmonary edema that develops. The role of the bronchial circulation in increased permeability edema needs further study, but some evidence has demonstrated an important contribution of the bronchial circulation in acute aspiration or inhaled lung injury.

Pleural effusions occur in both hydrostatic and increased permeability edema; most of the pleural fluid originates from the lung edema, although elevated systemic venous pressures can delay the removal of the pleural fluid by the parietal pleural lymphatics.

The clearance of the excess liquid and protein in the lung following either hydrostatic or increased permeability edema was investigated in several recent studies. Interestingly, lung lymphatics play a minor role in the clearance of the edema fluid. The pulmonary circulation appears to be the primary pathway for the removal of excess liquid and protein, but in the absence of pulmonary blood flow, the bronchopulmonary anastomatic flow removes over 50% of the excess liquid and protein. Also, the bronchial blood flow is adequate to nourish and maintain normal alveolar epithelial function in the absence of pulmonary blood flow. In addition, there is circumstantial evidence that the bronchial circulation, which drains to the right side of the heart, is an important pathway for the removal of edema fluid in the extraalveolar compartment.

Future research efforts need to be targeted to the role of the bronchial circulation in the development of increased permeability edema following inhalational injuries, gastric aspiration, and bronchopneumonia in which the conducting airways are involved. Also, more work should be done on the supportive role of the bronchial circulation in the presence of acute lung injury, especially after major reductions in pulmonary blood flow.

Acknowledgment

I thank Sanja Djukic for her invaluable assistance in the preparation of this manuscript. This work was supported in part by NIH Grants HL19155 and HL25816.

References

Aberle, D. R., Wiener-Kronish, J. P., Webb, W. R., and Matthay, M. A. (1988). Diagnosis of hydrostatic versus increased permeability pulmonary edema on the basis of chest radiographic criteria in critically ill patients. *Radiology* **168**:73–79.

Agostoni, P. G., Deffebach, M. E., Kirk, W., Lakshminarayan, S., and Butler, J. (1987). Upstream pressure for systemic to pulmonary flow from bronchial circulation in dogs. *J. Appl. Physiol.* **63**:485–491.

Allen, S. J., Drake, R. E., Katz, J., Gabel, J. C., and Saine, G. A. (1987). Elevation of superior vena caval pressure increases extravascular lung water after endotoxemia. *J. Appl. Physiol.* **62**:1006–1009.

Allen, S. J., Laine, G. A., Drake, R. E., and Gabel, J. C. (1988). Superior vena caval pressure elevation causes pleural effusion formation in sheep. *Am. J. Physiol.* **255**:H492–H495.

Allen, S. J., Drake, R., and Gabel, J. (1989). Left atrial hypertension causes pleural effusion formation in unanesthetized sheep. *Am. J. Physiol.* **257**:H690–H692.

Ando, F., Arakawa, M., Kambara, K., Miyazaki, H., Segara, T., and Hirakawa, S. (1990). Effect of superior vena caval hypertension on alloxan-induced lung injury in dogs. *J. Appl. Physiol.* **68**:478–483.

Bassadre, J. P., Sugi, K., Traber, D. C., Niehaus, G. D., and Herndon, D. N. (1988). The effect of leukocyte depletion on smoke inhalational injury in sheep. *Surgery* **104**:208–215.

Berthiaume, Y., Staub, N. C., and Matthay, M. A. (1987). Beta-adrenergic agonists increase lung liquid clearance in anesthetized sheep. *J. Clin. Invest.* **79**:335–343.

Berthiaume, Y., Broaddus, V. C., Gropper, M. A., Tanita, T., and Matthay, M. A. (1988). Alveolar liquid and protein clearance from normal dog lungs. *J. Appl. Physiol.* **65**:585–593.

Berthiaume, Y., Albertine, K. H., Grady, M., Fick, G., and Matthay, M. A. (1989). Protein clearance form the air spaces of unanesthetized sheep over 144 hours. *J. Appl. Physiol.* **67**:1887–1897.

Bland, R. D., Hansen, T. N., Haberken, C. M., and Bressack, M. (1982). Lung fluid balance in lambs before and after birth. *J. Appl. Physiol.* **53**:992–1004.

Broaddus, V. C., Wiener-Kronish, J. P., Berthiaume, Y., and Staub, N. C. (1988). Removal of pleural liquid and protein by lymphatics in awake sheep. *J. Appl. Physiol.* **64**:384–390.

Broaddus, V. C., Wiener-Kronish, J. P., and Staub, N. C. (1990). Clearance of lung edema into the pleural space in anesthetized sheep. *J. Appl. Physiol.* **68**:2623–2630.

Bruner, H. D., and Schmidt, C. F. (1947). Blood flow in the bronchial artery of the anesthetized dog. *Am. J. Physiol.* **148**:648–653.

Charan, N. B., Turk, G. M., and Dhand, R. (1984). Gross and subgross anatomy of bronchial circulation in sheep. *J. Appl. Physiol.* **57**:658–664.

Charan, N. B., Turk, G. M. and Hey, D. H. (1985). Effect of increased bronchial venous pressure on lung lymph flow. *J. Appl. Physiol.* **59**:1249–1253.

Cole, W. R., Witte, M. H., Kash, S. L., Rodger, M., Bleisch, V. R., and Muelheims, G. H. (1967). Thoracic duct-to-pulmonary vein shunt in the treatment of experimental right heart failure. *Circulation* **36**:539–543.

Courtice, F. C., and Simmonds, W. J. (1949). Absorption from the lungs. *J. Physiol. (Lond.)* **109**:103–116.

Dash, H., Lipton, M. J., Chatterjee, K., and Parmley, W. W. (1980). Estimation of pulmonary arterial wedge pressure from the chest radiograph in patients with chronic congestive cardiopulmonary and ischemic cardiomyopathy. *Br. Heart J.* **44**:322–329.

Deffebach, M. E., and Butler, J. (1989). Bronchial circulation and lung edema. In *Lung Biology in Health and Disease* Vol. 42. Edited by B. M. Sharf and S. S. Cassidy. *Marcel* New York, Dekker.

Drinker, C. R., and Hardenbergh, E. (1947). Absorption from the pulmonary alveoli. *J. Exp. Med.* **86**:7–18.

Gee, M. H., and Spath, Jr., J. A. (1980). The dynamics of the lung fluid filtration system in dogs with edema. *Circ. Res.* **46**:796–801.

Goodman, B. E., Fleisher, R. S., and Crandall, E. D. (1983). Evidence for active sodium transport by cultured monolayers of pulmonary alveolar epithelial cells. *Am. J. Physiol.* **245**:C78–C83.

Hutchinson, A. A., Bernard, G. R., Snapper, J. R., and Brigham, K. L. (1984). Effect of aerosol histamine on lung lymph flow in awake sheep. *J. Appl. Physiol.* **56**:1090–1098.

Jayr, C., and Matthay, M. A. (1991). Alveolar and lung liquid clearance in the absence of pulmonary blood flow. *J. Appl. Physiol.* **71**:in press.

Jerome, H., Broaddus, V. C., Arakawa, M., Osorio, O., Neuberger, M., and Staub, N. C. (1989). Evidence for mediastinal clearance of interstitial pulmonary edema. *FASEB J.* **3**:8374A.

Kowalski, T. F., Doershuk, C. M., Lakshmi, S., English, D., and Butler, J. (1989). The bronchial circulation in neutrophil delivery to streptococcal pneumonia in rabbits. *FASEB J.* **3**:A567.

Laine, G. A., Allen, S. J., Katz, J., Gabel, J. C., and Drake, R. E. (1986). Effect of systemic venous pressure elevation on lymph flow and lung edema formation. *J. Appl. Physiol.* **61**:1638.

Lakshminarayan, S., Kowalski, T. F., Kirk, W., and Butler, J. (1991). The effect of bronchial venous pressure on pulmonary edema in the dog. In press.

Lauweryns, J. M., and Baert, J. H. (1977). Alveolar clearance and the role of the pulmonary lymphatics. *Am. Rev. Respir. Dis.* **115**:625–683.

Magno, M., and Szidon, J. P. (1976). Hemodynamic pulmonary edema in dogs with acute and chronic lymphatic ligation. *Am. J. Physiol.* **231**:1772–1782.

Maron, M. B. (1982). Differential effects of histamine on protein permeability in dog lung and forelimb. *Am. J. Physiol.* **242**:H565–H572.

Mason, R. J., William, M. C., Widdicombe, J. H., Sanders, M. J., Misfeldt, D. S., and Berry, L. C. (1982). Transepithelial transport by pulmonary alveolar type II cells in primary culture. *Proc. Natl. Acad. Sci. U. S. A.* **79**:6033–6037.

Matthay, M. A., Landolt, C., and Staub, N. C. (1982). Differential liquid and protein clearance from the alveoli of anesthetized sheep. *J. Appl. Physiol.* **53**:96–104.

Matthay, M. A., Eschenbacher, W. L., and Goetzl, E. (1984). Elevated concentration of leukotriene D_4 in the pulmonary edema fluid of patients with the adult respiratory distress syndrome. *J. Clin. Immunol.* **4**:479–483.

Matthay, M. A., Berthiaume, Y., and Staub, N. C. (1985). Long-term clearance of liquid and protein from the lungs of anesthetized sheep. *J. Appl. Physiol.* **59**:928–934.

Matthay, M. A., and Wiener-Kronish, J. P. (1990). Intact epithelial barrier function is critical for the resolution of alveolar edema in man. *Am. Rev. Respir. Dis.* **142**:1250–1257.

Mellins, R. B., Levine, D. R., and Fishman, A. P. (1970). Effect of systemic and pulmonary venous hypertension on pleural and pericardial fluid accumulation. *J. Appl. Physiol.* **29**:564–569.

Miller, W. C., Wimi, W. W., and Rice, D. L. (1978). Contribution of systemic venous hypertension to the development of pulmonary edema in dogs. *Circ. Res.* **43**:598–600.

Murray, J. F. (1986). *The Normal Lung* 2nd ed. Philadelphia; W. B. Saunders, p. 42.

Nakahara, K., Ohkuda, K., and Staub, N. C. (1979). Effect of infusing histamine into the pulmonary or bronchial artery on sheep pulmonary fluid balance. *Am. Rev. Respir. Dis.* **120**:875–882.

Ohkuda, K., Nakahara, K., Binder, A., and Staub, N. C. (1981). Venous air emboli in sheep: Reversible increase in lung microvascular permeability. *J. Appl. Physiol.* **51**:887–894.

Paré, P. D., Brooks, L. A., and Baile, E. M. (1981). Effect of systemic venous hypertension on pulmonary function and lung water. *J. Appl. Physiol.* **51**:592–597.

Pietra, G. G., and Magno, M. G. (1978). Pharmacological factors influencing permeability of the bronchial circulation. *Fed. Proc.* **37**:2466–2470.

Pietra, G. G., Szidon, J. P., Leventhal, M.M., and Fishman, A. P. (1971).

Histamine and interstitial pulmonary edema in the dog. *Circ. Res.* **29**:323–337.

Pietra, G. G., Szidon, J. P., Carpenter, H. A., and Fishman, A. P. (1974). Bronchial venular leakage during endotoxin shock. *Am. J. Pathol.* **77**:387–406.

Raj, U. J., and Bland, R. D. (1986). Lung luminal liquid clearance in newborn lambs. *Am. Rev. Respir. Dis.* **134**:305–310.

Rippe, B., Allison, R. C., Parker, J. C., and Taylor, A. E. (1984). Effects of histamine, serotonin and norepinephrine on circulation of dog lungs. *J. Appl. Physiol.* **57**:223–232.

Smedira, N., Gates, L., Hastings, R., Jayr, C., Sakuma, T., Pittet, J. F., and Matthay, M. A. (1991). Alveolar liquid clearance in anesthetized rabbits. *J. Appl. Physiol.* **70**:1827–1835.

Staub, N. C. (1974). Pulmonary edema. *Physiol. Rev.* **54**:678–811.

Turino, G. M., Edelman, N. H., Senior, R. M., Richards, E. C., and Fishman, A. P. (1968). Extravascular lung water in cor pulmonale. *Bull. Physiol-Pathol-Respir.* **4**:47–64.

Wegria, R., Zehert, H., Walter, K. E., Entrup, R. W., Schyrver, C. D., Kennedy, W., and Paiewonsky, D. (1963). Effect of systemic venous pressure on drainage of lymph flow from thoracic duct. *Am. J. Physiol.* **204**:284–288.

Wiener-Kronish, J. P., Matthay, M. A., Callen, P. W., Filly, R. A., Gamsu, G., and Staub, N. C. (1985). Relationship of pulmonary hemodynamics to pleural effusions in patients with heart failure. *Am. Rev. Respir. Dis.* **32**:1253–1257.

Wiener-Kronish, J. P., Goldstein, R., Matthay, R., Biondi, J. W., Broaddus, V. C., Chatterjee, K., and Matthay, M. A. (1987). Lack of association of pleural effusions with chronic pulmonary and right atrial hypertension. *Chest* **92**:967–970.

Wiener-Kronish, J. P., and Matthay, M. A. (1988a). Pleural effusions associated with hydrostatic and increased permeability pulmonary edema. *Chest* **93**:852–858.

Wiener-Kronish, J. P., Broaddus, V. C., Albertine, K., Gropper, M. A., Matthay, M. A., and Staub, N. C. (1988b). The relationship of pleural effusions to increased permeability pulmonary edema in anesthetized sheep. *J. Clin. Invest.* **82**:1422–1429.

13

Airway Gas Exchange

MICHAEL P. HLASTALA and ERIK R. SWENSON

University of Washington School of Medicine
Seattle, Washington

I. Introduction

The conventional approach to the analysis of pulmonary ventilation deals with the airways as a dead space that participates in no gas exchange and acts simply as a conduit for the passage of air between the outside environment and the alveoli. In reality, however, inspired air undergoes some change during its trans-airway passage. The relatively cool and dry air is heated and humidified, a process that is most important since it protects the delicate lower airway epithelium from thermal and desiccation injuries. During inspiration, relatively dry and cool air passes through the nasal cavity (or mouth) and pharynx and into the airways. After moving into the airways of the lung, the air encounters a branching network of airways with progressively narrower diameters. The increasing total cross-sectional area of all the airways of a succeeding generation results in a lower linear velocity of convective movement. Along the way the airway surface is lined with a moist mucous layer with which air exchanges water, heat, and soluble gases. This airway exchange process would eventually cool and deplete the mucosa of water if it were not for the existence of the bronchial circulation.

Ventilating air exchanges gases with the airway surface during both inspiration and expiration. If soluble gases are present in either the inspirate or the expirate, they dissolve in the airway mucosa. The amount dissolved depends on the gas solubility as well as mass transport-limiting factors. A greater solubility implies a greater interaction with the airways. The bronchial circulation also plays a role in this airway gas-exchange process. Because this book deals with the bronchial circulation, this chapter focuses on the exchanges that occur within the airways. Research dealing with exchange within the mouth or nasal cavity (which are not perfused by the bronchial circulation) is not included.

II. Airway Exchange

Progressing into the airways, bifurcation occurs more and more frequently, so the air encounters narrower and shorter airways while moving toward the alveoli. The increased cross-sectional area results in a slower convective velocity and hence a greater time for interaction with the surface. In addition, the smaller airways have a greater surface-to-volume ratio, and the mean distance from the gas to the airway surface decreases, increasing the surface interaction. Airway wall tissue contains a rich supply of blood vessels from the bronchial circulation, as well as lymph vessels and nerves. Mucous glands supply the mucus that lines the airways. Ciliated epithelial cells line the airway surface and continually move the mucus toward the pharynx.

A general representation of airway gas exchange is shown in schematic form in Fig. 1. Air moves through the airway by a combination of convection and diffusion. The relative contribution of each depends on the position within the airway tree, convection being dominant in the large airways and diffusion in the small airways. At any point in the airways, air can exchange gas, heat, and water with the mucous layer lining the airway. The mucus then exchanges with the surrounding tissue. The tissues encountered during the outward movement are initially epithelium followed by perfused tissue and/or cartilage. Gases or heat eventually diffuse to the blood vessels and are carried away (or delivered) by the bronchial blood flow or by the bronchial and pulmonary blood flow from the intrapulmonary airways. The relative balance among these processes depends on the location (generation number) within the airways and the breathing conditions.

A complete discussion of the heating and humidification of the inspirate can be found in Chap. 9. If any soluble gas is present in the inspired air, some dissolves in the mucosa. The distance of penetration into the airway tree before complete loss of the soluble gas depends on the gas solubility β. A

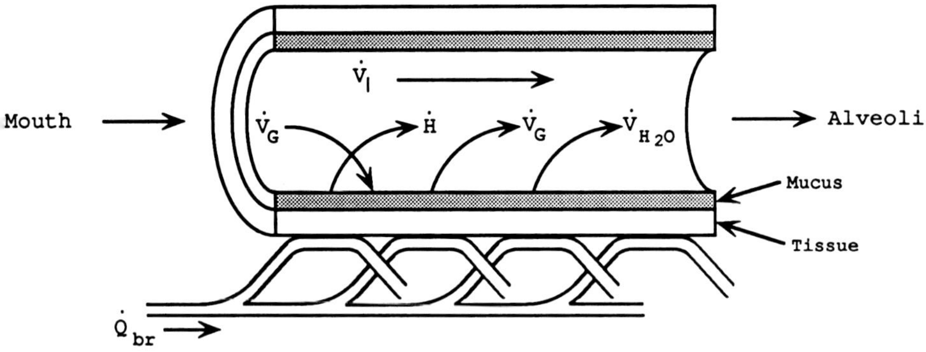

Figure 1 The heat-, water-, and gas-exchange processes in the airways. Curved arrows show the exchange directions during inspiration. $\dot{V}_I$, Inspired flow rate; $\dot{Q}_{br}$, bronchial blood flow rate; H, $\dot{V}_G$, and $\dot{V}_{H_2O}$, fluxes of heat, gas, and water, respectively.

greater fraction of higher solubility gas is absorbed by the airway tissue earlier in the passage from the mouth to the alveoli. If soluble gas is absent from the inspired air but present in the mucus (for example, soluble gases eliminated by the lungs and deposited on the airway mucosa by the previous exhalation), the gas desorbs and is added to the inspired gas. This latter process is identical to the heating and humidification of the inspired air.

An interesting aspect of both heat and gas exchange in the airway is their interaction. This is one of the factors that differentiates airway gas exchange from the constant-temperature alveolar gas exchange. A decrease in mucosal temperature increases inert gas solubility (Henry's law; see subsequent discussion), which increases inert gas absorption (or decreases gas exchange toward the gas phase). Ventilation causes the airways to be progressively cooler toward the mouth. Also, during inspiration, the heating and humidification of inspired air result in cooling of the mucosa. During each expiration, the opposite occurs as the mucosa is warmed, decreasing inert gas solubility and increasing gas loading into the expirate.

Exhaled air is cooled and dehumidified as the warm, moist, exhaled alveolar air passes through the cooler, larger airways. Because the vapor pressure of water over a cold liquid is less than over a warm liquid, some water condenses onto the mucous surface as the air cools. Any soluble gas from the alveoli present in the exhaled air interacts with the mucosa. Under normal circumstances, mouth-exhaled air is cooler and has lower soluble gas and water contents than air leaving the alveoli.

A. Modeling

Mathematical modeling of the respiratory system necessarily requires simplification. The purpose is not to reproduce the real system in detail but to include the main aspects of the real system that influence the processes of interest. A model is essentially a bookkeeping system designed to organize one's understanding of the system and allow numerical estimation of a particular process. Two alternative approaches have been used to model heat, water, and soluble gas transport in the human airways: detailed continuity and energy balance equations (Davidson and Schroter, 1983; Saidel et al., 1983; Gard et al., 1984), and control volume analysis (Hanna and Scherer, 1986; Ingenito et al., 1986; Tsu et al., 1988). The control volume analysis has several advantages: detailed knowledge of the velocity flow field is not required; complicated geometries are more easily handled; semi-empirical expressions for the rates of heat and mass transport can be used; and greater detail can be incorporated into later versions of the model.

The absorption of a gaseous solute by the respiratory tract involves entry of the solute into some or all of the tissue. For a simple solution of one solute in one solvent, there is a unique relation between the concentration of solute and its pressure within the solution. For inert gases, the partial pressure of each solute is uniquely related to its concentration (Henry's law):

$$P_X = \beta_X C_X \tag{1}$$

where P_X is the partial pressure of inert gas X, β_X is the capacitance coefficient (Piiper et al., 1971) of gas X, and C_X is the content of gas X. The relative degree of interaction depends on the solubility (or partition coefficient). Solubility data (expressed as an Ostwald partition coefficient) for a partial list of high solubility gases are presented in Table 1. In most cases blood solubility is listed. In some cases, however, blood solubility is not available, in which case water solubility is listed.

Inspired soluble gases eventually diffuse beyond the respiratory mucosa and enter the bronchial vasculature. With some gases, the transport from mucus or alveolar lining to other fluid compartments is great; for others, the transport is small and only the alveolar compartment need be considered. The effect of these secondary compartments on the apparent equilibrium depends on the solubility, inspired concentration, and reactivity of the gas, so that each set of conditions must be evaluated separately.

An example of a cylindrical control volume approach is shown in Fig. 2 for an airway with radius R positioned axially at a distance z from the airway entrance. The airway is radially divided into three regions: the airway lumen, a thin mucous layer of thickness ΔR_1 coating the airway wall and an underlying nonperfused tissue layer of thickness ΔR_2. A capillary bed lies beyond the nonperfused tissue layer and has an assumed temperature profile $T_c(z)$ and

Table 1 Soluble Gases[a]

Gas	λ water	Temperature (°C)	λ blood	Temperature (°C)	Reference
Halothane			3	37	Young and Wagner, 1979
Chlorine	4	30			Morgan and Frank, 1977
Benzene			8	37	Sato and Nakajima, 1979
Trichloroethylene			9	37	Åstrand and Övrum, 1976
Diethyl ether			11	37	Young and Wagner, 1979
Toluene			16	37	Sato and Nakajima, 1979
Xylene			31	37	Ogata and Tomokuni, 1970
Sulfur dioxide	36	30			Morgan and Frank, 1977
Styrene			52	37	Sato and Nakajima, 1979
Ethyl acetate			75	37	Schrikker et al., 1989
Acetaldehyde	79	25			Morgan and Frank, 1977
Methyl ethyl ketone			200	37	Sato and Nakajima, 1979
Formaldehyde	316	25			Morgan and Frank, 1977
Acetone			330	37	Young and Wagner, 1979
Butyl alcohol			1200	37	Åstrand et al., 1976
Ethyl alcohol			1756	37	Jones, 1983b
Phenol	3115	25			Morgan and Frank, 1977
Acetic acid			20,000	37	Schrikker et al., 1989
HCl	2,800,000	25			Morgan and Frank, 1977

[a] λ is the Ostwald partition coefficient (dimensionless).

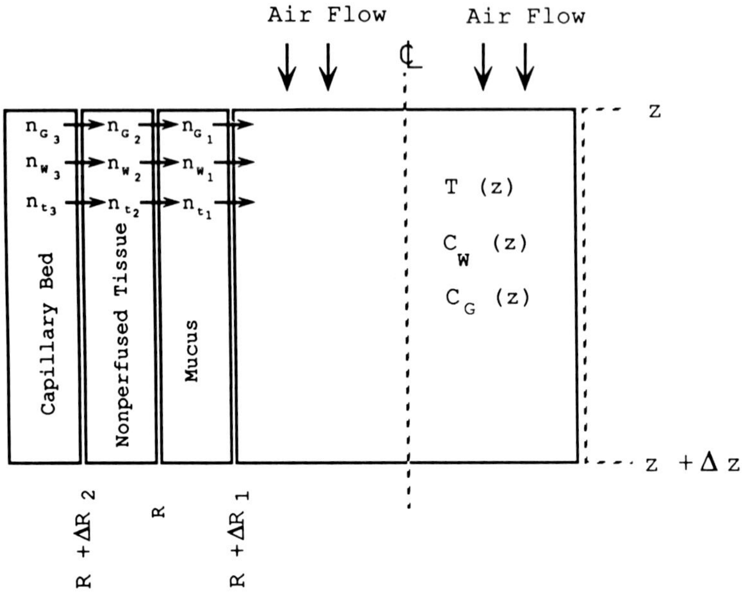

Figure 2 The control volume used in the modeling of exchange in the airway. The temperature and concentration variables shown represent bulk-average values for each region: airway lumen, mucus, and nonperfused tissue layer. T, C_W, and C_G are temperature and concentrations of water and gas, respectively, in the control volume gas phase; n_g, n_w, and n_t are the fluxes of gas, water, and heat, respectively. Z is axial position, and R is the control volume radius. ΔR_1 and ΔR_2 are the mucus and nonperfused tissue thicknesses, respectively.

soluble gas partial pressure $P_g(z)$. The variable describing temperature and concentration in each regions are bulk-average values for the entire regions. The gas in the airway is treated as a ternary system of dry air, water vapor, and one soluble gas and is assumed to behave in an ideal manner. Heat and mass-transfer coefficients are used to calculate the exchange rates of heat ($\dot{Q}_{sens}$, sensible heat flux) and mass ($\dot{V}_i$) between the mucosal surface and gas in the airway. From the known geometry of an airway in each generation, the heat, water, and soluble gas transfer can be calculated.

The control volume approach allows the prediction of heat, water, and soluble gas exchange with the airways during tidal ventilation. The heat-exchange and the mass-exchange processes are highly analogous. Not only do heat, water, and gas exchange occur simultaneously, but they also interact. Heating and cooling of the airway surface and mucous lining affect both evaporative water and soluble gas exchange by virtue of the temperature-dependent change in solubility of the gas in the airway tissue. Water evaporation provides a major source of heat exchange. With model parameters giving the best fit to experimental data, the model shows: (1) substantial heat recovery in the upper airways on exhalation, (2) overall respiratory heat and water loss to the environment, (3) low average mucous temperatures, and (4) significant inspiration to expiration change in mucous thickness. Warming of air continues through the generations of the airway tree all the way to the terminal bronchioles. Figure 3 shows that predictions from this control volume approach (Tsu et al., 1988) match very well experimental data from McFadden et al. (1985). With increased ventilation the warming of air shifts more distally into the airways as the mean temperature decreases at any axial position in the airway tree.

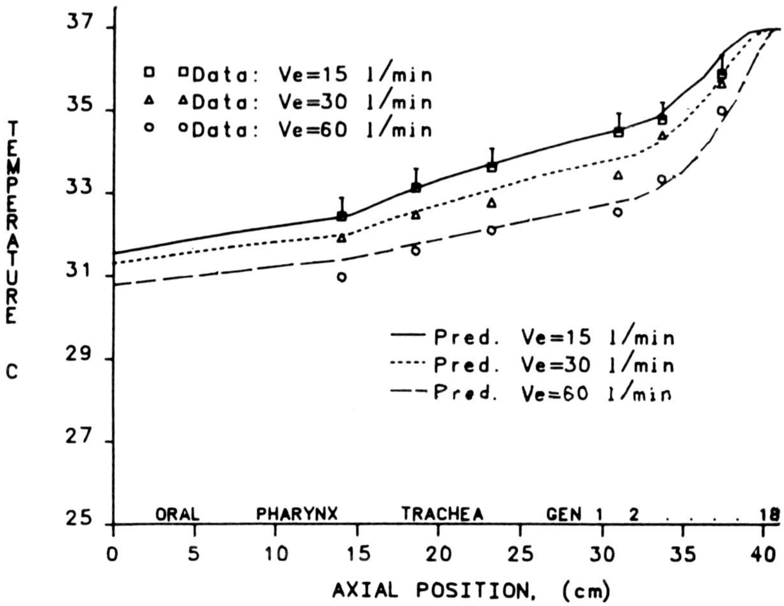

Figure 3 Comparion of simulated mean airway temperature with experimental data from McFadden et al. (1985). Data are shown for ventilations of 15, 30, and 60 L/min. (Reprinted with permission from the *Annals of Biomedical Engineering*; Volume 16; M. E. Tsu, A. L. Babb, D. D. Ralph, and M. P. Hlastala, Dynamics of heat, water, and soluble gas exchange in the human airways. I. A model study. Copyright 1988 by Pergaman Press, Inc.)

B. Surface Exchange

The interaction of soluble gases with the airways has been recognized for quite a long time. An early study of soluble gas exchange by Cander and Forster (1959) demonstrated unusually high end-tidal concentrations of ether and acetone during washin of these gases. These authors concluded that soluble gases dissolved in the respiratory dead space tissue during inspiration and revaporized during expiration. A similar conclusion was reached by Wigaeus et al. (1981) in their studies of the uptake and elimination of acetone. The relative uptake of inspired inert gas by the airways depends on the tissue solubility and inspired flow rate (Yokoyama and Frank, 1972; Aharonson et al., 1974; Davies, 1985). In addition, SO_2 is highly reactive and its airway absorption is dependent on concentration (Frank et al., 1969). Absorption through the respiratory tract of solvents, such as toluene (Carlson and Lindquist, 1977), trichloroethylene (Åstrand and Övrum, 1976), butyl alcohol (Åstrand et al., 1976), and xylene (Åstrand et al., 1978), can be substantial in the work environment.

A more detailed evaluation of these interaction phenomena was carried out by Schrikker et al. (1985, 1989). These authors performed short duration washin and washout experiments with the soluble gases diethyl ether ($\lambda \cong 13$), ethyl acetate ($\lambda \cong 75$), and acetone ($\lambda \cong 340$). The excretion (P_E/P_V) values for acetone were lowest of the three, an observation that is inconsistent with simple alveolar gas exchange from parallel compartments (Farhi, 1967). Analysis of the gas tension at the mouth during a single exhalation shows that, for acetone, the volume of gas expired before the beginning of phase II (the rapid rise phase of the exhaled inert gas partial pressure profile), a volume considered to represent anatomic dead space, is considerably smaller than that found for ether. This observation is consistent with airway solution of the more soluble gas, acetone. In their second study (Schrikker et al., 1989), a washin method was used to quantitate the excretion values for four soluble gases: ethyl acetate ($\lambda \cong 75$), acetone ($\lambda \cong 340$), ethyl alcohol ($\lambda \cong 2000$), and acetic acid ($\lambda \cong 20{,}000$). Using even more soluble gases than in the earlier study, it was shown that the excretion values were lower for the more soluble gases, an observation consistent with a substantial interaction of respired gas with the airway epithelial tissue. During inhalation, the gases evaporate from the airway surface and are inspired. During exhalation, the soluble gases are lost from the exhalate onto the airway surface. The relative elimination of the gas is thus decreased because of this airway interaction.

In another paper from the same group, Zwart et al. (1986) expressed concern about some experimental observations (Dueck et al., 1980) of acetone excretion values that were lower than the simultaneous ether excretion values. To explain this, Zwart constructed a mathematical model to account for airway mucosal solution of the inert gas. With tidal breathing, lower excretion values were calculated for the high-solubility gas, acetone, than expected from extrapolation of the excretion measurements of other lower solubility gases. This observation supports the contention that the solution of inert gas in the wall of the airway results in a lower than expected elimination and greater effective dead space for the inert gas, an effect that depends directly on the gas solubility. Similar findings were reported by Guenard et al. (1985). This high-solubility gas-airway interaction has important implications regarding the use of the multiple inert gas elimination technique (MIGET) (Wagner et al., 1974), which analyzes acetone elimination during tidal breathing. As a practical note, it is worth emphasizing that unexpectedly low acetone excretion values are seen only occasionally. However, Zwart points out that only a few of the MIGET publications show raw data and suggests that the significance of the airway interaction is minimized in the curve-fitting approach used in dealing with MIGET data.

C. Soluble Inert Gas Exchange

Often the study of $\dot{V}_A/\dot{Q}$ distribution with the multiple inert gas elimination technique is complicated by the finding of unexpectedly high or low excretion values of soluble inert gases during exercise or other conditions associated with large minute ventilations, such as high-frequency ventilation. These results, which can vary a great deal from individual to individual, may well be related to interactions between airway cooling, airway drying, and changes in bronchial blood flow. Highly soluble gases interact with the airway mucosa during inhalation and exhalation, causing an alteration in the elimination properties of these gases. Some authors (DeVries et al., 1982; Schrikker et al., 1985; Zwart et al., 1986) have concluded that interaction of the highly soluble gases (ether and acetone) with the airways explains their low excretion values. An implication of this interaction with the airways is that consideration of parallel alveolar compartments is inappropriate when interpreting MIGET data because of the influence of the large series compartment of the airway tissue on the soluble gas elimination.

The airways are thought to have a particularly important influence on the exchange of soluble inert gas during high-frequency ventilation (HFV). An explanation of this phenomenon incorporates the interaction of the mucosal liquid with the high degree of airway mixing (McEvoy et al., 1982). Tracheal temperature during HFV can be 3–5°C above body temperature (Robertson et al., 1982). The gradual heating of the airways, due to viscous energy dissipation, during HFV could cause a transient elevation in exhaled soluble gas as the increasing mucosal temperature and, thus, decreasing mucosal inert gas solubility drives off previously dissolved soluble gas into the air.

D. Alcohol

Ethyl alcohol is the highest solubility gas ($\lambda \sim 1756$ at 37°C), studied in detail for the relationship between its partial pressure in breath and blood. Over the years, a large number of studies have attempted to validate the use of end-exhaled alcohol as representative of alveolar, and hence blood, alcohol concentration. The major concern with these results has been the surprisingly large variability in the ratio of breath alcohol concentration (BrAC) to blood alcohol concentration (BAC). This averages about 2100. It is highly significant that there is a large intrastudy variation in the mean values and the range of variation (see Mason and Dubowski, 1975). The large variation is likely to be due to the substantial airway interaction and the lack of any control of the affecting physiological parameters during measurements of the blood-breath ratios.

The single-breath alcohol test is applied with very little control of ventilation parameters. Typical instructions to a subject are to "take in a breath and exhale all the way into the machine." Although some "breath test instrument operators" use different subjective criteria for deciding whether a test is suitable, there are no controls on pretest ventilatory pattern, preinspiratory lung volume, inspiratory flow rate, end-inspiration lung volume, end-inspiration breath-holding time, expiratory flow rate, or expiratory volume. Most alcohol breath test instruments are designed to sample end-exhalation breath, and most of the newer infrared instruments require exhalation for a minimal time or volume before a sample can be taken; presumably this is to avoid anatomic dead space contamination from the early part of the exhalate.

The interaction of alcohol with the airways is so strong because the high water/air and blood/air partition coefficients for alcohol mean that the exhaled alcohol concentration can be changed by the breathing pattern, the inspired air temperature, and its humidity (Jones, 1982a–c). Ventilation appears to have its effect through changes in airway mucosal temperature. Jones (1982b) showed that hyperventilation for 30 s (cooling the airway surface) results in an 11% decrease in exhaled BrAC. He also showed a 16% rise in BrAC after a 30 s breath hold (warming the airway surface). Ohlsson et al. (1990) recently confirmed these results qualitatively by showing a 6% drop after a three-breath hyperventilation and a 9% increase after a 15 s breath hold. In addition, because of the increasing BrAC with exhaled volume (Jones, 1982c; Ohlsson et al., 1990), the breath test values also depend on exhaled volume.

The control volume mathematical modeling approach can also be used to predict alcohol-airway exchange during normal breathing. This is done by adding a soluble gas (alcohol) flux term to the model shown in Fig. 2 (Tsu et al., 1990). The model predicts that during inspiration, because of the alcohol flux from the airway mucosa, an equilibrium concentration of alcohol is attained in the inspired air before the respiratory bronchioles are reached (Fig. 4). During exhalation, much of this alcohol is reabsorbed into the airway mucosa. With oral breathing, the alcohol flux shifts more distally into the airways compared with nasal breathing. The degree of airway interaction with soluble gas is thus directly dependent on its water solubility, explaining the observations of Schrikker et al. (1985, 1989) and Zwart et al., (1986).

If the airway interaction is minimized by rebreathing, then it should be possible theoretically to obtain a truer sample of alveolar alcohol. Jones (1983a) and Ohlsson et al. (1990) used rebreathing with a heated rebreathing bag and were able to obtain alveolar samples that were closely correlated with blood alcohol concentration. In each study, rebreathed air alcohol concentration was greater than single-breath end-tidal alcohol concentration, irrespective

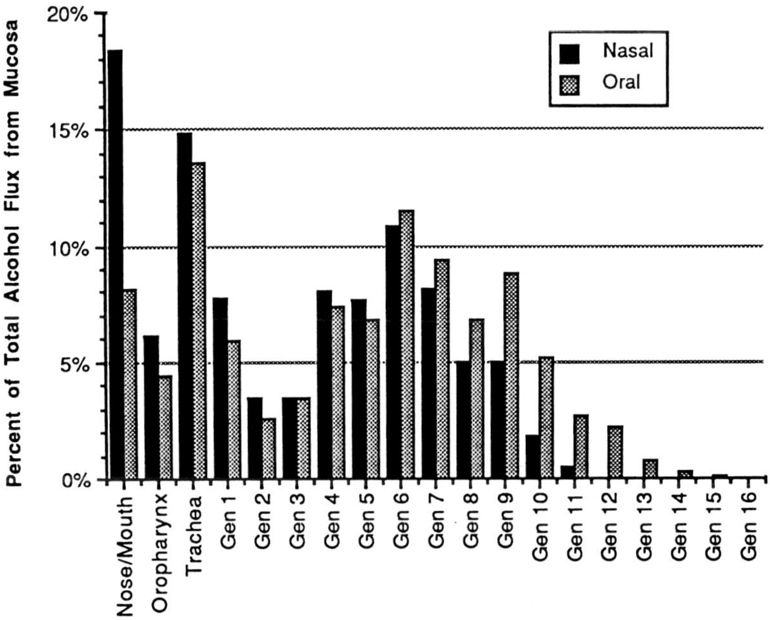

Figure 4 Longitudinal distribution of alcohol flux from the airway mucosa. Calculated values are shown for nasal and oral breathing. From Tsu et al., 1990).

of the breathing pattern (Fig. 5). The conclusion from these studies is that alcohol is always lost to the airways from exhaled air during the single-breath test. This loss varies among different individuals and even from time to time in the same individual, accounting for the variability in blood-breath ratio that depends on the pattern of breathing.

E. Bolus Experiments

A more quantitative assessment of airway gas-to-mucosa interaction has been made using indicator dilution principles. A bolus of gas passing along an airway disperses because of diffusion-convection interaction mechanisms in the gas phase as well as solution in the airway tissue. If a bolus containing two indicator gases is introduced into the airway and sampled at another location in the airway after convective movement, the relative volume of dilution of the bolus can be determined from the dispersion of the bolus. Using one gas with low solubility that remains in the gas phase and another with high solubility that also dissolves in the tissue, the tissue volume (the difference in volume of dispersion of the two gas boli) is determined from the separation of mean transit times of the two boli.

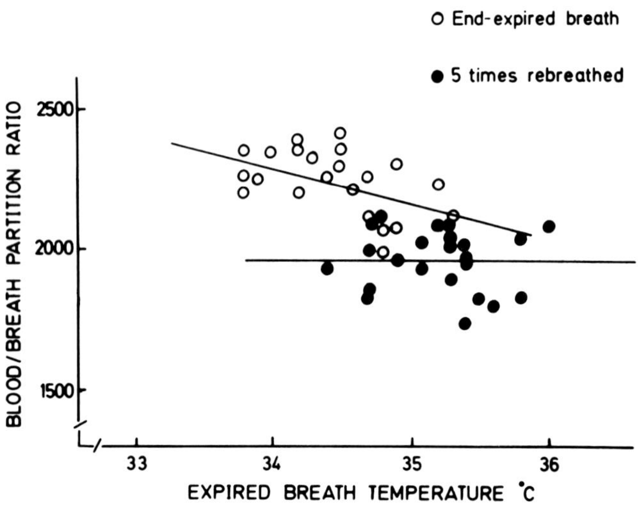

Figure 5 Blood/breath partition ratio versus breath temperature. Data are shown for rebreathed air and for single-breath end-tidal air samples. A higher blood/breath partition ratio reflects a lower breath alcohol concentration. End-tidal alcohol is lower than rebreathed alcohol. (From Jones, 1983a, with permission from the *Journal of Applied Physiology*.)

Ralph and Hlastala (1983) made bolus measurements using diethyl ether as the soluble gas and krypton as the insoluble gas. These gases were chosen because of their similar molecular weights (84 and 74, respectively), minimizing the possibility of separation of gases due to diffusion-related dispersion mechanisms (Ultman, 1981). The difference in volume of dispersion of the two gases indicated a depth of penetration into the mucosal tissue ranging from 28 to 56 μm. The variability may have reflected a variation in drying of the mucous lining of the airways as the depth of penetration of a gas depends on its diffusivity in the mucosal tissue and mucous water (Hlastala, 1974).

Baier et al. (1986) used a double-indicator method, with helium as the low solubility gas and dimethyl ether as the high solubility gas. Because the test gases used by Baier had quite different molecular weights, it may be that airway gas mixing affected these data. In the trachea of conscious adult sheep, the measurable water volume of the wall over a 15 cm length ranged between 0.50 and 0.70 ml. The corresponding penetration depth ranged between 63 and 82 μm. Changes in bronchial blood flow had no consistent influence on tissue volume, indicating a lack of significant movement of gas to the bronchial circulation. Baier et al. found that intravenous injection of histamine increased mean water depth by between 22 and 34% suggesting an increase in water. Intravenous injection of carbachol had no effect on water depth. If more mucus is present within the airways (as in asthma and bronchitis), there may be a greater interaction of soluble gases with the airways. However, there is also an increase in bronchial vascular blood flow in bronchitis.

III. Gas Exchange with the Bronchial Circulation

A. Oxygen and Carbon Dioxide

The contribution of the bronchial circulation to total oxygen uptake, CO_2 elimination, and inert gas exchange has been exceedingly difficult to measure. In the normal lung, bronchial blood flow is only a small fraction (1–3%) of total lung perfusion, and on these grounds alone, its role in quantitative gas transfer is likely to be very small. To further complicate the analysis, one must consider that gas flux to and from the bronchial arterial derived blood may occur either across the bronchial epithelium lining the airways or the alveolar epithelium, since anastomoses occur between the bronchial and the pulmonary vasculature at a precapillary or capillary level (anastomotic bronchial systemic-to-pulmonary flow). It is difficult to see how one could study separately the contributions of these two sites in the intact animal. In fact, it may be somewhat artificial to separate the two, at least on a physiological basis, since the bronchial epithelium at the terminal bronchiolar level represents an ever-increasing surface area of decreasing thickness perfused more and more by the pulmonary blood flow. Although the more proximal airways constitute a much smaller surface area with a thicker barrier, gas exchange at this level is enhanced somewhat by its exposure to the full ambient partial pressure during inspiration of fresh air.

Experimental protocols designed to study the contribution of the bronchial circulation to overall gas exchange suffer from many deviations from the normal state. Since any contribution is difficult to measure in the presence of parallel pulmonary perfusion, it is necessary either to stop pulmonary perfusion or to isolate a segment of the tracheobronchial tree. Both involve considerable changes in normal ventilation and blood flow patterns. Furthermore, it is not possible to predict whether either method over- or underestimates the gas-exchange contribution of the bronchial circulation. Gas exchange across the bronchial vasculature during pulmonary blood flow occlusion could be changed because there would be no contribution of the pulmonary flow to alter the gas tensions and driving pressure for gas elimination or uptake across the airways. On the other hand, the airways below the trachea may receive a considerable degree of pulmonary blood flow (approaching 50% of total measured airway perfusion) (Barman et al., 1988) and the loss of this contribution could result in an underestimation of normal gas transfer across the airways. Isolation of a segment of the tracheobronchial tree from the lung parenchyma eliminates the contribution of alveolar gas exchange but alters the normal partitioning of airway and bronchial-pulmonary anastomotic flow. Last, a distinction must be made between studies after acute and chronic obstruction of the pulmonary artery, since a chronic absence of pulmonary blood flow stimulates marked increases in bronchial blood flow.

Studies involving acute unilateral pulmonary artery obstruction in the sheep show remarkable O_2 and CO_2 transfer (8 and 20% of total O_2 uptake and CO_2 output, respectively) from a lung perfused only by the bronchial circulation (Charan and Carvalho, 1989). Negligible O_2 uptake from air rose to 10% on ventilation with 100% O_2 (Mandelbaum and Giammona, 1966). The CO_2 output by both lungs of dogs undergoing cardiopulmonary bypass averaged 3–5% of total CO_2 output. Similarly, in humans during cardiopulmonary bypass, CO_2 outputs approaching 10% of total CO_2 production have been measured (Deal et al., 1968). These data reflect larger than normal bronchial blood flows resulting from long-standing lung and heart disease in these patients (Baile et al., 1985). They probably represent the maximum gas transfer attributable to the bronchial blood flow, since it is likely that in the absence of pulmonary perfusion a greater fraction of it will traverse anastomotic pathways into the pulmonary vasculature. Under conditions in which there is no pulmonary blood flow, gas exchange presumed to be due to the bronchial circulation could reflect contributions from other sources, however. These include alveolar gas transfer resulting from retrograde pulmonary venous flow (Butler et al., 1989) and, at least in the case of CO_2, lung tissue metabolism and transpleural CO_2 diffusion (Sheppard et al., 1981). The fraction of bronchial blood draining into the pulmonary circulation has been estimated as high as 77% in acute studies (Schoedel et al., 1962), but it is not likely that the majority of this flow actually traverses the alveolar capillary bed. The studies just cited show that, despite extremely low end-tidal gas P_{CO_2} values (1–2 mmHg), the P_{CO_2} of blood draining into the left atrium remains close to the initial arterial values (15–20 mmHg) during cardiopulmonary bypass. These findings indicate a marked inefficiency of bronchial circulation gas exchange, as noted by Robertson et al. (1984) using inert gases in the dog lung. This suggests that gas exchange occurs principally across the airways since the normal postpulmonary capillary-alveolar P_{CO_2} difference is less than 1 mmHg. It should be remembered that the bronchial circulation is exquisitively sensitive to temperature changes and that its response over a wide range of cooling and heating is not a simple linear relationship (Agostoni et al., 1987). Thus all studies involving cardiopulmonary bypass or pulmonary artery obstruction (Solway et al., 1986) that result in airway cooling may entail large deviations in bronchial blood flow from those at normal body temperature.

With chronic loss of pulmonary perfusion, bronchial blood flow may increase by one to two orders of magnitude (Deffebach et al., 1987). In such cases, the bronchial blood flow contributes substantially to gas exchange. In humans, CO_2 output from a lung with either congenital absence of a pulmonary artery or following surgical ligation ranges from 25 to 37% of total CO_2 production. Little or no oxygen uptake occurs except under conditions of systemic hypoxemia or selective inhalation of hyperoxic gas into the affected lung (Tabakin et al., 1960; Viola and Abbate, 1973). Similar data have been reported in dogs (Bloomer et al., 1949; Lilker and Nagy, 1975) and in sheep, except that O_2 uptake by the affected lung was as high as 20% of the total O_2 consumption of the sheep (Charan and Carvalho, 1989). The marked augmentation of the bronchial circulation is likely to cause a significant perfusion of the alveolar capillary bed with greater gas-exchange efficiency than seen acutely in the absence of pulmonary artery perfusion. The only inert gas-exchange data relevant to this question are those of Kapitan et al. (1989) in patients with chronic thromboembolism studied before thromboendarterectomy. Many of these patients have greatly increased bronchial blood flows, but pulmonary perfusion, although low, is still present in some regions. Kapitan et al. found a high dead space fraction and increased heterogeneity of $\dot{V}_A/\dot{Q}$ distribution but no significant shunt. This is in contrast to the studies of Robertson et al. (1984) in acute pulmonary artery obstruction, in which the shunt fractions were between 3 and 20%. In modeling the effect of high bronchial blood flows (10–20% of cardiac output), Kapitan (1987), assuming no diffusion limitation, concluded that such flows reduce the apparent perfusion going to shunt and low $\dot{V}_A/\dot{Q}$ units by permitting a fraction of the cardiac output to undergo second and subsequent passes through the lungs. The effect is to improve both arterial P_{O_2} and P_{CO_2}.

Attempts to measure the contribution of the bronchial circulation to gas exchange in the presence of normal pulmonary perfusion have only been made in the isolated trachea. Swenson et al. (1986) found the CO_2 output by the in situ dog trachea amounted to 0.25–0.50% of the animal's CO_2 production. Using the dog lung morphological data of Horsfield and Cumming (1976), they calculated that total tracheobronchial CO_2 output could be as high as 10% of CO_2 production, assuming a direct relationship of surface area to gas exchange. These figures agree surprisingly well with those measured when the pulmonary circulation has been acutely occluded.

Acknowledging the limited data and experimental problems, it appears that bronchial gas exchange in the normally perfused lung is small for CO_2 and negligible for O_2 because total bronchial blood flow is low and normally perfuses only the airways. Under conditions of chronic loss of pulmonary perfusion, expansion of the bronchial circulation with resulting high anastomotic flow into the alveolar capillaries results in vitually normal CO_2 output but much less than normal O_2 uptake.

B. Inert Gases

Inert gas exchange in a diffusion-limited system is difficult to analyze, particularly with the added complexities of a cross-current exchange (see Fig. 1) and heterogeneity of the distribution of the membrane-diffusing capcity to bronchial blood flow ratio. A simplified analytic approach for a single gas compartment with ventilation $\dot{V}$ exchanging gas with an unventilated (stagnant) gas compartment through a gas diffusion barrier (with diffusive conductance D') and through a tissue diffusion barrier (with diffusive conductance D_m) to a perfusion bed with constant blood flow $\dot{Q}$ has been described by Hlastala (1987) (Fig. 6). The equations for retention and excretion of inert gases are

$$R = \frac{P_v}{P_a} = \frac{\lambda FG + \dot{V}/\dot{Q}(1 - G)}{\lambda FG + \dot{V}/\dot{Q}} \tag{2}$$

$$E = \frac{P_A}{P_a} = \frac{\lambda G}{\lambda FG + \dot{V}/\dot{Q}} \tag{3}$$

where $F = 1 + \beta g\dot{V}/D'$ and $G = 1 - e^{-D_m/Q\beta_b}$. R and E are inert gas retention and excretion, respectively, P_v is gas partial pressure in the blood coming

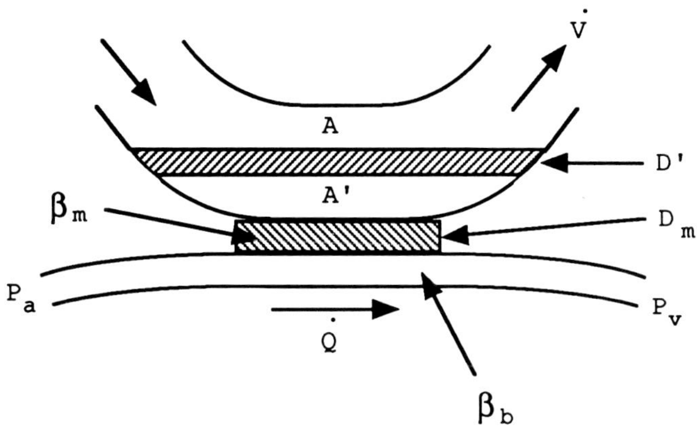

Figure 6 Diffusion limitation model of airway with ventilation ($\dot{V}$) and perfusion ($\dot{Q}$). Airway compartment A exchanges gas by convection and by diffusion with compartment A′ through gas-phase diffusive conductance (D′). Compartment A′ exchanges gas with blood by diffusion through membrane diffusion conductance (D_m). β_b, effective solubility in blood; β_m, solubility of gas in membrane; P_a, partial pressure of gas in the incoming blood; P_v, partial pressure of gas in the effluent blood.

into the gas-exchanging unit, P_a is gas partial pressure in the blood leaving the gas-exchange unit, P_A is gas partial pressure in the mixed gas leaving the gas-exchanging unit, β_b is the capacitance coefficient of the gas in blood (the same as Bunsen solubility coefficient), and β_g is the capacitance coefficient of the gas in the gas phase [for all ideal gases, equal to 1.16 ml (STPD)/L (BTPS)/torr at 37°C; see Piiper et al., 1971].

F represents diffusion limitation within the gas phase that may play a role in the airways with axial streaming in laminar flow regimes. With turbulence, D′ approaches ∞ and F approaches 1.0. G represents diffusion limitation within the mucus and the unperfused tissue layer and plays a role in larger airways. As the diffusion distances decrease with smaller airways, D_m approaches ∞ and G approaches 1.0. For gas exchange from the bronchial circulation, both solubility dependence and molecular weight dependence are expected.

Robertson et al. (1984) assessed inert gas exchange with the bronchial circulation utilizing the partially isolated left lower lobe (LLL) with occluded pulmonary circulation in the anesthetized dog. The only source of blood flow to the LLL came from the intact bronchial circulation and, possibly, a component of reversed venous blood flow (Butler et al., 1989). Since the bronchial arteries in the dog arise from the thoracic intercostal arteries, trace quantities of six inert gases dissolved in saline were infused into the bronchial circulation via the left atrium. The LLL was alternately ventilated with either air or 95% N_2 and 5% CO_2. On air, the shunt fraction determined by exchange of sulfur hexafluoride (SF_6) varied between 0.03 and 0.20, associated with a lobar bronchial blood flow of 3–8 ml/min. When the lobe was ventilated with N_2 and CO_2, bronchial flow increased two- to threefold in response to the alveolar hypoxia and the SF_6 shunt fraction increased to between 0.14 and 0.23. The degree of deoxygenation of blood flowing through the LLL ventilated with N_2 and CO_2 was highly variable among animals, although the O_2 shunt was always larger than that predicted from the SF_6 data. This observation suggests that, although the bronchial circulation participates in gas exchange, its gas-exchange pathways have a significant tissue diffusion limitation.

To evaluate gas exchange in larger airways, Swenson et al. (1986) carried out similar experiments with an isolated, bronchial circulation-perfused, tracheal preparation. Anesthetized dogs had tracheostomies just above the carina and were supported with a piston pump ventilator. The distal 20 cm segment of the trachea was ventilated unidirectionally with warm humidified air, and the exhaled gas from the isolated segment was collected in a mixing box. The six inert gases used for MIGET were infused into the left atrium, and inert gas concentrations in the arterial blood and mixed expired gas were measured and expressed as excretions ($E = P_E/P_a$). Inert gas exchange could be demonstrated to take place in the trachea, with excretions ranging from 3×10^{-5} for SF_6 to 0.92 for acetone. The diffusive component of this exchange process can be quantitated after transforming the data. The transformed Eq. (3) for excretion in a gas-exchanging unit with all the diffusive resistance in the tissue phase ($F = 1$) is

$$\ln \frac{1 - E}{E} = \ln \frac{\dot{V}}{\dot{Q}} + \ln \frac{1}{G} + \ln \frac{1}{\lambda} \tag{4}$$

For a homogenous lung unit, Eq. (4) predicts a linear relationship between $\ln[(1 - E)/E]$ and $\ln 1/\lambda$. Gases with differing $D_m/Q\beta_b$ ratios have different G values and fall on different lines displaced vertically (Fig. 7).

The data of Swenson et al. (1986) follow such a relationship (Fig. 7). Gases with the two highest molecular weights (SF_6 and halothane) had lower excretions [higher $(1 - E)/E$ ratio] than predicted from solubility alone. Separate measurements with acetylene (MW = 26), Freon 22 (MW = 86.5), and Forane (MW = 184), three inert gases with similar partition coefficients but disparate molecular weights (MW), showed a 39% difference (data not shown in Fig. 7) between the elimination of acetylene and Forane. This molecular weight dependence of inert gas elimination from the isolated trachea is much larger than that reported from the intact lung (Robertson et al., 1986), but the effect of airway gas exchange is not large enough to account for the

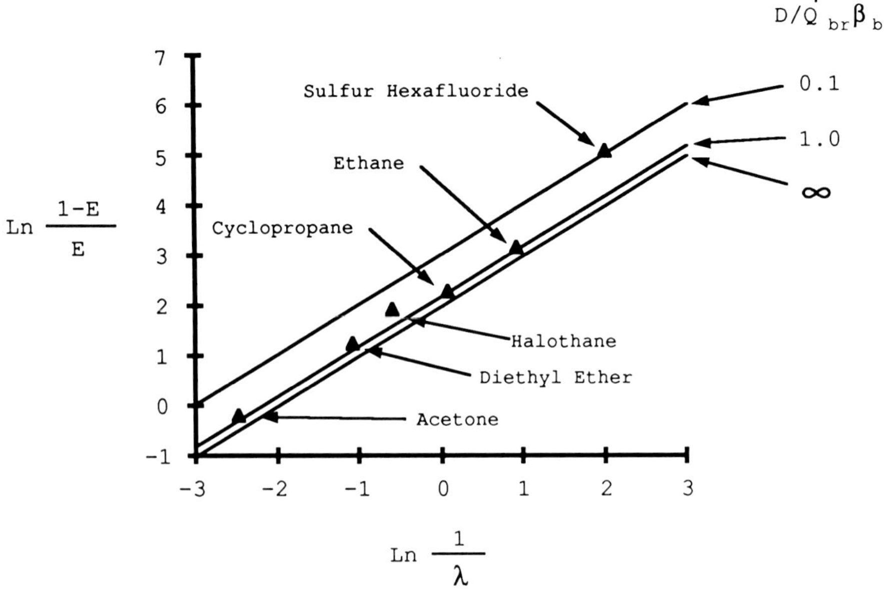

Figure 7 Transformed excretion plot: $\ln[(1-E)/E]$ is plotted against $\ln 1/\lambda$ for theoretical data from a homogenous airway unit with mean $\dot{V}_A/\dot{Q} = 100$. Lines are shown for three units with $D_m/\dot{Q}_{br}\beta_b$ of ∞, 1.0, and 0.1. Data points are for tracheal segment gas excretion in one dog (Swenson et al., 1986). Symbols are as defined in Fig. 1 and 6; E is inert gas excretion.

magnitude of the molecular weight effect seen in the whole lung, which demonstrates a slight increase in the retention of Forane compared with acetylene (after correction for solubility dependence).

These studies show that conducting airways have measurable inert gas exchange but that this demonstrates a large degree of diffusion limitation, presumably because the gases leaving the bronchial circulation must diffuse through a significant layer of tissue, water, and mucus before reaching the airway lumen.

IV. Summary

The image of the airways as passive conduits carrying air between the outside environment and alveoli is changing. In the earlier stages of respiratory physiology, the role of the airways as passive conduits to the gas-exchanging regions adequately described the process of exchanging O_2 and CO_2. However, now that more soluble gases are becoming important for the assessment of gas exchange using MIGET and for the evaluation of the protective effect of the airways against soluble pollutant gases, the interaction of gases with the airway has become a significant part of gas-exchange analyses. For this exchange, the bronchial circulation plays a critical role in delivery gas, heat, and water to or eliminating them from the airway tissue.

Under normal circumstances, the bronchial circulation makes a negligible contribution to the exchange of normal respiratory gases, O_2 and CO_2. With hypertrophy of the bronchial circulation in lung diseases, such as chronic pulmonary embolism, the bronchial circulation exchange can become a means of exchange of O_2 and CO_2 in the affected portion of the lung. For soluble gases, it is likely that the bronchial circulation usually plays a major role in gas exchange.

Inhaled pollutant gases deposit on the airways during inspiration, decreasing the amount delivered to the alveolar regions, where they can more readily be taken up by the blood. The pollutants are then added to the expired gas as it passes through the airways. The resulting "protective effect" decreases the relative absorption of these pollutant gases by the body, an effect directly related to the solubility of the gas in the airway mucosa.

In the future, experiments must be undertaken to define more carefully the role of the bronchial circulation in soluble gas exchange in both the normal lung and in the diseased lung.

References

Agostoni, P. G., Deffebach, M. E., Kirk, W., and Brengelmann, G. L. (1987). Temperature dependence of intraparenchymal bronchial blood flow. *Respir. Physiol.* **68**:259–267.

Aharonson, E. F., Menkes, H., Gurtner, G., Swift, D. L., and Proctor, D. F. (1974). Effect of respiratory airflow rate on removal of soluble vapors by the nose. *J. Appl. Physiol.* **37**:654–657.

Åstrand, I., and Övrum, P. (1976). Exposure to trichloroethylene. I. Uptake and distribution in man. *Scand. J. Work Environ. Health* **4**:199–211.

Åstrand, I., and Övrum, P., Lindqvist, T., and Hultengren, M. (1976). Exposure to butyl alcohol. Uptake and distribution in man. *Scand. J. Work Environ. Health* **3**:165–175.

Åstrand, I. Engström, J., and Övrum, P. (1978). Exposure to xylene and ethylbenzene. Uptake, distribution and elimination in man. *Scand. J. Work Environ. Health* **3**:185–194.

Baier, H., Moas, R., Yerger, L., and Wanner, A. (1986). In vivo estimation of tracheal wall water: Effects of histamine and carbachol. *J. Appl. Physiol.* **60**:1680–1685.

Baile, E. M., Ling, H., Heyworth, J. R., Hogg, J. C., and Paré, P. D. (1985). Bronchopulmonary anastomotic and noncoronary collateral blood flow in humans during cardiopulmonary bypass. *Chest* **87**:749–754.

Barman, S. A., Ardell, J. L., Parker, J. C., Perry, M. L., and Taylor, A. E. (1988). Pulmonary and systemic blood flow contributions to upper airways in canine lungs. *Am. J. Physiol.* **255**:H1130–H1135.

Bloomer, W. E., Harrison, W., Lindskog, G. E., and Liebow, A. A. (1949). Respiratory function and blood flow in the bronchial artery after ligation of the pulmonary artery. *Am. J. Physiol.* **157**:317–328.

Butler, J., Kowalski, T. F., Willoughby, S., and Lakshminarayan, S. (1989). An alternative nutrient blood supply after pulmonary artery occlusion. *FASEB J.* **3**:A567.

Cander, L., and Forster, R. E. (1959). Determination of pulmonary parenchymal tissue volume and pulmonary capillary blood flow in man. *J. Appl. Physiol.* **14**:541–551.

Charan, N. B., and Carvalho, P. (1989). Gas exchange with the bronchial circulation. *Am. Rev. Respir. Dis.* **139**:A445.

Davidson, M. R., and Schroter, R. C. (1983). A theoretical model of absorption of gases by the bronchial wall. *J. Fluid Mech.* **129**:313–335.

Davies, C. N. (1985). Absorption of gases in the respiratory tract. *Ann. Occup. Hyg.* **29**:13–25.

Deal, C. W., Louis, E., Kerth, W. J., Osborn, J. J., and Gerbode, F. (1968). Bronchopulmonary precapillary blood flow during cardiopulmonary bypass. *Am. Heart J.* **75**:43–48.

Deffebach, M. E., Charan, N. B., Lakshminarayan, S., and Butler, J. (1987). The bronchial circulation: Small, but a vital attribute of the lung. *Am. Rev. Respir, Dis.* **135**:463–481.

DeVries, W. R., Luijendijk, S. C. M., and Zwart, A. (1982). Inert tracer gas washout from mixed venous blood: The sloping alveolar plateua. *Respir. Physiol.* **50**:283–297.

Dueck, R., Young, I., Clausen, J., and Wagner, P. D. (1980). Altered distribution of pulmonary ventilation and blood flow following induction of inhalation anesthesia. *Anesthesiology* **52**:113–125.

Farhi, L. E. (1967). Elimination of inert gases by the lung. *Respir. Physiol.* **3**:1–11.

Frank, N. R., Yoder, R. E., Brain, J. D., and Yokoyama, E. (1969). SO_2 (^{35}S-labeled) absorption by the nose and mouth under conditions of varying concentration and flow. *Arch. Envion. Health* **18**:315–322.

Gard, R. J., Hlastala, M. P., and Babb, A. L. (1984). Heat and water exchange in an airway tissue model. *Physiologist* **27**:259.

Guenard, H., Manier, G., Castaing, Y., and Varene, N. (1985). Series dead space for inert gases in healthy subjects. *Pflugers Arch.* **403**:384, 387.

Hanna, L. M., and Scherer, P. W. (1986). Regional control of local airway heat and water vapor loses. *J. Appl. Physiol.* **61**:624–632.

Hlastala, M. P. (1974). Transient-state diffusion in rat subcutaneous tissue. *Aerospace Med.* **45**:269–273.

Hlastala, M. P. (1987). Diffusing capacity heterogeneity. In: *Handbook of Physiology*, Section 3. *The Respiratory System*, Vol. IV, *Gas Exchange*. Edited by L. E. Farhi and S. M. Tenney. Washington, D. C., American Physiological Society, pp. 217–232.

Horsfield, K., and Cumming, G. (1976). Morphology of the bronchial tree in the dog. *Respir. Physiol.* **26**:173–182.

Ingenito, E. P., Solway, J., McFadden, Jr., E. R., Pichurko, B. M., Carvalho, E. G., and Drazen, J. M. (1986). Finite difference analysis of respiratory heat transfer. *J. Appl. Physiol.* **61**:2252–2259.

Kapitan, K. S. (1987). Effects of the bronchial circulation on inert and respiratory gas exchange. *Fed. Proc.* **46**:94.

Kapitan, K. S., Buchbinder, M., Wagner, P. D., and Moser, K. M. (1989). Mechanisms of hypoxemia in chronic thromboembolic pulmonary hypertension. *Am. Rev. Respir. Dis.* **139**:1149–1154.

Jones, A. W. (1982a). Effects of temperature and humidity of inhaled air on the concentration of ethanol in a man's exhaled breath. *Clin. Sci.* **63**:441–445.

Jones, A. W. (1982b). How breathing technique can influence the results of breath-alcohol analysis. *Med. Sci. Law* **22**:275–280.

Jones, A. W. (1982c). Quantitative measurements of the alcohol concentration and the temperature of breathing during a prolonged exhalation. *Acta Physiol. Scand.* **114**:407–412.

Jones, A. W. (1983a). Role of rebreathing in determination of the blood-breath ratio of expired ethanol. *J. Appl. Physiol.* **55**:1237–1241.

Jones, A. W. (1983b). Determination of liquid/air partition coefficients for dilute solutions of ethanol in water, whole blood, and plasma. *J. Anal. Toxicol.* **7**:193–197.

Lilker, E. S., and Nagy, E. J. (1975). Gas exchange in the pulmonary collateral circulation of dogs: Effects of alveolar hypoxia and systemic hypoxemia. *Am. Rev. Respir. Dis.* **112**:615–619.

Mandelbaum, I., and Giammona, S. T. (1966). Bronchial circulation during cardiopulmonary bypass. *Ann Surg.* **164**:985–989.

Mason, M. F., and Dubowski, K. M. (1975). Breath-alcohol analysis: Uses, methods, and some forensic problems—review and opinion. *J. Forensic Sci.* **21**:9–41.

McEvoy, R. D., Davies, N. J., Mannino, E. L., Prutow, R. J., Schumacker, P. T., Wagner, P. D., and West, J. B. (1982). Pulmonary gas exchange during high-frequency ventilation. *J. Appl. Physiol.* **52**:1278–1287.

McFadden, E. R., Pichurko, B. M., Bowman, H. F., Ingenito, E., Burno, S., Dowling, N., and Solway, J. (1985). Thermal mapping of the airways in humans, airway temperature during respiration. *J. Appl. Physiol.* **58**:564–570.

Morgan, M. S., and Frank, R. (1977). Uptake of pollutant gases by the respiratory system. In: *Respiratory Defense Mechanisms, Part 1.* Edited by J. D. Brain, D. F. Proctor, and L. M. Reid. Marcel Dekker, New York, pp. 157–189.

Ogata, M., and Tomokuni, Y. (1970). Urinary excretion of hippuric acid and M- or P-methylhippuric acid in the urine of persons exposed to vapors of toluene and M- or P-xylene as a test of exposure. *Br. J. Ind. Med.* **27**:43–50.

Ohlsson, J., Ralph, D. D., Mandelkorn, M. A., Babb, A. L., and Hlastala, M. P. (1990). Accurate measurement of blood alcohol concentration with isothermal rebreathing. *J. Stud. Alcohol* **51**:6–13.

Piiper, J., Dejours, P., Haab, P., and Rahn, H. (1971). Concepts and basic quantities in gas exchange physiology. *Respir. Physiol.* **13**:292–304.

Ralph, D. D., and Hlastala, M. P. (1983). Interaction of soluble gases with tracheal airway mucosa. *Physiologist* **26**:A68.

Ralph, D. D., Babb, A. L., and Hlastala, M. P. (1985). Interaction of ethanol with airway mucosa during exhalation. *Prog. Artificial Organs* 1119–1121.

Robertson, H. T., Coffey, R. L., Standaert, T. A., and Truog, W. E. (1982). Respiratory and inert gas exchange during high-frequency ventilation. *J. Appl. Physiol.* **52**:683–689.

Robertson, H. T., Jindal, S., Lakshminarayan, S., Albert, R., Kirk, W., Hlastala, M. P., and Butler, J. (1984). Gas exchange properties of the bronchial circulation in a dog lobe maintained in zone I conditions. *Am. Rev. Respir. Dis.* **129**:A229.

Robertson, H. T., Whitehead, J., and Hlastala, M. P. (1986). Diffusion-related differences in the elimination of inert gases from the lung. *J. Appl. Physiol.* 61:1162–1172.

Saidel, G. M., Kruse, K. L., and Primiano, Jr., F. P. (1983). Model simulation of heat and water transport dynamics in an airway. *J. Biomech. Eng.*

105:189–193.

Sato, A., and Nakajima, T. (1979). Partition coefficients of some aromatic hydrocarbons and ketones in water, blood and oil. *Br. J. Ind. Med.* **36**:231–234.

Schoedel, W., Kusachi, R., Piiper, J., and Rezai, S. (1962). Differenzierung des broncho-pulmonalen Bluteinstroms in einen Prä-, intra- und postcapillären Anteil. *Pflugers Arch.* **275**:534–538.

Schrikker, A. C. M., deVries, W. R., Zwart, A., and Luijendijk, S. C. M. (1985). Uptake of highly soluble gases in the epithelium of the conducting airways. *Pflugers Arch.* **405**:389–394.

Schrikker, A. C. M., deVries, W. R., Zwart, A., and Luijendijk, S. C. M. (1989). The excretion of highly soluble gases by the lung in man. *Pflugers Arch.* **415**:214–219.

Shepard, Jr., J. W., Minh, V. D., and Dolan, G. F. (1981). Gas exchange in nonperfused dog lungs. *J. Appl. Physiol.* **51**:1261–1267.

Solway, J., Leff, A. R., Dreshaj, I, Munoz, N. M., Ingenito, E. P., Michaels, D., Ingram, R. H., and Drazen, J. M. (1986). Circulatory heat sources for canine respiratory heat exchange. *J. Clin. Invest.* **78**:1015–1019.

Swenson, E. R., Robertson, H. T. R., and Hlastala, M. P. (1986). Gas exchange in the in situ isolated trachea. *Am. Rev. Respir. Dis.* **133**:A27.

Tabakin, B. S., Hanson, J. S., Adhikari, P. K., and Miller, D. B. (1960). Physiologic studies in congenital absence of the left main pulmonary artery. *Circulation* **22**:1107–1111.

Tsu, M. E., Babb, A. L., Ralph, D. D., and Hlastala, M. P. (1988). Dynamics of heat, water, and soluble gas exchange in the human airways. I. A model study. *Ann. Biomed. Eng.* **16**:547–571.

Tsu, M. E., Babb, A. L., Sugiyama, E. D., and Hlastala, M. P., (1991) Dynamics of soluble gas exchange in the airways. II. Effects of breathing conditions. *Respir. Physiol.* **83**:261–276.

Ultman, J. S. (1981). Gas mixing in the pulmonary airways. *Ann. Biomed. Eng.* **9**:513–527.

Viola, A. R., and Abbate, E. H. (1973). Respiratory function and effective collateral flow 8 years after ligation of the left pulmonary artery. *Am. Rev. Respir. Dis.* **108**:1216–1220.

Wagner, P. D., Saltzman, H. A., and West, J. B. (1974). Measurement of continuous distribution of ventilation-perfusion ratio: Theory. *J. Appl. Physiol.* **36**:588–599.

Wigaeus, E., Holm, S., and Åstrand, I. (1981). Exposure to acetone. Uptake and elimination in man. *Scand. J. Work Environ. Health* **7**:84–94.

Yokoyama, E., and Frank, R. (1972). Respiratory uptake of ozone in dogs. *Arch. Environ. Health* **25**:132–138.

Young, I., and Wagner, P. D. (1979). Solubility of inert gases in homogenates of canine lung tissues. *J. Appl. Physiol.* **46**:1207–1210.

Zwart, A., Luijendijk, S. C. M., and deVries, W. R. (1986). Excretion-retention data of steady state gas exchange in tidal breathing. I. Dependency on the blood-gas partition coefficient. *Pflugers Arch.* **407**:204–210.

14

Plasma Exudation from Tracheobronchial Microvessels in Health and Disease

CARL G. A. PERSSON

University Hospital of Lund
Lund, Sweden

I. Introduction

In airway defense and inflammation a large number of tissue responses occur. Many of these, including increased muscle tone, secretion, blood flow, and pooling of blood, are graded increments of normal baseline functions. In contrast, plasma exudation is a specific tissue defense and inflammatory response unrelated to the normal capillary exchange of solutes. The increased vascular permeability that results in plasma exudation is a profound change, with gap formation in the wall of postcapillary venules (Fig. 1). Locally, the transmural colloidal osmotic pressure gradient is abolished by this mechanism. Plasma exudation in the airways is executed by permeability mechanisms in the subepithelial microvessels and those in the epithelial lining. Exudation permeability is distinct from the absorption permeabilities that regulate fluxes of small and large solutes from the airway lumen and into the circulation.

Plasma exudation is used in this text to describe the mediator-induced extravasation of plasma from postcapillary venules. Plasma exudation into the airway lumen is the further passage across the epithelial lining of the plasma exudate (containing extravasated plasma, plasma-derived peptides, and an

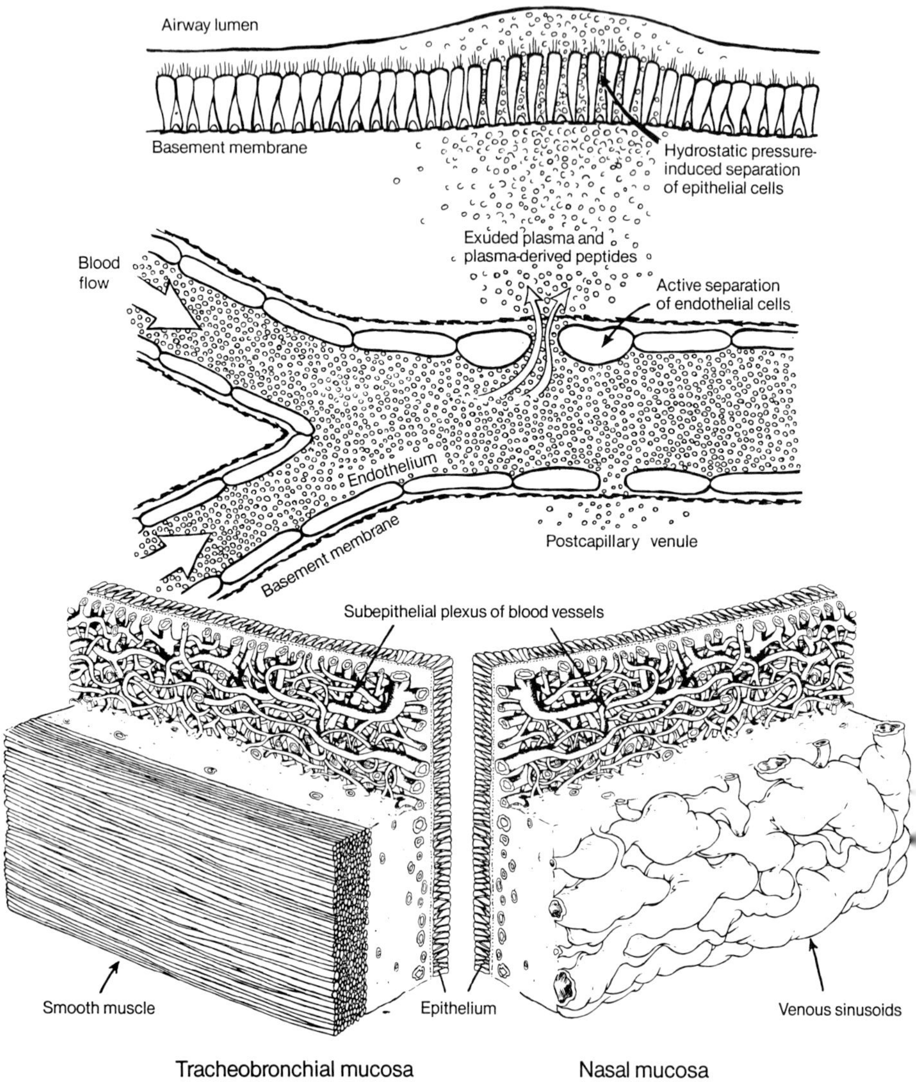

Figure 1 The proposed mechanism of exudation of plasma through microvascular-mucosal barriers, which are similar in tracheobronchial and nasal airways. However, deeper tissue components which are directly involved in obstruction of the airway passages are greatly different.

increased volume of fluid). The word *transudation* is avoided because medical dictionaries, as well as the current literature, seem to use "transudation" interchangeably to describe both the passive flux of protein-poor watery fluid out of capillaries (and across the mucosa) and the inflammatory stimulus-induced flow of proteinaceous fluid from postcapillary venules across the mucosa. The latter exudative process is an integrated response of the airway mucosa and microcirculation and has been termed "mucosal exudation" (Persson, 1991).

Strategically positioned just beneath the airway epithelium there is a copious plexus of capillary-venular tracheobronchial microvessels (Miller, 1947; Sobin et al., 1963; Laitinen et al., 1987). After mucosal provocation with inflammatory stimuli, the venules respond promptly with extravasation of plasma. Exuded plasma distributes in the interstitial spaces of the airway tissue and is slowly cleared by the lymphatic system. A small degree of reabsorption into airway microvessels may also occur. A much more important distribution of extravasated plasma in the airways is out across the epithelial lining to mix with the mucosal secretions. As demonstrated in guinea pig tracheobronchial airways and human nasal airways, significant amounts of plasma exudate, enough to replace the periciliary fluid layer or even more, appear promptly on the airway surface after mucosal provocation (e.g., Persson and Erjefält, 1986; Erjefält and Persson, 1989; Baumgarten et al., 1986; Greiff et al., 1990b). This could be an important defense mechanism to wash away toxic substances and allow the potent protein systems of blood plasma, including circulating immunoglobulins, to operate immediately on the airway mucosal surface at the very site where the insult occurs (Persson et al., 1991). If exaggerated, the airway plasma exudation process is pathological and one of the major mechanisms in asthma, bronchitis, and rhinitis (Persson, 1986, 1989c; Persson and Pipkorn, 1989).

It is understandable that such a dramatic effect as plasma exudation has been difficult to accept as a well-controlled mechanism. In particular in the airways, where exuded plasma macromolecules also appear on the mucosal surface, this has been thought to be an event that could only occur secondarily to tissue injury with epithelial disruption. In accordance with this notion, the current literature on mucosal and respiratory defense ignores the role of plasma exudation. However, experimental data obtained in animal and human airways indicate that the vascular endothelial and the mucosal epithelial change that allows the passage of plasma macromolecules is a noninjurious, fully reversible process that is under the influence of mediators, autacoids, hormones, and drugs. The present overview discusses some developments in the role of plasma exudation in airway diseases. Furthermore, it is proposed that plasma exudation has important roles in the mucosal defense of normal airways.

II. Historical Notes on Exudative Airway Disease

A humoral hypothesis of airway symptoms in asthma and rhinitis can be traced to Hippocrates and his disciples in ancient Greece 450 years BCE (Adams, 1938). The evil humor was thought to arise in the brain from which it descended into nasal and bronchial airways. Aretaeus and Galen (about 100–200 CE) considered asthma a disease caused by a viscid, irritating humor in the airways. Galen logically maintained that purging the naval cavities was a remedy for asthma. Unfortunately, Aretaeus' chapter on the treatment of asthma has been lost.

It took a long time before the anatomic impossibility of the origin of respiratory catarrhs from the brain was demonstrated. In 1672, Richard Lower wrote in the introduction to his book *De Catarrhis*:

> But since the opinion has generally persisted amongst learned doctors everywhere that catarrh and every kind of flux come from the cerebrum, I shall at this point attempt to prove the contrary. People claim that the fluid collected in the ventricles of the brain oozes down into the nostrils solely by the cribriform plate, and into the palate by the pituitary gland; but I shall prove that the structure of these parts is such that neither is possible.

There was an immediate precedent to this discussion by Lower. In 1660, Schneider (see Sakula, 1988) made an equally strong case against the idea of cerebral catarrhs. Unfortunately, this advance did not result in improved therapy. According to Lower (1672), there was now an even better rationale for frequent employment of bloodletting since "the substance of the catarrh is derived from the fluid of the blood."

The view that asthma is caused by abnormal airway humors also found many supporters during the eighteenth and nineteenth centuries. As quoted by Kahn (1928), John Millar wrote in 1769; "the superfluous serum, which ought to be thrown out by expiration, is accumulated; the fibres become turgid and edematous; and the organs of respiration are weakened." Robert Bree (1807) stated that the clinical manifestation of asthma was "merely an extraordinary effort to get rid of some peccant and irritating matter existing in the air-tubes" (Kahn, 1928). Bree was corrected on this point by the brilliant expert on asthma, Henry Hyde Salter (1868): "The fact is, Dr. Bree mistook the effect for the cause."

Salter recognized the inflammatory nature of asthma. He was probably the first to emphasize that it is the bronchial, not the pulmonary microcirculation that takes part in the airway disease processes. He reasoned that asthmatic hemoptysis must come from bronchial microvessels and this made him realize (Salter, 1868):

> ... what I never could well understand before, the invariable bronchial mucous exudation upon any form of protracted attack of asthma; for that which would produce bronchial hyperemia, even though passive, would necessarily produce an increase of the bronchial secretion.

A number of Austrian, German, and French workers of the nineteenth century considered that swelling of the bronchial mucous membrane was responsible for the asthmatic attack. In 1872, Weber expanded on this theme and reasoned that the swelling resulted from vasomotor turgescence (see Schultz, 1924). This view may have erred in overstressing the similarities between nasal and bronchial mucosal vasomotor mechanisms (Persson, 1989a). Stoerk (1875) could have been the first to actually observe the airway during an asthmatic attack (see Kahn, 1928). Through his "bronchoscope" he saw the narrowing of the airways lumen and concluded that mucosal swelling (and exudations) contributed significantly to the obstruction in asthma. Whereas Stoerk could only observe the largest airways, Curschmann focused on exudations in the smaller airways. In his classic study on asthma (1883), Curschmann preferred to call the disease "bronchiolitis exudativa."

It was demonstrated before Curschmann's observations that extravasation of protein-rich plasma is a cardinal sign of inflammation in general. In 1882, Cohnheim pointed out that plasma exudation occurs between endothelial cells that are directly affected by an inflammatory factor. It can be concluded from Cohnheim's further observations and writings that he believed that plasma exudation and leukocyte extravasation are distinct processes and that in mucosal lined cavities the exuded plasma enters the lumen to mix with the secretions.

During the first half of the twentieth century, progress in research on plasma exudation mechanisms was slow. Beyond the frequent observations by pathologists (e.g., Huber and Koessler, 1922; Rigler and Koucky, 1938; Dunnill et al., 1969) that asthmatic airways contain thick and proteinaceous material, there are few hints of the occurrence and importance of airways plasma exudation. In 1932, Florey and associates demonstrated the cholinergic control of airways secretions. They also observed that when evaporative demands on airway fluids to humidify inhaled air were high, secretions did not suffice. The increase of mucosal fluid that was induced by exposure of the feline trachea to dry air was not reduced by atropine. Florey et al. (1932) observed epithelial alterations; the submucosa was edematous and its blood vessels dilated. Hence, the dry air caused an acute inflammation and the production of considerable amounts of fluid, "being the product of vascular transudation rather than secretion from the glands." However, this inflammatory stimulus-induced effect is not mentioned among the eight points in the summary of the report by Florey et al. (1932). Also, in the four editions of Florey's famous *General Pathology* there are excellent chapters on inflammation of mucous membranes but Florey (1970) only mentions in passing that a plasma exudate may seep through the mucosa.

In 1949, Ingelstedt and Ivstam suggested that the source of human nasal "secretions" under inflammatory conditions was mostly a plasma exudate. In the same year the first report on the treatment of asthma and rhinitis with glucocorticoids appeared (Bordley et al., 1949). This milestone in the medical history of airway diseases (Persson, 1989a) focused on the fact that sputum production ceased and the pale edematous mucosa with thick coverings, as observed by nasal inspections, became normal soon after the start of treatment with adrenocorticotropic hormone (ACTH). The results of this study already inferred that exudations might be significant in the pathogenesis of asthma and rhinitis. It now seems well established that glucocorticoids are effective on that component of airway fluid that is not a secretory product but a plasma exudate (Persson, 1989b). There are several ways in which the exuded plasma and its products may contribute to the pathology of asthma (Dunnill et al., 1969; Persson, 1986, 1988a).

During the 1950s and 1960s, several investigators (Miles and Wilhelm, 1960; Spector and Willoughby, 1963; Willoughby and Spector, 1968) studied plasma exudation as an intriguing mechanism of defense and inflammation. Airways were not examined so any thought of a primary role of plasma exudation for defense soon gave way to more fundamental hypotheses that claimed to explain the causal pathways of the inflammatory process itself. During the last few decades, the discovery of many new biochemical and cellular aspects of inflammation have dominated the discussion. The rapid developments in these fields have found their way into complex schemes eclipsing the plasma exudation mechanism. Airway plasma exudation, if mentioned at all, has been downgraded to a secondary line of defense and the view most widely disseminated is that luminal entry of plasma exudate occurs only after frank damage has been inflicted upon the mucosa.

Microcirculation research underwent a different development, Cohnheim's interest in active vascular leakage mechanisms during inflammation was replaced by more mechanical and mathematical approaches. Different pore sizes should explain not only the normal exchange of fluid and solutes between interstitium and capillaries, but also the inflammatory leakage. In 1961, Majno and Palade provided an ultrastructural basis for plasma exudation between systemic venular endothelial cells. They also championed Cohnheim's original theory of direct endothelial effects and suggested that a contractile endothelial mechanism caused these cells to separate actively. The study of inflammatory macromolecular vascular leakage became a rapidly growing section of microvascular research. Although plasma exudation was downplayed by inflammatory researchers, it became an increasingly popular topic among the microcirculationists. The latter workers, though, maintained their somewhat mechanical approach: plasma exudation was merely linked with edema formation and with various calculations of protein transport.

Despite that supporting data have been available for a long time, the multipotential roles of plasma exudation in the pathogenesis of airway diseases have only recently been emphasized (Persson, 1986, 1988a). The plasma exudation aspect of asthma ties nicely into the early humoral hypotheses of this airway disease. A few passages in Salter's book on asthma come to mind, spelling out the importance of making observations in a nondogmatic way, or of: "reading real nature rather than the journal *Nature*."

III. Methods Used to Study Plasma Exudation

Thus far there have been surprisingly few studies of airways plasma exudation. This is due, in part, to a scarcity of specific methods.

A. Particulate Tracers

Early observations on inflammatory vascular permeability were made with particulate tracers, such as mercuric sulfide (Arnold, 1875) and carbon particles (Pietra et al., 1971, 1974; Hurley, 1983). If injected into the systemic circulation just before administration of an inflammatory mediator, the carbon particles map out those microvessels that have become leaky. The particulate tracer passes through the endothelial gaps but is then trapped because it cannot pass the basement membrane of the endothelium. Thus the particle tracer technique has been used to show that inflammatory permeability changes take place in postcapillary venules and, furthermore, that the tracheobroncial microvessels react to mediators of the inflammation of asthma, whereas the pulmonary microvessels do not (Pietra et al., 1971, 1974; Hurley, 1983). By giving histamine to the lungs of dogs by aerosol and by direct injection in the parenchyma, Pietra et al. (1971) demonstrated that carbon was trapped in bronchial but not in pulmonary microvessels. Histamine and other mediators that are inflammatory in the airways have been given to isolated lungs, perfused through the pulmonary artery, without causing signs of pulmonary edema (Hurley, 1983; Persson et al., 1982).

McDonald (1988a, b) admirably demonstrates the usefulness of another particular tracer, monastral blue, in his work on inflammation in the rat trachea. He uses this method to relate the neurogenic vascular permeability response to changes in white cells and in the epithelium adjacent to leaky microvessels. Most interestingly, he has also demonstrated that viral infection increases the vascular permeability response and that this abnormality remains after the detectable pathology of the infection has disappeared (McDonald, 1988b).

Particulate tracers cannot be used to estimate the extent of plasma exudation or the distribution of the exudate, however. They provide only a single measurement and cannot be given to humans. A more significant limitation is perhaps the observation that particle tracer measurement can show an apparently normal vessel when there is nevertheless an ongoing plasma exudation. For instance, the late-phase (over 5 h) airways plasma exudation induced in the guinea pig tracheal mucosa and submucosa by topical platelet actuating factor (PAF) was not detectable with the carbon particle method. The immediate phase was, however (O'Donnell et al., 1990). One can only speculate about why the more sustained aspects of vascular permeability may not be detected by particulate tracers. Perhaps the gaps are only initially sufficiently wide. A diminished gap size, together with other impediments, such as adhering thrombocytes and neutrophils, may prevent the particulate trapping in the late phase, although, there is still significant extravasation of plasma.

B. Solute Tracers

The choice of a solute tracer is not trivial. Albumin is the most common but may not always provide specific information about a plasma exudation process. Albumin is a rather small plasma protein that is normally present in airway liquids. In vitro studies also suggest that albumin may be actively secreted by the mucosa (Webber and Widdicombe, 1989), but in vivo this appears to be a mechanism of only marginal importance (Raphael et al., 1988). Albumin is an important component of an inflammatory exudate, but its use as a tracer may be limited by the fact that it may accumulate in bronchial liquids under baseline conditions. It also needs emphasizing that dye tags and radiolabeling of albumin, which are frequently used, need careful validation.

In acute mucosal inflammation there is an obvious bulk exudation of plasma into the lumen. Similarly after topical provocation, along with native tracers like albumin, fibrinogen, and α_2-macroglobulin, injected plasma tracers, such as macromolecular dextrans, appear on the mucosal surface. (Erjefält and Persson, 1989; Svensson et al., 1989; Baumgarten et al., 1986; and unpublished observations by Alkner, Persson, Pipkorn, and Svensson). Since plasma can appear promptly on a mucosal surface that has an intact epithelial lining (Persson et al., 1987; Luts et al., 1990), one must assume that the mucosal crossing is almost exclusively by paracellular routes (Figs. 1 and 2). This assumption is supported by the likelihood that the epithelial cells

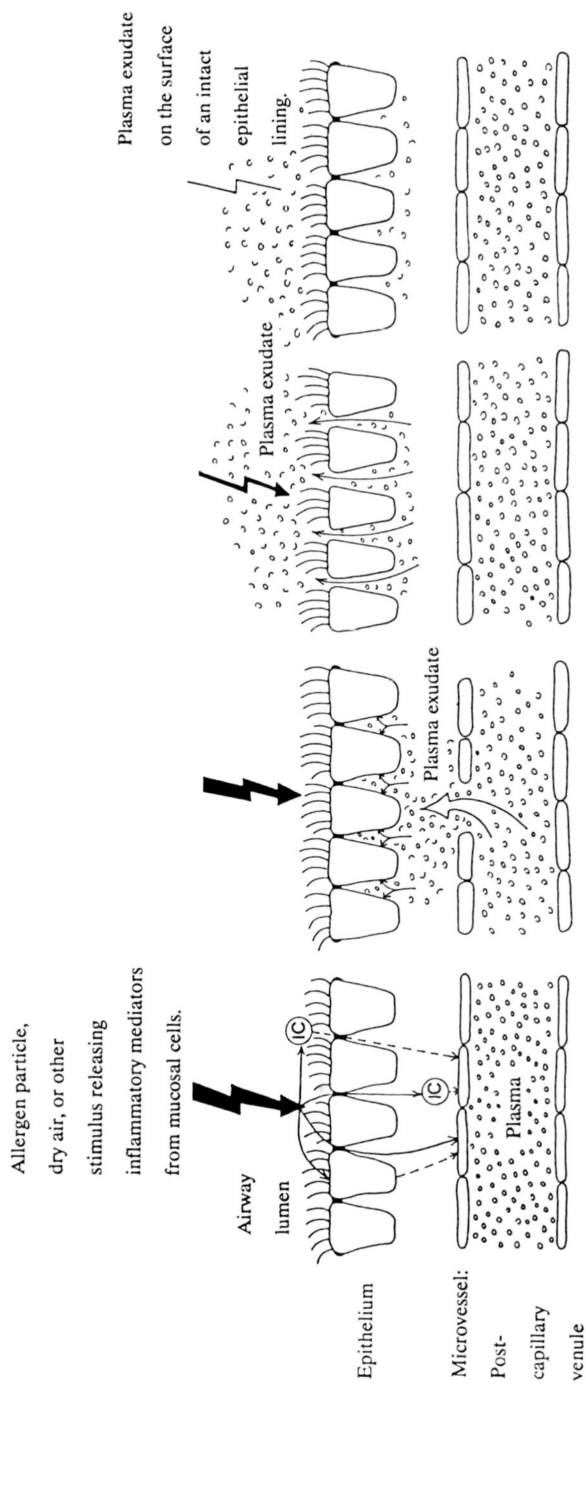

Figure 2 The proposed mechanism for plasma exudation from subepithelial microvessels to the mucosal surface (see text). IC, inflammatory cells in and on the mucosa (including mast cells and epithelial cells).

could not have survived a rapid transcellular passage of such large amounts of blood plasma.

During the late-phase plasma exudation after toluene diisocyanate exposure, Erjefält and Persson (1989) observed that the airway wall-to-lumen ratio of fibrinogen concentrations was larger than that for albumin. This finding may be due to a greater size selectivity of the epithelial compared to the vascular barrier during sustained exudative responses. It is perhaps more likely, however, that fibrin formation in the inflamed airway tissue hindered the passage of fibrinogen across the epithelial lining.

Electrical charge is another determinant of the ability of macromolecules to pass a variety of barriers in the airways (endothelial and epithelial cell linings and their basement membranes). Fluorescein-labeled dextran macromolecules (FITC-D) of 70,000 of 156,000 daltons have less charge than the native proteins, and despite its greater size, FITC-D 156,000 passes the mucosal barrier more readily than albumin (Persson and Erjefält, 1986; Erjefält and Persson, 1989). Again, these data support the notion of an unfiltered flow of plasma exudate into the airway lumen.

C. The Blood Pool

The measurement of plasma exudation in tissue samples requires the intravascular plasma content of the tracer to be known so that it can be subtracted from the total to give the extravascular amount. The blood pool of tissue samples can be quantitated by various techniques so that its total tissue plasma content can be reduced (Erjefält et al., 1985). It has been claimed that by flushing saline through the aorta (and the pulmonary artery) the airway tissue blood pool is readily eliminated (Sheppard et al., 1986; Lundberg and Saria, 1983; Boschetto et al., 1989). This is not well supported by actual data. It is, in fact, not possible to wash out more than about half the blood pool of the airway microvessels with these flushing techniques (Erjefält and Persson, 1991a). Measurements of the remaining blood pool would be particularly important under inflammatory conditions when more blood may be trapped in newly recruited and dilated microvessels. Recent work from Widdicombe's laboratory has demonstrated the presence of large venous sinuses in the submucosa of tracheobronchial tissue obtained from animals and humans. This intriguing finding makes the blood pool measurements even more important.

Observations of a consistently good correlation between the content of plasma exudate in the airway tissue and the airway lumen, respectively (see Fig. 2) (Erjefält and Persson, 1989), indicate that the problem of variations in the blood pool can be circumvented by sampling and assaying the airway mucosal surface material as indicated subsequently.

D. Mucosal Surface Liquids

Sputum analyses have provided information on plasma exudation in asthmatic and bronchitic patients but can only be employed in patients who regularly produce sputum.

Bronchoalveolar lavage retrieves alveolar lining fluid to an unknown extent, and the alveolar fluid may be up to 100 times as large as the airway fluid component (Reynolds, 1987). There are other limitations to bronchoalveolar lavages, including exudates due to trauma, the necessity of using premedications, large and unknown variabilities in total and lavaged mucosal surface areas, and risks to the patient, raising ethical problems. Interestingly, considering that the alveolar is so much larger than the bronchial surface, Lam et al. (1985) observed no difference between normal and asthmatic subjects in the plasma protein content of bronchoalveolar lavage fluids, whereas in material sampled by a small-volume lavage of a main bronchus, asthmatic patients had 10-fold greater levels of plasma proteins than nonasthmatic subjects.

In animal tracheal and nasal and human nasal airways, absorbing disks of filter paper are being used both to expose a defined surface area to mediators or allergens and to sample its liquids. However, fluid and solutes extracted from airway tissue rather than surface liquids are probably sampled by these disks (Erjefält and Persson, 1990).

By carrying out nontraumatic retrograde lavage of the trachea from an adjoining main bronchus after sacrifice, a defined large airway surface liquid has been sampled after in vivo provocation (Fig. 3) (Persson and Erjefält, 1986; Erjefält and Persson, 1989). It has thus been possible to correlate the amount of exuded plasma in the airway lumen with that in the underlying tissue. The data suggest that the plasma tracer components of the surface liquids faithfully reflect the mucosal and submucosal inflammatory plasma exudation process, its intensity, and time course (Persson and Erjefält, 1986; Erjefält and Persson, 1989).

E. Guinea Pig Tracheobronchial Superfusions

Erjefält et al. (1985) developed a technique whereby the mucosal surface of the large tracheobronchial airways in guinea pigs can be exposed to various concentrations of mediators, tracers, and drugs. A small catheter is introduced orally and positioned in the tracheal lumen at about the level of the cricoid cartilage. The catheterization is carried out without surgery, and measurements in catheterized and noncatheterized airways show that the method does not cause a disturbance of the baseline levels of plasma tracers (Erjefält et al., 1985; Persson et al., 1986). Since plasma exudation into the airway lumen occurs at the slightest provocation (for example just by touching the mucosa) these findings suggest that the procedure is nontraumatic. The intratracheal catheter is used for the administration of inflammatory factors (such as mediators, allergen, and occupational agents) to specifically provoke the mucosa of the tracheobronchial airways. Clearly, only small volumes of liquid can be introduced through the catheter without causing effects on breathing or producing foam in the airways. By infusion at a low rate (0.02 ml/min) for 2–10 min (occasionally for 30 min), these problems have been largely avoided. Potent provocations cause breathing difficulties due to both bronchoconstrictor effects and effects on volume and composition of the airway surface liquids. In the latter instances the small infusion volume per se is only a small contributory factor (Fig. 3).

A major asset of the present technique is the specific distribution of the superfusate on tracheobronchial mucosal surfaces, sparing the bronchoalveolar region (beyond the fifth generation of bronchi). This selective distribution has been determined by analyses of superfused tracer macromolecules in postsacrifice samples of tissue (Erjefält and Persson, 1991b). It has been confirmed by gamma camera recordings obtained in vivo during and after superfusion of fluid containing ^{99m}Tc-DTPA (Greiff et al., 1990a). The latter technique has also demonstrated that mucociliary transport does not move the superfused liquid away from the tracheobronchial area. A most significant finding is that applied inflammatory stimuli do not appreciably alter the distribution of material infused through the tracheal catheter (Erjefält and Persson, 1991b).

The technique is also well suited for studies of absorption of luminal material, under control conditions as well as during plasma exudation processes. It allows the deposition of absorption tracers specifically on to the tracheobronchial mucosa. This cannot be accomplished by inhalation procedures because the material is then also deposited in the bronchoalveolar region. Furthermore, by coadministration in the tracheal superfusate one can be certain of an equal airway distribution of both the tracer for absorption and the inflammatory factor. By taking advantage of these possibilities, Erjefält and Persson (1991b) and Greiff et al. (1991b) have now demonstrated that absorption of both small and large solutes is not altered by the plasma exudation process induced by mediators and allergen. This distinction between inward and outward airway mucosal permeabilities is also seen in human nasal airways (Greiff et al., 1991a). The one-way traffic aspect of airway plasma exudation is an important consideration in discussions of the role of this process in health and disease. Absorption versus exudation across the airway mucosa is treated in more detail elsewhere (Persson et al., 1991).

The local superfusion technique can be combined with the introduction into the tracheal lumen of a probe for measurement of mucosal blood flow by

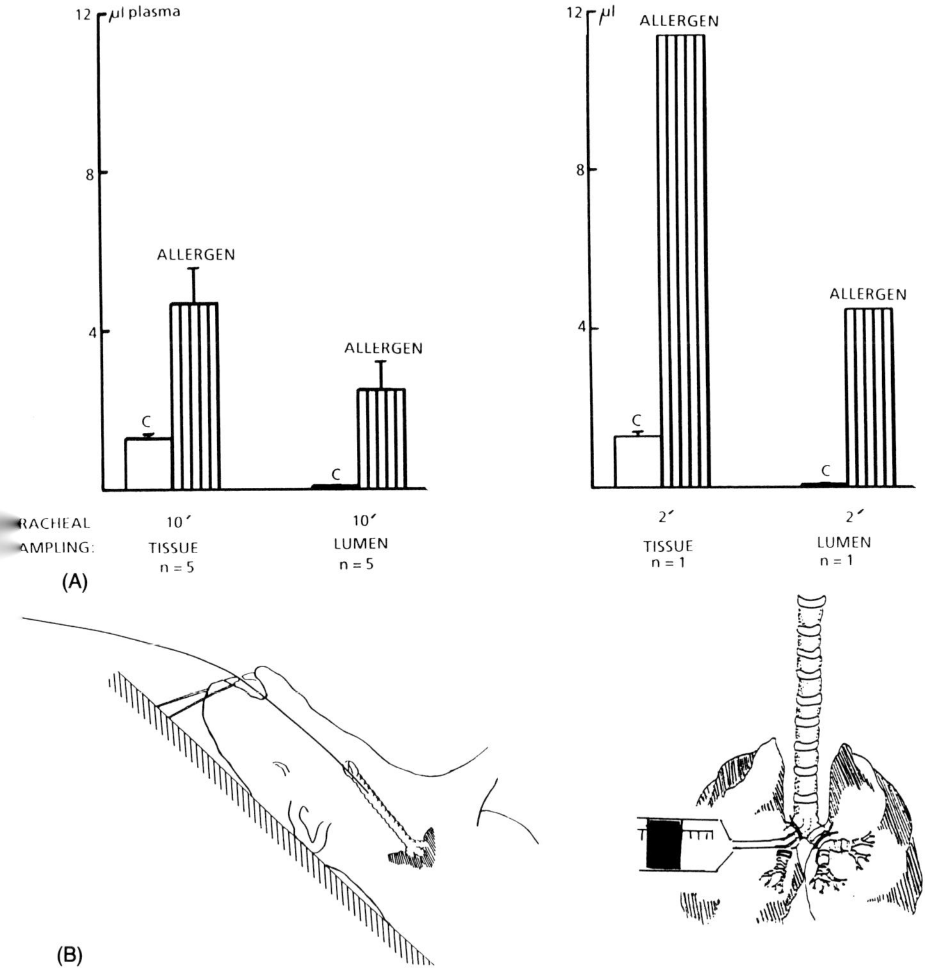

(A)

(B)

Figure 3 (A) Allergen challenge-induced airway plasma exudation responses in tracheobronchial airways of guinea pigs previously sensitized to produce IgE antibodies. Within 10 min after the provocation, plasma is exuded into airway tissue and lumen (left). In one animal (right) that reacted strongly to the allergen, a very pronounced exudation response was evident within 2 min after exposure (C, background control values). On the ordinate is μl plasma determined in 50 mg airway tissue (TISSUE) or in fluid recovered after lavaging the lower portion of the trachea (LUMEN). (B) Guinea pig tracheobronchial superfusion. (Left) A thin catheter, passed through the mouth and down the trachea to the level of the cricoid cartilage, is used to infuse small volumes of agents and tracers. (Right) Retrograde lavage of the trachea from a main bronchus after sacrifice following in vivo provocation.

the laser Doppler method (Erjefält and Persson, 1991a). Such measurements are of interest because in theory blood flow may affect the plasma exudation response. Probably because the airway mucosa and submucosa are so well perfused with blood (Parsons et al., 1985), moderate changes in blood flow seem to have little effect on the plasma exudation process (Erjefält and Persson, 1991a; Svensson et al., 1990). Topical application of large doses of epinephrine on cat tracheal microvessels, however stopped both blood flow and inflammatory stimulus-induced plasma exudation (Erjefält and Persson, 1982). However, the conditions of this latter experiment may be considered extreme and grossly abnormal.

IV. Inducers of Plasma Exudation

By superfusing the airway mucosa with minute volumes of fluid with or without "active" solutes for various periods of time, the influence of different concentrations of mediators, drugs, and other factors on airway surface liquids has been examined. It seems important to use local application of inflammatory agents. Given systemically, they may produce severe extraairway effects that indirectly influence airway responses (Erjefält and Persson, 1989).

A. Effects of Cellular Mediators

As evidenced by the prompt vascular response to a topically applied mediator, penetration across the epithelial lining to the subepithelial microvessels is readily achieved with small molecules. It does not seem to matter whether the mediator is a peptide, amine, or phospholipid product. However, details of how the epithelial penetration of these agents occur remain unknown. One can assume that luminal-to-subepithelial concentration gradients may vary greatly depending on the physicochemical properties of the mediator. With allergens and certain mediators, indirect mechanisms are involved. Inflammatory cells on or in the mucosa, or the epithelial cells themselves, are the first targets of these agents. This interaction results in the cellular production and release of inflammatory mediators that reach the subepithelial microvessels, where plasma exudation is induced (Fig. 2).

The endothelial cells of postcapillary venules harbor receptors for mediators, hormones, and drugs that control the leakiness of the venular wall (Grega et al., 1988). Through direct effects the endothelial cells are made to separate and close, respectively, by exudative and antiexudative agents. These effects can be prevented by drugs that are specific pharmacological antagonists to the active agents at the cell surface receptor level.

In my own work with Ingrid Erjefält and others, a selection of inflammatory factors has been examined. Histaminic mediators, including bradykinin and leukotrienes, have been studied because their effects may give a generally valid picture of the acute plasma exudation response. They may also be involved in disease processes in the airways, after being released, by the effect on inflammatory cells of allergens or other factors (see Fig. 2).

We have examined the effects of allergens and capsaicin, the latter substance a neurogenic stimulus that exerts exudative effects, particularly in the airways of guinea pigs and rats. We have also looked for provocations that produce more sustained exudative responses, thinking that this would be more relevant to chronic disease conditions. Toluene diisocyanate (TDI) seems to have these "desirable" properties. TDI is also of interest because it may be the most common culprit in causing occupational asthma among workers in the paint and plastic industries.

Cellular mediators, such as histamine, leukotrienes C_4 and D_4, and platelet activating factor (PAF), produced prompt and dose-dependent plasma exudation into guinea pig tracheobronchial airways tissue and lumen (Persson et al., 1986, 1987, Erjefält and Persson, 1989). The present mucosal superfusion technique showed that the leukotrienes were 50 or more times more potent than suggested by other techniques for local application of mediators to the guinea pig trachea (Persson et al., 1986; Woodward et al., 1983).

The plasma exudation response is induced within 1 or 2 min of provocation (Fig. 3), and with the histaminic mediators the duration of the response is normally very brief. The whole exudation process may be over within 5–15 min. The transient nature of the process is also evident when the active concentration of a mediator applied to the airway mucosa is maintained for prolonged periods of time (Greiff et al., 1990b). Human nasal airway studies have demonstrated that the histamine-induced plasma exudation response is fully reversible in the sense that a second and a third provocation carried out at 30 min intervals produced the same exudative effect (Svensson et al., 1989).

PAF produced not only an immediate response in guinea pig tracheobronchial airways but also, after a decline in the exudation, a second peak of plasma exudation at 5 h (Persson et al., 1987; Erjefält and Persson, 1989). The mechanism involved in the development of the PAF-induced late-phase exudative effect is not known. Both the immediate and the late-phase responses were inhibited by a PAF antagonist given to the animals before the PAF. Similarly, the late-phase response is inhibited by giving a short-acting xanthine derivative, enprofylline, before PAF (O'Donnell et al., 1990). The short-lived nature of PAF itself, together with the pharmacology of the inhibitory drugs, suggests that the late exudative phase is secondary to events induced immediately by the PAF. Even more sustained late-phase exudation responses are seen after allergen and low-molecular-weight chemical "sensitizers," such as TDI (see later).

Other cellular mediators, such as prostaglandins, may also produce airway plasma exudation. LTB_4 was not effective, however (Persson et al., 1986). Adenosine is both a cellular and a neural mediator. No exudative effect was detected after superfusing guinea pig airways with adenosine (unpublished observations by Erjefält, Lundblad, and Persson).

B. Neural Actions

The cholinergic transmitter substance acetylcholine and its analogs are without plasma exudation effects in the airways. Near lethal bronchoconstricting doses of carbachol were associated with only marginal increases in plasma tracers in superfused guinea pig airways (Erjefält and Persson 1989), and part of the small amount of [^{131}I]albumin that appeared on the mucosal surface may in fact have been the result of a carbachol-induced secretory response (Webber and Widdicombe, 1989).

The airways also contain peptidergic nerves (Lundberg and Saria, 1983; Karlsson and Persson, 1989). Of these, the tachykinin nerves have been implicated in plasma exudation responses. In 1981, Erjefält et al. originally reported that the "prototype" tachykinin undecapeptide, substance P, increased the intravascularly administered Evans blue dye content of airway tissue. In this study in cat trachea as well as in many of the later studies in rodent airways (Lundberg and Saria, 1983), changes in the blood pool were not examined. Actual assessment of neurogeinc extravasation and exudation in rodent airways was done by Erjefält and coworkers (see below). McDonald (1988a, b) used particulate monastral blue to show the leaky sites in the airway microvasculature. Lundberg and Saria (1983) reported that the airway tissue became diffusely fluorescent with protein-bound Evans blue dye. Using fluorescence and electron microscopy, Sundler and coworkers (Persson et al., 1987; Luts et al., 1990) demonstrated the distribution of extravasated fluorescein-isothiocyanate–labeled dextrans (MW 150,000) in the lamina propria and on the surface of the airway mucosa after topical provocation with capsaicin.

The stimulation of tachykinergic nerves with capsaicin produces exudation of different plasma tracers into the airway interstitium and lumen as a very consistent response in guinea pig superfusion experiments (Persson et al., 1985, 1986; Persson and Erjefält, 1988; Erjefält and Persson, 1989). Also, tachykinin antagonists given locally in doses several times below those required by the intravenous route inhibited the neurogenic plasma exudation response in guinea pig airways (Persson et al., 1985). It has been claimed that several types of airway provocation in guinea pigs are in part mediated through tachykinin innervation. Topical tachykinin antagonism was without effect on the plasma exudation induced by superfusion of histamine (Persson et al., 1985), however, and similarly, local anesthesia, which prevented the effect of capsaicin, did not reduce the exudative action of bradykinin or allergen (Erjefält and Persson, 1991a). These findings agree with observations in human airways in which allergen, bradykinin, and histamine induce plasma exudation but tachykinin-mediated vascular permeability responses have not been demonstrated. Indeed, in human airways both substance P and capsaicin seem to be without plasma exudation effects (Malm and Petersson, 1985; Bascom et al., 1988).

The β_2-agonist, terbutaline, increased the airway tissue blood pool, whereas at the same time it attenuated the neurogenic and other mediator-induced plasma exudation (Persson et al., 1986). Further, terbutaline dose dependently reduced capsaicin-, bradykinin-, and histamine-induced plasma exudation into the lumen of guinea pig trachea (Erjefält and Persson, 1991a). Terbutaline exerted this antiexudative action despite the fact that concomitantly it increased the mucosal-submucosal blood flow (Erjefält and Perrson, 1991a).

This β-agonist drug-induced effect could have an endogenous counterpart in the effects of released epinephrine. Thus epinephrine, released or given systemically, has antiexudative effects through activation of β-adrenoceptors (Persson et al., 1982). Grega et al., (1980) demonstrated that vasoactive and inflammatory mediators, such as bradykinin and histamine, must be given locally to produce plasma exudation in canine forelimbs. If given systemically these mediators reduce blood pressure and release epinephrine, which, through activation of β-receptors, inhibits the plasma exudation.

C. Allergic and Occupational Agents

In guinea pigs sensitized to produce IgE antibodies, allergen provocations produce an immediate plasma exudation response that appears to correlate well with the intensity of the allergic reaction. In strongly responding animals, plasma exudation is profuse within 2 min. of provocation (Fig. 3). The late-phase reaction after allergen provocation is associated with significant plasma exudation. Glucocorticoid (budesonide) treatment inhibits both the late exudation and obstructive effects (Andersson and Persson, 1988).

TDI is a major causative agent in occupational asthma. Two unsaturated isothiocyanate groups make TDI a highly reactive chemical capable of producing complex inflammatory effects on the airway mucosa. When superfused in minute amounts (0.003–0.03 μl), TDI produced dose-dependent and very sustained plasma exudation into the tracheobronchial lumen of guinea pigs (Erjefält and Persson, 1989). In airways previously exposed twice to TDI, as little as 0.3 nl TDI produced an exudative inflammation that lasted longer than 17 h (Erjefält and Perrson, 1992). TDI was dissolved in olive oil in a concentration of 10^{-8} M, and far lower concentrations than this would be present in the airway tissue in these experiments. The maximally allowed exposure of workers to TDI is 15 μg/kg per workday (maximal inhaled dose).

V. Tracheobronchial Plasma Exudation as a Primary Mucosal Defense

That the airway epithelium is considered a tight barrier severely restricting the traffic or macromolecules has probably been a significant obstacle for any thought of plasma exudation as a primary defense reaction. The prevailing view has been that frank destruction of the epithelial lining is required to allow exuded plasma to enter the airway lumen. Plasma exudation is therefore not treated as a primary mechanism in current textbooks on mucosal and respiratory defense mechanisms, if it is mentioned at all in this literature. However, the restriction of a tight epithelial lining is not valid for exudation processes (Persson, 1989c, 1991) that occur in the opposite direction to mucosal absorption from the lumen.

The amount of plasma exudate that reached the mucosal surface 10 min or less after an inflammatory provocation of guinea pig tracheobronchial airways could be more than the calculated periciliary fluid volume (Persson and Erjefält, 1986). Furthermore, the epithelium appeared histologically intact after such a provocation (Persson et al., 1987; Luts et al., 1990). Erjefält and Persson (1989, 1991b) and Greiff et al. (1991b) observed that large and small tracers, present in the airway lumen during mediator- or allergen-induced plasma exudation, were absorbed at an unchanged rate compared with normal control conditions. This unidirectional passage of plasma exudate into the lumen could not be a secretory process, because a variety of nonsecreted plasma tracers, including fluorescein-labeled dextrans (70,000 and 156,000 dalton) and fibrinogen, concomitantly entered the lumen during the exudation. Indeed, a persistent passage of plasma tracers into the lumen with different kinds and doses of inflammatory mediators, together with the unidirectional route, suggested the following possible mechanism (see Fig. 2).

It was hypothesized that the plasma exudate in the tissue constitutes an osmotic and mechanical pressure force from beneath whereby epithelial cells transiently separate, allowing the luminal entry of exudate along a hydrostatic pressure gradient (Persson, 1989c; Erjefält and Persson, 1989). This hypothesis was tested in an isolated preparation of the guinea pig trachea in which hydrostatic pressure differences between serosal and mucosal sides could be regulated. Only a slight increase in serosal hydrostatic pressure (5 cmH_2O) was required to cause a significant flow of a macromolecular solute (dextran, 70,000 daltons) from the serosal to the mucosal surface in these isolated airways (Fig. 4) (Persson et al., 1990). As with the mucosal crossing of plasma in vivo, the in vitro response was reversible and repeatable. The presence of bradykinin, histamine, or carbachol on the luminal surface of the in vitro preparations did not increase the pressure-induced epithelial passage of macromolecules from the serosa, nor did terbutaline reduce it, suggesting that the action of mediators and drugs on epithelial cells may not be a significant part of this process. From histology and measurements of the release of lactate dehydrogenase, it appeared that the isolated and pressure-exposed tracheal mucosa remained normally viable during the course of these in vitro experiments (Persson et al., 1990).

The hydrostatic pressure-induced mucosal crossing of macromolecules in vitro was not associated with an increased absorption permeability of the mucosa (Gustafsson and Persson, 1991). Hence, both in vitro and in vivo the luminal entry of exudate was a unidirectional process. These observations are consistent with electron microscopy findings (Luts et al., 1990) and suggest that functional epithelial tight junctions are reassembled immediately after the passage of the exudate. It was concluded that airway exudation is an integrated respiratory defense mechanism of the mucosa and the subepithelial microcirculation.

VI. Exudation and Hypersecretion as Distinct Processes

Asthma and chronic bronchitis are both characterized as inflammatory airway diseases with hypersecretion (Pride, 1987) or, rather, hypersecretion and hyperexudation (Persson, 1988a, b) as one of the significant disturbances. Airway epithelial and glandular secretory processes have been examined extensively for many years. Several excellent reviews describe the recent progress in the neural control, structural and molecular biology aspects, and the pharmacology of airway secretions (Lopez-Vidreiro and Reid, 1978; Sturgess, 1984; Nadel and Holtzmann, 1984; Kaliner et al., 1986; Marin, 1986; Richardson and Peatfield, 1987; Basbaum et al., 1988). The role of inflammation in hypersecretion has been particularly addressed. Despite a vast literature on the subject, the role of bronchial secretions in the pathogenesis of asthma has been difficult to define.

Sputum production is elevated, especially in severe asthma (Salter, 1868; Turner-Warwick and Openshaw, 1987). Clinical improvement is associated with a reduced sputum production, in particular during treatment with antiinflammatory drugs, including glucocorticoids, cromoglycate, and terbutaline (Bordley et al., 1949; Keal, 1971; Heilpern and Rebuck, 1972; Sadoul et al., 1981; Moretti et al., 1984; Turner-Warwick and Openshaw, 1987). A con-

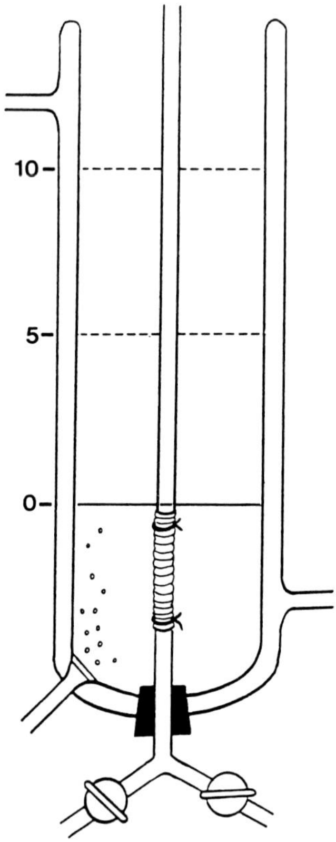

(A)

Figure 4 (A) Guinea pig tracheal preparation to set hydrostatic pressure differences between serosal and mucosal sides. (B) Unidirectional passage of FITC dextran (70,000 daltons) from serosal to mucosal side of isolated tracheal preparation showing effect of slight increase in serosal hydostatic pressure (upper figure = 5 cmH_2O; lower figure = 10 cmH_2O) in increasing flow. Ordinate = FITC dextran (arbitrary units).

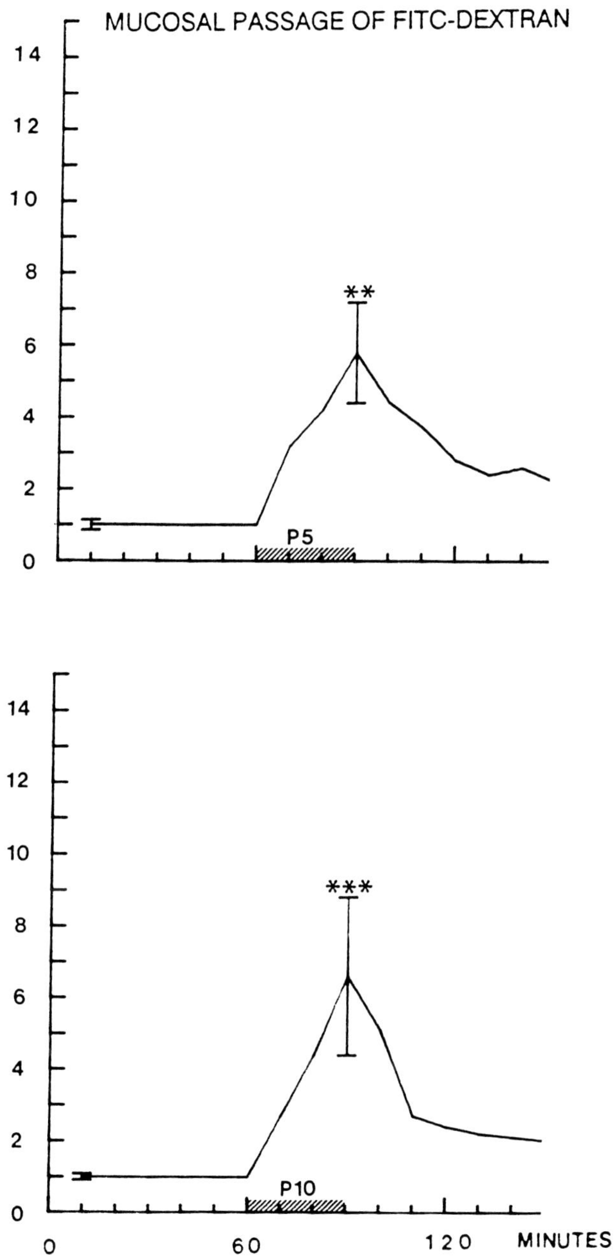
MUCOSAL PASSAGE OF FITC-DEXTRAN
14
12
10
8
6
4
2
0
**
P5
14
12
10
8
6
4
2
0
***
P10
0
60
120
MINUTES

(B)

sistent effect seems to be a reduction in the plasma exudate component of the sputum. Keal (1971) looked for changes in chemical tracers to indicate secretion during the glucocorticoid-induced reduction in sputum volumes in asthma. No reduction but, in contrast, an increase in the sputum concentration of secretory tracers was observed, and Keal (1971) suggested that the effect of steroid therapy "lies in the reduction of transudate rather than any change in mucosal gland secretion." This inference was later supported by data reported by Moretti et al. (1984), who analyzed a variety of markers of secretion and plasma proteins in sputum from 19 subjects with asthmatic bronchitis. Thus 2 weeks of glucocorticoid treatment reduced albumin levels to one-fifth of starting values, but the levels of fucose and *N*-acetylneuraminic acid remained virtually unchanged. No information was provided on changes in sputum volumes (Moretti et al., 1984).

In human airways in vitro, the presence of glucocorticoids has only marginal effects on mucus secretion induced by histamine and 5-monohydroxyeicosatetraenoic acid (Maron et al., 1985). On the other hand, there is abundant experimental support for the antiplasma leakage effects of antiasthma drugs, in particular the glucocorticoids (Persson, 1988a; Andersson and Persson, 1988). Serum has been demonstrated to be a potent stimulus of airways glycoprotein secretion (Richardson and Peatfield, 1987). Hence, a glucocorticoid-induced reduction in vivo of mucus secretion may be secondary to inhibition of plasma exudation.

The possibility of a pathogenic role in asthma for the component of airway "hypersecretion" that by definition, is not a secretion but a plasma exudate is thus supported by the composition of airway liquids in asthma and by the effects of clinically effective drugs on that composition.

If the concentration of albumin in asthmatic and bronchitic sputum represented only undiluted plasma exudate, this volume would constitute less than 10% of the sputum volume (Brogan et al., 1971; Honda et al., 1988). Besides grandular secretion, however, a large volume of fluid from vessels and tissue is likely to result from the exuded plasma. For example, the inflammatory break down of extravasated proteins increases the number of small molecules and, hence, increases interstitial osmotic pressure, which attracts fluid from the vessels. A more diluted exudate may therefore become a major component of airway luminal liquids in inflammatory airway diseases. Unfortunately, the volume and composition of tracheobronchial lining fluid cannot be determined easily.

It is thought that under normal baseline conditions plasma proteins up to a molecular weight of 300,000 daltons slowly diffuse into the airway lumen (Reynolds, 1987). Thus, native albumin in sputum and lavage samples would have accumulated on the mucosal surface for an unknown period of time.

Based on in vitro observations, it has been claimed that albumin also enters by mucosal secretory processes (Webber and Widdicombe, 1989). When there is plasma exudation as a defense or an inflammatory reaction, however, the amount of secreted albumin is probably negligible in comparison with what has been exuded. This view is supported by animal and human data. In the guinea pig tracheobronchial airways, provocation-induced exudation of "plasma" into the lumen appears equally large or even larger when a non-secreted molecule, such as FITC dextran 150,000, is used as a plasma tracer and compared with albumin. Such drugs as β_2-agonists have been demonstrated to reduce the exudation of albumin and infused dextran (Persson et al., 1986; Erjefält and Persson, 1991b), although they increase the secretion of albumin (Webber and Widdicombe, 1989). Carbachol also increases the secretion of albumin in vitro (Webber and Widdicombe, 1989). However, the amount of albumin appearing on the mucosal surface in vivo in response to near lethal doses of carbachol is trivial and barely significant; it cannot be compared with the albumin that is exuded into the airway lumen after inflammatory provocation (Erjefält and Persson, 1989). Also, large doses of methacholine (25 mg) produced only a small "secretion" of albumin in human nasal airways (Raphael et al., 1988).

Human nasal mucosa responds to moderate doses of histaminc with significant, reproducible exudations of albumin, fibrinogen, and TAME-esterase activity (α_2-macroglobulin) (Svensson et al., 1989). Of importance is that the ratio between albumin and fibrinogen in the mucosal surface exudate was about the same as that in the blood (unpublished work by Alkner, Persson, Pipkorn, and Svensson), demonstrating that there is probably a bulk exudation of plasma proteins across the vascular-mucosal barriers of human airways. Raphael et al. (1989) confirmed the nonsecretory nature of the albumin that appears in nasal washings after histamine provocation and demonstrated that even at very large histamine doses (10 mg) the secreted amount of albumin is marginal.

Albumin levels in sputum and bronchial lavage liquids in asthma and bronchitis are elevated along with IgG and a variety of other plasma proteins (Ryley and Brogan, 1973; Stockley et al., 1979; Moretti et al., 1984). Since the epithelial barrier has been widely considered a tight and size-selective barrier, attempts have been made to make the data fit into such restricted diffusion characteristics in which mucosal surface concentrations of plasma proteins should be inversely related to their molecular sizes. When a larger molecule, such as IgG (150,000 daltons); appeared with a sputum-serum ratio that was the same as that for albumin (67,000 daltons) either this caused only confusion or it was taken as evidence for the local production of IgG (Ryley and Brogan, 1973; Stockley et al., 1979). Even during exacerbations of airway diseases, this size-dependent analysis was attempted despite that the actual data on a variety of proteins from albumin to α_2-macroglobulin (900,000 daltons) gave ratios in the sputum that were not far from those in the plasma (Stockley et al., 1979). It seems much more likely that, after laboratory and natural provocations, there is a bulk exudation of plasma into the airway tissue and lumen as described earlier.

VII. Conclusion

As an airways defense mechanism, plasma exudation has several important characteristics. It is induced promptly and at mild to moderate stimuli. It is a brief process, because the spontaneous closure of the vascular exudation sites is very effectively carried out even in the presence of active mediator concentrations. A major asset of this defense is the swift passage of the plasma exudate into the airway lumen, occurring without damage to the epithelial lining and without making this barrier abnormally permeable to the absorption of solutes present on the airway mucosal surface. Hence, a primary defense is carried out by a small burst of multipotent plasma protein systems immediately appearing on the mucosal site where the insult takes place. This dramatic but localized change is fully reversible, and the process is compatible with the view that the epithelial lining is a tight barrier that poorly absorbs macromolecules. When the insult to the airways is of a more severe nature, as is the case with TDI, plasma exudation is more sustained. Even so, the response may be reversible and the epithelial lining may remain largely intact (Persson et al., 1992).

The volume of "unchanged plasma" that is cleared into the airway lumen can be calculated based on the luminal content of specific macromolecular plasma tracers. However, actual exuded plasma, through activation and breakdown of its numerous protein systems is expected to increase its content of solutes severalfold. To an as yet unknown extent, the exudate that reaches the lumen attracts a much larger volume of fluid than that corresponding to the original plasma volume. In normal, localized defense reactions the luminal appearance of the plasma exudate or transudate may not cause problems but be cleared by mucociliary transport and coughing. The increased amount of plasma fluid exudate may not only be protective but also aid in the conditioning of inhaled cold dry air when the demand is high during the hyperpnea of exercise.

In asthma, plasma exudation is probably pathogenetical in several ways. The abundant venular system beneath the epithelial lining may not only be a large fluid reservoir but also a giant source of inflammatory mediators for "release" after a variety of mucosal provocations. Besides physical effects as increased amounts and altered properties of luminal material, the plasma exudate thus releases all kinds of potent agents, such as kinins, complement fragments, and coagulation, fibrinolysis, and other peptides. The pathophysiology of the plasma exudate and its pharmacology suggest that the significant "hypersecretion" in asthma is not only a secretion but largely a plasma exudate. In asthma and other inflammatory airways diseases, exuded plasma in the wall and the lumen could potentially contribute to both the physical and the physiological abnormalities.

References

Adams, F. (1938). Works of Hippocrates. *Med. Classics* **3**:1–380.

Andersson, P. T., and Persson, C. G. A. (1988). Developments in anti-asthma glucocorticoids. In *Directions for New Antiasthma Drugs.* Edited by S. R. O'Donnell and C. G. A. Persson, Basel, Birkäuser, pp. 239–260.

Arnold, J. (1875). Ueber das Verhalten der Wandrungen der Blutgefässe bei der Emigration weisser Blutkörper. *Virchows Arch.* [*A*] **62**:487–503.

Basbaum, C., Carlson, D., Davidson, E., Verdugo, P., and Gail, D. G. (1988). Cellular mechanisms of airway secretion. *Am. Rev. Respir. Dis.* **137**:479–485.

Bascom, R., Green, S., Kagey-Sobotka, A., and Proud, D. (1988). Effect of intranasal capsaicin on symptoms and mediator release. *Am. Rev. Respir. Dis.* **137**:375.

Baumgarten, C. R., Nichols, R. C., Naclerio, R. M., Lichtenstein, L. M., Norman, P. S., and Proud, D. (1986). Plasma kallikrein during experimentally induced allergic rhinitis: Role in kinin formation and contribution to tame-esterase activity in nasal secretions. *J. Immunol.* **137**:977–982.

Bordley, J. E., Carey, R. A., Harvey, A. M., Howard, J. E., Kattus, A. A., Newman, E. V., and Winkenwerder, W. L. (1949). Preliminary observations on the effect of adenocorticosteroid hormone (ACTH) in allergic disease. *Bull. Johns Hopkins Hosp.* **85**:396–398.

Boschetto, P., Roberts, N. M., Rogers, D. F., and Barnes, P. J. (1989). Effect of anti-asthma drugs on microvascular leakage in guinea-pig airways. *Am. Rev. Respir. Dis.* **139**:416–421.

Brogan, T. D., Ryley, H. C., Neale, L., and Yassa, J. (1975). Soluble proteins of bronchopulmonary secretions from patients with cystic fibrosis, asthma, and bronchitis. *Thorax* **30**:72–79.

Cohnheim, J. (1882). *Vorlesungen ueber allgemeine Pathologie I.* Berlin, August Hirschwald, pp. 232–367.

Curschmann, H. (1883). Ueber Bronchiolitis exsudativa and ihr Verhaltniss zum Asthma nervosum. *Deutsch Arch. Klin. Med.* **32**:1–34.

Dunnill, M. S., Massarella, G. R., and Anderson, J. A. (1969). A comparison of the quantitative anatomy of the bronchi in normal subjects, in status asthmaticus in chronic bronchitis, and in emphysema. *Thorax* **24**:176–179.

Erjefält, I., and Persson, C. G. A. (1982). Effects of adrenaline and terbutaline on mediator-increased vascular permeability in the cat trachea. *Br. J. Pharmacol.* **77**:399P.

Erjefält, I., and Persson, C. G. A. (1989). Inflammatory passage of plasma macromolecules into airway tissue and lumen. *Pulm. Pharmacol.* **2**:93–102.

Erjefält, I., and Persson, C. G. A. (1990). On the use of absorbing discs to sample airway surface liquids. *Clin. Exp. Allergy* **20**:193–197.

Erjefält, I., and Persson, C. G. A. (1991a). Pharmacological control of plasma exudation in guinea-pig lower airways. *Am. Rev. Respir. Dis.* **143**:1008–1014.

Erjefält, I., and Persson, C. G. A. (1991b). Plasma exudation into the airway lumen in a "one-way traffic." Effects of topical provocations on absorption and exudation across the mucosa in guinea-pig tracheobronchial airways. *Clin. Exp. Allergy.* **21**:217–224.

Erjefält, I., and Persson, C. G. A. (1992). Increased airways sensitivity to toluene-diisocyanate and effects of xanthines and a glucocorticoid. *Clin. Exp. Allergy.*

Erjefält, I., Persson, C. G. A., and Saldeen, T. (1981). Effects of fibrinopeptides and substance P on airway plasma. *Acta Soc. Med. Suec. Hyg.* **90**:RÄ 3P.

Erjefält, I. A. L., G.-Wagner, Z., Strand, S. E., and Persson C. G. A. (1985). A method for studies of tracheobronchial microvascular permeability to macromolecules. *J. Pharmacol. Methods* **14**:275–283.

Florey, H. W. (1970). *General Pathology*, 4th ed. London, Lloyd-Luke.

Florey, H., Carleton, H. M., and Wells, A. Q. (1932). Mucus secretion in the trachea. *Br. J. Exp. Pathol.* **13**:269–284.

Grega, G. J., Maciejco, J. J., Raymond, R. M., and Sak, P. D. (1980). The interrelationship among histamine, various vasoactive substances, and macromolecular permeability in the canine forelimb. *Circ. Res.* **46**:264–275.

Grega, G. J., Persson, C. G. A., and Svensjö, E. (1988). Endothelial cell reactions to inflammatory mediators assessed in vivo by fluid and solute flux analysis. In: *Endothelial Cells.* Edited by U. S. Ryan, Boca Raton, FL, CRC Press, pp. 103–122.

Greiff, L., Wollmer, P., Erjefält, I., Pipkorn, U., and Persson, C. G. A. (1990a). Clearance of ^{99m}Tc-DTPA from guinea-pig nasal, tracheobronchial, and bronchoalveolar airways. *Thorax* **45**:881–885.

Greiff, L., Pipkorn, U., Alkner, U., and Persson, C. G. A. (1990b). The "nasal pool-device" applies controlled concentrations of solutes on human nasal airway mucosa and samples its surface exudations/ secretions. *Clin. Exp. Allergy* **20**:253–259.

Greiff, L., Wollmer, P., Pipkorn, U., and Persson, C. G. A. (1991a). Unaffected absorption of ^{51}Cr-EDTA during histamine-induced plasma exudation. *Thorax.* In press.

Greiff, L., Erjefält, I., Wollmer, P., Pipkorn, U., and Persson, C. G. A. (1991b). Different patterns of inflammatory effects on airway barriers: Plasma exudation with and without increased absorption of small or large luminal solutes. *Thorax.* In press.

Gustafsson, B., and Persson, C. G. A. (1991). Asymmetrical effects of hydrostatic pressure-induced movement of macromolecules across the airway mucosa. *Clin. Exp. Allergy,* **21**:121–126.

Heilpern, S., and Rebuck, A. S. (1972). Effect of disodium cromoglycate (Intal) on sputum protein composition. *Thorax* **27**:726–728.

Honda, I., Shimura, S., Sasaki, T., Sasaki, H., Takishima, T., and Nakamura, M. (1988). Airway mucosal permeability in chronic bronchitics and bronchial asthmatics with hypersecretion. *Am. Rev. Respir. Dis.* **137**:866–871.

Huber, H. L., and Koessler, K. K. (1922). The pathology of bronchial asthma. *Arch. Intern. Med.* **30**:689–760.

Hurley, J. V. (1983). *Acute Inflammation*, 2nd ed. Edinburgh, Churchill-Livingstone.

Ingelstedt, S., and Ivstam, B. (1949). The source of nasal secretion in infectious allergic and experimental conditions. *Acta Otolaryngol (Stock.)* **37**:451–456.

Kahn, M. H. (1928). Historical survey of our knoweldge of bronchial asthma. *Med. Life* **35**:108–162.

Kaliner, M., Shelhamer, J. H., Borson, B., Nadel, J., Patow, C., and Marom, Z. (1986). Human respiratory mucus. *Am. Rev. Respir. Dis.* **134**:612–621.

Karlsson, J. A., and Persson, C. G. A. (1989). Novel peripheral neurotransmitters and control of the airways. *Pharmacol. Ther.* **43**:397–423.

Keal, E. E. (1971). Biochemistry and rheology of sputum in asthma. *Postgrad. Med. J.* **47**:171–177.

Laitinen, L. A., Laitinen, A. and Widdicombe, J. G. (1987). Effects of inflammatory and other mediators on airway vascular beds. *Am. Rev. Respir. Dis.* **135**:567–570.

Lam, S., Leriche, J. C., Kijek, K., and Phillips, R. T. (1985). Effect of bronchial lavage volume on cellular and protein recovery. *Chest* **88**:856–859.

Lopes-Vidrerio, M. T., and Reid, L. (1978). Chemical markers of mucous and serum glycoproteins and their relation to viscosity in mucoid and purulent sputum from various hypersecretory diseases. *Am. Rev. Respir. Dis.* **117**:465–477.

Lower, R. (1672) *De Catarrhis*. Translated by R. Hunter and I. Macalpine. London, Dawsons, 1963.

Lundberg, J. M., and Saria, A. (1983). Capsaicin induced desensitization of the airway mucosa to cigarette smoke, mechanical and chemical irritants. *Nature* **302**:251–253.

Luts, A., Sundler, F., Erjefält, I., and Persson, C. G. A. (1990). The airway epithelial lining is intact promptly after the mucosal crossing of a large amount of plasma exudate. *Int. Arch. Allergy Appl. Immunol.* **91**:385–388.

Majno, G., and Palade, G. E. (1961). Studies on inflammation I. *J. Biophys. Biochem. Cytol.* **11**:571–605.

Malm, L., and Petersson, G. (1985). Tachykinins and nasal secretion. In *Tachykinin Antagonists*. Edited by R. Håknsson and F. Sundler. Amsterdam, Elsevier-North Holland.

Marin, M. G. (1986). Pharmacology of airway secretion. *Pharmacol. Rev.* **38**:273–289.

Maron, Z., Shelhamer, J., Alling, D., and Kaliner, M. (1984). The effects of corticosteroids on mucous glycoprotein secretion from human airways in vitro. *Am. Rev. Respir. Dis.* **129**:62–65.

McDonald, D. M. (1988a). Neurogenic inflammation in the trachea. I. Changes in venules, leukocytes, and epithelial cells. *J. Neurocytol.* **17**:583–603.

McDonald, D. M. (1988b). Respiratory tract infections increase susceptibility to neurogenic inflammation in the rat trachea. *Am. Rev. Respir. Dis.* **137**:1432–1440.

Miles, A. A., and Wilhelm, D. L. (1960). The activation of endogenous substances inducing pathological increases of capillary permeability. In *The Biochemical Response to Injury*. Edited by H. B. Stoner and C. J. Threlfall. Oxford, Blackwell, pp. 51–83.

Miller, W. S. (1947). *The Lung*. Springfield, IL, Charles C. Thomas, pp. 74–88.

Moretti, M., Giannico, G., Marchioni, C. F., and Bisetti, A. (1984). Effects of methylprednisolone on sputum biochemical components in asthmatic bronchitis. *Eur. J. Respir. Dis.* **65**:365–370.

Nadel, J. A., and Holtzmann, M. J. (1984). Regulation of airway responsiveness and secretion: role of inflammation. In *Asthma* Edited by A. B. Kay, K. F. Austen and L. M. Lichtenstein. London, Academic Press, pp. 129–153.

O'Donnell, S. R., Erjefält, I., and Persson, C. G. A. (1990). Early and late tracheobronchial plasma exudation to PAF administered to the airway mucosal surface in guinea pigs: Effects of WEB 2086 and enprofylline. *J. Pharmacol. Exp. Ther.* in press.

Parsons, G. H., Kramer, G. C., Link, D. P., Lantz, B. M. T., Gunther, R. A., Green, J. F., and Cross, C. E. (1985). Studies of reactivity and distribution of bronchial blood flow in sheep. *Chest* **87**:1805–1825.

Persson, C. G. A. (1986). Role of plasma exudation in asthmatic airways. *Lancet* **2**:1126–1129.

Persson, C. G. A. (1988a). Plasma exudation and asthma. *Lung* **166**:1–23.

Persson, C. G. A. (1988b). Sputum albumin in obstructive airways. *Am. Rev. Respir. Dis.* **138**:1646–1647.

Persson, C. G. A. (1989a). On the medical history of asthma and rhinitis. In *Rhinitis and Asthma. Similarities and Differences.* Edited by N. Mygind, U. Pipkorn and R. Dahl. Copenhagen, Munksgaard, pp. 9–20.

Persson, C. G. A. (1989b). Plasma leakage in inflamed airways. What glucocorticoids tell us about obstructive airway disease. In *Glucocorticoids and Mechanisms of Asthma*. Edited by F. E. Hargreave, J. C. Hogg, J.-L. Malo, and J. M. T. Toogood. Amsterdam, Excerpta Medica, pp. 232–242.

Persson, C. G. A. (1989c). Permeability changes in obstructive airway diseases. In *Bronchitis IV*. Edited by H. J. Sluiter and R. Van Der Lende. Assen, Van Gorcum, pp. 236–248.

Persson, C. G. A. (1991). Plasma exudation in the airways. Mechanisms and function. *Eur. Respir. J.* In press.

Persson, C. G. A., and Erjefält, I. (1986). Inflammatory leakage of macromolecules from the vascular compartment into the tracheal lumen. *Acta Physiol. Scand.* **126**:615–616.

Persson, C. G. A., and Pipkorn, U. (1989). Pathophysiology and pharmacology of asthma and rhinitis. In *Rhinitis and Asthma. Similarities and Differences*. Edited by N. Mygind, U. Pipkorn, and R. Dahl, Copenhagen, Munksgaard, pp. 275–288.

Persson, C. G. A., Erjefält, I., Grega, G. J., and Svensjö, E. (1982). The role of β-receptor agonists in the inhibition of pulmonary edema. In *Lung Microvascular Injury.* Edited by A. B. Malik and N. C. Staub, *Ann. N. Y. Acad. Sci.* **384**:544–557.

Persson, C. G. A., Erjefält, I., and Karlsson, J. A. (1985). Effects of tachykinins and tachykinin antagonists on the tracheobronchial microcirculation. In *Tachykinin Antagonists.* Edited by R. Håkanson and F. Sundler. Amsterdam, Elsevier–North Holland, pp. 171–179.

Persson, C. G. A., Erjefält, I., and Andersson, P. (1986). Leakage of macromolecules from guinea pig tracheobronchial microcirculation. Effects of allergen, leukotrienes, tachykinins, and anti-asthma drugs. *Acta Physiol. Scand.* **127**:95–106.

Persson, C. G. A., Erjefält, I., and Sundler, F. (1987). Airway microvascular and epithelial leakage of plasma induced by PAF-acether and capsaicin. *Am. Rev. Respir. Dis.* **135**:A401.

Persson, C. G. A., Erjefält, I., Gustafsson, B., and Luts, A. (1990b). Subepithelial hydrostatic pressure may regulate plasma exudation across the mucosa. *Int. Arch. Allergy Appl. Immunol.* in press.

Persson, C. G. A., Erjefält, I., Alkner, U., Baumgarten, C., Greiff, L., Gustafsson, B., Luts, A., Pipkorn, U., Svensson, C., and Wollmer, P. (1991). Plasma exudation as a first line mucosal defense. *Clin. Exp. Allergy* **21**:17–24.

Persson, C. G. A., Gustafsson, B., Luts, A., Sundler, F., and Erjefält, I. (1992). Toluene diisocyanate produces an increase in airway tone that outlasts the inflammatory exudation phase. *Clin. Exp. Allergy.* In press.

Pietra, G. G., Szidon, J. P., Leventhal, M. M., and Fishman, A. P. (1971). Histamine and interstitial pulmonary edema in the dog. *Circ. Res.* **29**:323–330.

Pietra, G. G., Szidon, J. P., Carpenter, H. A., and Fishman, A. P. (1974). Bronchial venular leakage during endotoxin shock. *Am. J. Pathol.* **77**:387–402.

Pride, N. B. (1987). Epidemiology of bronchial hypersecretion: recent studies. *Eur. J. Respir. Dis.* **71**(Suppl. 153):13–18.

Raphael, G., Druce, H., Baraniuk, J., and Kaliner, M. (1988). The pathophysiology of rhinitis. I. Assessment of the sources of protein in methacholine-induced nasal secretion. *Am. Rev. Respir. Dis.* **138**:413–420.

Raphael, G. D., Meredith, S. D., Baraniuk, J. N., Druce, H. M., Banks, S. M., and Kaliner, M. A. (1989). The pathophysiology of rhinitis. II. Assessment of the sources of protein in histamine-induced nasal secretions. *Am. Rev. Respir. Dis.* **139**:791–800.

Reynolds, H. Y. (1987). State of the art. Broncho-alveolar lavage. *Am. Rev. Respir. Dis.* **135**:250–263.

Richardson, P. S., and Peatfield, A. C. (1971). The control of airway mucus secretion. *Eur. J. Respir. Dis.* (Suppl. 153):43–51.

Rigler, L. G., and Koucky, R. (1938). Roentgen studies of the pathological physiology of bronchial asthma. *Am. J. Roentgenol.* **39**:353–362.

Ryley, H. C., and Brogan, T. D. (1973). Quantitative immunoelectrophoretic analysis of the plasma proteins in the sol phase of sputum from patients with chronic bronchitis. *J. Clin. Pathol.* **26**:852–856.

Sadoul, P., Puchelle, E., Zahm, J. M., Jacquot, J., Aug, J., and Polu, J. M. (1981). Effect of terbutaline on mucociliary transport and sputum properties in chronic bronchitis. *Chest* **80**:885–889.

Sakula, A. (1988). A history of asthma. *J. R. Coll. Physicians Lond.* **22**:36–44.

Salter, H. H. (1868). *On asthma, Its Pathology and Treatment,* 2nd ed. London, Churchill.

Schultz, W. (1924). Asthma bronchiale. *Erge. Med.* **5**:557–599.

Sheppard, D., Scypinski, L., Horn, J., Gordon, T., and Thompson, J. E. (1986). Granulocyte-mediated airway edema in guinea pigs. *J. Appl. Physiol.* **60**:1213–1220.

Sobin, S. S., Frasher, W. G., Tremer, H. M., and Hadley, G. G. (1963). The microcirculation of the tracheal mucosa. *Angiology* **14**:165–170.

Spector, W. G., and Willoughby, D. A. (1963). The inflammatory response. *Bacteriol. Rev.* **27**:117–154.

Stockley, R. A., Mistry, M., Bradwell, A. R., and Burnett, D. (1979). A study of plasma proteins in the sol phase of sputum from patients with chronic bronchitis. *Thorax* **34**:777–782.

Stoerk, K. (1875). *Asthma bronchiale.* Stuttgart, Ferdinand Enke, pp. 1–102.

Sturgess, J. M. (1984). Structure of human airway mucosa. *Semin. Respir. Med.* **5**:301–307.

Svensson, C., Baumgarten, C. R., Pipkorn, U., Alkner, U., and Persson, C. G. A. (1989). Reversibility and reproductibility of histamine-induced plasma leakage in the human nasal airways. *Thorax* **44**:13–18.

Svensson, C., Persson, C. G. A., Baumgarten, C. R., Alkner, U., and Pipkorn, U. (1990). Topical α-adrenoceptor stimulation may not reduce histamine-induced plasma leakage in human nasal airways. Thesis, Lund, pp. 89–101.

Turner-Warwick, M., and Openshaw, P. (1987). Sputum in asthma. *Postgrad. Med. J.* **63**(Suppl. 1):79–82.

Webber, S. E., and Widdicombe, J. G. (1989). The transport of albumin across the ferret in vitro whole trachea. *J. Physiol. (Lond.)* **408**:457–472.

Willoughby, D. A., and Spector, W. G. (1968). Inflammation in agranulocytotic rats. *Nature* **219**:1258.

Woodward, D. F., Weichman, B. M., Gill, C. A., and Wasserman, M. A. (1983). The effect of synthetic leukotrienes on tracheal microvascular permeability. *Prostaglandins* **25**:131–142.

Part VI

CLINICAL ASPECTS

15

Clinical Aspects of the Bronchial Circulation

JOHN BUTLER

University of Washington School of Medicine
Seattle, Washington

I. Introduction

This is a brief review of clinical circumstances in which alterations of the bronchial circulation influence symptoms and disability or offer therapeutic guidance. In part the information explains our great interest in, and justifies the myriad investigations of this relatively obscure regional circulation. Other chapters pursue the clinical correlations to greater depth.

A. Clinical Anatomy

We define the bronchial circulation as the systemic circulatory supply to the intrathoracic airways and lung. Although this supply is mostly from the anatomic bronchial arteries, it often comes from other arteries, particularly in disease. The upper, extrathoracic trachea is supplied by nonbronchial arteries (see Chap. 8), although its lower part may receive some branches from the intrathoracic bronchial vasculature. Within the thorax that part of the bronchial circulation supplying the lower trachea and airways outside the lung substance drains mostly into the right atrium. That supplying the intrapulmonary airways and the rest of the lung drains into the left atrium. The rich mucosal vasculature from the bronchial circulation links the pulmonary venous bed (left atrium) with the systemic venous bed (right atrium). The vasculature in and around the airways also forms a continuous network from the upper trachea to the respiratory bronchioles. This network anastomoses freely with the pulmonary circulation, which, although preferring mainly the smaller airways, provides some blood supply to larger airways as well (Barman et al., 1988).

B. Physical Examination

Since the bronchial circulation is so small and so deeply hidden in the chest it is no surprise that it is normally undetectable on clinical examination or chest x-ray. However, it is capable of rather enormous hypertrophy in some chronic conditions. When this occurs hypertrophy can be suspected if there is (Fig. 1)

1. Such a chronic lesion
2. Hemoptysis

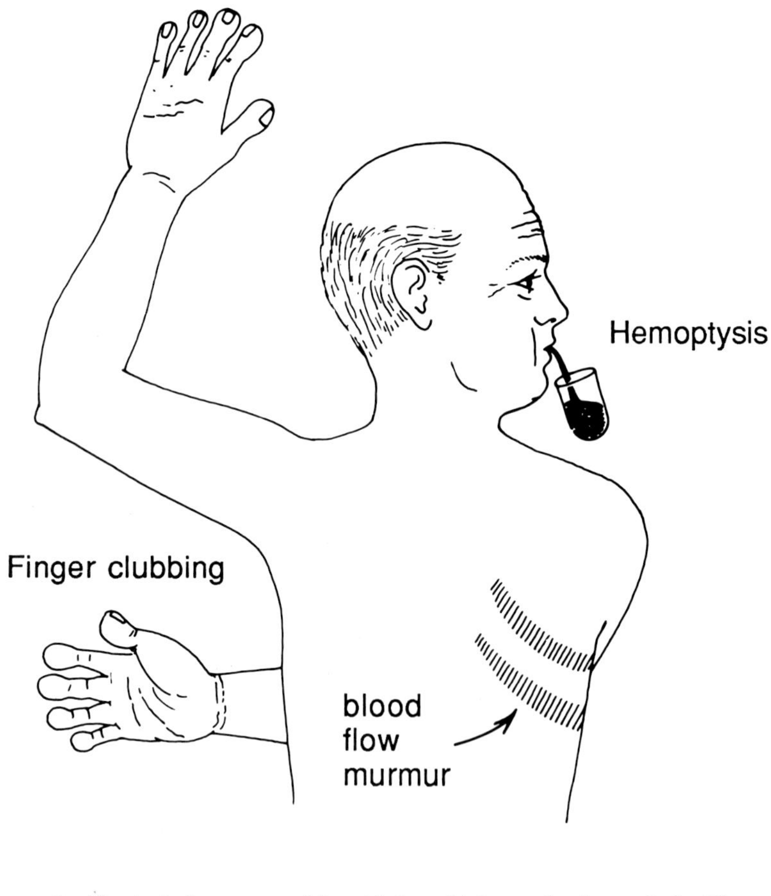

Figure 1 Physical signs compatible with bronchial vascular hyperplasia. These are nonspecific.

3. Finger clubbing
4. A flow murmur, usually over the upper chest at the back, that is unaltered by inhalation
5. Cyanosis associated with congenital heart disease or hypoventilation (see Chap. 21.)

C. Chest X-ray

Like the physical examination, the chest x-ray does not reveal the bronchial circulation under normal conditions. Hypertrophy can be suspected if there is (Fig. 2):

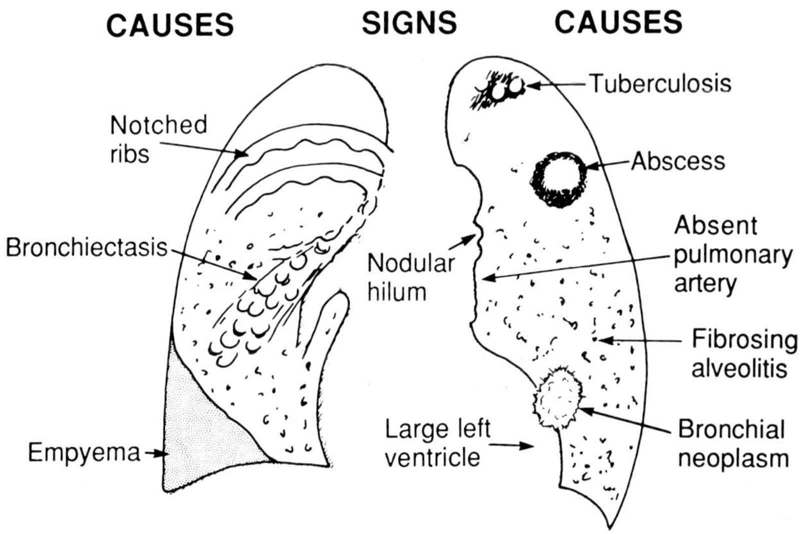

Figure 2 Chest x-ray showing signs compatible with bronchial vascular hyperplasia: notched ribs (hypertrophied subcostal arteries), nodular shadows at the hilum (hypertrophied branches of bronchial artery), and enlarged left ventricle (large increase in bronchial blood flow). Some of the chronic causes leading to bronchial vascular hypertrophy are also shown.

1. One of the associated risk conditions
2. Notching of the ribs
3. A nodular hilar shadow
4. Posterior indentations of the barium-filled esophagus
5. Apical pseudofibrosis

II. Airway Problems

A. Asthma

In asthma, bronchial blood flow is increased, particularly to the mucosa, which becomes hyperemic during asthmatic attacks (Baier et al., 1985). The hyperemia leads to edema and swelling of the mucosa and usually an increased exudation onto the luminal surface. This reduces the caliber, particularly if the smaller airways are involved, and so increases airway resistance and the work of breathing. Because of this reduction in caliber, the effect of smooth muscle bronchoconstriction is exaggerated (James et al., 1989). At the same time the inflammatory response (which may be partly a neurogenic inflammatory edema; see Chap. 17) increases airway irritability and potentiates coughing. It is interesting that hyperventilation alone causes a similar mucosal hyperemia in normal subjects and much more markedly in asthmatic individuals (McFadden, 1983; Gilbert et al., 1987). This is because air, unless fully humidified and warmed to body temperature, cools the mucosa and increases the osmolality of the mucus lining, both of which increase bronchial blood flow. Cold also causes bronchospasm. It is thought that this reaction, accompanying the tachypnea of exercise, is responsible for exercise-induced asthma.

Bronchospasm is always associated with an increase in the bronchial blood flow to the airway smooth muscle. Such a vasodilatory change can occur in the absence of mucosal hyperemia as a response to alterations in the autonomic nervous system or to the action of autonomic drugs, such as methacholine (Long et al., 1985).

Certain therapeutic suggestions arise from these considerations. Since part of the asthmatic response is due to bronchial vascular hyperemia, such vasoconstrictor drugs as epinephrine along with bronchodilators should increase airway caliber better than β-agonist drugs alone, which only relax the smooth muscle spasm. Thus a drug that combines vasoconstrictor α-agonist and a bronchodilator β-agonist action, such as epinephrine, should be best for decreasing the resistance to airflow; indeed, subcutaneous epinephrine remains a most useful, perhaps the most useful, drug for the emergency treatment of asthma. Further supporting the role of the inflammatory ("eosinophilic bronchitis") hyperemia of the bronchial vasculature in asthma in causing the breathlessness and wheezing is the long-term improvement that follows steroidal and nonsteroidal antiinflammatory and antihyperemic agents (see Chap. 16).

B. Bronchitis

Acute bronchitis is also associated with vasodilation of the bronchial mucosal vessels (Stothert et al., 1990). This may follow the inhalation of toxic gases, particularly cigarette smoke, fluid aspirations, trauma, such as that due to intubation, and infections, particularly viral infections of the upper respiratory tract. Chronic bronchitis, due to repeated injury to the airway from cigarette smoke, leads to more localized and chronic vasodilation and vascular hypertrophy (Nakamura et al., 1961). Again, steroids have been used to suppress the chronic inflammatory reaction and appear to be useful, a least temporarily.

The rich and continuous vascular network in the mucosa means that aerosolized drugs deposited anywhere on the mucosa can affect all parts of the bronchial tree (Kowalski et al., 1989). This is important because although higher concentrations are likely to be present locally at the site of deposition, the aerosol drugs can reach airways that are blocked, or have little ventilation, via the bronchial vasculature. Thus efforts to localize the site of action by altering the speed of inhalation or the size of the particle are not likely to be clinically essential (Cushley et al., 1983). Similarly, it is evident that therapeutic or toxic chemical aerosols or gases that are inhaled can reach the right heart although most of an intrapulmonary dose is absorbed into the pulmonary venous blood.

C. Lung Transplantation

The pulmonary circulation normally helps to perfuse the bronchial vasculature of the smaller airways and, to a diminishing extent, the larger airways up to the lower trachea. This pulmonary blood flow is augmented if the pressure in the bronchial vasculature falls, as it must after airway and systemic arterial transection for lung transplantation. Ischemic necrosis of the airways at the site of the bronchial anastomosis, attributed to the loss of nutrition from the bronchial blood flow, has been the main cause of morbidity and mortality following transplantation (see Chap. 23). During lung transplantation the numerous tiny bronchial vessels cannot be reanastomosed like the pulmonary vessels (Fig. 3). Instead, revascularization is encouraged by pulling a loop of omentum through the diaphragm and wrapping it around the airway anastomotic site. Recently the danger of ischemia of a tracheal anastomosis in double-lung transplantation was contrasted with the success that has attended anastomosing the airways closer to, or actually within, the lung substance (Patterson et al., 1990). These airways are nourished by larger pulmonary arterial contributions. Combined

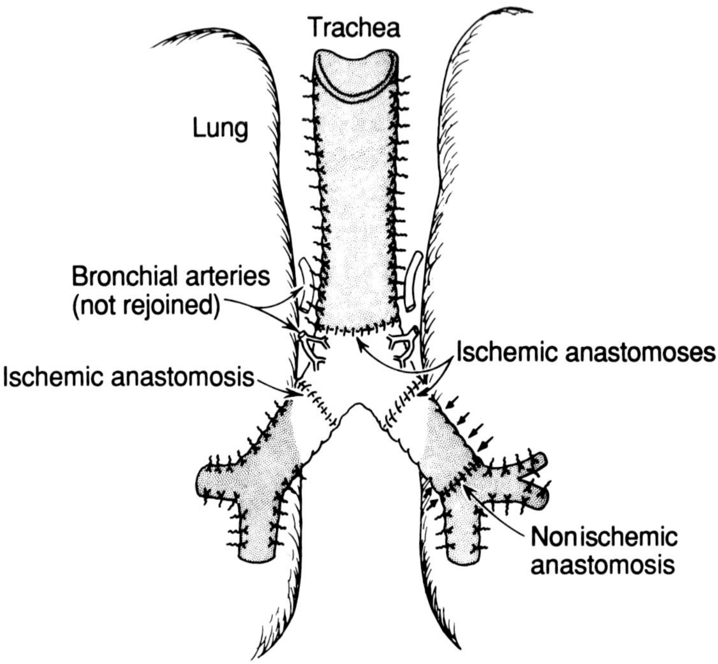

Figure 3 Lung transplantation. The shaded airways are vascularized from the small vascular branches (bronchial and pulmonary) depicted around them. The small arrows suggest new vessels from the reanastomosed pulmonary vasculature within the lung (nonischemic anastomosis). No such source of blood flow is available outside the lung (ischemic anastomosis).

heart-lung transplantation has been associated with fewer airway necrosis problems, probably because nutritive bronchial vessels frequently arise from the coronary arteries.

D. Bronchial Bleeding

Lesions of the airways are the usual cause of hemoptysis, so the expectorated blood generally comes from the bronchial circulation. Occasionally it comes from the pulmonary circulation when the parenchyma is damaged in early infarction, alveolar hemorrhage in pulmonary edema, or erosion of pulmonary vessels in Rasmussen's aneurysm of tuberculosis. However, it is the hyperplastic bronchial circulation that bleeds later after infarction and when vascular granulomatous tissue ulcerates in bronchiectasis, cystic fibrosis, tuberculosis, or lung abscesses in continuity with the airways.

Hemoptysis also occurs when the bronchial arterial bed, including that in the airway walls, is greatly enlarged because pulmonary blood flow is absent or diminished as a result of acquired or congenital heart disease. Such situations may occur, for instance, in Fallot's tetralogy.

Bleeding in mitral stenosis and other causes of chronic pulmonary venous pressure elevation also seems to come from the abnormally rich bronchial vasculature of the airways. In these conditions bronchial venous return by the pulmonary veins is impeded so it reverses and flows into the right atrium, which is at a lower pressure. In these conditions the bronchial venous plexus in the mucosa is markedly increased and is thought to be the source of the hemoptysis (Ferguson et al., 1944). Other causes of bleeding in patients with mitral valve disease are pulmonary infarctions, which are frequent, and alveolar hemorrhage in association with pulmonary edema.

Of particular concern to the clinician, of course, is that the hemoptysis could be coming from the exuberant bronchial vessels supplying an ulcerating bronchial neoplasm: blood streaking of the sputum is frequently the first sign of this dreaded lesion.

The treatment of bronchial bleeding is considered in detail in Chap. 22. Our current approach depends on its severity. When the hemoptysis is massive and could lead to death from asphyxia (which is commoner than death from exsanguination), bronchoscopy, preferably with a wide-lumen (rigid) bronchoscope, is indicated to suck the blood out and open the airway. This sometimes localizes the side and even the lobe from which the bleeding is coming. Bronchial angiography, performed as an emergency, can then be better directed. The blood is aspirated everywhere, however, and recognition even of the side it comes from is often impossible. Under these circumstances and in less severe bleeding, angiography is the preferred procedure (Fig. 4). The abnormal vessels are usually evident, and efforts are made to occlude the bleeding vessel with thrombogenic materials. The possibility that the bleeding comes from a pulmonary arterial aneurysm rather than the bronchial vessels is important to remember (see Chap. 22). After the bleeding has been staunched surgical resection can be performed with less risk.

When the bleeding is not severe, bronchoscopy is indicated to search for bronchial neoplasm. It is dangerous to attribute hemoptysis to simple bronchitis.

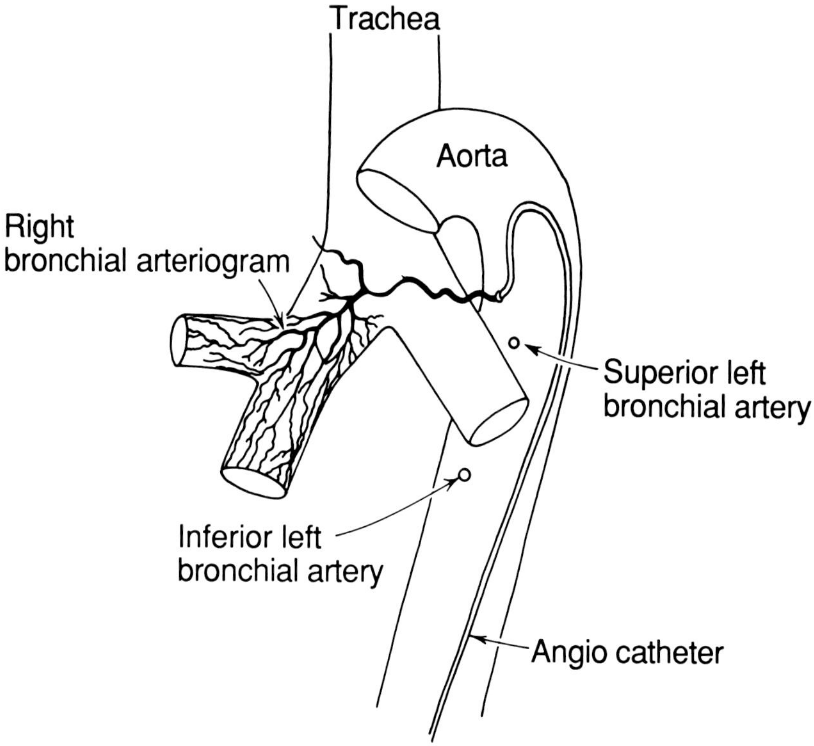

Figure 4 Bronchial angiography. A catheter shaped like a shepherd's crook is used to inject contrast medium into the aortic arch so that bronchial arterial vessels are shown. The catheter is then wedged selectively in the vessel shown to serve the vascular bed of interest and a high-contrast angiogram performed.

III. Parenchymal Disease

Chronic inflammatory disease of the parenchyma, whether due to specific infections, collagen diseases, immunological diseases, or "idiopathic" interstitial pneumonitis, is usually associated with an increased bronchial circulation (Turner-Warwick, 1963; Müller and Bordt, 1980). Acute flare-ups occur in many of these diseases, and, particularly if cavitation occurs, either the bronchial or the pulmonary circulation can be the source of the blood in the sputum. In patients with the acquired immunodeficiency syndrome (AIDS), pneumocystis infection is the most common cuase of hemoptysis, but other infections and neoplasms, such as Kaposi's sarcoma, may be responsible. The bronchial circulation is enlarged in patients with pneumonia (Cudkowicz, 1952). Pneumococcal pneumonia not infrequently causes hemoptysis, but the blood in the sputum is often dark and altered, suggesting its inflammatory origin. The pulmonary circulation to the diseased areas is cut off by hypoxic vasoconstriction, thrombotic obstruction, and pressure on the pulmonary vessels from the inflammation. Although the acute leukocytic response in pneumococcal pneumonia in rabbits is from the pulmonary circulation (Kowalski et al., 1989), the bronchial circulation appears to supply the inflammatory response in aspiration types of acute lung injury in dogs (Kowalski et al., 1988). The high rate of metabolism of the inflamed lung, packed with leukocytes, is such that any remaining pulmonary blood flow, as well as the bronchial blood flow, becomes depleted of oxygen and, because it drains into the left atrium, causes a right-to-left shunt effect. A similar abnormality can occur in the adult respiratory distress syndrome (ARDS).

The bronchial blood flow supplies the cells and other factors necessary for chronic inflammation in the lungs, as discussed earlier in considering hemoptysis and in Chap. 18. It enlarges, sometimes to a surprising extent, in the chronically inflamed region. For instance, in bronchiectasis, the rate of bronchial arterial blood flowing through anastomoses into the pulmonary vascular bed can be sufficient to reduce and even reverse the local pulmonary blood flow. This is useful in directing the pulmonary flow to more normal, ventilated regions. Arterialized blood may be sampled from a catheter floating in the pulmonary artery to the diseased lung (Fig. 5).

Since the bronchial circulation is important for the inflammatory response and subsequent healing of the lung, therapeutic maneuvers should not jeopardize it. Sustaining the bronchial blood flow means that excessive positive end-expiratory pressure (PEEP) should be avoided in such conditions as ARDS since a positive alveolar pressure diminishes bronchial blood flow (Modell et al., 1981). Systemic arterial pressures should be maintained by transfusions and related techniques since bronchial flow diminishes with falling

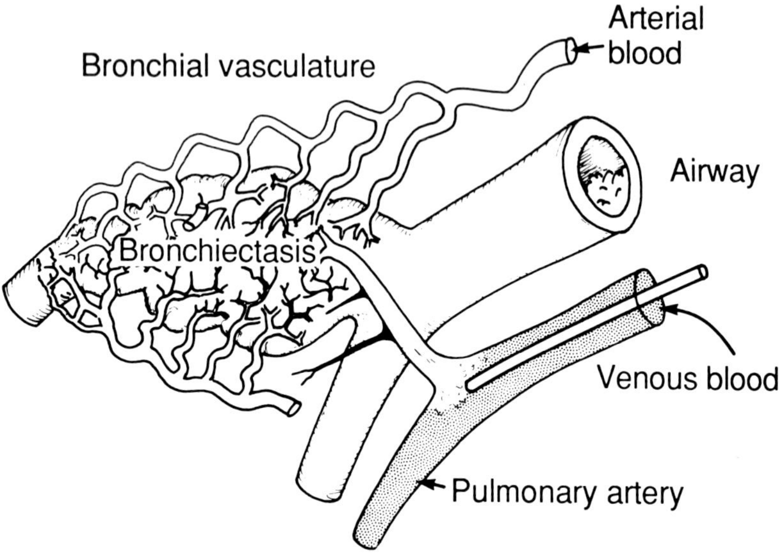

Figure 5 Bronchial vascular hyperplasia in bronchiectasis. Arterialized blood (light colored) reverses the normal systemic venous blood in the pulmonary artery (dark colored). A blood sample via a cardiac catheter may show arterialized blood in a branch of the pulmonary artery serving the bronchiectatic region.

blood pressure (State et al., 1957). It ceases altogether in dogs when systemic arterial pressures fall below 40 mmHg (Auld et al., 1960). Since the distribution of bronchial blood flow is not sensitive to decubitus position like the pulmonary flow, nursing the patient in the lateral position with the bad lung up offers no disadvantage.

IV. Vascular Alterations

Systemic vessels from the aorta, including the bronchial arteries, enlarge, sometimes very substantially, when there is pulmonary artery atresia or stenosis due to congenital heart disease. The nutrition of the lung parenchyma is thereby assured. The systemic blood in these vessels can provide some gas-exchange function through anastomoses with the pulmonary vasculature. These anastomoses occur between the bronchial vasculature and the pulmonary arteries as well as the capillaries and veins. The ratio of ventilation to perfusion in the lungs of these patients is always high, so CO_2 can be cleared from the systemic arterial blood. This systemic arterial blood is hypoxic in cyanotic congenital heart disease, so a little O_2 uptake can also occur. In some patients CO_2 clearance is so good that it leads to a diminution of ventilatory drive and hypoxia due to underventilation akin to that seen in patients undergoing renal dialysis. Obviously, in patients in whom the bronchial circulation is sufficiently developed to partially compensate for the lack of a pulmonary inflow, surgical shunt operations, such as the Taussig shunt, may not be required (Lintermans et al., 1966). If a complete surgical repair is to be carried out, the patency of the central pulmonary arteries must be assured. This can require highly tailored angiography as described in Chap. 21.

Large left-to-right shunts, for instance in ventricular septal defect, lead to severe pulmonary vascular disease associated with pulmonary hypertension and multiple obstructions in the small vessels. There is hyperplasia of the bronchial vasculature, and proximal bronchopulmonary anastomoses become very evident. Pulmonary arterial blood at high pressure is postulated to flow through these anastomoses and then back into the pulmonary vessels downstream of the obstructing lesions to reach the alveolar capillaries (Yaginuma et al., 1990).

Acquired pulmonary artery occlusion is usually due to embolism. In the acute stage there is little risk of lung necrosis because ventilation assures tissue oxygenation as long as the airways remain patent, and substrate deficiency is prevented by the bronchial circulation and, particularly in the early stages, by reverse flow in the pulmonary veins (see Chap. 15). Since the bronchial flow remains so small at first, it could be important to encourage reverse pulmonary venous flow at this time by deep breathing (see Chap. 15). Acquired, chronic pulmonary artery occlusion leads to hyperplasia of the bronchial circulation and an increase in systemic blood flow, which suffices to nourish the tissues and may take part in gas exchange. The pulmonary vasculature distal to the obstruction is very abnormal, however, showing the changes of severe pulmonary hypertension, including plexogenic arteriopathy (see Chap. 20). Unfortunately, therefore lung biopsy cannot distinguish this disease from Primary Pulmonary Hypertension. This arteriopathy may be why there is little resumption of pulmonary blood flow after thromboendarterectomy and edema almost always occurs. This type of "reperfusion edema," occurring from abnormal, hypertrophied vessels, is obviously different from that occurring in lungs reperfused after short periods of ischemia have damaged the normal tissues. The abnormalities clear with time, however, and lung perfusion increases and becomes more uniform.

Bronchopulmonary sequestration is characterized by sequestrated lung tissue that has no pulmonary blood flow. A systemic artery from the descending aorta is its sole blood supply. Therefore, when hemoptysis occurs from a sequestered lobe, angiographic obstruction of the main bronchial arterial supply could lead to its necrosis.

V. Pleural Disease

The bronchial circulation supplies the visceral pleura in the human. The parietal pleura is also supplied by the systemic circulation from the intercostals. In chronic pleural infections, such as empyema, bronchial vessels hypertrophy, sometimes very markedly. Since this takes time, decortication, when performed early, is much less likely to be marred by difficult bleeding problems. In the initial phases of pleural infection, when the metabolic demands of the inflammatory reaction and the accumulated leukocytes are high, additional oxygen may improve bacterial clearance (Carvalho et al., 1989). It is postulated that there is hypoxia within the mass of leukocytes and that bacteriocidal power improves if this lack of oxygen is corrected, since oxygen is necessary for the "metabolic burst" of the leukocytes when they destroy bacteria.

VI. Unusual Problems

In some patients who have a markedly hypertrophied bronchial circulation, its supply from the coronary arteries can lead to a "coronary steal" syndrome. This may be so severe as to lead to angina when the patient exercises, or even to myocardial infarction (Kawasuji et al., 1984; Stefas et al., 1990).

The diagnostic and therapeutic aspects of the bronchial circulatory supply of lung neoplasms have been explored (see Chap. 19). Bronchial angiography was formerly used to establish the presence of a bronchial neoplasm when other techniques yielded equivocal results. The images were seldom tissue specific, however, and the method was dismissed for this purpose. Likewise, the infusion of chemotherapeutic substances into the bronchial artery serving the tumor, although of great interest in the 1960s, is rarely used these days. The ability to achieve relatively high concentrations of antineoplastic agents with newer techniques using agents linked to tumor-specific antibodies is evoking renewed interest, however. With these materials the problems of low concentrations because of perfusion of the neoplasm from multiple sources, or of potential damage from chemicals to the spinal cord via spinal arteries arising from the bronchial artery, are no longer as worrisome.

VII. Summary

The bronchial circulation is normally hidden from physical examination and chest x-ray. It can become evident after undergoing marked hyperplasia in chronic infections, however, and in congenital and chronic acquired vascular abnormalities associated with restriction of pulmonary arterial blood flow. Then physical signs (finger clubbing, flow murmurs over the lungs, and hemoptysis), although not specific, suggest its hypertrophy, and chest x-ray changes (notched ribs, nodular hilar shadows, and enlarged left ventricle) heighten suspicion. Angiography is necessary for confirmation.

The bronchial circulation plays a significant role in several clinical problems. The hyperemia of the airway mucosa in asthma and bronchitis tends to cause mucosal swelling and to narrow the smaller airways. Aerosolized bronchial vasoconstrictors could be helpful in reducing the airway resistance. Most hemoptysis comes from the bronchial circulation, and this bleeding is now treatable by bronchial artery embolization.

Parenchymal inflammatory changes and their healing depend on the bronchial rather than the pulmonary circulation, so efforts to protect the bronchial rather than pulmonary circulation seem rational. Pulmonary vascular lesions, both congenital and acquired, often lead to hyperplasia of the bronchial circulation, which takes over the nutrition of the alveolar tissues and sometimes a modicum of gas exchange. Pleural inflammation requires hyperemia and, if chronic, hyperplasia of the systemic arteries involved. Decortication after empyema may be easier if undertaken early before such hypervascularization develops.

Further details of these and other clinical problems are found in the subsequent chapters dealing with the role of the bronchial circulation in lung diseases.

References

Auld, P. A. M., Rudolph, A. M., and Golinko, R. J. (1960). Factors affecting bronchial collateral flow in the dog. *Am. J. Physiol.* **198**:1166–1170.

Baier, H., Long, W. M., and Wanner, A. (1985). Bronchial circulation in asthma. *Respiration* **48**:199–205.

Barman, S. A., Ardell, J. L., Parker, J. C., Perry, M. L., and Taylor, A. E. (1988). Pulmonary and systemic contributions to upper airways in canine lung. *Am. J. Physiol* **255**(24):H1130–H1135.

Carvalho, P., Nielson, C. P., Kirk, W., and Charan, N. B. (1990). The effects of oxygen on bacterial clearance from the pleural space in sheep. *Am. Rev. Respir. Dis.* **141**:A766.

Cudkowicz, L. (1952). Some observations of the bronchial arteries in lobar pneumonia and pulmonary infarction. *Br. J. Tuberc.* **46**:99–102.

Cushley, M. J., Lewis, R. A., and Tattersfield, A. E. (1983). Comparison of three techniques of inhalation on the airway response to terbutaline. *Thorax* **38**:908–913.

Ferguson, F. C., Kobilak, R. E., and Deitrick, J. E. (1944). Varices of the bronchial veins as a source of hemoptysis in mitral stenosis. *Am. Heart. J.* **328**:445–456.

Gilbert, I. A., Fouke, J. M., and McFadden, E. R. (1987). Heat and water flux in the intrathoracic airways and exercise induced asthma. *J. Appl. Physiol.* **63**:1681–1691.

James, A. L., Paré, P. D., and Hogg, J. C. (1989). The mechanism of airway narrowing in asthma. *Am. Rev. Respir. Dis.* **139**:242–246.

Kawasuji, M., Murakami, S., Watanabe, X., and Iwa, T. (1949). Coronary artery steal via a large antastomosis between the coronary and bronchial arteries successfully treated by surgical division. *J. Thorac. Cardiovasc. Surg.* **32**:119–121.

Kowalski, T. K., Lakshminarayan, S., Kirk, W., Graham, M. M., and Butler, J. (1988). The role of the bronchial circulation in the leucocyte response to acute lung injury. *Am. Rev. Respir. Dis.* **137**:368A.

Kowalski, T. F., Doerschuk, C., Lakshminarayan, S., English, D., and Butler, J. (1989). The bronchial circulation in neutrophil delivery to streptococcal pneumonia in rabbits. *FASEB J.* **3**:A567.

Kowalski, T. F., Kirk, W., Graham, M. M., Lakshminarayan, S., and Butler, J. (1990). The drainage route of the bronchial vasculature. *Respir. Physiol.* **82**:65–74.

Lintermans, J. P., Guntheroth, W. G., and Figley, M. M. (1966). Extensive accessory pulmonary arteries in the presence of relatively normal primary pulmonary arteries. *Am. Heart J.* **71**:527–532.

Long, W. M., Yerger, L. D., Martinez, H., Codias, E., Sprung, C. L., Abraham, W. M., and Wanner, A. (1985). Effects of histamine on bronchial artery blood flow and bronchomotor tone. *J. Appl. Physiol.* **59**:254–261.

McFadden, E. R. (1983). Respiratory heat and water exchange: Physiologic and clinical implications. *J. Appl. Physiol.* **54**:331–336.

Modell, H. L., Beck, K., and Butler, J. (1981). Functional aspects of canine bronchial-pulmonary vascular communication. *J. Appl. Physiol.* **50**:1045–1051.

Müller, K. M., and Bordt, J. (1980). Der Bronchialarteriienkreislauf untel Krankhaften Verülterissen. *Prax. Pneumol.* **34**:324–331.

Nakamura, T., Katori, R., Miyazawa, K., Ohtomo, S., Watanabe, T., Miuura, Y., and Takizawa, T. (1961). Bronchial blood flow in patients with chronic pulmonary disease and its influence upon respiration and circulation. *Dis. Chest* **39**:193–206.

Patterson, G. A., Todd, T. R., Cooper, J. D., Pearson, F. G., Winton, T. L., and Maurer, J. (1990). Airway complications after double lung transplantation. *J. Thorac. Cardiovasc. Surg.* **99**:14–21.

State, D., Salisbury, P. F., and Weil, P. (1957). Physiologic and pharmacologic studies of collateral blood flow. *J. Thorac. Surg.* **34**:599–608.

Stefas, L., Assayag, P., Aubrey, P., Brochet, E., Faraggi, M., Gamerman, G., and Valere, P. E. (1990). Coronary to bronchial artery anastomosis with bronchial steal syndrome demonstrated by thallium-201 myocardial tomoscintigraphy. *Eur. Heart J.* **11**:275–279.

Stothert, J. C., Ashley, K. D., Traber, L. D., Deubel-Ashley, K., Kramer, G. C., Herridon, D. N., and Traber, D. L. (1990). Systemic blood flow to the lung after smoke inhalation and bronchial artery occlusion. *FASEB J.* **4**:A1074.

Turner-Warwick, M. (1963). Precapillary systemic-pulmonary anastomoses. *Thorax* **18**:225–237.

Yaginuma, G., Mohri, H., and Takahashi, T. (1990). Distribution of arterial lesions and collateral pathways in the pulmonary hypertension of congenital heart disease: A computer-aided study. *Thorax* **45**:586–590.

16

Airways
Asthma, Bronchitis, and Emphysema

ADAM WANNER

University of Miami
and Mt. Sinai Medical Center
Miami Beach, Florida

WILLIAM M. LONG

North Dakota Medical School
Grand Forks, North Dakota

I. Introduction

The mechanisms of airflow obstruction in bronchial asthma, chronic bronchitis, and emphysema, the three principal types of obstructive lung disease, have been studied extensively. Airway smooth muscle contraction, airway hypersecretion, and permanent disruption of the peripheral airway and alveolar architecture have received special attention, and their respective roles in airflow limitation have been well characterized. Much less information has been obtained on the role of the circulation of the airways in obstructive lung disease.

Theoretically, the circulation of the airways could be of importance because the disease processes in bronchial asthma and chronic bronchitis involve primarily the conducting airways whose blood supply is derived from the tracheal and bronchial circulations, because vascular responses typically participate in inflammation, a feature of bronchial asthma and chronic bronchitis, and because the bronchial circulation may provide blood flow to the lung tissue in emphysema, when the pulmonary circulation is compromised. Although the airway circulation is difficult to study in human subjects because of the invasiveness of the required experimental techniques, circumstantial evidence of the participation of the airway circulation in the pathophysiology of bronchial asthma, chronic bronchitis, and emphysema is available. This evidence has been derived either indirectly from observations in humans or from direct observations in animal models of human airway disease. The validity of both approaches can justifiably be questioned. Unfortunately, they must suffice until new methods are developed that are feasible for use in human subjects.

Some of the currently available information on the bronchovascular adaptations that relate to airway disease is summarized in this chapter; other relevant bronchovascular responses, such as those to airway cooling and drying, changes in arterial blood gas composition, infections, and inflammation, are addressed in other chapters. Given the scarcity of human data, it is difficult totally to avoid speculation when discussing the role of the airway circulation in airway disease. This chapter is no exception.

II. Acute Bronchovascular Responses

There is increasing evidence suggesting that inflammation plays a prominent role in mediating the response of the airway to physical and chemical injury as well as antigens and infectious agents. Clinically, this response may present as bronchial asthma and acute bronchitis. The three major vascular manifestations of inflammation, hyperemia, endothelial hyperpermeability, and tissue edema, have been demonstrated in models of airway injury, and some of the mechanisms responsible for the observed alterations have been elucidated. These mechanisms include the actions of leukocytes and inflammatory mediators and of neurotransmitters and neuropeptides on vascular endothelial and smooth muscle cells. Most of the available information on vascular responses has been derived from observations in animal models. To what extent these findings can be extrapolated to patients with bronchial asthma is unresolved.

A. Morphological Evidence

Mast cells, granulocytes, and peptidergic neurons have been demonstrated in the vicinity of vessels in the airway wall (Sheppard et al., 1986; Burnstock, 1986), and each of these cells probably plays a role in the inflammatory vascular responses to airway irritation. The leukocytes could be present in the perivascular regions before airway injury (e.g., tissue mast cells) or be secondarily recruited into the vessel wall in response to airway injury (Bjork et al., 1982; Issekutz et al., 1980). Lebargy et al. (1987) reported histological changes occurring in the tracheal mucosa of sensitized rats within 60 min following inhalation challenge with antigen. They found subepithelial edema and increased amounts of luminal secretions in the bronchi in 9 of 15 animals tested. They also found a decrease in the number of toluidine blue-stainable mast cells and interpreted this finding as an expression of mast cell degranulation. Subepithelial edema and capillary engorgement have also been reported in the tracheobronchial tree of sensitized rats and guinea pigs during systemic anaphylaxis (Lee et al., 1985; Dixon and Warren, 1950). Thus, the allergic reaction in the lower airways seems to be associated with two morphological stigmata of inflammation, vascular hyperemia and tissue edema. Other forms of airway injury may also be characterized by vascular congestion and edema in the bronchial wall. The technical difficulties involved in the morphometric assessment of tissue edema, however, particularly in the trachea and larger bronchi, may preclude the detection of the microvascular changes.

B. Physiological Evidence

The major functional characteristics of the vascular response to injury in the airway are increased blood flow and microvascular hyperpermeability. The increased blood flow in the inflamed airway is generally thought to result from dilatation of small bronchial arteries. Changes in venomotor tone can also influence the local vascular response to inflammation, however, especially relative to the interaction between microvascular perfusion and permeability. For example, the increased vascular permeability caused by bradykinin can be further augmented by the concomitant administration of the vascoconstrictor serotonin, presumably by an increased hydrostatic microvascular pressure (Weiner and Altura, 1967). Inflammation-linked leakage of macromolecules from the microvasculature can occur through endothelial pores and vesicles or through the formation of intercellular gaps. In the dog paw, the permeability of the microvascular endothelium for molecules, as determined by their plasma-lymph ratio, was found to depend on their molecular weight, configuration, and charge (Alksne, 1959). The data were interpreted as fitting transport through small pores (40 Å), large pores (>1600 Å), and vesicles. Histamine and bradykinin increased all three transport processes. Endothelial gaps, mainly in postcapillary venules, are now thought to constitute an important site for microvascular leakage during inflammation (Majno et al., 1969).

Histamine, other chemical mediators, and sensory autonomic nerve stimulation can produce intercellular gaps in postcapillary venules (Gabbiani et al., 1970; Majno and Palade, 1961; McDonald, 1987; Svensjo and Grega, 1986). It has been shown in the rat tracheal mucosa that in response to sensory autonomic nerve stimulation the intercellular gaps form rapidly, measure 1.5 μm in diameter, and close within minutes (McDonald, 1987). To maintain open gaps, sequential mediator actions may be required (Grega et al., 1985). The physiological response is probably brought about by the effects of the inflammatory mediators, including neuropeptides, on contractile elements in endothelial cells and pericytes (Miller and Sims, 1986). Interestingly, the endothelial hyperpermeability for morphological markers is not shared by the basement membranes; such particles tend to become trapped by the basement membrane (Alksne, 1959; Renkin et al., 1974).

Permeability for macromolecules may be increased by inflammatory mediators to such an extent that a colloid-oncotic pressure gradient across the vessel wall is no longer present (Grega et al., 1986). Whether hydraulic conductivity, that is, the ease with which water fluxes occur across the vascular endothelium, is also increased is less clear. Hydraulic conductivity may be more related to intravascular hydrostatic pressure than macromolecular permeability (Renkin et al., 1974).

Since the exact relationship between the rate of water and macromolecular extravasation and the magnitude of tissue edema formation is unclear, a change in one of the two parameters should not be equated with a concomitant change in another. The rate of extravascular volume change during hyperpermeability states is governed by the rates of net fluid extravasation, lymphatic drainage, and transepithelial liquid transport into the airway lumen. Attempts should therefore be made to characterize perfusion, permeability, and edema in the airway wall independently when assessing the vascular component of airway inflammation.

Airway anaphylaxis in animals has been the best studied model of the bronchovascular responses in airway disease, notably bronchial asthma. In allergic sheep, inhalation challenge with specific antigen leads to an increase in total bronchial arterial blood flow measured by an electromagnetic flowmeter, which corresponds with an immediate increase in airflow resistance (Fig. 1). Pharmacological blockade studies showed that changes in blood flow were independent of the bronchoconstriction (Long et al., 1988). Mucosal blood flow, measured by a soluble gas uptake method, also participates in this response (Csete et al., 1989). The allergic hyperperfusion may be accompanied by macromolecular hyperpermeability as demonstrated by Persson et al. (1986; Persson and Erjefalt, 1986), who found increased macromolecular transport from the airway vasculature to the airway lumen in allergic guinea pigs as early as 5 min following local antigen challenge. Similarly, intravenously administered ovalbumin has been shown to cause Evan's blue extravasation in the conducting airways of sensitized guinea pigs (Evans et al., 1988). In contrast to the lower airways, mucosal blood flow in the nose has been reported to decrease after local antigen challenge (Holmberg et al., 1988). The differential responses may be due to differences in vascular anatomy and control at the two sites.

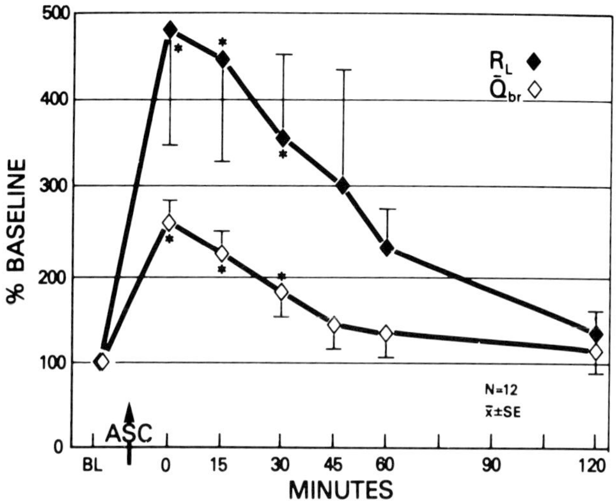

Figure 1 Effect of aerosolized *Ascaris suum* antigen (ASC) on pulmonary airflow resistance (R_L) and bronchial blood flow ($\bar{Q}_{br}$, electromagnetic blood flowmeter) in allergic sheep. BL = baseline. 0 = immediately after the antigen challenge. (From Long et al., 1988, with permission from the *Journal of Applied Physiology.*)

C. Role of Inflammatory Mediators

Amines, kinins, lipid metabolites, and other inflammatory mediators have been tested with respect to their airway vascular effects. The vasodilator effect of histamine in the peripheral systemic vascular bed has been known for some time, and both H_1 and H_2 histamine receptors seem to be involved (Chipman and Glover, 1976; Duff et al., 1953). In the human forearm, the initial response to the intraarterial infusion of histamine has been reported to be H_1-receptor dependent followed by an H_2-receptor-dependent phase as assessed by specific histamine antagonists (Chipman et al., 1976). It has also been suggested that histamine receptor stimulation may have opposing effects on vasomotor tone depending upon the intravascular pressure. In the guinea pig heart, for instance, infused histamine causes coronary vasodilation at a perfusion pressure of 40 mmHg but vasoconstriction at 65 mmHg (Kang et al., 1987; Merrill et al., 1987). Infused histamine lowers tracheal vascular resistance in dogs, and inhaled histamine increases bronchial blood flow measured by different methods and tracheal mucosal blood flow (soluble gas uptake method) in sheep (Fig. 2) (Chediak and Wanner, 1991; Laitinen et al., 1987a; Long et

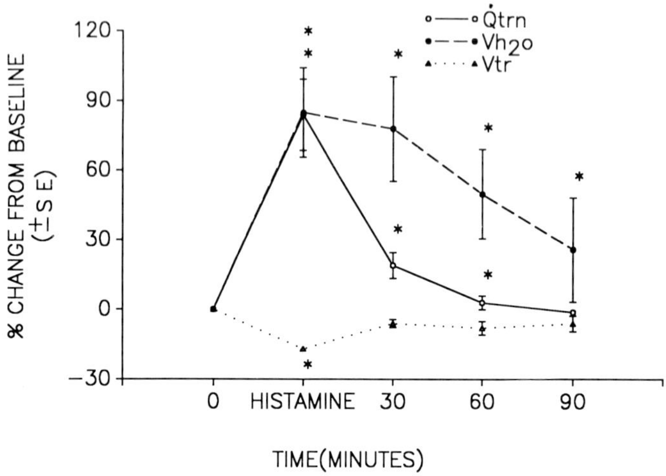

Figure 2 Effects of aerosolized histamine (0.9 mg) on tracheal mucosal perfusion normalized for carotid artery pressure ($\dot{Q}_{trn}$), mucosal water content (Vh_2O), and tracheal air volume (V_{tr}) as an index of airway smooth muscle tone. Mean value of six adult conscious sheep. *$p < 0.05$ compared to respective time control (not shown). Note different time courses among the three parameters. (From Chediak et al., *Resp. Physiol.*, 1991; with permission.)

al., 1985). In the sheep, the increase in both total and mucosal airway blood flow after histamine aerosol challenge is mainly H_2-receptor mediated, possibly with a sequential activation of H_1-receptors in the mucosa.

Histamine not only increases airway blood flow but typically produces intercellular gaps in postcapillary venular endothelium and promotes the extravasation of macromolecules into subepithelial airway tissues (Gabbiani et al., 1970; Majno and Palade, 1961; Majno et al., 1969). Infused histamine was used in these studies, and the histamine liberator 48/80 was also effective (Pietra et al., 1971). The respective roles of H_1- and H_2-histamine receptors in macromolecular hyperpermeability have not been characterized in the airway, but based on observations made in the skin, H_1 histamine receptors could predominate. For example, Ahmed et al. (1983) found in allergic sheep that the response (wheal) to intracutaneous histamine was blunted by the H_1-antagonist chlorpheniramine but not by the H_2-antagonist metiamide.

Baier et al. (1986) have shown that in addition to causing macromolecular hyperpermeability, histamine is also capable of increasing airway mucosal water volume in the intact sheep. They found that for a comparable degree of bronchoconstriction, inhaled histamine but not inhaled methacholine produced a small increase (15%) in tracheal mucosal water volume as determined with a soluble gas uptake method. Subsequently it was shown that this mucosal edema induced by the administration of histamine in the airway lumen is almost entirely H_1 histamine receptor-mediated (Chediak and Wanner, 1991).

Bradykinin is a potent vasodilator and increases permeability in systemic vascular beds, including those in the airways (Gabbiani et al., 1970; Majno and Palade, 1961; Svensjo et al., 1977). As with histamine, venular endothelial gap formation seems to play an important role in the bradykinin-induced vascular hyperpermeability.

The lipoxygenase and cyclooxygenase products of arachidonic acid and platelet activating factor have also been shown to influence the airway vasculature. In the trachea, the sulfidopeptide leukotrienes have been shown to have variable effects on vascular resistance in different animal species (Austen and Orange, 1975; Lee et al., 1985; Peck et al., 1981) and to increase bronchial microvascular permeability (Peck et al., 1981). Prostaglandin E_1 and F_2 and prostacyclin are vasodilators with little effect on permeability (Higgs et al., 1979; Knight et al., 1986; Laitinen et al., 1987a; Svensjo, 1978). Vasodilator prostanoids also contribute significantly to the increase in bronchial blood flow that accompanies allergic bronchoconstriction in sheep (Long et al., 1988).

The bronchovascular effects of platelet activating factor are to increase blood flow and permeability (Bjork and Smedegard, 1983; Laitinen et al., 1987b). In guinea pigs, the injection of platelet activating factor has been reported to lead to Evan's blue extravasation in the trachea and bronchi, which was blocked by an antagonist of platelet activating factor but not by platelet depletion or cyclooxygenase and lipoxygenase inhibitors (Evans et al., 1987). This suggests a direct effect of platelet activating factor on microvascular permeability without the need for platelet activation. Interestingly, the presence of platelets seems to be required for platelet activating factor-induced vascular hyperpermeability in other systemic vascular beds in other species. For example, platelet activating factor causes macromolecular hyperpermeability in the hamster cheek pouch and rat skin only when platelets are available (Hwang et al., 1985; Bjork and Smedegard, 1983). Arachidonic acid metabolites produced by the activated platelets seem to be secondary vascoactive mediators in these animals.

Toxic oxygen radicals generated by polymorphonuclear granulocytes may also participate in the macromolecular hyperpermeability associated with airway injury and inflammation. For example, inhaled toluene diisocyanate-induced Evan's blue extravasation in guinea pig airways has been shown to be inhibited by catalase (Lewis and Granger, 1986; Sheppard et al., 1986). It is possible, of course, that the blocking effect of catalase could have been due to actions other than hydrogen peroxide scavenging.

D. Role of Neural Pathways

The autonomic nervous system, although playing an important role in the response of the airways to physiological stimuli, may also participate in pathophysiological responses, including those associated with bronchial asthma. The autonomic innervation of the airway circulation varies among different species (Doidge and Satchell, 1982; Mann, 1971). Adrenergic nerves appear to be generally more numerous in association with bronchial vessels than cholinergic nerves (Partanen et al., 1982). The presence of peptidergic nerves in the vicinity of bronchial vessels has also been established in humans and several other mammals (Barnes, 1987).

The role of the cholinergic nervous system in the control of the airway vasculature is controversial. In the sheep trachea, intravenous atropine sulfate does not appear to affect tracheal mucosal blood flow (Barker et al., 1988). Likewise, the local administration of methacholine aerosol has been shown not to alter tracheal mucosal blood flow significantly, even after precontraction of the vasculature by intravenous vasopressin (Barker et al., 1988). Inhaled methacholine, at a concentration sufficient to cause bronchoconstriction, has also been shown to have only a negligible effect on bronchial blood flow in sheep (Long et al., 1988). Possibly, the level of cholinergic control of the airway vasculature shows interspecies variability, and the response to exogenous cholinergic agonists depends on the mode of administration, that is, aerosol versus systemic. A difference between aerosol and intravenous administration may be related to the fact that acetylcholine-induced vasodilation has been shown to be mediated by endothelium-derived relaxant factors. The endothelium is probably more accessible to circulating than inhaled cholinergic agonists. Differences in parasympathetic neural control and responsiveness may also exist among different airway generations.

In keeping with the failure of atropine to alter tracheal mucosal blood flow, Laitinen et al. (1987c) also observed only minimal changes in tracheal vascular resistance in dogs after vagal transection. In contrast to the sheep studies, however, vagal nerve stimulation produced a decrease in tracheal vascular resistance in dogs, an effect that was partially blocked by atropine. Intraarterial infusion of acetylcholine or methacholine was also reported to increase total tracheal blood flow and decrease tracheal vascular resistance in dogs, again an atropine-blockable effect (Himori and Taira, 1986; Laitinen et al., 1987a).

Analogous to the cholinergic nervous system, the adrenergic tone controlling baseline airway blood flow appears to be negligible as suggested by the inability to change tracheal mucosal blood flow in sheep with the α-adrenergic blocking agent phentolamine and the β-adrenergic blocking agent propranolol (Barker et al., 1988). In contrast, the airway circulation shows typical vasoconstrictor and vasodilator responses to locally administered α- and β-adrenergic agonists, respectively (Barker et al., 1988). Similar observations have been made in the trachea and bronchi of dogs using the β-adrenergic agonists isoproterenol and albuterol and the α-adrenergic agonists norepinephrine and phenylephrine (Himori and Taira, 1976; Laitinen et al., 1987a; Lung et al., 1976).

Several neuropeptides have potent vascular effects in the airways. Laitinen et al. (1987c) showed that, in dogs, atropine pretreatment only partially blocked the decrease in tracheal vascular resistance during vagal nerve stimulation and that this was not blocked by hexamethonium. This suggests antidromic vagal vasodilation, presumably mediated by neuropeptides. The same authors showed that vascoactive intestinal peptide, substance P, and several other neuropeptides lowered tracheal vascular resistance, with neurokinin A the most potent (Laitinen et al., 1987d). Of all the peptides tested, only the neuropeptide tyrosine was found to be a vasoconstrictor. Noncholinergic, vagally induced vasodilation in the bronchial tree was also reported by another group of investigators (Martling et al., 1985). The possibility therefore exists that local axon reflexes, via the release of vasoactive neuropeptides, control airway mucosal blood flow.

In addition, intravenously administered substance P has been shown to increase vascular permeability in the trachea and central bronchi of rats, but not in peripheral bronchi (Sertl et al., 1988). It is therefore likely that peptidergic nerves participate in pathological vascular responses in the airway wall (neuro-inflammation). Whether cholinergic and adrenergic responses, if present during airway inflammation, modify vascular responses remains to be explored. The demonstration that β-adrenergic agonists inhibit mediator- and capsaicin-induced macromolecular permeability in the airway suggests a homeostatic role of the sympathetic nervous system in airway inflammation (Dabney et al., 1981; Grega et al., 1981; Persson et al., 1986). Possibly, the mechanism by which sympathomimetics counteract microvascular hyperpermeability for macromolecules is by preventing venular endothelial cell contraction and hence gap formation.

The pathogenetic roles of leukocyte products and products released from autonomic nerves in the vascular manifestations of airway inflammation seem to be firmly established based on the various observations in animals. This suggests that the inflammatory mediators and neuropeptides that have been shown to contract airway smooth muscle (bronchospasm) and alter epithelial secretory function (hypersecretion) also increase airway blood flow and microvascular permeability (edema). Thus, most of the features of bronchial asthma

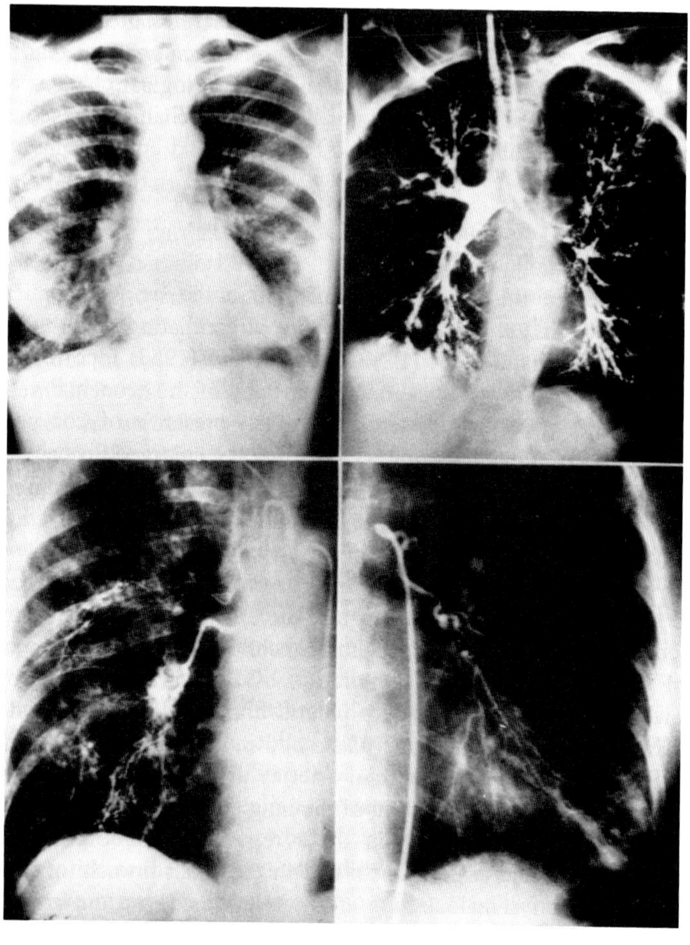

Figure 3 Chest roentgenogram (top left), bronchogram (top right), right bronchial arteriogram (bottom, left), and left bronchial arteriogram (bottom right) in a patient with chronic bronchitis, emphysema, and localized right lower lobe bronchiectasis. Note bronchiectatic dilation of right lower lobe bronchi, rarefaction of small bronchi in other parts of the lung (bronchogram), corresponding hypertrophy and tortuosity of right lower lobe bronchial arteries, and atrophy of bronchial arteries in the remainder of the lung periphery (bronchial arteriogram). (Courtesy of Manual Viamonte, M.D., Mount Sinai Medical Center, Miami Beach, FL.)

possibility that there is a nonuniform distribution of bronchial blood flow in these patients with decreases in emphysematous regions and increases in uninvolved regions.

C. Mechanisms

In contrast to bronchial asthma, the pathogenesis of the abnormal bronchial circulation in chronic bronchitis and emphysema is unknown. However, several investigators have attempted to answer the question of whether the bronchovascular changes are the cause or consequence of pulmonary emphysema by using animal models. Ricketts and Carrington (1968) attempted to produce experimental emphysema in sheep by injecting a radiopaque silastic compound to occlude the major bronchial arteries. None of the animals developed anatomic evidence of pulmonary emphysema. Likewise, Ellis et al. (1951) found no emphysematous changes in dogs after obliteration of all bronchial branches with a diameter greater than 35 μm. In contrast, injection of a sclerosing substance into the bronchial arteries has been reported to cause emphysematous changes in the horse (Edwards, 1961). Because the bronchial arteries were reduced in proportion to general tissue loss on a regional basis and some of the bronchial arteries were enlarged in uninvolved areas of the lung (McLaughlin and Edwards, 1966), it is possible that the sclerosing agent caused emphysema directly, with secondary adaptations of the bronchial circulation rather than primary bronchovascular obliteration leading to destruction of lung parenchyma. Taking all the evidence together, it is therefore unlikely that the bronchial circulation plays a pathogenic role in the development of pulmonary emphysema. The causes and physiological consequences of the secondary changes of the bronchial circulation in emphysema remain to be elucidated.

IV. Clinical Implications

Increased airway blood flow and microvascular hyperpermeability appear to be the principal manifestations of bronchovascular dysfunction. It is therefore worth examining the possible role of hyperperfusion and hyperpermeability in the airway in the pathophysiology and treatment of airflow obstruction. Some of the proposed interactions between the airway circulation and airflow have been subjected to the scrutiny of experimentation; others remain hypothetical, waiting to be tested (Table 1). Without question, critical data, especially human data, are still missing. Unless this void is filled, the clinical implications of the bronchovascular manifestations in airway disease remain speculative.

Table 1 Proposed and Demonstrated Effects of the Airway Circulation on Airflow Resistance

Congestion and edema
Airway narrowing due to mechanical effects (airflow obstruction in small airways)
Hyperperfusion
Increased influx of inflammatory cells causing airway narrowing by mediator generation
Preferential distribution of circulating homeostatic factors (e.g., epinephrine) to narrowed airway
Blunting of airway smooth muscle contraction by increased clearance of locally released mediators
Endothelial cell activation or injury
Release of endothelium-derived substances with airway smooth muscle effects

A. Airflow Obstruction

The possibility that vascular congestion, airway wall edema, or fluid accumulation in the airway lumen resulting from hyperperfusion and microvascular hyperpermeability in airway disease increases airflow resistance is important. In a morphometric study of the airway circulation of sheep, Mariassy et al. (1991) conducted a morphometric analysis of the vascular compartment in the wall of the trachea and of 1.0 and 0.5 mm bronchioles. The lungs were fixed by bronchial and pulmonary artery perfusion with glutaraldehyde in three experimental conditions: bronchial artery pressure of 100 mmHg and pulmonary artery pressure of 20 mmHg (control); bronchial artery pressure of 100 mmHg and pulmonary artery pressure of 40 mmHg (pulmonary hypertension); bronchial artery pressure of 100 mmHg, pulmonary artery pressure of 40 mmHg, and pharmacological vasodilation with sodium nitroprusside (pulmonary hypertension plus vasodilation). Under control conditions, the microvascular volume fraction comprised 11, 19, and 12% of the subepithelial tissue in the trachea and 1 mm and 0.5 mm bronchioles, respectively. Pulmonary hypertension doubled the microvascular volume fraction in the 0.5 mm bronchiole but had no effect on the microvasculature in the trachea and 1 mm bronchiole. Pulmonary hypertension plus vasodilation doubled the microvascular volume fraction in the trachea and 0.5 mm bronchiole and increased it to a lesser extent in the 1 mm bronchiole. Pulmonary hypertension with or without vasodilation increased the mean wall thickness in the 0.5 and 1 mm bronchioles and decreased the airway cross-sectional area in the 1 mm bronchiole (Table 2). These observations demonstrate that the microvasculature comprises a considerable volume fraction of the subepithelial airway tissue and that vascular congestion can narrow the bronchiolar lumen.

This morphological study suggests that hemodynamic changes in the airway circulation can influence airway function. Experimental data supporting this are scarce, however. Hardy et al. (1988) made the observation that inhalation of prostaglandin I_2 decreases FEV_1 and V_{max30} (but not SGaw) in human subjects and attributed this to vascular congestion in peripheral airways. By using a surface probe, Kyle et al. (1985) examined the effect of various locally infused vasoactive agents on tracheal mucosal thickness in dogs. There was a mean baseline total thickness of the mucosa (down to the cartilage) of 660 ± 43 μm, an increase between 12 and 134 μm with vasodilators, and a decrease of 27 μm with the vasoconstrictor phenylephrine. The experimental setup did not permit differentiation between intravascular or extravascular (edema) volume changes, but the rapidity with which the changes occurred suggested changes in vascular volume. The magnitude of these changes is probably insufficient to alter airflow resistance in the trachea but could have a noticeable effect on airflow resistance in peripheral airways.

We tested this possibility in conscious sheep by measuring peripheral airflow resistance (R_p) with the aid of a cuff-tipped dual-channel fiberoptic bronchoscope placed in a lobar or segmental bronchus. Forced sinusoidal oscillations of air (5 Hz) were applied through one of the inner channels of the bronchoscope. Flow at the proximal end of this channel and pressure in the occluded airway (measured through the other inner channel) were related to each other after high-pass filtering to calculate R_p. Local instillation of carbachol produced a dose-dependent increase in R_p that was reversible with atropine. Local instillation of nitroglycerin caused a transient increase in R_p, and vasopressin a transient decrease followed by an increase in R_p. These observations suggest that carbachol increases R_p by contracting airway smooth muscle via the stimulation of muscarinic receptors; the vascular smooth muscle relaxant nitroglycerin increases R_p by vascular congestion since a relaxation of airway smooth muscle by nitroglycerin would have an opposite effect on R_p. The biphasic effect of vasopressin on R_p could be explained by vasoconstriction (decrease in R_p) followed by bronchoconstriction (increase in R_p).

The local generation of endothelium-derived substances with airway smooth muscle effects is another mechanism by which the airway circulation could affect airway function. Endothelial cells in culture have been shown to release into the medium potent vasoconstrictor polypeptides (O'Brien et al., 1987; Hickey et al., 1985). Recently, Yanagisawa et al. (1988) successfully sequenced and cloned a 21-residue peptide from large-vessel endothelium,

Table 2 Effect of Vascular Congestion on Bronchiolar Wall Thickness and Lumen in Sheep[a]

	Experimental condition	1 mm Bronchiole		0.5 mm Bronchiole	
Mean wall thickness/shortest airway radius, μm/μm	PH	0.12 ±0.02[b]	(0.08 ±0.02)	0.11 ±0.02[c]	(0.07 ±0.03)
	PH+V	0.12 ±0.01[b]	(0.08 ±0.02)	0.14 ±0.01[b]	(0.09 ±0.02)
Airway cross-sectional area/basement membrane length, $\mu m^2/\mu m$	PH	297 ±30[d]	(352 ±11)	158 ±15	(143 ±30)
	PH+V	315 ±27[b]	(348 ±24)	168 ±31	(160 ±25)

[a] Mean ± SD of five small airways, each matched by basement membrane length comparisons. Matching control values in parentheses. PH = pulmonary hypertension. PH + V = pulmonary hypertension plus vasodilation. The experimental conditions were created by fixation by vascular perfusion at different perfusion pressures: systemic arterial pressure at 100 mmHg and pulmonary arterial pressure at 20 mmHg (control); systemic arterial pressure at 100 mmHg and pulmonary arterial pressure at 40 mmHg (PH); systemic arterial pressure at 100 mmHg, pulmonary arterial pressure at 40 mmHg, and infusion of sodium nitroprusside (PH + V). Transpulmonary pressure was 5 cmH_2O and left atrial pressure 0 mmHg under all experimental conditions. Indicated values are significantly different compared to matching control values.

[b] $p < 0.05$.

[c] $p = 0.05$.

[d] $p < 0.01$.

which they called endothelin. Endothelin is a potent constrictor of vascular smooth muscle. Likewise, medium conditioned by contact with endothelial cells in culture has also been shown to produce prolonged contraction of tracheal smooth muscle in vitro (Glassberg et al., 1989). Bovine coronary artery rings and trachealis muscle strips both responded in a dose-dependent fashion to endothelium-conditioned medium, although the smooth muscle reactivity of the coronary rings was greater than that of trachealis muscle. These effects were shown to be present regardless of whether the endothelium was derived from large vessels or the microcirculation. Considering the close proximity of the airway smooth muscle to the subepithelial microvasculature, endothelium-derived factors could theoretically regulate smooth muscle tone in vivo as well. This remains to be demonstrated experimentally, however. Likewise, the possibility that this regulatory function of the microvascular endothelium is disturbed in airway disease, such as bronchial asthma and chronic bronchitis, remains hypothetical.

Fluid accumulation in the airway wall and airway lumen, as observed in pulmonary edema, has been shown to increase airflow resistance (Hogg et al., 1972; Issekutz et al., 1980; Michel et al., 1987). Whether airway edema associated with the inflammatory component of airway disease has similar effects on airflow has not been directly examined, although this is a likely possibility.

B. Influence of Airway Blood Flow on Local Inflammatory Process

If airway blood flow is increased in bronchial asthma or other forms of airway inflammation as suggested by the observations in animal models, this hemodynamic response could facilitate the influx of inflammatory cells into the airway wall, the distribution of homeostatic circulating factors (e.g., epinephrine) to the airway, and the clearance of locally released chemical mediators. There is indirect experimental evidence that an increase in airway blood flow increases the clearance of mediators from the airway wall. Thus, the recovery from peripheral airway constriction caused by histamine has been found, using airflow through a wedged bronchoscope, to depend equally on bronchial and pulmonary blood flow in dogs, with a decrease in either flow prolonging the bronchial response to histamine (Kelly et al., 1986). In keeping with this observation, Csete et al. (1989) showed that preventing the increase in musosal blood flow after antigen challenge prolongs the duration of airway narrowing in allergic sheep. The notion that airway blood flow is a determinant of the clearance of substances from tissue is also supported by the demonstration that an increase in nasal mucosal blood flow resulting from the local application of histamine increases the uptake of intranasal desmopressin (Olanoff et al., 1987).

The augmented airway blood flow in bronchial asthma could be advantageous or disadvantageous. On the one hand, the increased circulation may accelerate the recovery from the local inflammatory process and promote delivery of systemic drugs to the diseased airway tissue. On the other hand, the increased blood flow could reduce the magnitude and shorten the duration of the local action of inhaled absorbable drugs and enhance their systemic side effects. When treating airway disease with aerosols, the actions of the inhaled drug on the airway circulation may therefore be worth considering. For example, combining an inhaled β-adrenergic agonist with a vasoconstrictor with negligible airway smooth muscle effects could theoretically enhance the magnitude and duration of bronchodilation (Fig. 4).

V. Summary

Structural and functional changes in the bronchial circulation are present in bronchial asthma and chronic obstructive pulmonary disease (chronic bronchitis and emphysema) as demonstrated by in vivo and postmortem investigations. In chronic bronchitis and emphysema, the most striking finding is an

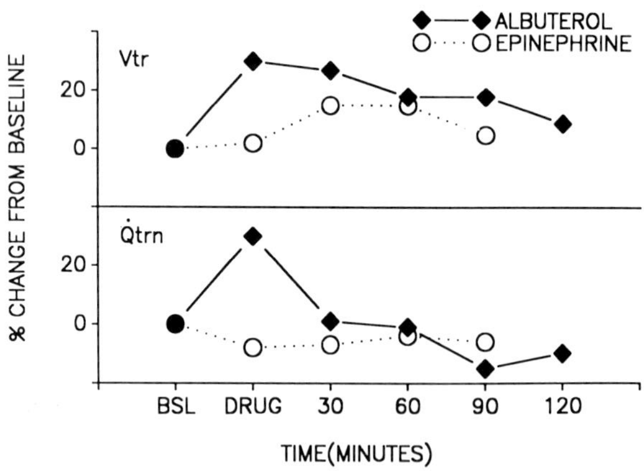

Figure 4 Effects of nebulized albuterol (200 μg) and racemic epinephrine (600 μg) on tracheal dead space (V_{tr}) and normalized mucosal blood flow ($\dot{Q}_{trn}$) in sheep. BSL = baseline, DRUG = immediately after aerosol administration. Both the β-adrenergic agonist albuterol and the combined α- and β-adrenergic agonist epinephrine dilate the trachea, but only the β-adrenergic agonist increases mucosal blood flow. (Courtesy of A. D. Chediak, M.D. and M. E. Csete, M.D.)

uneven distribution of the bronchial circulation with atrophy in regions of lung destruction (emphysema) and hypertrophy in regions with intact lung tissue but abnormal bronchi (chronic bronchitis, bronchiectasis). The functional consequences of these vascular lesions are unknown.

In bronchial asthma, the typical morphological changes of the bronchial circulation are hyperemia and edema in the airway wall. Animal studies suggest that the functional correlates of these lesions are an increase in bronchial blood flow and microvascular hyperpermeability for macromolecules. Both leukocyte-mediated inflammation and neuroinflammation seem to participate in the pathogenesis of the increased perfusion and permeability of the bronchial circulation. On the one hand, the increased blood flow and edema formation could obstruct peripheral bronchi by increasing the thickness of the airway wall. On the other, the increased blood flow could limit the magnitude and duration of the inflammatory process and hence bronchoconstriction and epithelial hypersecretion by rapidly clearing locally released chemical mediators in the airway wall. With respect to therapy, the increased bronchial blood flow in asthma could be of advantage by enhancing the delivery of systemic drugs to the diseased airway or of disadvantage by promoting clearance of inhaled drugs from the diseased airway.

References

Ahmed, T., Krainson, J. P., and Yerger, L. D. (1983). Functional depression of H_2 histamine receptors in sheep with experimental allergic asthma. *J. Allergy Clin. Immunol.* **72**:310–320.

Alksne, J. F. (1959). The passage of colloidal particles across the dermal capillary wall under the influence of histamine. *Q. J. Exp. Physiol.* **44**:51–66.

Austen, K. F., and Orange, R. P. (1975). Bronchial asthma: The possible role of the chemical mediators of immediate hypersensitivity in the pathogenesis of subacute chronic disease. *Am. Rev. Respir. Dis.* **11**:423–436.

Baier, H., Moas, R., Yerger, L., and Wanner, A. (1986). In vivo estimation of tracheal wall water: Effects of histamine and carbachol. *J. Appl. Physiol.* **60**:1680–1685.

Barker, J. A., Chediak, A. D., Baier, H. J., and Wanner, A. (1988). Tracheal mucosal blood flow responses to autonomic agonists. *J. Appl. Physiol.* **65**:829–834.

Barnes, P. (1987). Neuropeptides in human airways: Function and clinical implications. *Am. Rev. Respir. Dis.* **136**:S77–S83.

Bjork, J., and Smedegard, G. (1983). Acute microvascular effects of PAF-acether, as studied by intravital microscopy. *Eur. J. Pharmacol.* **96**:87.

Bjork, J., Hedqvist, P., and Arfors, K. E. (1982). Increase in vascular permeability induced by leukotriene B_4 and the role of polymorphonuclear leukocytes. *Inflammation* **6**:189–199.

Botenga, A. S. J. (1970). *Selective Bronchial and Intracostal Arteriography.* Baltimore, Williams & Wilkins.

Burnstock, G. (1986). The changing face of autonomic neurotransmission. *Acta Physiol. Scand.* **126**:67–91.

Chediak, A. D., and Wanner, A. (1991). Effects of histamine on tracheal mucosal perfusion, water content and airway smooth muscle in sheep. *Respir Physiol.* **84**:231–243.

Chipman, P., and Glover, W. E. (1976). Histamine H_2-receptors in the human peripheral circulation. *Br. J. Pharmacol.* **56**:494–496.

Csete, M. E., Chediak, A. D., and Wanner, A. (1989). Mucosal blood flow influences the duration of allergic airway smooth muscle contraction in the trachea. *Am. Rev. Respir. Dis.* **139**(4):A228.

Cudkowicz, L. (1980). Bronchial arterial circulation in men: Normal anatomy and responses to disease. In: *Pulmonary Vascular Diseases,* Vol. 14. Edited by K. Moser. New York, Marcel Dekker, pp. 112–232.

Cudkowicz, L., and Armstrong, J. B. (1953). The bronchial artery in pulmonary emphysema. *Thorax* **8**:46–58.

Dabney, J., Premen, A., Soika, C., and Dobbins, D. (1981). Aminophylline attenuates the edemogenic action of histamine. *Physiologist* **24**(4):107.

Dixon, F. J., and Warren, S. (1950). Antigen tracer studies and histologic observations in anaphylactic shock in the guinea pig. *Am. J. Med. Sci.* **219**:414–421.

Doidge, J. M., and Satchell, D. G. (1982). Adrenergic and nonadrenergic inhibitory nerves in mammalian airways. *J. Auton. Nerv. Syst.* **5**:83–99.

Duff, F., Greenfield, A. D. M., Shepherd, J. T., and Thompson, I. D. (1953). A quantitative study of the response to acetylcholine and histamine of the blood vessels of the human hand and forearm. *J. Physiol. (Lond.)* **120**:160–170.

Edwards, D. W. (1961). A summary of the third conference on research in emphysema: Air pollution and chronic pulmonary insufficiency. Answer to question 5. *Am. Rev. Respir. Dis.* **83**:581–582.

Ellis, F. H., Gringlay, J. H., and Edwards, J. E. (1951). The bronchial arteries. I. Experimental occlusion. *Surgery* **30**:810–826.

Evans, T. W., Chung, K. F., Rogers, D. F., and Barnes, P. J. (1987). Effect of platelet-activating factor on airway vascular permeability: Possible mechanisms. *J. Appl. Physiol.* **63**:479–484.

Evans, T. W., Rogers, D. F., Aursudkij, B., Chung, K. F., and Barnes, P. J. (1988). Inflammatory mediators involved in antigen-induced airway microvascular leakage in guinea pigs. *Am. Rev. Respir. Dis.* **138**:395–399.

Fick, R. B., Jr., Metzger, W. J., Richerson, H. B., Zavala, D. C., Moseley, P. L., Schoderbek, W. E., and Hunninghake, G. W. (1987). Increased bronchovascular permeability after allergen exposure in sensitive asthmatics. *J. Appl. Physiol.* **63**:1147–1155.

Gabbiani, G., Badonnel, M. C., and Majno, G. (1970). Intra-arterial injections of histamine, serotonin, or bradykinin: A topographic study of vascular leakage. *Proc. Soc. Exp. Biol. Med.* **135**:447–452.

Glassberg, M. K., Nolop, K. B., Jackowski, J. T., Abraham, W. M., Wanner, A., and Ryan, U. S. (1989). Endothelial cells produce a constrictor of airway smooth muscle. *Am. Rev. Respir. Dis.* **139**(4):A229.

Grega, G. J., Svensjo, E., and Adamski, S. (1981). Macromolecular permeability of the microvascular membrane: Physiological and pharmacological regulation. *Microcirculation* **1**(4):325.

Grega, G. J., Adamski, S. W., and Svensjo, E. (1985). Is there evidence for venular large junctional gap formation in inflammation? *Microcirc. Endothelium Lympathics* **2**:211–233.

Grega, G. J., Adamski, S. W., and Dobbins, D. E. (1986). Physiological and pharmacological evidence for the regulation of permeability. *Fed. Proc.* **45**:96–100.

Hardy, C. C., Bradding, P., Robinson, C., and Holgate, S. T. (1988). Bronchoconstrictor and antibronchoconstrictor properties of inhaled prostacyclin in asthma. *J. Appl. Physiol.* **64**:1567–1574.

Hickey, K. A., Rubanyi, G., Paul, R. J., and Highsmith, R. F. (1985). Characterization of a coronary vasoconstrictor produced by cultured endothelial cells. *Am. J. Physiol.* **248**:C550–C556.

Higgs, G. A., Cardinal, D. C., Moncada, S., and Vane, J. R. (1979). Microvasculatory effects of prostacyclin (PGI_2) in the hamster cheek pouch. *Microvasc. Res.* **18**:245–254.

Himori, N., and Taira, N. (1976). A method for recording smooth muscle and vascular responses of the blood-perfused dog trachea in situ. *Br. J. Pharmacol.* **56**:293–299.

Hogg, J. C., Agarawal, J. B., Gardiner, A. J. S., Palmer, W. H., and Macklem, P. T. (1972). Distribution of airway resistance with developing pulmonary edema in dogs. *J. Appl. Physiol.* **32**:20–24.

Holmberg, K., Bake, B., and Pipkorn, U. (1988). Nasal mucosal blood flow after intranasal allergen challenge. *J. Allergy Clin. Immunol.* **81**:541–547.

Hwang, S.-B., Li, C.-L., Lam, M.-H., and Shen, T. Y. (1985). Characterization of cutaneous vascular permeability induced by platelet-activating factor in guinea pigs and rats and its inhibition by a platelet-activating factor receptor antagonist. *Lab. Invest.* **52**:617–630.

Issekutz, A. C., Movat, K. W., and Movat, H. Z. (1980). Enhanced vascular permeability and haemorrhage-inducing activity of rabbit C5a: Probable role of polymorphonuclear leukocyte lysosomes. *Clin. Exp. Immunol.* **41**:512–520.

Kang, Y. H., Wei, H. M., Fisher, H., and Merrill, G. F. (1987). Histamine-induced changes in coronary circulation and myocardial oxygen consumption: Influences of histamine receptor antagonists. *FASEB J.* **1**:483–490.

Kelly, L., Kolbe, J., Mitzner, W., Spannhake, E. W., Bromberger-Barnea, B., and Menkes, H. (1986). Bronchial blood flow affects recovery from constriction in dog lung periphery. *J. Appl. Physiol.* **60**:1954–1959.

Knight, K. R., Collopy, P. A., and O'Brien, B. M. (1986). Response of the rabbit cutaneous microcirculation to prostanoid modifiers as determined by laser dopler flowmetry. *Microvasc. Res.* **31**:197–202.

Kyle, H., Robinson, N. P., and Widdicombe, J. G. (1985). Changes in mucosal thickness in the dog trachea. *J. Physiol. (Lond.)* **362**:13P.

Laitinen, L. A., Laitinen, A., and Widdicombe, J. (1987a). Effects of inflammatory and other mediators on airway vascular beds. *Am. Rev. Respir. Dis.* **135**:S67–S70.

Laitinen, L. A., Laitinen, M. A., and Widdicombe, J. G. (1987b). Dose-related effects of pharmacological mediators on tracheal vascular resistance in dogs. *Br. J. Pharmacol.* **92**:703–709.

Laitinen, L. A., Laitinen, M. V. A., and Widdicombe, J. G. (1987c). Parasympathetic nervous control of tracheal vascular resistance in the dog. *J. Physiol. (Lond.)* **385**:135–146.

Laitinen, L. A., Laitinen, A., Salonen, R. O., and Widdicombe, J. G. (1987d). Vascular actions of airway neuropeptides. *Am. Rev. Respir. Dis.* **136**:S59–S64.

Lebargy, F., Lenormand, E., Pariente, R., and Fournier, M. (1987). Morphological changes in rat tracheal mucosa immediately after antigen challenge. *Bull. Eur. Physiopathol. Respir.* **23**:417–421.

Lee, T. H., Austen, K. F., Leitch, A. G., Israel, E., Robinson, D. R., Lewis, R. A., Corey, E. J., and Drazen, J. M. (1985). The effects of fish-oil-enriched diet on pulmonary mechanics during anaphylaxis. *Am. Rev. Respir. Dis.* **132**:1204–1209.

Lewis, R. E., and Granger, H. J. (1986). Neutrophil-dependent mediation of microbascular permeability. *Fed. Proc.* **45**:109–113.

Long, W. M., Sprung, C. L., El-Fawall, H., Yerger, L. D., Eyre, P., Abraham, W. M., and Wanner, A. (1985). Effects of histamine on bronchial artery blood flow and bronchomotor tone. *J. Appl. Physiol.* **59**:254–261.

Long, W. M., Yerger, L. D., Martinez, H., Codias, E., Sprung, C. L., Abraham, W. M., and Wanner, A. (1988). Modification of bronchial blood flow during allergic airway responses. *J. Appl. Physiol.* **65**:272–282.

Lopez-Vidriero, M. T., and Reid, L. (1983). Pathological changes in asthma. In *Asthma,* 2nd Ed. Edited by T. J. H. Clark and S. Godfrey. London, Chapman and Hall, pp. 79–98.

Lung, M. A. K. Y., Wang, J. C. C., and Cheng, K. I. K. (1976). Bronchial circulation: An auto-perfusion method for assessing its vasomotor activity and the study of alpha- and beta-adrenoreceptors in the bronchial artery. *Life Sci.* **19**:577–580.

Majno, G., and Palade, G. E. (1961). Studies on inflammation. I. The effect of histamine and serotonin on vascular permeability: An electron microscopic study. *J. Biophys. Biochem. Cytol.* **11**:571–605.

Majno, G., Shea, S. M., and Levelthal, M. (1969). Endothelial contraction induced by histamine-type mediators. *J. Cell Biol.* **42**:647–672.

Mann, S. P. (1971). The innervation of mammalian bronchial smooth muscle: The localization of catecholamines and cholinesterases. *Histochem. J.* **3**:319–331.

Mariassy, A. T., Gazeroglu, H., and Wanner, A. (1991). Morphometry of the subepithelial circulation in sheep airways: Effect of vascular congestion. *Am. Rev. Respir. Dis.* **143**:162–166.

Martling, C.-R., Anggard, A., and Lundberg, J. M. (1985). Non-cholinergic vasodilation in the tracheobronchial tree of the cat induced by vagal nerve stimulation. *Acta Physiol. Scand.* **125**:343–346.

McDonald, D. M. (1987). Neurogenic inflammation in the respiratory tract: Actions of sensory nerve mediators on blood vessels and epithelium of the airway mucosa. *Am. Rev. Respir. Dis.* **136**:S65–S72.

McLaughlin, R. F., and Edwards, D. W. (1966). Naturally occurring emphysema, the fine gross and histopathologic counterpart of human emphysema. *Am. Rev. Respir. Dis.* **93**:22–25.

Merrill, G. F., Kang, Y. H., Wei, H. M., and Fisher, H. (1987). Pressure-dependent vasoactive effects of histamine in the coronary circulation. *FASEB J.* **1**:308–311.

Michel, R. P., Zocchi, L., Rossi, A., Cardinal, G. A., Ploy-Song-Sang, Y., Poulsen, R. S., Milic-Emili, J., and Staub, N. C. (1987). Does interstitial lung edema compress airway and arteries? A morphometric study. *J. Appl. Physiol.* **62**:108–115.

Miller, F. N., and Sims, D. E. (1986). Contractile elements in the regulation of macromolecular permeability. *Fed. Proc.* **45**:84–88.

Nagaishi, C., Nagasawa, N., Okada, Y., Yamashita, M., and Inaba, N. (1972). *Functional Anatomy and Histology of the Lung.* Baltimore, University Park Press.

Nakamura, T., Katori, R., Miyazawa, K., Ohtomo, S., Watanabe, T., Miuura, Y., and Takizawa, T. (1961). Bronchial blood flow in patients with chronic pulmonary disease and its influence upon respiration and circulation. *Dis. Chest* **39**:193–206.

O'Brien, R. F., Robbins, R. J., and McMurtry, I. F. (1987). Endothelial cells in culture produce a vasoconstrictor substance. *J. Cell. Physiol.* **132**:263–270.

Olanoff, L. S., Titus, C. R., Shea, M. S., Gibson, R. E., and Brooks, C. D. (1987). Effect of intranasal histamine on nasal mucosal blood flow and the antidiuretic activity of desmopressin. *J. Clin. Invest.* **80**:890–895.

Partanen, M., Laitinen, A., Hervonen, A., Toivanen, M., and Laitinen, L. A. (1982). Catecholamine- and acetylcholinesterase-containing nerves in human lower respiratory tract.*Histochemistry* **76**:175–188.

Peck, M. J., Piper, P. J., and Williams, T. J. (1981). The effect of leukotrienes C_4 and D_4 on the microvasculature of guinea-pig skin. *Prostaglandins* **21**:315.

Persson, C. G. A., and Erjefalt, I. (1986). Airway microvascular permeability to large molecules. *Bull. Eur. Physiopathol. Respir.* **22**(Suppl. 7):23–31.

Persson, C. G. A., Erjefalt, I., and Andersson, P. (1986). Leakage of macromolecules from guinea-pig tracheobronchial microcirculation. Effects of allergen, leukotrienes, tachykinins, and anti-asthma drugs. *Acta Physiol. Scand.* **127**:95–105.

Pietra, G. G., Szidon, J. P., Leventhal, M. M., and Fishman, A. P. (1971). Histamine and interstitial pulmonary edema in the dog. *Circ. Res.* **29**:323–337.

Renkin, E. M., Carter, R. D., and Joyner, W. L. (1974). Mechanism of the sustained action of histamine and bradykinin on transport of large molecules across capillary walls in the dog paw. *Microvasc. Res.* **7**:49–60.

Ricketts, H. J., and Carrington, C. B. (1968). Experimental bronchial artery occlusions in sheep. In *Proceedings of the 11th Aspen Emphysema Conference*. Bethesda, U.S. Dept. HEW, pp. 187–189.

Schulmon, E. S., MacGlashan, D. W., Jr., Peters, S. P., Schleimer, R. P., Newball, H. H., and Lichtenstein, L. M. (1982). Human lung mast cells: Purification and characterization. *J. Immunol.* **129**:2662–2667.

Sertl, K., Wiedermann, C. J., Kowalski, M. L., Hurtado, S., Plutchok, J., Linnoila, I., Pert, C. B., and Kaliner, M. A. (1988). Substance P: The relationship between receptor distribution in rat lung and the capacity of substance P to stimulate vascular permeability. *Am. Rev. Respir. Dis.* **138**:151–159.

Sheppard, D., Scypinski, L., Horn, J., Gordon, T., and Thompson, J. E.

(1986). Granulocyte-mediated airway edema in guinea pigs. *J. Appl. Physiol.* **60**:1213–1220.

Svensjo, E. (1978). Bradykinin and prostaglandin E_1, E_2, and F_2-induced macromolecular leakage in the hamster cheek pouch. *Prostaglandins Med.* **1**:397.

Svensjo, E., Persson, C. G. A., and Rutili, G. (1977). Inhibition of bradykinin induced macromolecular leakage from post-capillary venules by a β_2-adrenoreceptor stimulant, terbutaline. *Acta Physiol. Scand.* **101**:504–506.

Weiner, R., and Altura, B. M. (1967). Serotonin-bradykinin synergism in the mammalian capillary bed. *Proc. Soc. Exp. Biol. Med.* **124**:494.

Woods, D. A., and Miller, M. (1938). The role of the dual pulmonary circulation in various pathologic conditions of the lung. *J. Thorac. Surg.* **7**:649–670.

Yanagisawa, M., Kurihara, H., Kimura, S., Tomobe, Y., Kobayashi, M., Mitsui, Y., Yazaki, Y., Goto, K., and Masaki, T. (1988). A novel potent vasoconstrictor peptide produced by vascular endothelial cells. *Nature* **332**:411–415.

17

Neurogenic Inflammation of the Airways and Acute Lung Injury

S. LAKSHMINARAYAN

Veterans Administration Medical Center
and University of Washington School of Medicine
Seattle, Washington

I. Introduction

The large surface area of the airspaces, which are constantly exposed to the external environment via inspired air, and their large internal vascular area, constantly exposed to the total cardiac output via the right heart, make the lung a prime target for injury from inhaled or blood-borne toxins. In chronic inflammatory states, such as lung abscesses (see Chap. 18), it has been recognized for a long time that the pulmonary circulation is almost absent in the diseased regions and that their major blood supply is from the bronchial circulation. However, the role of the bronchial circulation in acute lung inflammation or injury is not well known. This chapter reviews pertinent studies that have been done and discusses their implications for the role of the bronchial circulation in acute lung injury.

II. Neurogenic Inflammation of the Airways

It is now known that the airways have a rich supply of sensory nerves. Sensory nerves play a key role in the vasodilation and increased vascular permeability that occur in response to irritant stimuli in several organs, such as the skin, the eye, and the joints.

This local tissue response has been called neurogenic inflammation. In a seminal paper, Lundberg and Saria (1983) demonstrated in rats that increased permeability of the naso-tracheobronchial vessels occurred in the mucosa of the nose, larynx, trachea, and major bronchi in response to a variety of stimuli, including cigarette smoke, ether, formalin, and capsaicin. They also noticed that local chemical irritation (histamine and bradykinin) and vagal nerve stimulation induced an increase in vascular permeability leading to edema in the subepithelial region in the rat trachea. Stimulation of the cervical vagus nerve also evoked neurogenic inflammation in the trachea and bronchi of the guinea pig and the rat (Lundberg and Saria, 1982). Further, they showed that the increase in vascular permeability was reduced or abolished in animals in which C fiber afferents in the respiratory tract had degenerated by pretreating the animals with capsaicin (Lundberg et al., 1983a). Stimulation of the sensory (afferent) axons that innervate the airway via the stellate ganglion also causes neurogenic inflammation in guinea pigs (Saria et al., 1984).

The role of the vagus in the development of neurogenic inflammation is complex. Efferent fibers (motor axons in the vagus nerves) are not responsible for the neurogenic vasodilation because the neurogenic inflammatory effect of vagal stimulation is not blocked by hexamethonium (a blocker of synaptic efferent transmission in autonomic ganglia) or atropine (a blocker of the muscarinic effects of cholinergic nerves) (Lundberg and Saria, 1982). McDonald et al. (1988) showed that the neurogenic inflammation is not mediated by preganglionic efferent axons in the vagus nerve. It is also known that rats receiving capsaicin from the second day of life to deplete the sensory nerves of substance P and destroy the myelinated sensory axons show a decreased bronchial vascular vasodilatory response to nonspecific irritants and to mediators such as histamine and bradykinin (Gamse et al., 1980). This suggests that both specific and nonspecific stimuli can evoke vasodilation, due at least in part to sensory nerves.

Generally, studies have utilized two major techniques to quantitate the increase in permeability of the vessels that is produced by an inciting stimulus. Earlier studies used the amount of Evan's blue that diffused out of the vascular lumen into the tissues (Saria and Lundberg, 1983). Evan's blue binds to plasma albumin, so the use of Evan's blue shows the permeability of blood vessels to molecules approximately 60 kD in size. However, since the extravasated Evan's blue moves rapidly through the vessel wall to the interstitial connective tissue and to the lymphatics, the precise site of the extravasation of the dye through the vascular endothelium cannot be ascertained. To solve this problem, McDonald et al. (1987) used Monastral blue (Joris et al., 1982), a copper phthalocyanine pigment that is a particulate and hence is too large to cross the intact endothelium or the basal lamina in the blood vessels. McDonald (1988) produced neurogenic inflammation in the trachea and bronchi in rats by electrically stimulating the superior laryngeal and the vagus nerves and showed that within 2–5 min of vagal stimulation, the postcapillary venules and collecting venules 7–80 μm in diameter were the sites of increased endothelial permeability; capillaries, arterioles, and larger venules did not show any evidence of increased permeability. Using electron microscopy they also showed that gaps as wide as 1.5 μm could be seen between endothelial cells in the postcapillary venules. These venules were subepithelial and were present between the cartilaginous rings in the trachea. In the extrathoracic trachea the posterior membranous portion showed evidence of increased permeability; however, in the intrathoracic trachea the posterior membranous portion did not (McDonald, 1988).

In another set of experiments, Brokaw and McDonald (1988) showed that vagal stimulation caused up to a fivefold increase in the amount of dye extravasation that began within 30 s of the onset of vagal stimulation and lasted for 3–5 min. Tachyphylaxis developed after stimuli as brief as 15 s and reduced the dye extravasation produced by a subsequent period of vagal stimulation for as long as 4 h.

In addition to the increase in vascular permeability, white blood cells, primarily monocytes and neutrophils but also erythrocytes and platelets, adhere to the endothelium of the abnormally permeable venules in neurogenic inflammation (McDonald, 1988). Since it is known that the increase in vascular permeability seen in several inflammatory states requires the presence of neutrophils, Bethel and colleagues (1988) investigated the role of the neutrophil and other blood components in the increase in vascular permeability induced by substance P. Using a rat preparation in which the aorta, and therefore all the upper tracheal vessels, were perfused with blood-free Krebs-Henseleit solution containing albumin and Monastral blue, they noted that intravenous substance P or electrical stimulation of the vagus nerve still increased the amount of extravasated Monastral blue. They concluded that the adherence of neutrophils and monocytes to endothelium was more an effect of the neurogenic inflammation than a cause.

McDonald et al. (1988) demonstrated that only a few sensory nerves were located near the affected venules and no nerves were within 1 μm of the walls of the venules. However, the epithelium and the arterioles of the airway mucosa were densely innervated so that all intraepithelial nerves were within 0.1 μm of the epithelial cells. They therefore raised the interesting idea that the neuropeptides from the sensory nerves may evoke the release of secondary mediators from the epithelial cells that subsequently contribute to the increase in vascular permeability.

It is also known that the mediators of neurogenic inflammation also cause substantial changes in airway epithelial permeability. In addition to the morphological data provided by McDonald et al., Persson and Erjefalt (1985) showed that the application of capsaicin to the luminal surface of the guinea pig trachea increases the movement of fluorescinated dextran and ^{131}I albumin from the blood into the airway lumen. In addition, neurogenic inflammation caused the secretory granules in the serous and mucus cells of the airway epithelium to move to the cell apex and subsequently discharge their contents into the lumen, suggesting that sensory nerves also influence the production of mucus by epithelial secretory cells (McDonald, 1987).

Several factors modify neurogenic inflammation (Lundberg et al., 1983b). It is diminished or abolished by transection of the vagus nerve; prior treatment with capsaicin, either systemically or by topical application to the vagus nerve; application of local anesthetics to the tracheal lumen; and systemic injections of substance P antagonists. (See also Chap. 8.) In addition, McDonald (1987) showed a striking increase in sensitivity to neurogenic inflammation of the trachea in rats with a history of naturally occurring airway infections caused by a variety of pathogens, including *Mycoplasma pulmonis,* rat coronovirus, and Sendai virus, at a time when the animals are clinically well. One may speculate that the hyperreactivity of the blood vessels and muscles of the airways seen in humans after viral or upper respiratory infections could be mediated by a similar mechanism. Much more needs to be known about the modulators and the significance of neurogenic inflammation.

III. Airway Mucosal Injury and Inflammation

Kramer et al. (1989) studied the effect of the inhalation of cotton smoke on airway blood flow in sheep. They measured bronchial blood flow, using the microsphere method, for up to 30 h after the inhalation of cotton smoke. Though the inhalation injury had little effect on cardiac output or blood flow to peripheral systemic tissues, airway blood flow was increased ninefold in the trachea, eightfold in the mainstem bronchi, and 12-fold in the intraparenchymal bronchi. Since systemic arterial pressures were unchanged, they concluded that the increased airway blood flow was due to selective vasodilatation of the airway vasculature. They went on to hypothesize that this increased airway blood flow could lead to increased filtration of fluid from the bronchial microvasculature and thus contribute to the pulmonary edema seen in inhalation injury. Similarly, Schelegle et al. (1990) showed a dose-dependent increase in mucosal bronchial blood flow following exposure to 4 parts per million of ozone for 4 h when measured by a Doppler flow probe.

In a canine preparation of inflammatory edema induced by the inhalation of acrolein deposited on carbon particles, histological examination using Monastral blue as the tracer revealed increased permeability of the bronchial vessels down to small bronchioles (0.5 mm innerdiameter, ID) (Hales et al., 1989). Ligation of the bronchial arteries delayed the onset and lessened the magnitude of the edema around the affected airways. Since acrolein inhalation also caused edema in the lung after the pulmonary artery was ligated, the authors concluded that the bronchial circulation can be a major source of fluid leakage. Using a lymph fistula preparation in sheep, Walsh et al. (1988) showed that inhalation of cotton smoke increased lung lymph flow fourfold after 24 h and that bronchial arterial occlusion caused an attenuation of this increased lung lymph flow.

Thus, there is now an increasing body of evidence that the bronchial circulation is important in acute lung injury in that its blood flow rises and contributes to the increased exudation of fluid. This increase in the bronchial blood flow could be beneficial insofar as inflammation must precede healing. It could provide the factors necessary for the inflammation of the local region as well as aid in the removal of inflammatory debris and edema that must occur to allow the recovery and repair of the injured lung.

IV. Pneumonia

It has been known for many years that the pulmonary blood flow is reduced in regions of pneumonia and that this reduction in blood flow matches the area of radiographic density. This has been demonstrated in the human by pulmonary angiography as well as perfusion lung scans using macroaggregated radiolabeled albumin (Wagner et al., 1964; Cudkowicz, 1968). It has also been inferred from the results of other methods. For instance, in 25 patients with verified lobar pneumonia, it was shown using the technique of cinedensigraphy to measure the presence of the pulmonary arterial pulse that pulmonary blood flow was absent or greatly decreased over the pneumonic area (Standertskjold-Nordenstam, 1965). In early pneumonia in the human, conventional pulmonary angiography showed diminished filling of the lobar branches of the pulmonary artery (Cicero et al., 1968). In an experimental study of distemper bronchopneumonia in dogs, Mathes et al. (1932) found poor filling of the large branches of the pulmonary artery; the terminal arterioles of the pulmonary circulation appeared blunted and pruned, suggesting thromboses. However, it is interesting that they noted that the bronchial arteries and the lymphathics were dilated and patent. As early as 1912, Karsner and Ash proposed that the "red hepatization" seen in classic pneumococcal lobar pneumonia was due to an augmented bronchial arterial blood flow distal to the occluded pulmonary arteries. They further suggested that the red cells in the alveoli stem from the high inflow pressure of the bronchial circulation.

Using postmortem arteriography, Cudkowicz (1952) showed dilation and an increase in the number of bronchial blood vessels to regions of lobar pneumonia in four patients who died from overwhelming pneumonia. In several instances the lobar pulmonary artery was occluded, presumably from thrombi. The peripheral branches of the pulmonary circulation filled in a retrograde fashion from communicating bronchial arteries. He also proposed that the restoration of the pulmonary circulation in lobar pneumonia is slow and speculated that it proceeds concurrently with a slow regression of the bronchial circulation. In humans, perfusion lung scanning has shown that the reduced pulmonary blood flow to an area of lobar pneumonia persists long after clinical resolution of the pneumonia.

The mechanisms that control the increase in bronchial blood flow following pneumonia are unknown. The time at which the bronchial vasculature dilates following the onset of pneumonia is also not known, although Mathes et al. (1932) noted dilated bronchial vessels in the early stages of distemper bronchopneumonia in dogs.

Kowalski et al. (1989) studied the relative contributions of the bronchial and pulmonary circulations to the delivery of neutrophils as well as inflammatory edema in a rabbit preparation of pneumococcal pneumonia. They occluded the left pulmonary artery of rabbits and compared the inflammatory exudate and edema response to the local instillation of *Streptococcus pneumoniae* into the experimental left lower lobe (supplied by the bronchial circulation only) with that of the right lower lobe, which had both the pulmonary and bronchial circulations intact. They used technetium-99m-labeled erythrocytes and ^{125}I-labeled albumin to measure extravascular lung water and protein accumulation and quantitative morphometry to assess neutrophil accumulation 6 h after instillation of the organisms. When pulmonary blood flow was absent, there was less extravasation of protein and almost no emigration of neutrophils in the pneumonic area. They therefore concluded that in the very early response to bacterial challenge, the pulmonary, not the bronchial circulation, was primarily responsible for both the inflammation and the delivery of neutrophils.

It seems clear that, in established pneumonia, while the bronchial circulation to the region increases, the pulmonary circulation decreases after reacting to the initial inflammatory response. It is tempting to speculate that the increase in the bronchial circulation provides the blood supply to aid in the recovery from pneumonia, although no data are available to prove this.

V. Adult Respiratory Distress Syndrome

Unlike the regionally limited inflammation in pneumonia, the damage to the lung after a variety of blood-borne or inhaled agents is widespread. It is now well recognized that different underlying diseases predispose many patients to develop the widespread lung injury commonly called the adult respiratory distress syndrome (ARDS) (Pepe, 1986). The most notable of these are sepsis, shock, multiple trauma, aspiration, and toxic gas inhalation. The increased permeability of the pulmonary microvessels results in the leakage of a protein-rich edema fluid from the damaged intravascular compartment to the interstitial and intraalveolar spaces. This syndrome results in inflammatory edema that involves most regions of the lung, although the damage is patchy.

The role of the bronchial circulation in this inflammatory (increased permeability) edema has been investigated in two ways. First, is the bronchial circulation a site of the fluid leak in uremic edema? Borgstrom et al. (1960) hypothesized that the central distribution of pulmonary edema, with clear peripheral lung zones seen radiographically in patients with uremic pneumonitis, was because a toxic substance or substances in uremia increased the permeability of the bronchial vessels. In the anesthetized dog they injected a 0.2–0.8% solution of a bile salt (sodium deoxycholate) into a major bronchial artery and found that this produced the perihilar pattern of edema seen in patients with uremic pneumonitis. Histologically, they noted distended bronchial vessels with perivascular hemorrhage and edema. They also found an inflammatory reaction in these regions although the periphery of the lung was normal. However, when the same bile salt (with the dosage adjusted for the different volume of the pulmonary blood flow) was injected into the pulmonary circulation, a more generalized pattern of edema was seen. Histology revealed alveolar hemorrhage and edema but the peribronchial areas were normal. They therefore concluded that, at least in their preparation, the bronchial circulation was the site of leakage in central uremic pulmonary edema.

A similar approach to the study of the role of the bronchial circulation in the formation of pulmonary edema has been to investigate the effects of other chemicals known to mediate inflammation. Histamine has been the agent most often studied, and the results are complex. Pietra and colleagues (1971) noted that in dogs, histamine administration, intravascularly or as an aerosol, increased the permeability of bronchial veins but not that of the pulmonary microvessels. This was shown by the leakage of colloidal carbon through the bronchial venous intercellular junctions. Subsequently these authors showed similar effects with intravenous endotoxin (Pietra et al., 1974). In contrast to these studies, Brigham et al. (1976) found that, in sheep, histamine infused in the pulmonary artery was twice as effective at increasing lung lymph flow and lymph protein concentration compared to when it was infused into the left atrium and thus the bronchial circulation. In a similar study, Nakahara et al. (1979) demonstrated that equal doses of histamine infusion into the bronchial artery and pulmonary arteries of sheep caused similar increases in lung lymph and protein flow. They concluded that the site of action of histamine was probably the pulmonary microcirculation because the local concentration of histamine, when infused in the bronchial circulation, was much greater than when it was infused into the pulmonary circulation because the blood flows were so different. More recent studies using an isolated dog forelimb preparation have shown that histamine increases the permeability of systemic blood vessels (Maron, 1982). The bronchial vasculature is a systemic bed within the lungs. Recent results of histamine administration by intravenous infusion (Bernard et al., 1984) or by aerosol (Hutchison et al., 1984) suggest that it has only a transient effect on pulmonary vascular permeability. These effects of histamine are likely to be a result of two mechanisms. One is the increase in the permeability of the bronchial venules. The other is the increase in pulmonary artery pressure caused by histamine, so there is a recruitment of the pulmonary vascular bed and thus an increase in the lymph flow because the surface area available for fluid flux is increased.

Other studies have now shown that histamine increases the permeability of the tracheal microvessels to large tracer molecules, such as dextran (Erjefalt et al., 1985; Kramer et al., 1988). In studying the effects of histamine on bronchovascular as well as smooth muscle responses in sheep, Long et al. (1985), using an electromagnetic flow probe around the bronchial artery, showed that, following aerosolized histamine, bronchial blood flow rose 2½ times and airway resistance increased even more. The bronchial blood flow response was blocked by H_2-antagonists; the airway bronchoconstrictor response was blocked by H_1-antagonists. They concluded that the smooth muscle and the vascular responses were mediated by different sets of receptors. Kramer and associates (1988), using a lymph fistula preparation in the sheep, showed that intravenous histamine increased lung lymph flow by three- to fourfold within 1 h. Bronchial arterial occlusion had no effect on normal lung lymph flow but reduced the histamine-induced increase in lymph flow by one-third. Thus, the majority of evidence suggests that histamine increases the permeability of the bronchial vessels. The contribution of this to the increased extravascular water found in inflammatory edema remains to be elucidated. Other mediators of inflammation, such as bradykinin, some of the leukotrienes, and antigen challenge in sensitized animals, have similar effects on the tracheal bronchial circulation (Persson and Erjefalt, 1985).

In humans with ARDS, premortem and postmortem pulmonary angiograms have shown pulmonary vascular obstructions, obliterations, and thromboses (Greene et al., 1981; Snow et al., 1982). Early in the course of

ARDS, thombotic obliteration of the pulmonary vasculature is commonly seen in patients who die within the first 10–14 days. In those who survive longer than 10–12 days, fibrocellular proliferation of the intima leading to pulmonary vascular obliteration is commonly seen. In situ thombosis due to decreased flow, hypoxic pulmonary vasoconstriction, and compression of pulmonary vessels by perivascular cuffs of edema have all been hypothesized as the cause of the early changes. Despite the diffuse injury in ARDS and the restriction of pulmonary perfusion, healing, which depends on an adequate blood flow, is usually very good. The survivors show remarkably good pulmonary function upon recovery (Lakshminarayan et al., 1976). It could be that the bronchial circulation provides an alternative blood supply to the regions of injury where the pulmonary circulation was cut off.

Acute increases in anastomotic bronchial flow have been observed in the dog using an *in situ,* isolated, perfused, left lower lobe preparation of diffuse lung injury induced by either the vascular route (oleic acid or α-naphthylthiourea) or the airway route (HCl or glucose-glucose oxidase aspiration; Figs. 1 and 2) (Lakshminarayan et al., 1987). That this effect was not due to the presence of edema alone was shown because hydrostatic edema of a

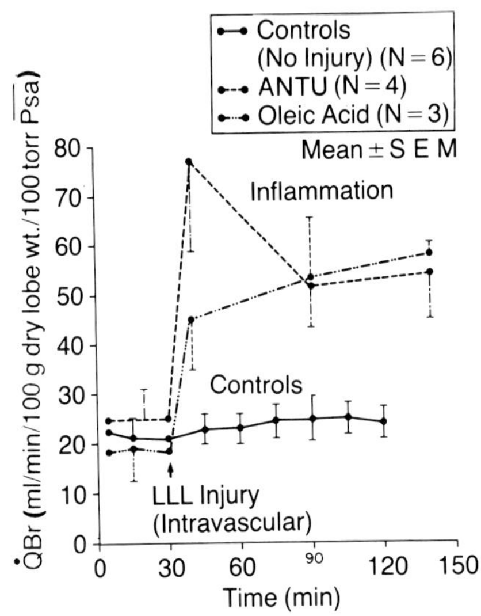

Figure 1 Increase in anastomotic bronchial blood flow after pulmonary vascular injury with α-naphthylthiourea or oleic acid. Controls represent the animals with no intervention. Values shown are mean ± standard error of the mean (SEM). (Modified from Lakshminarayan et al., 1987, with permission from the *Journal of Applied Physiology.*)

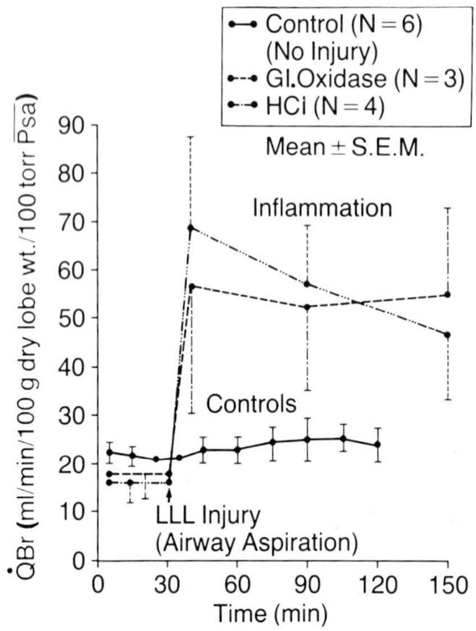

Figure 2 Increase in anastomotic bronchial blood flow following aspiration injury via the airways with glucose-glucose oxidase or hydrochloric acid (HCl) aspiration. Values shown are mean ±SEM. (Modified from Lakshminarayan et al., 1987, with permission from the *Journal of Applied Physiology*.)

similar degree did not cause an increase in anastomotic blood flow (Lakshminarayan et al., 1987). Thus the increase in bronchial blood flow could have been due to the inflammatory mediators known to be present in inflammatory, but not in hydrostatic, edema. Subsequently, Deffebach and his colleagues (1987) studied some of the mediators involved in this response. Since arachidonic acid metabolites are responsible for many of the inflammatory events observed after lung injury, they hypothesized that the cyclooxygenase products of arachidonic acid metabolism may be important regulators of the bronchovascular response to acute lung injury. Using the same form of injury as Lakshminarayan et al. (1987), they showed that when cyclooxygenase inhibition was achieved before the stress of the surgery and lung injury, the bronchial blood flow was markedly decreased compared with that in controls blocked after a surgical preparation without lung injury. Subsequent lung injury increased the blood flow by an amount similar to the lung injury in the control animals. They therefore concluded that the increase in bronchial blood flow after a nonspecific stress, such as surgery, is caused by the cyclooxygenase products, but that other mediators and factors are responsible for the inflammatory increase after acute lung injury (Fig. 3) (Deffebach et al., 1987).

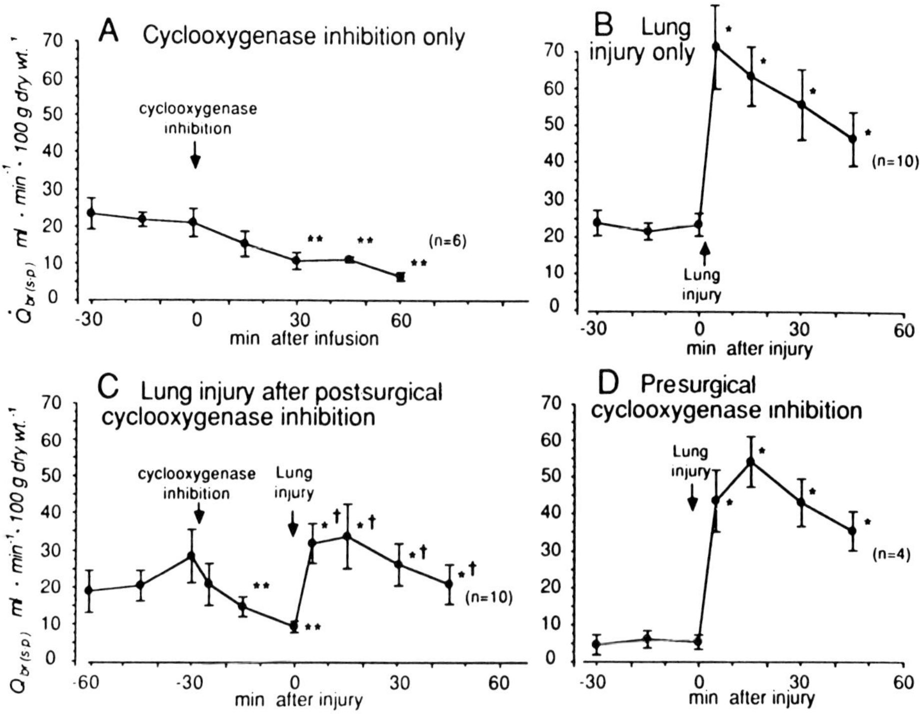

Figure 3 Anastomotic bronchial blood flow [$\dot{Q}_{br(s\text{-}p)}$] after cyclooxygenase inhibition and injury with α-napthylthiourea or glucose-glucose oxidase. Cyclooxygenase inhibition followed 30 min of stable $\dot{Q}_{br(s\text{-}p)}$, except in group D, which received cyclooxygenase inhibition before surgical preparation. Values shown are means + SEM. $^*P < 0.05$ compared with preinjury values of same experimental group. $^{**}P < 0.05$ compared with precyclooxygenase inhibition values in the same group. $P < 0.05$ compared with injury only group at the same time after injury. (From Deffebach et al., 1987, with permission from the *Journal of Applied Physiology*.)

VI. Summary

A new area of study is that of neurogenic inflammation of the tracheobronchial tree. The increase in permeability that occurs following neurogenic inflammation occurs predominantly around the postcapillary and collecting venules. The mediators and mechanisms involved are now the object of much investigation and, it is hoped, will lead to new therapeutic strategies. The implications of neurogenic inflammation in terms of the inflammatory component of asthma also need clarification.

Although it is well known that the pulmonary blood flow decreases to a region of acute inflammation, it has not been widely appreciated that the bronchial blood flow increases. This is time dependent and can eventually be quite considerable. It happens in both localized inflammation (such as lobar pneumonia) and generalized patchy lung injury, such as ARDS. Experimental studies suggest that this increase occurs within the first few hours to days following the injury and that it persists throughout the course of the injury. In injury due to inhaled noxious agents, such as smoke, the increased bronchial blood flow has been shown to contribute to the formation of edema around the airways as well as to increased lung lymphatic flow. The mechanisms involved in this compensatory increase of the bronchial blood flow merit further study. The role of the bronchial circulation in coping both with an acute inflammation and with the subsequent repair are also not known.

References

Bernard, G. R., Snapper, J. R., Hutchinson, A. A., and Brigham, K. L. (1984). Effects of left atrial presure elevation and histamine on lung lymph in awake sheep. *J. Appl. Physiol.* **56**:1083–1089.

Bethel, R. A., Brokaw, J. J., Evans, T. W., Nadel, J. K., and McDonald, D. M. (1988). Substance P-induced increase in vascular permeability in the rat trachea does not depend on neutrophils or other components of circulating blood. *Exp. Lung Res.* **14**:769–779.

Borgstrom, K. E., Ising, U., Linder, E., and Lunderquist, A. (1960). Experimental pulmonary edema. *Acta Radiol.* **53**:97–119.

Brigham, K. L., Bowers, R. E., and Owen, P. J. (1976). Effects of antihistimines on the lung vacular response to histamine in unanesthetized sheep. Diphenhydramine prevention of pulmonary edema and increased permeability. *J. Clin. Invest.* **58**:391–398.

Brokaw, J. J., and McDonald, D. M. (1988). Neurally mediated increase in vascular permeability in the rat trachea: Onset, duration, and tachyphylaxis. *Exp. Lung Res.* **14**:757–767.

Cicero, R., Cardosa, J. M., and Del Castillo, H. (1968). Selective angiography of the bronchial arteries in pulmonary tuberculosis. *Am. Rev. Respir. Dis.* **98**:623–633.

Cudkowicz, L. (1952). Some observations of the bronchial arteries in lobar pneumonia and pulmonary infarction. *Br. J. Tuberc.* **46**:99–102.

Cudkowicz, L. (1968). *The Human Bronchial Circulation in Health and Disease.* Baltimore, Williams & Wilkins, pp. 158–173.

Deffebach, M. E., Lakshminarayan, S., Kirk, W., and Butler, J. (1987). Bronchial circulation and cyclooxygenase products in acute lung injury. *J. Appl. Physiol.* **63**:1083–1088.

Erjefalt, I., Wagner, F., Strand, S. E., and Persson, C. G. A. (1985). A method for studies of tracheal microvascular permeability to macromolecules. *J. Pharmacol. Methods* **14**:275–283.

Gamse, R., Holzer, P., and Lembeck, F. (1980). Decrease of substance P in primary afferent neurons and impairment of neurogenic plasma extravasation by capsaicin. *Br. J. Pharmacol.* **68**:207–213.

Greene, R., Zapol, W. M., Snider, M. T., Reid, L., Snow, R., O'Connell, R. S., and Novelline, R. A. (1981). Early bedside detection of pulmonary vascular occlusion during acute respiratory failure. *Am. Rev. Respir. Dis.* **124**:593–601.

Hales, C. A., Barkin, P., Jung, W., Lamborghini, D., and Burke, J. (1989). Bronchial artery ligation modifies pulmonary edema after exposure to smoke with acrolein. *J. Appl. Physiol.* **67**:1001–1006.

Hutchison, A. A., Bernard, G. R., Snapper, J. R., and Brigham, K. L. (1984). Effect of aerosol histamine on lung lymph in awake sheep. *J. Appl. Physiol.* **56**:1090–1098.

Joris, I., Wortham, D., and Majno, G. (1982). Vascular labeling with Monastral blue B. *Stain Technol.* **57**:177–183.

Karsner, H. T., and Ash, H. E. (1912). Studies in infarction. II. Experimental bland infarction of drugs. *J. Med Res.* **27**:205–223.

Kowalski, T. F., Doerschuk, C. M., Lakshmi, S., English, D., and Butler, J. (1989). The bronchial circulation in neutrophil delivery to streptococcal pneumonia in rabbits. *Fed. Proc. Voc.* **3**(3):A567.

Kramer, G. C., and Gunther, R. A. (1988). Relative contributions of the bronchial and pulmonary circulations to lung lymph flow during histamine infusion. *Am. Rev. Respir. Dis.* **13**:368A.

Kramer, C. G., Lindsey, D. C., Wu, C. H., Russell, L. A., and Gross, C. E. (1988). Airway blood flow distribution and lung edema after histamine infusion in awake sheep. *J. Appl. Physiol.* **65**:1847–1854.

Kramer, G. C., Herndon, D. N., Linares, H. A., and Traber, D. L. (1989). Effects of inhalation injury on airway blood flow and edema formation. *J. Burn Care Rehabil.* **10**:45–51.

Lakshminarayan, S., Stanford, R. E., and Petty, T. L. (1976). Prognosis after recovery from adult respiratory distress syndrome. *Am. Rev. Respir. Dis.* **113**:7–16.

Lakshminarayan, S., Jindal, S. K., Kirk, W., and Butler, J. (1987). Acute increases in anastomotic bronchial systemic to pulmonary blood flow due to generalized lung injury. *J. Appl. Physiol.* **62**:2358–2361.

Long, W. M., Sprung, C. L., El-Fawall, H., Yerger, L. D., Eyre, ?, Abraham, W. M., and Wanner, A. (1985). Effects of histamine on bronchial artery blood flow and bronchomotor tone. *J. Appl. Physiol.* **59**:254–261.

Lundberg, J. M., and Saria, A. (1982). Capsaicin-sensitive vagal neurons in control of vascular permeability in rat trachea. *Acta Physiol. Scand.* **115**:521–523.

Lundberg, J. M., and Saria, A. (1983). Capsaicin-induced desensitization of airway mucosa to cigarette smoke, mechanical and chemical irritants. *Nature* **302**:251–253.

Lundberg, J. M., Brodin, E., and Saria, A. (1983a). Effects and distribution of vagal capsaicin-sensitive P neurons with special reference to the tracheal and lungs. *Acta Physiol. Scand.* **119**:243–252.

Lundberg, J. M., Saria, A., Brodin, E., Rosell, S., and Folkers, K. (1983b). A substance P antagonist inhibits vagally induced increase in vascular permeability and bronchial smooth muscle contraction in the guinea pig. *Proc. Natl. Acad. Sci. U S A* **80**:110–1124.

Maron, M. B. (1982) Differential effects of histamine on protein permeability in dog lung and forelimb. *Am. J. Physiol.* **242**(11):H565–572.

Mathes, M. E., Holman, E., and Reichert, F. L. (1932). A study of the bronchial pulmonary and lymphatic circulations of the lung under various pathologic conditions experimentally produced. *J. Thorac. Surg.* **I**:339–362.

McDonald, D. M. (1987). Neurogenic inflammation in the respiratory tract; actions of sensory nerve mediators on blood vessels and epithelium of the airway mucosa. *Am. Rev. Respir. Dis.* **136**:S65–S72.

McDonald, D. M. (1988). Neurogenic inflammation in the rat trachea. I. Changes in venules, leukocytes and epithelial cells. *J. Neurocytol.* **17**:583–603.

McDonald, D. M., Mitchell, R. A., Gabaella, G., and Haskell, A. (1988). Neurogenic inflammation of rat trachea. II. Identity and distribution of nerves mediating the increase in vascular permeability. *J. Neurocytol.* **17**:605–628.

Nakahara, A., Ohkuda, K., and Staub, N. C. (1979). Effect of infusing histamine into pulmonary or bronchial artery on sheep pulmonary fluid balance. *Am. Rev. Respir. Dis.* **120**:875–882.

Pepe, P. E. (1986). The clinical entity of adult respiratory distress syndrome. In *Critical Care Clinics.* Edited by H. P. Weidemann, M. A. Matthay, and R. A. Matthay. Philadelphia, W. B. Saunders, pp. 377–403.

Persson, C. G. A., and Erjefalt, I. (1985). Inflammatory leakage of macraomolecules from the vascular compartment into the tracheal lumen. *Acta Physiol. Scand.* **126**:615–616.

Pietra, C. G., Szidon, J. P., Leventhal, M. M., and Fishman, A. P. (1971). Histamine and interstitial pulmonary edema in the dog. *Circ. Res.* **29**:323–337.

Pietra, C. G., Szidon, J. P., Carpenter, H. A., and Fishman, A. P. (1974). Bronchial venular leakage during endotoxin shock. *Am. J. Pathol.* **77**:387–406.

Saria, A., and Lundberg, J. M. (1983). Evans blue fluorescence: Quantitative and morphological evaluation of vascular permeability in animal tissues. *J. Neurosci. Methods* **8**:41–49.

Saria, A., Theodorsson-Norheim, E., Gamse, R., and Lundberg, J. M. (1984). Release of substance P and substance K-like immunoreactivities from the isolated perfused guinea pig lung. *Eur. J. Pharmacol.* **106**:207–208.

Schelegle, E., Gunther, R., Parsons, G., Colbert, S. R., Yousef, A. A., and Cross, C. (1990). Acute ozone exposure increases bronchial blood flow in conscious sheep. *Respir. Physiol.* **8**:325–336.

Snow, R., Davis, P., Pontoppidan, H., Zapol, W. M., and Rein, L. (1982). Pulmonary vascular remodeling in adult respiratory distress syndrome. *Am. Rev. Respir. Dis.* **126**:887–892.

Standertskjold-Nordenstam, C. G. (1965). The pulmonary circulation during pneumonia. A cinedenisgraphic study. *Acta Radiol. Suppl.* 239.

Wagner, H. N., Sabiston, D. C., Ilio, M., McAfee, J. G., Meylor, J. K., and Langan, J. K. (1964). Regional pulmonary blood flow in many by radioisotope scanning. *JAMA* **187**:601–603.

Walsh, J. C., Macquire, J., Herndon, D., Traber, L. D., Traber, D. L., and Kramer, G. C. (1988). The bronchial circulation contributes to lung lymph flow after inhalation injury. *Fed. Proc.* **2**:953.

18

The Bronchial Circulation in Chronic Lung Infections

NIRMAL B. CHARAN and PAULA G. CARVALHO

Veterans Administration Medical Center
Boise, Idaho

and University of Washington School of Medicine
Seattle, Washington

I. Introduction

It has long been known that the bronchial circulation is involved in chronic lung infections. As pointed out by Cudkowicz in Chap. 1, Leonardo da Vinci sketched human lungs detailing not only the bronchial arteries, but also a cavitary lesion surrounded by a dense plexus of bronchial vessels. It has been suggested that this drawing represents the earliest description of a tuberculous cavity supplied by bronchial arteries. Since that time, numerous studies have confirmed that the bronchial circulation hypertrophies in certain chronic lung infections. The mechanisms that produce hypertrophy of the bronchial circulation have not been investigated.

The bronchial circulation has been studied in a variety of chronic inflammatory lung diseases, including bronchiectasis, tuberculosis, lung abscess, and empyema. However, its role in fungal and parasitic lung infections has not yet been investigated.

II. Bronchiectasis

Among the various chronic pulmonary diseases, bronchiectasis is most commonly associated with hypertrophy of the bronchial arteries and the development of bronchopulmonary anastomoses.

In bronchiectasis the bronchial arteries enlarge and proliferate markedly. For example, Cudkowicz (1979) described a bronchial artery to the right lung that measured 6 mm in diameter, the normal diameter of the bronchial artery being less than 2 mm (Pump, 1972). Proliferation of the bronchial arteries was observed as early as 1938 by Wood and Miller (1938). They performed a series of postmortem studies in humans with various lung diseases by infusing Hill's mass (bismuth oxychloride in gum acacia) into the bronchial artery and taking roentgenograms of the lungs in their inflated state. Their series included one specimen of bronchiectasis from a young female adult that showed an extensive network of new bronchial arterial branches along the course of the bronchi and bronchioles in the diseased lobe. The main bronchial artery to this lobe was also slightly dilated and quite tortuous.

Bronchiectasis is also characterized by the presence of large bronchopulmonary anastomoses. Liebow and associates (1949) studied 18 lung specimens surgically removed from patients with bronchiectasis. At the time of surgical resection, the bronchial arteries were found to be greatly enlarged in 11 of the 18 specimens. Bronchovascular casts were prepared by injecting vinylite into the bronchial arteries in lungs inflated by negative pressure. When the plastic was injected into the bronchial arteries, it immediately flowed out from the pulmonary arteries at the hilum, but not from the pulmonary veins. The plastic utilized in this preparation was too viscid to penetrate the capillaries. Thus, these observations provided evidence for the development of large anastomoses between the bronchial and the pulmonary arteries in bronchiectasis. Detailed examination of the casts also confirmed significant bronchial arterial enlargement and the presence of bronchopulmonary anastomoses in 15 of 18 specimens.

From these studies, it is apparent that there can be numerous large anastomoses between the bronchial and pulmonary arteries in patients with bronchiectasis. Therefore, it is likely that the systemic arterial pressure may be partially transmitted to the pulmonary arteries, provided that the bronchial blood flow is sufficiently increased in the affected regions of lung. Thus the pressure in the pulmonary arteries may increase in areas of bronchiectatic lung tissue in which large bronchopulmonary anastomoses are present. This may result in an effective shunting of pulmonary arterial blood away from the anastomotic regions into areas of normal lung. Indeed, Noszkov et al. (1979) measured vascular pressures and determined oxygen saturation in the pulmonary trunk and terminal branches of the pulmonary artery in patients with bronchiectasis. They found locally increased pulmonary artery occlusion (wedge) pressures of 30–50 mmHg in bronchiectatic regions, but pressures were normal in the pulmonary trunk and its main branches. Oxygen saturation measured with an unwedged catheter in the pulmonary artery supplying the bronchiectatic region was equal to that measured in the systemic arterial circulation, whereas oxygen saturation measured in the pulmonary trunk was the same as that of venous blood.

The mechanisms responsible for the development of bronchopulmonary anastomoses in bronchiectasis are not well understood. Enlargement of the bronchial arteries in bronchiectasis is associated with the development of granulation tissue during the course of the organizing pneumonitis that precedes the changes of bronchiectasis. As the disease progresses, there is an increased production of granulation tissue. Because the bronchial circulation supplies blood to the airways, increased production of granulation tissue in the bronchi results in an increase in the bronchial blood flow. The bronchial blood flow then drains into the pulmonary circulation through increased numbers of bronchopulmonary anastomoses. Whether these bronchopulmonary anastomoses have a functional significance is not known; most likely, changes in the vasa vasorum provide this drainage route for blood from the bronchial to the pulmonary circulations.

Bronchopulmonary communications are usually located in the walls of the bronchiectatic sacs (Liebow et al., 1949). In half of the cases, the anastomoses can be as large as 1 mm in diameter. The bronchial arteries are spirally shaped before their junction with the pulmonary arteries. It is possible that the increase in resistance caused by this spiral configuration of the bronchial arteries reduces transmission of the systemic arterial pressure to the pulmonary arteries, thus preventing this factor in the development of pulmonary hypertension.

The bronchial circulation in bronchiectasis has also been examined by angiographic techniques. Miyazawa et al. (1970) performed selective bronchial artery catheterization in eight patients with bronchiectasis. Characteristic angiographic findings included an enlarged and tortuous proximal portion of the bronchial artery, which wound around ectatic bronchi and gave off numerous branches. There was marked hypervascularity from the large number of proliferated vessels in the bronchial inflammatory lesions. The fine network of peripheral vessels responsible for the bronchial capillary bed was relatively sparse, however. In this study, the pulmonary arteries were not visualized. One explanation for this is that contrast media injected into the bronchial artery became rapidly diluted by the pulmonary blood flow. The authors concluded from the study that the communications between the pulmonary and the bronchial arteries are present predominantly in the large vessels.

A study by Darke and Lewtas (1968) utilized both selective bronchial arteriography and thoracic aortography to study the bronchial arteries in various chronic lung disorders. A total of 23 patients with bronchiectasis were studied. In 50%, the contrast material was seen to pass from the aorta, through dilated bronchial arteries supplying the bronchiectatic segment and into the pulmonary artery. Two main patterns of flow emerged. In the first, contrast material passed freely into the pulmonary capillaries, then the pulmonary veins, and then into the left heart. This was termed "forward flow." In the second pattern, seen in only 3 patients, contrast flowed against the normal stream of the pulmonary artery and passed toward the hilum of the lung, a situation described as "reverse flow." Such reverse flow was thought to result from increased vascular resistance in the pulmonary capillary bed as the result of the chronic inflammatory changes and the increase in bronchopulmonary blood flow. This usually occurred in unilateral bronchiectasis when pulmonary artery pressures measured in the pulmonary trunk were normal. The presence of reverse flow may appear on a pulmonary angiogram as an occlusion of a lobar pulmonary artery and may be misdiagnosed as a pulmonary embolism. In these cases, when antegrade flow of contrast medium is absent, obtaining blood samples from the distal pulmonary artery for oxygen determination may be useful in confirming that the angiographic abnormality is due to increased bronchopulmonary blood flow, rather than to a pulmonary embolism.

In patients with severe bronchiectasis, selective pulmonary angiography may occasionally demonstrate rapid dilution of contrast material in the pulmonary artery, indicating a flow of systemic blood into the pulmonary artery (Tadavarthy et al., 1982).

Several investigators have attempted to estimate bronchial blood flow in patients with bronchiectasis. The most common method used has been to measure the right and left ventricular outputs. The difference between the higher left ventricular output and the lower right ventricular output is assumed to be due to the bronchial flow returning to the left ventricle through the bronchopulmonary anastomoses. This technique does not measure that portion of the bronchial blood flow that drains into the right side of the heart via the azygos system, but this amount is comparatively small.

Fishman and associates (1958) measured bronchial blood flow using the Fick principle in two patients with bronchiectasis. They found that bronchial blood flow in these patients was 315 and 382 ml/min, or approximately 4% of the cardiac output, the normal being less than 1%. Such a marked increase in bronchial blood flow is not uniformly present in all patients with bronchiectasis. For example, Nakamura et al. (1961) studied eight patients with bronchiectasis by simultaneously obtaining the right and left ventricular output curves with dye dilution methods. They found that the bronchial blood flow was increased in only half the patients and was quite variable. In this series, flows ranged between 200 and 700 ml/min. In one patient, however, the bronchial blood flow was greater than 6 L/min. The authors could not explain the reason for such high flows, and it is possible that a technical error existed. They also found that the increase in bronchial blood flow appeared to be related to the extent and type of disease. Blood flows were higher in cystic bronchiectasis than in cylindrical bronchiectasis.

Fritts et al. (1961) also indirectly measured bronchial blood flow by right and left ventricular dye dilution curves in 11 patients with bronchiectasis. They found variable blood flows with a mean value of 9.7% of the cardiac output, compared with flows of approximately 1.0% of the cardiac output in normal subjects. In 1 patient, bronchial blood flow equaled 35% of cardiac output. It is not clear why some patients with bronchiectasis have such markedly high flows. Cudkowicz (1970) found average bronchial blood flows of 17.9% of cardiac output in 9 patients with bronchiectasis. Miyazawa et al. (1970) measured the bronchial blood flow by angiographic dye dilution in 6 patients with bronchiectasis and varying degrees of parenchymal involvement. Flows ranged from 710 ml/min in a patient with bronchiectasis involving all lobes to 0 ml/min in another patient with only one lobe involved. These studies support the view that patients with limited disease tend to have less bronchial arterial flow compared with patients with extensive disease.

During pulmonary artery catheterization, arterialized blood can sometimes by withdrawn from an unwedged catheter in patients with bronchiectasis. This is thought to come from the enlarged bronchopulmonary anastomoses (Vaccarezza et al., 1966). Therefore, in the presence of bronchiectasis, the "mixed venous" oxygen data obtained from the pulmonary artery should be interpreted with caution. For instance, Roosenburg and Deenstra (1954) performed right heart catheterization in six patients with advanced bronchiectasis as part of a functional examination before resection. The catheter was inserted into the pulmonary artery supplying the diseased portion of the lung, and the blood oxygen saturation in that artery was measured. They found that the oxygen saturation in the bronchiectatic area of the lung was significantly higher compared with that in the normal lung. The oxygen saturation was indeed definitely higher than that in the mixed venous blood and, in many cases, was equal to the oxygen saturation in the systemic blood. These findings suggest that functional bronchopulmonary anastomoses occur on the pulmonary arterial side of the pulmonary capillaries. In fact, in many cases, an arterial pressure curve was recorded when the artery to the affected bronchiectatic area was occluded during catheterization. These pressure curves are likely to be caused by partial transmission of the systemic pressure in the dilated bronchial arteries via large anastomoses with the pulmonary arteries.

The histology of the pulmonary and the bronchial arteries in bronchiectasis was described by Cudkowicz (1952a). Severe intimal proliferation and atheromatous changes can occur in the proximal pulmonary arterial trunk. The presence of precapillary anastomoses between the pulmonary and aberrant bronchial arteries at the periphery of the lungs has been observed in histological sections.

III. Lung Abscess

The bronchial circulation has been studied in only a few patients with lung abscess. Marchand et al. (1950) found that the pulmonary arteries supplying the wall of the abscess are generally obliterated by infected thrombi; therefore, there is a minimal contribution from the pulmonary artery to the abscess cavity. In contrast, when Cudkowicz injected the bronchial artery with dye, he was able to demonstrate that the majority of the blood supply to the walls of the abscess cavity came from the bronchial circulation (Cudkowicz, 1952b). Wood and Miller (1938), using angiographic techniques in human autopsy studies, also noted alterations in the bronchial artery in cases of lung abscess. There was proliferation of new vessels surrounding the diseased area, and some dilatation of the smaller branches of the bronchial artery was present. Noszkov et al. (1979) performed selective angiography in one patient with a lung abscess. After contrast injection, they were able to demonstrate a fine, looplike pattern of bronchial arterial branches surrounding the abscess cavity. In this patient, all the bronchial arteries were normal in size and diameter.

Attempts have been made to measure the bronchial blood flow in patients with lung abscess. The bronchial blood flow was measured in four patients by Nakamura et al. (1961) and was found to be less than 1% of the cardiac output. These authors concluded that the bronchial blood flow is not increased in lung abscess.

From this limited information, it appears that the bronchial arteries supply the wall of the abscess cavity; however, the total bronchial blood flow may remain unchanged.

One recent animal study addressed the anatomy of the bronchial circulation in lung abscess. The bronchial blood flow was not measured, however. Charan et al. (1985) studied the bronchial circulation by corrosion casting techniques in sheep with naturally occurring lung abscesses. In this study, the vascular casts were prepared by infusing Batson's solution into the bronchoesophageal trunk, pulmonary artery, and, through the left atrium, into the

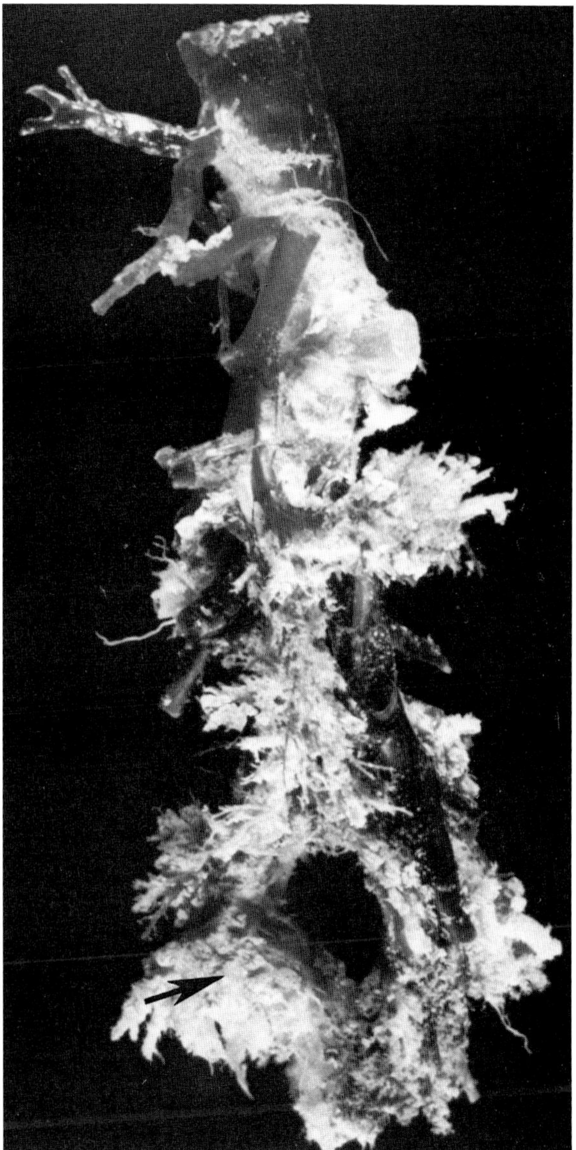

Figure 1 A dissected (pulmonary vasculature and airways removed) cast of the right lung of a sheep. In this specimen the bronchial artery, pulmonary artery, and pulmonary vein were infused with plastic of different colors. The arrow points to the abscess cavity, which is surrounded by the white bronchial vascular plexus.

pulmonary veins. In contrast to the results described in humans, the bronchial artery was found to be markedly dilated and hypertrophied (Figs. 1 through 3). The abscess cavities were surrounded by a dense microvascular plexus supplied exclusively by the bronchial arteries. Casting material that was infused into the pulmonary artery and into the pulmonary vein did not appear in the walls of the abscess cavities, indicating that the pulmonary circulation did not play a role in these lung infections. Scanning electron microscopy of the inner wall of the abscess cavities revealed a dense plexus of bronchial vessels with only a few isolated nests of alveolar capillaries remaining. Pulmonary capillaries were sparse and were entirely filled by the casting material injected into the bronchial artery. The bronchial capillaries were straight, and presumably their elongation was due to an increased pressure in the abscess cavity (Fig. 2). Communications were present between the pulmonary capillary and the

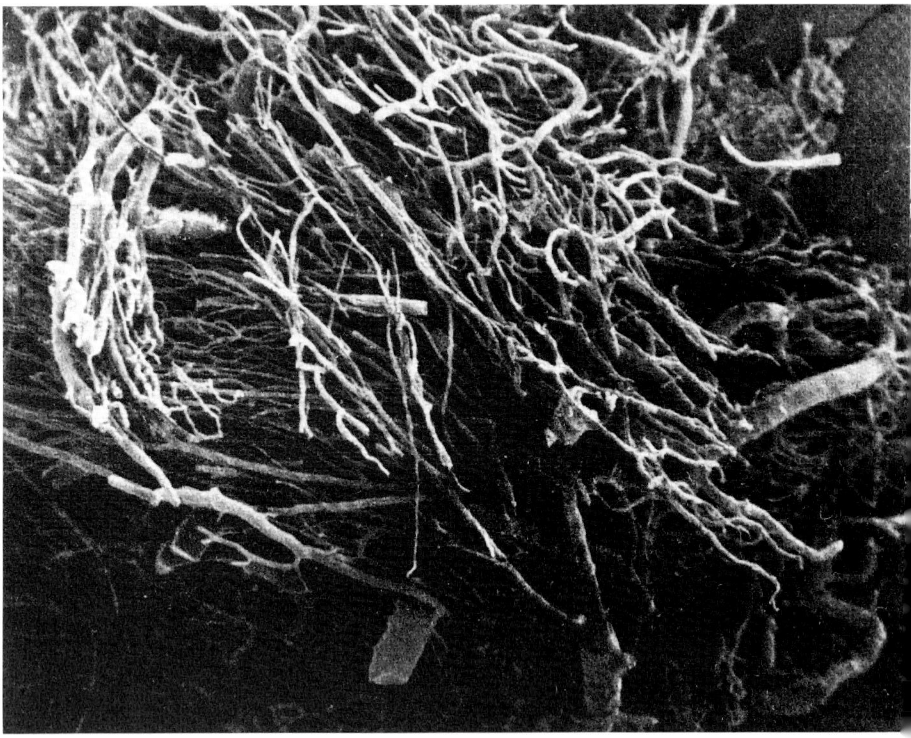

Figure 2 Scanning electron micrograph of the inner wall of an abscess cavity in the lung showing a rich plexus of bronchial vessels. These vessels are straight, perhaps caused by an increased pressure in the abscess cavity.

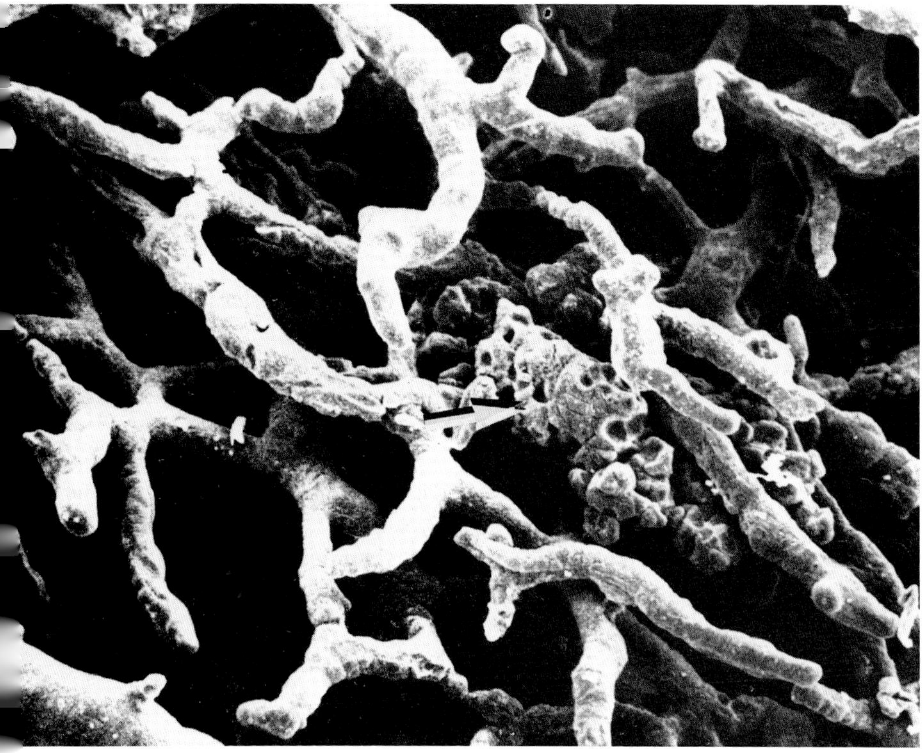

Figure 3 Scanning electron micrograph of the inner wall of an abscess cavity in the lung under higher magnification. The arrow points to the sparse pulmonary capillaries nestled in a network of bronchial capillaries, with a few interconnecting vessels present between the two circulations.

bronchial microvasculature. Because abscess cavities are uniformly associated with the airways, it is not surprising that the vascular supply to these lesions originates from the bronchial circulation. It is also possible that the hypertrophied bronchial circulation is necessary for the control of lung infection and repair.

IV. Tuberculosis

Gross enlargement of the bronchial arteries in tuberculosis was noted as early as 1845 by Guillot (1845). These changes were later confirmed by Wood and Miller (1938), who found in five patients with tuberculosis consistent and marked changes in the bronchial arteries in the tuberculous lung region. These vessels were dilated and tortuous and ramified extensively. The severity of disease correlated with the extent of vascular proliferation and hypertrophy. Residual changes were present in arrested cases of tuberculosis. Wood and Miller's angiographic studies indicated that an increase in the supply of oxygenated blood existed in and around the diseased areas of lung. When the tuberculous process was associated with silicosis and right ventricular hypertrophy, anastomotic channels were present between the bronchial and pulmonary circulations, possibly causing a further increase in the pulmonary artery pressure. This finding is interesting because nonsilicotic tuberculous cases rarely die of right-sided heart failure, whereas patients with silicotuberculosis frequently do.

This study also provides confirmation that hemoptysis in some patients with tuberculosis is of bronchial arterial origin. In some cases, Wood and Miller (1938) found that anastomotic bronchovascular channels developed through adhesions between the lobes. The authors thought that these new vessels could be involved in the continued hemorrhage following ligation of a lobar branch of the pulmonary artery in an attempt to arrest hemoptysis.

Steinberg et al. (1950) demonstrated that the pulmonary arteries supplying lung parenchyma with tuberculous changes are obliterated. Since the patients in this series underwent artificial pneumothoraces for the treatment of tuberculosis, however, it is difficult to conclude that tuberculosis was uniquely responsible for the obliterations.

Cudkowicz (1952b) performed angiographic and histological examinations at autopsy in five patients with tuberculosis. He demonstrated the presence of endarteritis and aneurysmal dilatations of the branches of the pulmonary arteries (Rasmussen's aneurysms) that were present in the walls of tuberculous cavities. The most uniform features observed in these lungs were the distortion, tortuosity, and remarkable proliferation of the bronchial arteries supplying caseating areas. Histologically, the pulmonary arteries were grossly obliterated as a result of intimal proliferation and thrombosis. The branches of the pulmonary artery did not supply blood to lung parenchyma containing caseating tuberculous lesions because they became thrombosed in the early stages of disease. In the branches of the pulmonary arteries proximal to tuberculous lesions, some recanalization had taken place by proliferation of the vasa vasorum. This was evidenced by the appearance in the pulmonary lumen of contrast medium initially injected into the bronchial artery. In the presence of pleural adhesions, the branches of the bronchial arteries showed massive medial hyperplasia and intimal proliferation. The systemic arteries from the parietal pleura also entered the adhesions. The bronchial arteries were dilated in the tuberculous regions and appeared to be largest in the walls of the cavities, but their muscular coats were quite thin. It is possible that it is these dilated bronchial arteries that, in the past, were considered aneurysmal dilatations of the pulmonary arteries. In this study, free anastomoses between the pulmonary and bronchial systems were not observed. It has been postulated that the obliterative changes in the pulmonary arteries could help to prevent pulmonary hemorrhage, whereas the compensatory proliferation of the bronchial circulation could produce bleeding.

Artificial pneumothorax therapy for pulmonary tuberculosis was thought to be beneficial in controlling, or "resting" the disease, presumably by decreasing the oxygen supply of the lung and thus curtailing the activity of tubercle bacilli. Tuberculous bacteria do not grow in closed, hypoxic cavities, as they depend on aerobic metabolism for their energy production. These bacteria proliferate at an accelerated rate when a tuberculous cavity ruptures into an aerated structure, such as a bronchus or vessel. It has been proposed that ligation of the pulmonary artery in unilateral tuberculosis may inhibit progression of the disease, but studies in primates showed that ligation of a pulmonary artery led to the opposite effect (Scott et al., 1950). In this same study, extensive tuberculous lesions were found in the ligated side, and this process was thought to be related to the high oxygen tensions in the blood reaching the lung, presumably via the bronchial circulation. Cudkowicz (1965) also postulated that the dilated bronchial arteries near areas of tuberculous caseous necrosis not in direct communication with patent bronchi may provide a source of oxygen for tubercle bacilli.

Studies have shown that the bronchial blood flow increases in pulmonary tuberculosis. Cudkowicz (1965) measured the bronchial blood flow by the indirect dye dilution method in patients with unilobar pulmonary tuberculosis and found it to be approximately 4% of the cardiac output. This measurement varied in some other studies using the same technique: Fritts et al. (1961) found a bronchial blood flow of 2.9% of the cardiac output, whereas Nakamura et al. (1961) found flows of 8.4% of the cardiac output.

Roosenburg and Deenstra (1954) measured the pulmonary arterial oxygen saturation during cardiac catheterization in five patients with advanced pulmonary tuberculosis. They found that the oxygen saturation in the pulmonary arteries of lungs or lobes showing extensive changes due to tuberculosis was quite close to the oxygen saturation seen in the systemic blood and much higher than the saturation in the mixed venous blood. They also found that the pressure in these pulmonary arteries was much higher than in the uninvolved lung. These findings suggest that there can be large anastomoses between the bronchial and the pulmonary arteries in tuberculosis.

V. Empyema

Since the visceral pleura is supplied by the bronchial circulation in many species, it is likely that the bronchial circulation is affected by the inflammation of the pleural space. However, the changes in the bronchial circulation with infections in the pleural space have not been studied in detail.

Wood and Miller (1938) studied the bronchial circulation in one case of chronic empyema. At autopsy, there was fibrous thickening of the pleura with a few small, calcified, pleural nodules. The bronchial arteries were dilated and could be followed much farther toward the periphery of the lung than in a normal lung. There was also a marked increase in the fine branching of the bronchial arteries and an extensive anastomosis with the pulmonary arteries. An increase in bronchopulmonary anastomoses was also present on the uninvolved side.

We conducted a preliminary study to investigate whether the bronchial circulation hypertrophies in pneumococcal empyema (Carvalho et al., 1990). *Streptococcus pneumoniae* was introduced into either the right or left pleural space in sheep. This resulted in an extensive inflammatory reaction within 6 h, as evidenced by an increase in neutrophil count, protein, and lactate dehydrogenase (LDH) in the pleural fluid samples. The animals were sacrificed at 72 h. On autopsy, a thick and fibrinous layer was found to cover and adhere to both pleural surfaces at the site of infection. Prominent adhesions were found between the two pleural surfaces, with empyema fluid loculated within these adhesions. The bronchial circulation was studied by infusing Batson's #17 casting solution into the common bronchial artery. The bronchial vessels lining the visceral pleura were more prominent and appeared to form a plexus compared with the contralateral, uninfected side (Fig. 4). Proliferation of the bronchial vessels was found in the visceral pleura, and these extended into the areas of inflammation where the pleural peel was forming. This preliminary study indicates that proliferation and hypertrophy of the bronchial circulation may occur very early in experimental empyema.

VI. Summary

Although the bronchial circulation has not yet been studied extensively in chronic lung infections, sufficient data are available to suggest that the bronchial vasculature proliferates and hypertrophies in such diseases as bronchiectasis, lung abscess, tuberculosis, and empyema. In some of these conditions, with the possible exception of lung abscess, the bronchial blood flow also increases. The mechanisms responsible for this vascular proliferation and the increase in blood flow in response to chronic lung infection are not known. It

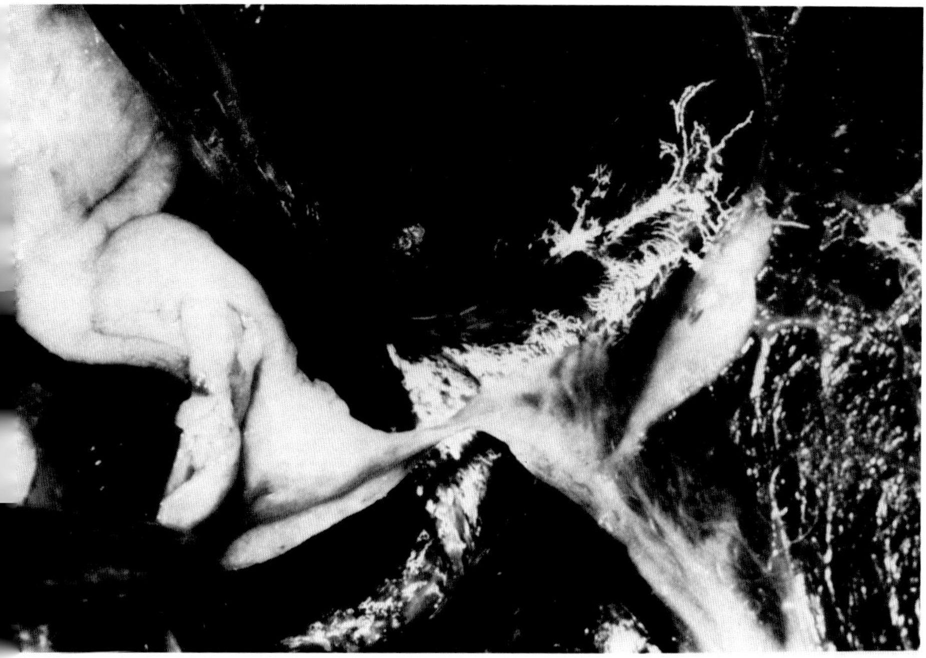

Figure 4 Photograph of the bronchial microvessels in the visceral pleura separated from the thick pleural peel of pus and debris following experimental empyema. The bronchial arteries were infused with white plastic. The bronchial blood supply to the contralaterial (noninfected) side was sparse.

can be speculated that these mechanisms are adaptive and are involved in resolution and repair after lung infection. Indeed, because the pulmonary circulation is obliterated in regions of disease, the bronchial circulation may play a very important role in defense against certain lung infections. If the bronchial circulation is important for resolution and repair following lung damage, it could have important implications in patients undergoing lung transplantation, as the bronchial blood flow may not be reestablished in the transplanted lung. Pneumonia appears to be common in patients who receive a lung transplant, and infection seems to be the major cause of death (Burke et al., 1984; Veith, 1978). It has been found that the reestablishment of bronchial blood flow during lung transplantation appears to prevent subsequent lung infections during the postoperative period (Mills et al., 1970). It is possible that the bronchial circulation is more important than the pulmonary circulation for host defense mechanisms in certain lung infections, especially in poorly ventilated areas of the lung. Further studies are required to elucidate the role of the bronchial circulation in lung infections.

References

Burke, C. M., Theodore, J., Dawkins, K. D., Yousem, S. A., Blank, N., Billingham, M. E., Kessel, A. B., Jamieson, S. W., Oyer, P. E., Baldwin, J. C., Stinson, E. B., Shumway, N. E., and Robin, E. D. (1984). Post-transplant obliterative bronchiolitis and other late lung sequelae in human heart-lung transplantation. *Chest* **86**:824–829.

Carvalho, P., Nielson, C. P., Kirk, W., and Charan, N. B. (1990). The effects of oxygen on bacterial clearance from the pleural space. *Am. Rev. Respir. Dis.* **141**:A766.

Charan, N. B., Turk, G. M., and Dhand, R. (1985). The role of bronchial circulation in lung abscess. *Am. Rev. Respir. Dis.* **131**:121–124.

Cudkowicz, L. (1952a). Some observations of the bronchial arteries in lobar pneumonia and pulmonary infarction. *Br. J. Dis. Chest* **46**:99–102.

Cudkowicz, L. (1952b). The blood supply of the lung in pulmonary tuberculosis. *Thorax* **7**:270–276.

Cudkowicz, L. (1965). Cardiorespiratory studies in pulmonary tuberculosis. *Can. Med. Assoc. J.* **92**:111–115.

Cudkowicz, L. (1970). The collaterial circulation of the lung and finger clubbing. A review. *Prog. Respir. Res.* **5**:436–449.

Cudkowicz, L. (1979). Bronchial arterial circulation in man. Normal anatomy and responses to disease. In *Pulmonary Vascular Disease.* Edited by K. M. Moser. Lung Biology in Health Disease, executive editor C. Lenfant, Vol. 14. New York, Marcel Dekker, pp. 111–232.

Darke, C. S., and Lewtas, N. A. (1968). Selective bronchial arteriography in the demonstration of abnormal systemic circulation in the lung. *Clin. Radiol.* **19**:357–367.

Fishman, A. P., Turino, G. M., Brandfonbrener, M., and Himmelstein, A. (1958). The effective pulmonary collateral blood flow in man. *J. Clin. Invest.* **37**:1071–1086.

Fritts, H. W., Harris, P., Chidsey, C. A., III, Clauss, R. H., and Cournand, A. (1961). Estimation of flow through bronchial-pulmonary vascular anastomoses with use of T-1824 dy. *Circulation* **23**:390–398.

Guillot, N. (1845). Recherches anatomique et pathologiques sur les amas de charbon products pendant la vie dans les organes respiratories de l'homme. *Arch. Gen. Med.* **7**:151–284.

Liebow, A. A., Hales, M. R., and Lindskog, G. F. (1949). Enlargement of the bronchial arteries and their anastomoses with the pulmonary arteries in bronchiectasis. *Am. J. Pathol.* **25**:211–231.

Marchand P., Gilroy, J. C., and Wilson, N. H. (1950). Anatomical study of the bronchial vascular system and its variations in disease. *Thorax* **5**:207–221.

Mills, N. L., Boyd, A. D., and Gheranpong, C. (1970). The significance of bronchial circulation in lung transplantation. *J. Thorac. Cardiovasc. Surg.* **60**:866–874.

Miyazawa, K., Katori, R., Ishikawa, K., Yamaki, M., Kobayashi, Y., Tsuiki, K., Matsunaga, K., and Nakamura, T. (1970). Selective bronchial arteriography and bronchial blood flow; correlative study. *Chest* **57**:416–422.

Nakamura, T., Katori, R., Miyazawa, K., Ohtomo, S., Watanbe, T., Watanbe, T., Miura, Y., and Takizawa, T. (1961). Bronchial blood flow in patients with chronic pulmonary disease and its influences upon respiration and circulation. *Dis. Chest* **39**:193–206.

Noszkov, A., Gulacsy, I., and Kiss, T. (1979). Angiography of the bronchial and pulmonary arteries in chronic non-specific lung diseases. *Acta Chir. Acad. Sci. Hung.* **20**:225–234.

Pump, K. K., (1972). Distribution of bronchial arteries in the human lung. *Chest* **62**:447–451.

Roosenburg, J. G., and Deenstra, H. (1954). Bronchial-pulmonary vascular shunts in chronic pulmonary affections. *Dis. Chest* **26**:664–671.

Scott, H. W. Jr., Hanlon, C. R., and Olson, B. J. (1950). Experimental tuberculosis (2). Effects of ligation of pulmonary arteries on tuberculosis in monkeys. *J. Thorac. Surg.* **20**:761–773.

Steinberg, I., McCoy, H. I., and Dotter, C. T. (1950). Angiocardiography in artificial pneumothorax. *Am. Rev. Tuberc.* **62**:353–359.

Tadavarthy, S. M., Klugman, J., Castaneda-Zuniga, W. R., Nath, P. H., and Amplatz, K. (1982). Systemic-to-pulmonary collaterals in pathological states. *Diagn. Radiol.* **144**:55–59.

Vaccarezza, R. F., Viola, A. R., Vaccarezza, D. A., Ugo, V. A., Vacario, D. J., and Zuffardi, E. A. (1966). Verification of the collateral systemic circulation in pulmonary pathology. *Dis. Chest* **49**:130–138.

Veith, F. J. (1978). Lung transplantation. *Surg. Clin. North Am.* **58**:357–364.

Wood, D. A., and Miller, M. (1938). The role of the dual pulmonary circulation in various pathologic conditions of the lungs. *J. Thorac. Surg.* **7**:649–670.

19

Circulation of Lung Neoplasms

RICHARD W. HYDE

University of Rochester Medical Center
Rochester, New York

I. Introduction

The rapid development of angiography after World War II made it practical to visualize the pulmonary and bronchial circulations. The increasing incidence of lung neoplasms coupled with effective chemotherapeutic agents for malignancies, such as lymphomas, stimulated many investigators to treat lung neoplasms by infusing these new agents into the pulmonary and bronchial circulation of experimental animals and humans. This chapter reviews these developments. Enthusiasm for this therapeutic approach has waned in recent years, but it has resulted in a detailed description of the interaction of lung tumors with the pulmonary and bronchial circulations.

II. Visualization and Description of Blood Supply to Lung Neoplasms

A. Early Experimental Studies

Physiological studies around the turn of the century provided important background for later studies of the circulation to lung tumors. Ghoreyeb and Karsner in 1913 reviewed earlier European reports describing the circulation to the lungs and called attention to the debate about the level of anastomoses between the bronchial and pulmonary circulations. Miller (1907) and others claimed anastomoses existed only at the capillary level; some investigators stated that there is an extremely free exchange of blood via rich anastomotic vessels between the two systems (Verloop, 1948). The experiments in living dogs reported by Ghoreyeb and Karsner in 1913 were prophetic for understanding later disputes about the source of the circulation to neoplasms of the lung. They clearly showed that the pressures maintained in the pulmonary and bronchial circulations determined the tissues labeled by the simultaneous injection of stained gelatins into the two circulations. For example, little admixture took place if physiological pressures were used for simultaneous injections of the bronchial and pulmonary circulations, but if the pressure in one circulation was reduced to zero, the circulation with pressure readily perfused both capillary beds. Failure to consider perfusion pressure present in vivo can explain many of the disputes that developed later when the circulation to neoplasms of the lung were studied in vitro with injections of contrast media into the bronchial and pulmonary circulations.

In 1938, Wright, an Australian pathologist, performed postmortem injections of the bronchial and pulmonary circulations in two patients with bronchogenic carcinoma accompanied by "secondary tumors" in both lungs. In addition, he injected seven specimens with a variety of metastatic tumors. For the most part, he heeded the advice of Ghoreyeb and Karsner and simultaneously injected his gelatin solutions at pressures of 180 mmHg into the aorta to perfuse the bronchial arteries and 70 mmHg into the pulmonary arteries. With few exceptions, all his tumors received blood flow from the bronchial circulation. However, small secondary tumor nodules of bronchogenic carcinoma that only involved "two alveoli" showed labeling from the capillaries of the adjacent alveolar septa. When several or more alveoli were involved, alveolar capillaries were reduced in number and labeling came from the bronchial arteries. The lung metastases from a malignant teratoma of the testes showed "lakes of gelatin which had escaped mainly from the pulmonary artery but in some cases from the bronchial arteries." He noted a collagenous stroma in the bronchial artery fields but not around the pulmonary arteries. This led him to speculate that the marked increase in the bronchial circulation perfusing lung tumors developed because excitation of these collagenous tissues around bronchial vessels permitted proliferation of the bronchial artery supply and lack of this collagenous matrix around pulmonary arteries prevented their proliferation. Later studies confirmed this remarkable inability of pulmonary arteries to show the hyperplastic growth of bronchial arteries perfusing tumors and inflammatory lesions (Milne, 1967).

Wood and Miller in 1938 reported conflicting results. They injected suspensions of radiopaque bismuth oxychloride into the blood vessels of an unspecified number of postmortem human lungs with malignancies and followed this by stereoscopic x-rays but did not inject the pulmonary and bronchial circulations simultaneously. Carcinomas of the bronchus showed dilated and tortuous bronchial vessels, and metastatic sarcomas showed normal bronchial vessels. They concluded that the bronchial arteries "remain uninvolved" in metastatic lung tumors, but the one figure of a metastatic lesion they printed showed nodules of increased radiodensity following bronchial artery injections. One can thus surmise that there were at least some connecting vessels between the bronchial circulations and the metastatic nodules. Unfortunately, they provided no data describing pulmonary artery injections so that there was no way to determine the principal blood supply to these metastatic tumors.

Two laboratories studied sarcoma transplanted into the lung of rabbits by intravenous injections of tumor cells or by direct injection of the cells into the lung parenchyma. In 1936, Asai concluded from microscopic observations and x-rays that, initially, vessels from the pulmonary artery enter the tumor, but later these vessels are occluded by tumor growth and blood supply comes from dilated and distorted, irregular, brush-shaped vessels at the edge of the tumor. He interpreted these findings to indicate nutrient supply via the bronchial circulation. Ogilvie and coworkers (1965), using a similar preparation, performed postmortem injections of India ink into the aorta of rabbits and concluded that tumors near the hilum, regardless of size, were always perfused by the bronchial circulation but peripheral tumors had to grow to 2–3 mm in diameter before being stained via the bronchial circulation. In addition, they visualized the lungs of five living animals by transilluminating the blood vessels after injecting India ink into the left ventricle. They observed the pulsatile flow of ink into peripheral metastatic tumors 3 mm or more in diameter 10 s before the ink appeared in the nearby pulmonary arteries. From these findings, they concluded that peripheral tumors did not develop a bronchial blood supply until greater than 2 mm in diameter. These studies in rabbits may not be representative of other species, however, because according to Asai the bronchial circulation of rabbits does not penetrate very deeply into the lung parenchyma compared with other species.

Jonas and Carrington in 1969 published a landmark contribution to the understanding of later studies in humans. They injected gelatin solution and vinylite of different colors into the pulmonary artery and aorta of dogs who died with a variety of primary and metastatic lung tumors. From their microscopic studies, serial sections enabled them to identify the origin of the blood vessels communicating with the tumors. Small metastatic tumors and occasionally the edge of large tumors showed infiltration of the alveolar spaces with

commonly had visualization with the pulmonary artery injections. However, he also briefly described studies of metastatic tumors in animals that showed, even in the same lung, some metastatic tumors with excellent visualization via the bronchial artery injection and others via the pulmonary artery injection. Compression of the perfusing bronchial artery by tumor growth followed by development of perfusion from the pulmonary artery via the collaterals could explain this variability. Milne concluded that the discrepancies in the literature about the blood supply of pulmonary metastases is real rather than an artifact of species selection or experimental technique.

Milne's studies provide a remarkably clear and elegant visualization of blood vessels to lung tumors, but the experimental method used does not allow one necessarily to conclude that the well-visualized vascular connections between the pulmonary artery and the vascular bed in the metastatic tumors represent the major perfusing vessels. First, his methodology did not permit simultaneous injections of the bronchial and pulmonary circulations at physiological pressures, so that the relative contribution of each vascular bed to the tumor is not known because the pressure in the two vascular beds did not duplicate their pressures present in vivo. Second, because of the extensive collateral circulation, bronchial blood flow into the tumor may drain into the pulmonary artery, reversing the direction of flow, as seen in inflammatory diseases. Evidence supporting reversed flow in the pulmonary arteries comes from in vivo pulmonary angiograms that show visualization of pulmonary arteries near tumors but no tumor "blush." While this lack of blush can result from reverse flow in the smaller draining pulmonary arteries, it may simply represent insufficient contrast media perfusing the pulmonary arteries to the lesion because the tumor has much less perfusion per volume of parenchyma compared to the surrounding lung tissue.

If Milne had also injected the pulmonary veins of his metastatic tumors and had shown an extensive vascular bed, similar to that demonstrated with the pulmonary arterial injections, the higher pressure in the pulmonary artery would make it impossible to refute his claim that the blood supply observed by pulmonary artery injections represented the major blood supply to the tumor. Miller and Rosenbaum (1967) performed injections of the pulmonary veins of lungs with metastatic tumors and frequently observed extensive networks of vessels between the pulmonary veins and the tumor. Therefore, if one combines the studies of Miller and Milne, one must conclude that sizable metastatic tumors may obtain their perfusion via the pulmonary circulation.

However, this conclusion does not mean that the pulmonary circulation has the ability seen in bronchial arteries to become larger and multiply. A consistent finding in Milne's angiograms is the preservation of the normal taper and distribution of the pulmonary arteries right onto the wall of the tumor. It seems as if the pulmonary arteries are passive observers, immune to growth factors from the tumor, and are only reluctantly attached to the aggressive hyperplastic vessels exuding from the tumor.

C. In Vivo Human Studies

Early efforts to visualize the bronchial blood supply to tumors evolved into a method in which a flexible hooked catheter was advanced into the femoral artery percutaneously by the Seldinger technique (Viamonte, 1964; Newton and Preger, 1965; Reuter et al., 1965). After the wire guide is removed, under fluoroscopic guidance the catheter is advanced into the aorta and the tip is moved up and down on the wall at the expected location of the origin of the bronchial arteries. Especially if the bronchial artery is enlarged by increased blood flow to a tumor or diseased area, the catheter readily enters the bronchial artery's orifice. Injection of a small test dose of 1–3 ml dye usually induces cough if the catheter is in the bronchial artery, and then 3–10 ml dye is injected to visualize the bronchial circulation (Fig. 1). In vivo studies in humans using this method essentially confirmed studies describing the circulation to lung tumors in animals and in resected or postmortem human specimens. Primary lung neoplasms demonstrate bronchial artery perfusion with a tumor blush in as many as 95% of patients. Failure to visualize the bronchial circulation has been attributed to occlusion of the bronchial artery by compression by the tumor, severe aortic athrosclerosis resulting in inability to identify the orifice to the bronchial artery, failure to isolate one of multiple bronchial arteries coming off the aorta, and an origin of the bronchial artery that does not directly arise from the descending aorta and cannot therefore be located (Fig. 2) (Cauldwell et al., 1948). Adenocarcinomas and anaplastic tumors showed a more prolific blood supply than observed in squamous cell carcinomas. Bronchial adenomas tend to have the richest blood supply seen in primary lung tumors (personal communication, Dr. Manuel Viamonte, Jr.). However, the vascular pattern of tumors is not sufficiently characteristic to predict tumor type or even distinguish between tumors and benign inflammatory lesions (see later) (Greenspan, 1971; Viamonte et al., 1965). Demonstration of the bronchial circulation to metastatic tumors was much less common, with the bronchial circulation appearing normal in four of the six patients studied by Newton and Preger (1965).

On the basis of 55 bronchial arteriograms in patients with malignant pulmonary neoplasms, Viamonte et al. (1965) classified a set of common abnormal vascular patterns:

1. Localized hypervascularity in a tumor. This takes various forms, such as tumor blush, increased number of small branches in the area

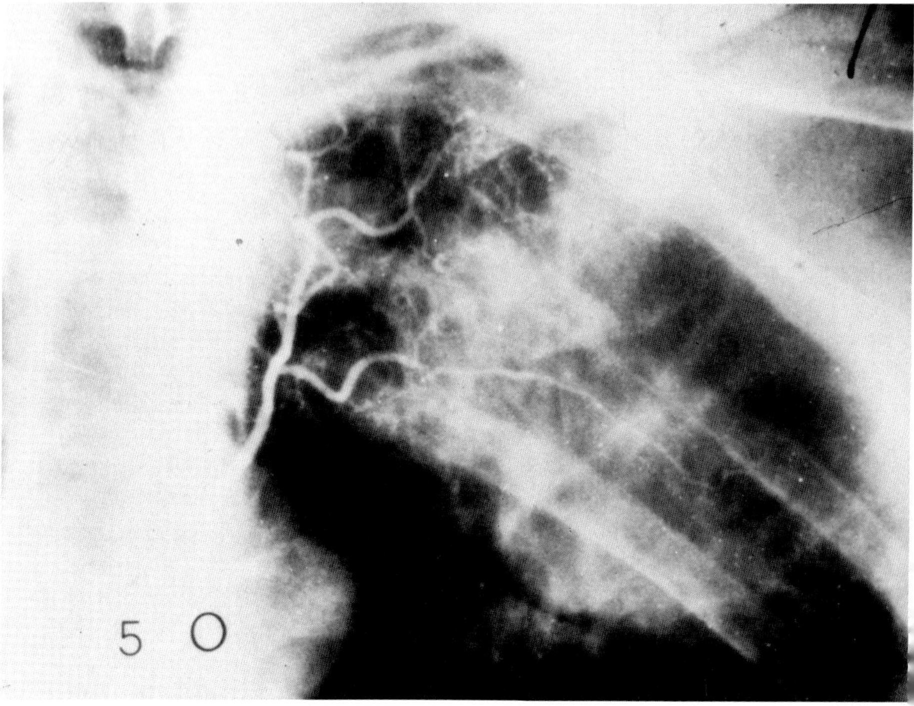

Figure 1 Bronchial arteriography of a large squamous cell carcinoma of the left upper lobe. The catheter used for injection of the dye was introduced into the femoral artery percutaneously by the Seldinger technique and then advanced into the thoracic arota. At the level of the fifth thoracic vertebra (label with the number 5), the hooked tip of the catheter entered the bronchial artery and contrast medium was injected. The tip of the catheter cannot be seen in this photograph of the x-ray but is located inside the circle to the right of the 5. Note the enlarged size of the bronchial artery feeding the tumor and the tortuous small blood vessels within the tumor, best seen in the upper, medial portions of the mass. (This figure was kindly provided by Dr. Manuel Viamonte, Jr., Mount Sinai Medical Center, Miami Beach, Florida.)

of the tumor, or ectatic or fusiform vessels with abnormal branching in an irregular distribution within the tumor. These hyperplastic vessels were rarely seen in squamous cell carcinoma but were common in other forms of primary lung cancer.

2. Sequestered forms. A very vascular tumor is readily visualized, but the feeding vessel and surrounding tissue show little or no visualiza-

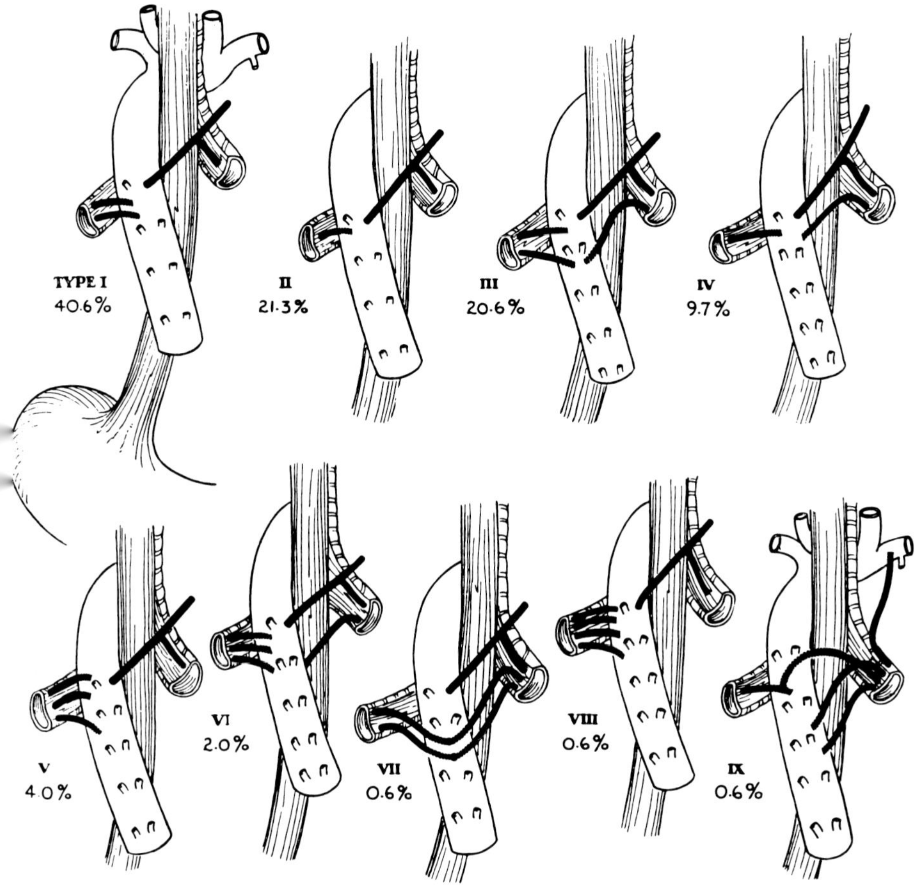

Figure 2 Types of bronchial artery supply to the lung determined from 150 human cadavers by Cauldwell and coworkers (1948). Note in type IX (lower right-hand corner) that some blood supply to the left lung originates from the left subclavian artery. In the text, the authors stated that 3% of specimens showed a bronchial artery arising from a subclavian artery. Early investigators reported origins from the internal mammary, intercostal, and innominate arteries. None of these arteries would be identified by the standard technique of bronchial arteriography with a hooked catheter placed in the descending aorta. (By permission of *Surgery, Gynecology, and Obstetrics*.)

tion, probably because the well-visualized high blood flow in the tumor makes the feeding blood vessels relatively inconspicuous.

3. Aberrant or dual vascular supply. Tumors may receive additional blood supply from intercostal or internal mammary arteries. Anastomotic channels may be seen between these systemic arteries as well as to the pulmonary, bronchial, and mediastinal veins. Other groups also noted the frequent occurrence of bronchial artery-to-pulmonary artery anastomoses (Cudkowicz and Armstrong, 1953; Miyazawa et al., 1970).
4. Avascular pattern. Lung carcinomas, especially squamous cell carcinoma, may show little or no visualization with injection of the neighboring bronchial artery or intercostal artery. However, the more sensitive method of injection of radiolabeled macroaggregates into the bronchial artery feeding the neoplasm shows perfusion on subsequent scans.
5. Bronchial hypervascularity of apparently uninvolved lung parenchyma. Unsuspected tumor invasion of lung parenchyma may be suspected by observing hypervascularity in the area of lung adjacent to the tumor.

D. Microscopic Studies

Microscopic anatomy of the endothelium of lung tumors has attracted little interest. Neyazaki and associates (1970) stated that in all types of pulmonary carcinomas, blood vessels from 10 to 300 μm in diameter have a thin-layered endothelium without elastic tissue. In these endothelial cells, pinocytotic and micropinocytotic vesicles were absent or few in number. Gaps and fenestrations in the endothelial walls were observed in many places. Intercellular junctions were tightly closed by the zonula adherens, which appear on electron microscopy as dense areas 300 Å in length and 100 Å in width. Unlike the continuous capillary endothelium in the pulmonary circulation, all these tumors had a fenestrated type of endothelium. These authors concluded that the more porous endothelium of tumors may favor the access of chemotherapeutic agents into the tumor while sparing normal lung tissue protected by its more continuous endothelium. However, these drugs also have ready access to such organs as liver, bone marrow, and spleen, where the endothelium is primarily a discontinuous layer with large pores.

Unlike metastatic tumors, primary lung carcinomas frequently form microscopic sinusoids or vascular lakes near the surface of the tumor just below the airway mucosa. Minor damage and subsequent leakage of blood from these vessels into the airway lumen cause hemoptysis. The presence of such sinusoids in primary lung neoplasm has been evoked to explain the clinical aphorism that hemoptysis in a patient with a lung tumor indicates a primary lung neoplasm rather than a metastatic tumor (Wood and Miller, 1938).

E. Differential Diagnosis of Lung Tumors from Bronchial Arterial Angiography

Early investigators proposed that the tumor blush and other dramatic irregularities of the bronchial vessels on bronchial arteriograms were specific for malignant neoplasms and would be clinically useful in distinguishing neoplasms from benign tumors and masses secondary to infectious processes, such as tuberculosis and fungal disease (Viamonte, 1964; Ikeda et al., 1968; Miyazawa et al., 1970). Further experience showed that these vascular changes were indicative of growth of both malignant and nonmalignant processes (Greenspan, 1971). For example, hamartomas have a vascular structure indistinguishable from that of bronchogenic carcinoma (Kahn et al., 1965). Some trends were noted, however. Adenocarcinomas of the lung tend to have a prominent vascular supply; squamous cell cancers are usually relatively avascular. Primary lung neoplasms rarely demonstrated perfusion via the pulmonary artery circulation, so demonstration of perfusion from the pulmonary artery to a mass suggests the diagnosis of pulmonary arteriovenous malformation or a metastatic lesion. Some investigators have proposed using bronchial arteriography for the diagnosis of neoplasms in the lungs of patients with malignant tumor cells found in the sputum, without a demonstrable lesion on the chest x-ray, in which the tumor blush or other abnormality of the perfusion pattern might identify the neoplasm. In recent years, however, computed tomography of the chest has markedly improved the ability to detect small lesions, so this indication for bronchial arteriography may now be obsolete.

III. Treatment of Lung Neoplasms with Regional Perfusion of Chemotherapeutic Agents

A. Development of Regional Perfusion of Antineoplastic Drugs for Treatment of Lung Neoplasms

In 1950, Klopp and coworkers introduced regional tumor chemotherapy in humans by infusing nitrogen mustard into the carotid, temporal, and iliac arteries of patients with epidermoid carcinomas of the head, gliobastomas, brain metastases from the breast, and a fibrosarcoma of the thigh. Complete and permanent relief of pain was claimed in each case, as well as frequent reduction of size of the tumor with softening and transient partial clearing of the tumor in the perfused vascular bed. Bierman et al. published an abstract in 1951 describing intraarterial infusions of nitrogen mustard in 92 patients with inoperable visceral metastases to the liver, spleen, stomach, colon, and "other viscera." They concluded that intraarterial chemotherapy is a practical adjuvant to the surgical and radiological attack on neoplasms, but the lack of subsequent detailed publications of these preliminary findings suggest they lost their initial enthusiasm for this therapeutic approach. Within a few years, several other groups published detailed reports describing poor responses with intraarterial chemotherapy to a variety of organs (Bonner et al., 1952; Grady et al., 1953). Despite these discouraging reports, in the late 1950s and well into the 1960s arterial infusions of chemotherapy for the treatment of lung tumors generated considerable enthusiasm and interest. Blades and Hall (1958) and Pierpont and Blades (1960) infused nitrogen mustard and TEPA (triethylene thiophosphoramide) through the distal port of a balloon-tipped catheter that temporarily occluded the main pulmonary artery of dogs for 15 min. With small doses, some of their animals survived. Morris and Goldberg (1961) treated 18 men with bronchogenic carcinoma by infusing nitrogen mustard via a cardiac catheter placed in the main pulmonary artery perfusing the tumor. Of 18 patients 10 had subjective benefit consisting of relief of pain or dyspnea. In 9 patients, the chest x-rays showed an objective reduction in the size of the tumor; 5 patients developed white counts below 1000 cells per mm^3, and 1 of these patients died 18 days after the injection of *Pseudomonas* pneumonia presumably secondary to the leukopenia.

Creech and coworkers (1958, 1959) reported performing regional perfusion of the pulmonary circulation of seven patients with primary carcinoma of the lung by using two pump oxygenators simultaneously. One of the pumps drew blood from the vena cava and returned it to the femoral artery to maintain whole-body oxygenation. The other circuit pumped blood from the left atrium into a catheter passed, via the right ventricular outflow tract, into the main pulmonary artery, where it was tied in place. Multiple doses of unspecified amounts of nitrogen mustard were then infused into this circuit over a 30 min interval. A detailed description of these patients was not published, but one patient regained ventilation to an atelectatic lung. The atelectasis was secondary to a squamous cell carcinoma that had occluded the right mainstem bronchus and extended into the trachea. Another patient died 4 days after perfusion from cerebral edema attributed to massive necrosis from an unsuspected cerebral metastases. Another patient died of an unspecified pulmonary complication on the third day after the operation. No further attempts to use this highly invasive technique have been published to my knowledge.

Other investigators at this time sought ways to gain access to the bronchial circulation in humans and deliver chemotherapy via the bronchial circulation. Neyazaki (1962) passed a catheter, with a balloon 6 cm from the tip, via the femoral artery into the aorta of dogs and humans. He inflated the balloon when it reached the level of the diaphragm to temporarily occlude the aorta. He then injected radiopaque material into the lumen to the distal port of the catheter and thereby visualized the bronchial arteries. He never reported using this method to deliver chemotherapy and abandoned it in favor of direct catheterization of bronchial arteries originating from the aorta (Neyazaki et al., 1969). Cliffton and Mahajan (1963) developed a quadruple-lumen catheter with two balloons (Fig. 3). When properly positioned in the aorta from the femoral artery, inflation of the balloons occluded the aorta just distal to the left subclavian artery and at a point 10 cm lower at the level of the eighth thoracic vertebra. After visualization of the bronchial arteries by injecting radiopaque dye into the channel that had an orifice between the two balloons, they then infused nitrogen mustard into this channel and 5 min later deflated the upper balloon. They collapsed the lower balloon 10 min later to restore the circulation. In seven patients with far advanced primary lung carcinomas, they reported palliation of severe symptoms, including cough, pain, and dyspnea in most of their patients, without serious complications.

A later report (Cliffton, 1969) described results in 21 patients. Cough was improved in 80% and pain present in 15 patients was at least partially relieved in 9. Average survival was 8 months in the treated patients and 1.8 months in 6 patients considered for perfusion but in whom it was not completed because of technical difficulties.

Rheinlander and coworkers (1962) perfused nitrogen mustard into the aorta of 12 patients with inoperable primary lung cancer during temporary occlusion of the lower thoracic aorta. In 6 patients, they temporarily clamped the lower thoracic aorta at the time of an exploratory thoracotomy. In the other 6 patients, they introduced an inflatable catheter into the lower thoracic aorta via the femoral artery with a technique similar to the method described by Neyazaki (1962). The authors stated that all but 1 patient had some form of transient clinical benefit, such as prompt relief of pain, control of underlying cough, relief from tracheal obstruction, and improvement in dyspnea. They stated there was no evidence to suggest prolongation of life. Their method did not prevent egress of chemotherapy to the arteries arising from the arch of the aorta, and they believe this explained partial or total deafness in 4 patients and persistent moderate to severe mental confusion in 3 patients.

Many groups have reported their experience of delivering cancer chemotherapeutic agents to the bronchial arteries of lung tumors via catheters

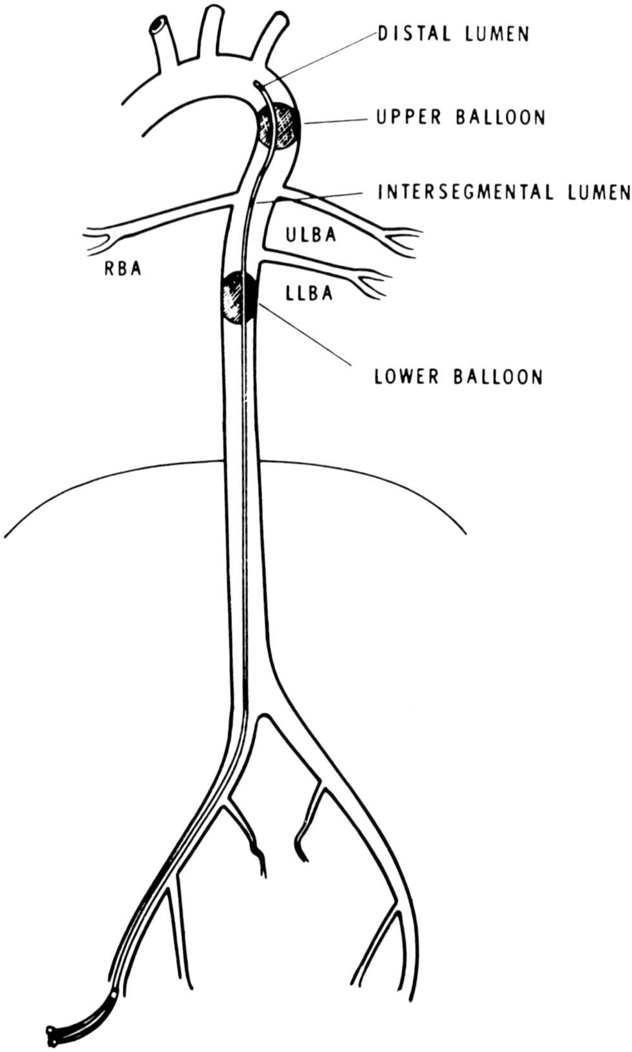

Figure 3 The quadruple-lumen, double-balloon catheter developed by Cliffton and Mahajan (1963). The catheter has been advanced from the femoral artery into the descending thoracic arota. Two lumina supply the balloons, which are inflated to isolate blood vessels arising from the fourth to the eighth thoracic vertabrae. Another lumen extends to the tip of the catheter, and the fourth lumen emerges between the balloons. Chemotherapeutic agents or dyes are injected into this lumen and then displaced from the enclosed segment of the aorta into the bronchial arteries by the volume of the injectate and by deflation of the upper balloon. The lower balloon is deflated 10 min later and the catheter withdrawn.

placed in the orifice of the bronchial arteries by the technique developed by Viamonte, European investigators, and others (Cliffton, 1969; Ekholm et al., 1983; Haller et al., 1966; Hellekant, 1979; Hellekant et al., 1978; Kahn et al., 1965; Kao and Yang, 1986; Neyazaki et al., 1969; Tate et al., 1968; Uchiyama et al., 1988; Wirtanen and Ansfeld, 1968). Compared with the earlier methods of perfusing chemotherapeutic agents into the bronchial circulation, this method is technically simpler and avoids introducing chemotherapy into other parts of the body, such as those perfused by the carotid, spinal, renal, femoral, and mesenteric circulations. These advantages are won at the expense of possible failure to cannulate and perfuse chemotherapy into bronchial vessels that have atypical anatomy or cannot be located for technical reasons.

The early report by Tate et al. in 1968, in which they infused either nitrogen mustard or cyclophosphamide into the bronchial arteries of 14 patients with primary lung neoplasms, proved to be prophetic. Only 3 of their patients had subjective improvement, and only 1 patient had objective improvement with shrinkage of size of the tumor, but he died with extensive metastatic disease 5 weeks later. Unlike other authors in previous and subsequent reports, they were frank enough to consider their results disappointing and recommended modification of the technique. Suggested modifications included using repetitive infusions or continuous infusions of chemotherapy over 1–2 weeks, combining therapy with radiotherapy, and perfusing with radioactive microspheres. Subsequent investigators frequently used multiple infusions or radiation therapy after the infusion. Some of these workers claimed subjective improvement in 75% or more of the patients (Uchiyama et al., 1988). Unfortunately, many of these studies did not determine if the beneficial effect could have been achieved by radiation therapy alone (Ekholm et al., 1983; Uchiyama et al., 1988). No groups have claimed long-term objective benefits in more than a small fraction of patients at best (Kao and Yang, 1986), and no investigative group has published long-term follow-up studies that claim bronchial artery infusions of cancer chemotherapy have a well-defined indication for the treatment of primary carcinoma of the lung.

Essentially complete abandonment of the early enthusiasm can be ascribed to a number of causes. Bronchial artery anatomy has proven to be just as variable as predicted by the early anatomic studies of Cauldwell et al. (1948) (Fig. 2), so that infusing chemotherapy into the bronchial arteries arising from the descending aorta likely misses cancerous tissue receiving its nutrition via the bronchial circulation from the intercostal arteries, internal mammary arteries, and arteries arising from the subclavian artery.

In approximately 20% of patients referred for bronchial artery infusions, radiologists cannot gain access to the vascular bed of the tumor for additional reasons, such as severe aortic atherosclerosis, inability to locate the perfusing artery, and occlusion of the initial perfusing bronchial artery by tumor growth.

The studies of Jonas and Carrington (1969) suggest that once a bronchial artery is occluded by tumor growth, perfusion may develop from pulmonary arteries via the collateral channels to the bronchial circulation. These tumors would therefore not respond to chemotherapy delivered through the remaining bronchial arteries.

The expanding edge of the tumor adjacent to the alveoli likely obtains its perfusion from the pulmonary circulation, so that total destruction of the tumor would require infusion of chemotherapy via both the pulmonary and bronchial artery circulations. Further evidence of possible significant perfusion of primary lung tumors via the pulmonary circulation comes from the older studies that infused chemotherapy distal to an obstructing balloon in the pulmonary artery perfusing the region of the tumor. According to Pierpont (1960), Morris and Goldberg (1961), and Creech and coworkers (1958, 1959), many of these patients obtained transient symptomatic relief so that some tumoricidal effect appears to have been achieved from the pulmonary artery injections. Alternatively, the clinical improvement may have resulted from the chemotherapy gaining access to the bronchial arteries after passing through the heart, reaching the aorta, and perfusing the bronchial circulation. Pulmonary artery infusions could also enter the bronchial circulation via precapillary or postcapillary anastomotic channels.

Many studies used radiation therapy in conjunction with bronchial artery perfusion so that there is no way to determine which mode of therapy resulted in the claimed clinical benefit.

Despite a large number of reports, no investigative team has undertaken a trial of bronchial artery infusions with an appropriate control population. This ideally would be saline infusions into the bronchial artery in place of chemotherapy accompanied by systemic administration of the chemotherapy at an appropriate dose. Cliffton (1969), using his double-balloon catheter in the aorta that temporarily stopped blood flow between the fourth and eighth thoracic intercostal arteries (Fig. 3), reported that infusions of nitrogen mustard into the occluded aorta resulted in an average survival of 8 months in 21 treated patients compared to only 1.8 months in 6 patients considered for perfusion but in whom treatment was not completed because of technical difficulties. Unfortunately, he gave no further information that characterized the two patient populations so that the appropriateness of his control subjects could not be evaluated.

Modification of earlier methods and the use of different kinds of chemotherapy have not improved long-term clinical results (Kao and Yang, 1986; Uchiyama et al., 1988). Investigators have used different perfusion schedules with multiple treatments and sometimes kept catheters in place for as long as 2 weeks (Wirtanen and Ansfield, 1968). Initially nitrogen mustard was the most popular agent, but others infused thio-TEPA and, more recently, mitomycin C. A recent innovative technique uses bronchial artery infusion of the short-acting agent cisplatin followed by the intravenous infusion of sodium thiosulfate 10 min later (Uchiyama et al., 1988). Sodium thiosulfate is known to reduce both the toxicity and tumor effect of cisplatin and thereby decreases the systemic toxicity from this agent (Fig. 4). Despite these trials of different agents with varying methods of perfusion, however, equally dismal results appear to have been obtained even with these later studies.

Because carcinoma of the lung so frequently has metastases beyond the chest at the time of diagnosis, any therapy focusing only on involvement of the lung and its immediate structures is doomed to failure in the majority of patients.* Thus, the whole concept of restricting chemotherapy to the region of the primary tumor must have limited goals: transient control of such symptoms as pain, cough, and hemoptysis. Debulking of tumor mass with regional perfusion to improve the efficacy of other forms of therapy may be an important approach if more effective forms of treatment are developed in the future.

B. Complications of Arterial Perfusion of Tumors with Chemotherapy

Initially there was considerable concern about significant morbidity and mortality from regional perfusion of lung tumors with chemotherapeutic agents. Fortunately, early investigators performed studies in dogs and other animals and worked out dose schedules that largely minimized the acute toxic effects of chemotherapy, such as severe chemical pneumonitis, sloughing of the skin on the chest wall, perforation of the aorta or esophagus, and transverse myelitis (Pierpont and Blades, 1960; Rheinlander et al., 1966). In addition, before attempts at regional perfusion with toxic agents, radiologists developed considerable experience with studies directed at providing selective angiograms of the bronchial and pulmonary circulation. These studies led to guidelines to avoid complications from injury to the spinal cord from the dye or chemotherapy (Di Chiro, 1974; Feigelson and Ravin, 1965; Kardjiev et al., 1974; Hellekant, 1979; Killen and Foster, 1966). For example, initial injection of dye is limited to only 1–3 ml, and care must be taken not to completely occlude the bronchial or spinal artery with the catheter so that flow is maintained during the injection. Use of a catheter with a tapered tip plus demonstration of free

---

*Most texts state 5 year cures for all patients with carcinoma of the lung is in the range of 5–12%, and 25% in patients able to undergo resection (Mountain, 1988; Silverberg et al., 1990). This suggests that 75–95% of patients have metastatic disease beyond the lungs at the time of their initial evaluation.

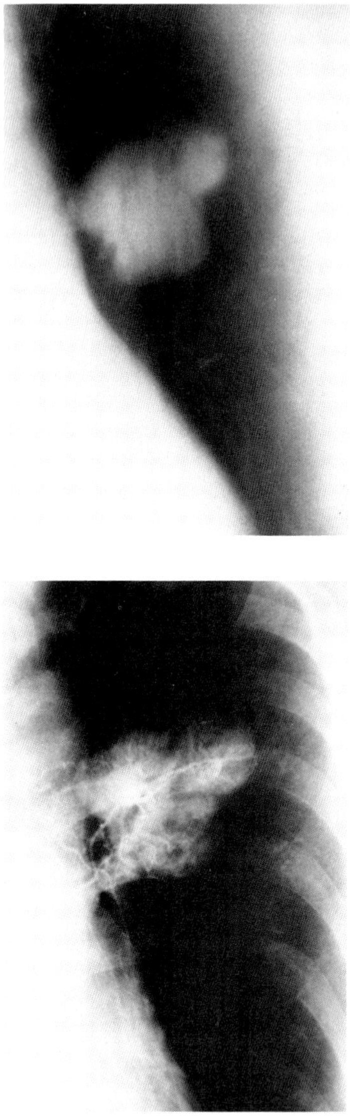

(a)

(b)

Figure 4 Multiple chest roentgenograms of a large cell pulmonary carcinoma in the left upper lobe of a 53-year-old woman with bone metastases treated with two courses of bronchial artery infusions of cisplatin and intravenous sodium thiosulfate rescue. (a) Anteroposterior (AP) tomogram before treatment. (b) Bronchial arteriogram demonstrating blood vessels in the tumor. (c) AP tomogram taken 2 weeks after initial cisplatin treatment. (d) AP tomogram after two courses of 100 mg cisplatin, 5 weeks after

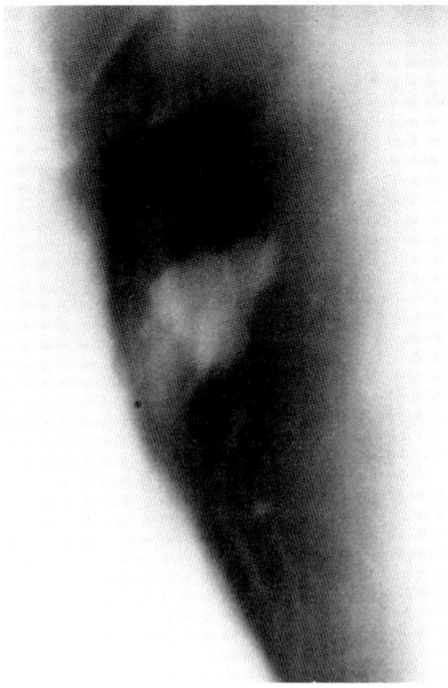

(c)

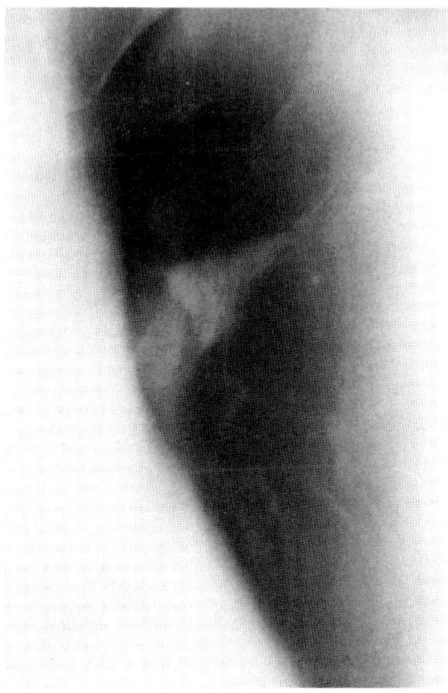

(d)

the first course of chemotherapy. Note that the size of the tumor decreased approximately 80%. The patient also received one course of combination chemotherapy including cyclophosphamide, thio-TEPA, and chromomycin A_3 for the treatment of multiple bone metastases. She died 8½ months after the initial bronchial infusion of cisplatin. (From Uchiyama et al., 1988.)

passage of blood through the catheter with suctioning are the usual techniques used to assure flow during the subsequent injection of 10–30 ml dye for visualization or infusion of chemotherapy. To my knowledge since the mid-1960s, no groups have reported transverse myelitis as a complication of bronchial artery chemotherapy. This has been attributed to the abandonment of contrast media, such as acetrizoate, that had a high rate of toxicity (Di Chiro, 1974). Several groups pointed out that toxic effects upon the spinal cord almost invariably resulted from injection of the fifth right intercostal artery (Feigelson and Ravin, 1965; Kardjiev et al., 1974; Hellekant, 1979). Caution in this region plus pilot injections of 1–3 ml dye to identify the bronchial artery before the use of large volumes of dye or chemotherapy are other likely explanations for the essential elimination of spinal cord injuries. If patients develop neurological symptoms in the legs, early investigators recommended a variety of interventions, including injecting diazepam or procaine into the spinal artery and performing lumbar puncture with multiple exchanges of 10 ml normal saline for spinal fluid to reduce the iodine concentration in the cerebrospinal fluid (Di Chiro, 1974; Feigelson and Ravin, 1965; Viamonte, 1964). However, the need for these heroic measures has not developed. Use of recently marketed nonionic contrast media would likely not help minimize the risk of spinal cord injury because this injury is now thought to be the result of mechanical blockage of the spinal artery resulting in hypoxic damage to the cord rather than a toxic effect of the dye.

Bronchial artery injections of chemotherapy are not without other severe complications from the chemotherapy. One recent series (Ekholm et al., 1983), reported that among 15 patients who received multiple bronchial artery injections of mitomycin C followed by radiation therapy, 4 developed swallowing difficulties, 3 had esophageal ulcers, including 1 tracheoesophageal fistula, 1 patient developed skin necrosis, and 3 patients died of hemoptysis several months after treatment. Fortunately, other investigators had fewer complications. A cursory review of 16 other reports published in English that describe a total of 364 patients reported only 11 serious complications. These complications included 1 tracheoesophageal fistula, 4 patients with deafness (1 complete) among 12 patients treated with hemibody nitrogen mustard during transient occlusion of the lower thoracic aorta with a balloon (Rheinlander et al., 1962), 4 patients with chemical pneumonitis, 5 patients with complications from trauma to the femoral artery at the site of introduction of the catheter inducing peripheral artery emboli, femoral artery thrombosis with palsy of the leg, occlusion of the left external iliac artery, and severe hematoma formation. A single patient exsanguinated from an aortic-eosphageal fistula 6 weeks after receiving a bronchial artery infusion of nitrogen mustard (Steckel et al., 1967), and one group had an unexplained death in a patient with severe obstructive lung disease 10 h after bronchial artery infusion of nitrogen mustard (Tate et al., 1968). Despite the technical challenge to the radiologists, however, major complications in the range of only 3% can be expected.

C. Growth Factors and Their Potential as Therapeutic Agents

In recent years, there has been an explosion in knowledge of vascular growth factors, also called angiogenic factors, their control, and relationship to neoplasms. One hypothesis proposes that solid tumors depend on the growth of capillaries, and every increase in the tumor cell population must be preceded by an increase in new capillaries to nourish the tumor (Folkman and Klagsbrun, 1987). Tumor cells can synthesize their own angiogenic factors, such as heparin binding endothelial cell growth factors, transforming growth factors, and fibroblast growth factors. These factors attract and activate macrophages and other cells that release angiogenic growth factors, secrete collagenases and heparinases that activate angiogenic factors normally sequestered in the extracellular matrix, and release vascular permeability factors that bring fibrinogen into the extracellular spaces. The resultant fibrin gel provides support for capillary growth. Despite this expansion of knowledge of angiogenesis, no specific biochemical hypotheses have come forth to explain the limited growth of the pulmonary circulation compared to the dramatic proliferation of the bronchial circulation. Suppression of angiogenic factors has already shown potential for treatment of paraneoplastic and neoplastic lung diseases. Progressive pulmonary hemangiomatosis in a 12-year-old boy was controlled by the administration of α-interferon, which is an inhibitor or proliferation of endothelial cells, fibroblasts, and collagen (White et al., 1989). Other interferons have shown some ability to cause regression of Kaposi's sarcoma (Real et al., 1986; Rios et al., 1985). The development of more potent and less toxic inhibitors of angiogenesis will likely lead to their application for the treatment of lung neoplasms. If these new agents prove to have a short half-life and potent systemic toxicity, regional perfusion via the bronchial, pulmonary, or both circulations may again attract interest.

IV. Comparison with Treatment of Tumors in Other Organs with Regional Perfusion

Regional perfusion of lung tumors has fallen into disfavor, but a number of investigators have expressed optimism about the efficacy of infusion of chemotherapy via the hepatic artery for the treatment of metastatic carcinoma of the liver (Stagg et al., 1984; Patt, 1988; Pettavel, 1988). Regional perfusion of the extremities, mainly for melanomas and sarcomas, has also attracted interest (Nachbur et al., 1988). For the extremities most protocals specify extracorporeal oxygenators attached to the femoral artery and veins accompanied by hyperthermia of the limb. Surgeons first performed hepatic artery infusions of chemotherapy with external infusion pumps attached to transcutaneous catheters placed surgically or transarterially via the femoral or brachial artery. Unfortunately, common complications included thrombosis of the hepatic and neighboring arteries, sepsis originating from the catheter site, and hemorrhage from the hepatic artery or from gastroduodenal ulcers. In a representative study, Reed et al. (1981) reported major complications in over half of 109 patients receiving hepatic artery infusions and a mortality of 7% from the procedure. This high complication rate is now largely avoided by the use of implantable subcutaneous pumps. The pump is refilled with chemotherapeutic agents delivered percutaneously through a diaphragm into the pump's reservoir. Sepsis from the transcutaneous catheter sites is avoided, thrombotic complications are markedly reduced, and the patient is mobile. Major complications are of the order of only 2% (Lightdale and Daly, 1987). This method permits the continuous infusion of chemotherapy over many weeks and has the theoretical advantage of allowing the chemotherapy to attack a larger percentage of tumor cells during the phase of synthesis of DNA when they are much more vulnerable to the effects of the drugs that interfere with cell proliferation.

The blood supply to the hepatic tumors is predominantly via the hepatic artery, but the portal system can at times supply a substantial fraction of the flow to small tumors as well as occasionally to larger tumors. This anatomic variability in perfusion appears to closely mimic the variable blood supply to lung tumors and has led to perfusion of the portal circulation with chemotherapy following resection of colon tumors in the hope of destroying microscopic metastases (Metzger, 1988). Hepatic artery ligation followed by portal vein infusions of chemotherapy for the treatment of well-established metastatic liver disease has been attempted but largely abandoned because of a mortality in the range of 10–15% (Lightdale and Daly, 1987).

Unfortunately, the clinical efficacy of these descriptions of regional perfusion of chemotherapy to the liver and extremities is difficult to determine. Studies claiming benefits suffer from the use of historical controls, the lack of controls receiving systemic therapy, and possible bias in the selection of subjects (Hartley and Fletcher, 1987; Ghussen et al., 1984; Reed et al., 1981). Certainly developments in the field of hepatic artery infusion deserve close observation because the techniques developed may be applicable to the bronchial artery perfusion of lung tumors. To date there have been no attempts, to my knowledge, to use implantable pumps for bronchial artery infusions. However, what is learned with hepatic artery infusions may not be transferable to the treatment of lung carcinomas. These lung tumors have such a high incidence of metastatic disease outside the chest that local control of the disease in the lungs may give little or no long-term benefit.

V. Summary

Experimental studies of infusion of material into the bronchial and pulmonary circulation of lung tumors in humans and other animals have essentially settled earlier disputes about the source of the blood supply to lung tumors. These tumors frequently have a complex and variable blood supply so that precise, predictable patterns of perfusion from the bronchial or pulmonary circulation are not possible. Primary carcinomas of the lung tend to receive most of their perfusion from bronchial arteries, and these arteries can show considerable increase in size. However, the advancing edge of the tumor appears to receive its blood supply from the pulmonary circulation. If the tumor blocks its own bronchial blood supply, blood flow through the commonly occurring collateral channels to the pulmonary arterial circulation is reversed so that branches of the pulmonary artery provide perfusion to large parts of the tumor. Metastatic tumors, when small, are perfused by the pulmonary circulation, but when larger, they frequently demonstrate perfusion via the bronchial circulation. Unlike the bronchial arteries, the pulmonary arteries adjacent to tumors show no vascular dilation or proliferation. Earlier claims that angiographic patterns may have diagnostic value have been discarded because tumor "blushes" and other perfusion patterns do not reliably establish types of tumors or even distinguish neoplasms from benign inflammatory lesions.

Enthusiasm for the regional perfusion of malignant lung tumors with chemotherapy via the pulmonary or bronchial circulation peaked in the 1960s and subsequently waned. No adequately controlled trials have shown lengthening of survival or diminished mortality. The high incidence of extrathoracic metastases from primary lung carcinomas has made efforts at controlling intrathoracic disease with regional perfusion an unrewarding undertaking. Rapid symptomatic control of cough, dyspnea, and pain has been frequently reported, however. Unfortunately, controlled trials have not demonstrated that this palliation requires the complexities of regional perfusion of the tumor compared to simpler forms of therapy, such as systemic chemotherapy or radiation therapy.

Many studies report a transient decrease in the bulk of tumors with regional perfusion of chemotherapy via the bronchial or pulmonary circulations. The development of more effective chemotherapeutic agents that have improved efficacy following reduction in the tumor burden may therefore lead to a resurgence in the use of regional perfusion of chemotherapeutic agents to the lungs.

References

Asai, T. (1936). Experimental study of nutrient vessel of sarcoma transplanted into the lungs of rabbits. *Gann* **30**:784–789.

Bierman, H. R., Byron, L. R., Jr., and Kelly, K. H. (1951). Therapy of inoperable visceral and regional metastases by intra-arterial catheterization in man (abstract). *Cancer Res.* **11**:236.

Blades, B., and Hall, E. R. (1958). Preliminary observations of the injection of potentially carcinolytic drugs into the pulmonary artery with temporary occlusion of the blood supply of the lung. *Am. Surg.* **24**:492–494.

Bonner, C. D., Thurman, A., and Homburger, F. (1952). A critical study of regional intraarterial nitrogen mustard therapy in cancer. *Ann. Surg.* **136**:912–918.

Cauldwell, E. W., Siekert, R. G., Lininger, R. E., and Anson, B. J. (1948). The bronchial arteries. An anatomical study of 150 human cadavers. *Surg. Gynecol. Obstet.* **86**:395–442.

Cliffton, E. E. (1969). Bronchial artery perfusion for treatment of advanced lung cancer. *Cancer* **23**:1151–1157.

Cliffton, E. E., and Mahajan, D. R. (1963). Technique for visualization and perfusion of bronchial arteries: Suggested clinical and diagnostic applications. *Cancer* **16**:444–452.

Creech, O., Jr., Krementz, E. T., Ryan, R. F., and Winblad, J. N. (1958). Chemotherapy of cancer: Regional perfusion utilizing an extracorporeal circuit. *Ann. Surg.* **148**:616–632.

Creech, O., Jr., Krementz, E. T., Ryan, R. F., Reemtsma, K., and Winblad, J. N. (1959). Experiences with isolation-perfusion technics in the treatment of cancer. *Ann. Surg.* **149**:627–640.

Cudkowicz, L., and Armstrong, J. B. (1953). The blood supply of malignant pulmonary neoplasms. *Thorax* **8**:152–156.

Di Chiro, G. (1974). Unintentional spinal cord arteriography: A warning. *Radiology* **112**:231–233.

Ekholm, S., Albrechtsson, U., and Tylen, U. (1983). Bronchial artery infusion of Mitomycin C in carcinoma. *Cardiovasc. Intervent. Radiol.* **6**:86–96.

Feigelson, H. H., and Ravin, H. A. (1965). Transverse myelitis following selective bronchial arteriography. *Radiology* **85**:663–665.

Folkman, J., and Klagsbrun, M. (1987). Angiogenic factors. *Science* **235**:442–447.

Ghoreyeb, A. A., and Karsner, H. T. (1913). A study of the relation of pulmonary and bronchial circulation. *J. Exp. Med.* **18**:500–506.

Ghussen, F., Nagel, K., Groth, W., Muller, J. M., and Stutzer, H. (1984). A prospective randomized study of regional extremity perfusion in patients with malignant melanoma. *Ann. Surg.* **200**:764–768.

Grady, E. D., Krantz, S., and Brown, P. F. (1953). Treatment of cancer by intermittent injection of nitrogen mustard via cannulated arteries. *Ann. Surg.* **137**:366–374.

Greenspan, R. H. (1971). Comments on bronchial arteriography (letter). *Chest* **59**:468.

Haller, J. D., Bron, K. M., Wholey, M. H., Poller, S., and Enerson, D. M. (1966). Selective bronchial artery catheterization for diagnostic and physiologic studies and chemotherapy for bronchogenic carcinoma. *J. Thorac. Cardiovasc. Surg.* **51**:143–152.

Hartley, J. W., and Fletcher, W. S. (1987). Improves survival of patients with stage II melanoma of the extremity using hyperthermic isolation perfusion l-phenylalanine mustard. *J. Surg. Oncol.* **36**:170–174.

Hellekant, C. (1979). Bronchial angiography and intraarterial chemotherapy with mitomycin C in bronchogenic carcinoma. *Acta Radiol. Diagn.* **20**:478–496.

Hellekant, C., Boijsen, E., and Svanberg, L. (1978). Preoperative infusion of mitomycin C in the bronchial artery in squamous cell carcinoma of the lung. *Acta Radiol. Diagn.* **9**:1045–1056.

Ikeda, M., Neyazaki, T., Chiba, S., Yoneti, M., and Suzuki, C. (1968). Bronchial vascular pattern of various pulmonary diseases, with particular emphasis on its diagnostic value in pulmonary cancer. *J. Thorac. Cardiovasc. Surg.* **55**:642–652.

Jonas, A. M., and Carrington, C. B. (1969). Vascular patterns in primary and secondary pulmonary tumors in the dog. *Am. J. Pathol.* **56**:79–87.

Kahn, P. C., Paul, R. E., and Rheinlander, H. F. (1965). Selective bronchial arteriography and intraarterial chemotherapy in carcinoma of the lung. *J. Thorac. Cardiovasc. Surg.* **50**:640–645.

Kao, E., and Yang, M. (1986). Selective bronchial arteriography and its therapeutic application. *J. Formosan Med. Assoc.* **85**:845–855.

Kardjiev, V., Symeonov, A., and Chankov, I. (1974). Etiology, pathogenesis, and prevention of spinal cord lesions in selective angiography of the bronchial and intercostal arteries. *Radiology* **112**:81–83.

Killen, D. A., and Foster, J. H. (1966). Spinal cord injury as a complication of contrast angiography. *Surgery* **59**:969–981.

Klopp, C. T., Alford, C., Bateman, J., Berry, G. N., and Winship, T. (1950). Fractionated intra-arterial cancer chemotherapy with methyl bis amine hydrochloride; a preliminary report. *Ann. Surg.* **132**:811–832.

Kulig, A., and Zielinski, K. W. (1982). Evaluation of blood vessel distribution in primary lung carcinomas in man in relation to histological type. *Pol. Przegl. Radiol. Med. Nukl.* **46**:249–255.

Lightdale, C. J., and Daly, J. (1987). Management of primary and metastatic cancer of the liver. In *Disease of the Liver,* 6th Ed. Edited by L. Schiff and E. R. Schiff. Philadelphia, J. B. Lippincott, pp. 1159–1170.

Metzger, U. (1988). Intraportal chemotherapy for colorectal hepatic metastases. *Antibiot. Chemother.* **40**:51–60.

Miller, B. J., and Rosenbaum, A. S. (1967). The vascular supply to metastatic tumors. *Surg. Gynecol. Obstet.* **125**:1009–1012.

Miller, W. S. (1907). The vascular supply of the pleura pulmonalis. *Am. J. Anat.* **7**:389–407.

Milne, E. C. (1967). Circulation of primary and metastatic pulmonary neoplasms. *Am. J. Roentgenol.* **100**:603–619.

Miyazawa, K., Katori, R., Ishikawa, K., Yamaki, M., Kobayashi, Y., Tsuiki, K., Matsunaga, A., and Nakamura, T. (1970). Selective bronchial arteriography and bronchial blood flow; correlative study. *Chest* **57**:416–422.

Morris, J. F., and Goldberg, L. M. (1961). Chemotherapy of bronchogenic carcinoma utilizing cardiac catheterization. *Am. J. Med. Sci.* **242**:527–533.

Mountain, C. F. (1988). Surgical treatment of non-small cell lung cancer. In *Pulmonary Diseases and Disorders,* 2nd Ed. Edited by A. P. Fishman. New York, McGraw-Hill, pp. 1991–2000.

Nachbur, B., Vogt, W., and Goldhirsch, A. (1988). Treatment of soft tissue malignancies of the extremities by regional perfusion. *Antibiot. Chemother.* **40**:77–93.

Newton, T. H., and Preger, L. (1965). Selective bronchial arteriography. *Radiology* **84**:1043–1051.

Neyazaki, T. (1962). A method for arteriography of the bronchial artery. *Jpn. Heart J.* **3**:523–536.

Neyazaki, T., Ikeda, M., Seki, Y., Egawa, N., and Suzuki, C. (1969). Bronchial artery infusion therapy for lung cancer. *Cancer* **24**:912–922.

Heyazaki, T., Ikeda, M., Mitsui, K., Kimuri, S., Suzuki, M., and Suzuki, C. (1970). Angioarchitecture of pulmonary malignancies in humans. *Cancer* **26**:1246–1255.

Ogilvie, R. W., Blanding, J. D., Wood, M. L., and Knisely, W. H. (1965). The blood supply to experimental metastatic rabbit lung tumors. *Bibl. Anat.* **7**:136–141.

Patt, Y. Z. (1988). Hepatic arterial infusion of chemotherapy for metastatic colorectal cancer in the liver: Why, how and what? *Antibiot. Chemother.* **40**:1–11.

Pettavell, J. (1988). Intra-arterial chemotherapy using a pump. *Antibiot. Chemother.* **40**:36–40.

Pierpont, H. (1960). Techniques of lung perfusion with cancer chemotherapeutic agents. *Cancer Chemother. Rep.* **10**:15–19.

Pierpont, H., and Blades, B. (1960). Lung perfusion with chemotherapeutic agents. *J. Thorac. Cardiovasc. Surg.* **39**:159–165.

Real, F. X., Oettgen, H. F., and Krown, S. E. (1986). Kaposi's sarcoma and the acquired immunodeficiency syndrome: Treatment with high and low doses of recombinant leukocyte A interferon. *J. Clin. Oncol.* **4**:544–551.

Reed, M. A. L., Vaitkevicius, V. K., Al-Sarraf, M., Vaughn, C. B., Singhakowinta, A., Sexon-Porte, M., Izbicki, R., Baker, L., and Straatsma, G. (1981). The practicality of chronic hepatic artery infusion therapy of primary and metastatic hepatic malignancies: Ten-year results of 124 patients in a prospective protocol. *Cancer* **47**:402–409.

Reuter, S. R., Olin, T., and Abrams, H. L. (1965). Selective bronchial arteriography. *Radiology* **84**:87–95.

Rheinlander, H. F., Miller, H. H., Moquin, R. B., and Deterling, R. A., Jr. (1962). Upper hemibody infusion with alkylating agents for advanced lung cancer. *J. Thorac. Cardiovasc. Surg.* **44**:801–810.

Rheinlander, H. F., Tamabe, T., and Paul, R. E., Jr. (1966). Selective infusion of bronchial arteries with mechlorethamine in dogs. *Surgery* **60**:1044–1050.

Rios, A., Mansell, P. W., Newell, G. R., Reuben, J. M., Hersh, E. M., and Gutterman, J. V. (1985). Treatment of acquired immunodeficiency syndrome-related Kaposi's sarcoma with lymphoblastoid interferon. *J. Clin. Oncol.* **3**:506–512.

Silverberg, E., Boring, C. C., and Squires, T. S. (1990). Cancer statistics, 1990. *CA* **40**:9–28.

Stagg, R. J., Lewis, B. J., Friedman, M. A., Ignoffo, R. J., and Hohn, D. C. (1984). Hepatic arterial chemotherapy for colorectal cancer metastatic to the liver. *Ann. Intern. Med.* **100**:736–743.

Steckel, R. J., Doppman, J. I., Rolley, R. T., and Martos, E. J. (1967). Rupture of the aorta after mechlorethamine HCl infusion of a bronchial artery. *JAMA* **199**:936–939.

Tate, C. F., Jr., Viamonte, M., Jr., and Agnew, J. R. (1968). Bronchial arterial perfusion with cytotoxic agents for bronchogenic carcinoma. *Am. Rev. Respir. Dis.* **97**:685–693.

Uchiyama, N., Kobayashi, H., Nakajo, M., and Shinohara, S. (1988). Treatment of lung cancer with bronchial artery infusion of cisplatin and intravenous sodium thiosulfate rescue. *Acta Oncol.* **27**:57–61.

Verloop, M. C. (1948). The arteriae bronchiales and their anastomoses with the arteria pulmonalis in the human lung; a micro-anatomical study. *Acta Anat. (Basel)* **5**:171–205.

Viamonte, M., Jr. (1964). Selective bronchial arteriography in man. *Radiology* **83**:830–839.

Viamonte, M., Jr., Parks, R. E., and Smoak, W. M., III (1965). Guided catheterization of the bronchial arteries. *Radiology* **85**:205–230.

White, C. W., Sondheimer, H. M., Crouch, E. C., Wilson, H., and Fan, L. L. (1989). Treatment of pulmonary hemangiomatosis with recombinant interferon alpha-2a. *N. Engl. J. Med.* **320**:1197–1200.

Wirtanen, G. W., and Ansfield, F. J. (1968). Bronchial artery infusion in bronchogenic carcinoma. *Cancer Chemother. Rep.* **52**:263–269.

Wood, D. A., and Miller, M. (1938). The role of the dual pulmonary circulation in various pathologic conditions of the lungs. *J. Thorac. Surg.* **7**:649–670.

Wright, R. D. (1938). The blood supply of abnormal tissues in the lungs. *J. Pathol. Bacteriol.* **47**:489–499.

20

The Bronchial Circulation in Pulmonary Vascular Obstruction

DEBORAH SHURE

University of California, San Diego
and Veterans Administration Medical Center
San Diego, California

I. Introduction

The bronchial circulation has been thought to be involved in preservation of lung tissue distal to an acute obstruction of a pulmonary artery since Virchow's observation (1847) of the rarity of pulmonary infarction after pulmonary embolism. This clinical observation, often noted since, was experimentally confirmed by Virchow by ligation of the left pulmonary artery in a dog. Maintenance of tissue viability in this setting of complete obstruction of pulmonary arterial flow to one lung was assumed to be due to bronchial arterial flow. Subsequent studies in more recent times found an increased incidence of pulmonary infarction with simultaneous pulmonary artery obstruction and decreased bronchial arterial flow (Goetz et al., 1965; Mathes et al., 1932), adding support to the hypothesis.

Since these observations, many studies have examined the remarkable expansion of the bronchial circulation that occurs after pulmonary vascular obstruction. Considerable anatomic information has been obtained through the use of angiography, vascular casts, and histology. Physiological studies have provided information about factors influencing the timing and degree of increase in flow after obstruction.

Despite this wealth of anatomic, histological, and physiological information, many important questions concerning the role of the bronchial circulation in pulmonary vascular disease remain unanswered. This chapter reviews what we know about the bronchial circulation in a number of diseases involving obstruction of the pulmonary arterial bed and addresses some of the interesting unanswered questions. Because of physiological and anatomic differences, obstructive pulmonary vascular diseases are considered in terms of acute and chronic obstructive processes, arbitrarily defined as obstruction of hours to 1 or 2 days versus obstruction of days to months.

II. Acute Pulmonary Artery Obstruction

A. Clinical Findings

The historical basis for the observed infrequency of lung infarction after pulmonary embolism has been noted. Da Vinci's assumption that the bronchial circulation provides the essential nutritive flow to the lung has been accepted as the reason for the preservation of lung tissue after complete cessation of pulmonary flow to a large area of lung (Deffebach et al., 1987). Many observers have noted that infarction after embolization is more common in the presence of left ventricular failure or mitral stenosis (Cudkowicz, 1952; Fisher et al., 1970; Malmstrom et al., 1954). These conditions are characterized by an increase in pulmonary venous pressure, which has been shown experimentally to cause a decrease in bronchial flow. This relation between bronchial arterial flow and pulmonary venous pressure has been demonstrated in dogs and sheep (Malmstrom et al., 1954; Goetz et al., 1965; Charan et al., 1985). Because of the difficulty of bronchial flow measurements in humans, corresponding clinical data are not available, but the physiology appears to be similar. Thus, the need for some form of elevated pulmonary venous pressure (and a corresponding decrease in bronchial flow) to develop pulmonary infarction after embolization suggests a role for the bronchial circulation in maintaining basic lung nutrition after acute obstruction of the pulmonary arterial flow. The possibility for a nutritive function of reverse pulmonary venous flow immediately after the blockage is considered in Chap. 11.

Although not strictly caused by primary pulmonary vascular disease, pulmonary blood flow is reduced or abolished in most acute parenchymal lesions.

B. Experimental Findings

No data exist on the measurement of bronchial arterial flow after acute embolization in humans, but measurements have been made of pulmonary arterial oxygen saturation or partial pressure of oxygen after acute balloon occlusion of a pulmonary artery (Julian et al., 1960; Nordenstrom et al., 1966). In these studies, the oxygen saturation and the partial pressure of oxygen measured distal to the occlusion acutely reflected systemic arterial values rather than pulmonary arterial values. Such findings have been used to support the hypothesis of an immediate increase in bronchial flow following unilateral pulmonary artery obstruction. Another possible interpretation, however, is that the increase in oxygen saturation reflects only the aspiration of blood from an area that has been exposed to alveolar gas or to pure bronchial flow. It does not provide evidence for a quantitative increase in flow.

Animal studies of the effects of acute obstruction have been performed in sheep and dogs with conflicting results. Studies of balloon occlusion in dogs similar to those performed in humans found an immediate increase in pulmonary arterial oxygen saturation to systemic values distal to a proximal occlusion (Cudkowicz, 1958; Carlens et al., 1951; Isawa et al., 1972; Severinghaus et al., 1961). Again, the assumption was that this increase reflects increased bronchial flow, but the same caveat applies with respect to quantitation of flow.

Jindal et al. (1984) studied the responses of bronchial flow to acute occlusion of a lobar pulmonary artery in a dog model. In this model, the left lower lobe was isolated in a sling with an attached strain gauge to measure weight changes during pulmonary artery occlusion. The bronchial circulation remained intact, with the lung in the surgically opened chest. The pulmonary artery and vein were cannulated, and the isolated vascular system of the left lower lobe was perfused through separate reservoirs. The bronchial flow before and after pulmonary artery occlusion was measured by changes in the reservoir volumes in relation to the weight of the lobe. In this system, bronchial flow increased immediately after snaring the lobar pulmonary artery, from 27 to 60 ml/min by 90 min.

In contrast, a study of microvascular occlusion in sheep found a decrease rather than an increase in bronchial flow in the first hour after embolization (Malik and Tracy, 1980). In this study, sheep were embolized with 100 μm glass beads. Bronchial flow was measured by the radiolabeled microsphere technique. Bronchial flow at baseline was 1.6% of cardiac output. It remained normal for 5 min after embolization, but then decreased to 40% of the baseline value (0.7% of cardiac output) and remained depressed for the duration of the study (1 h).

These two studies raise the question of a possible difference in the response of the bronchial circulation to large-vessel versus small-vessel occlusion. This interpretation remains a possibility, but two additional studies suggest that the response to large- and small-vessel occlusion is not different. Williams and Towbin (1955) studied the responses of the bronchial circulation in the dog to both acute and chronic pulmonary artery obstruction. In their model, the left pulmonary artery of the dog was snared or ligated. Bronchial flow was measured directly by cannulation of the pulmonary artery (distal to the obstruction) and snaring the pulmonary veins. With proximal obstruction of the pulmonary artery and temporary occlusion of the pulmonary veins, flow from the cannulated pulmonary artery could come only from bronchial flow. This flow was measured by the rate of flow from the cannula. In this setting, Williams and Towbin found that bronchial flow decreased in the 2–4 h period after pulmonary artery snaring.

The second study used the same canine isolated lobar model used by Jindal et al. (1984) but kept the entire system at body temperature (Agostoni et al., 1987). Under these conditions, bronchial flow decreased after acute pulmonary artery occlusion. The results of this study suggest that the earlier finding of an acute increase in bronchial flow was probably due to the response of the bronchial circulation to lung rewarming when perfusion with cold reservoir blood was stopped, rather than to the physiological response to pulmonary artery obstruction.

C. Why Is Infarction Rare?

Based on these studies, the response of the bronchial circulation to acute pulmonary artery obstruction appears to be a decrease in flow, not the increase in flow usually assumed, at least during the first 24 h after pulmonary artery occlusion. What, then, prevents infarction? This is an important question that remains unanswered.

It is possible that even the decreased bronchial flow is sufficient to maintain lung viability. Some damage may occur without frank infarction. For example, microatelectasis and some degree of edema have been described histologically after embolization (Huber and Edmunds, 1967; Naimark, 1966). Surfactant has been found to decrease in the first 24 h after pulmonary artery obstruction and then return to normal levels (Stunick and Soloff, 1967; Chernick et al., 1966; Baritussio and Clements, 1981; Said et al., 1968; Shepard et al., 1980), suggesting some degree of metabolic dysfunction. Minimal bronchial flow may be sufficient to prevent further damage before pulmonary arterial flow increases after resolution of the embolus or after dilatation of existing bronchial vessels and formation of new vessels with an increase in overall bronchial flow. Another possibility is that reverse flow in the pulmonary veins nourishes the region without pulmonary arterial inflow (Shepard et al., 1981).

It is also possible that clinical acute embolization does not correspond completely to the experimental conditions of ligation or glass bead embolization. Perhaps vasoactive factors released from platelets in thromboemboli or from the pulmonary artery wall itself have additional effects on bronchial flow. Unfortunately, we have no way to resolve this question since no techniques are currently available to measure small differences in bronchial flow in humans. It may be possible, however, to examine this question in a preparation of acute thromboembolism using the radiolabeled microsphere technique to measure the bronchial flow in an intact animal.

III. Chronic Pulmonary Artery Obstruction

A. Clinical Findings

Congenital absence of a pulmonary artery provides a unique physiological condition for examination of the effects of chronic absence of pulmonary flow on the formation of bronchial collateral vessels. In pure pulmonary artery agenesis not associated with congenital cardiac abnormalities, the lung without pulmonary arterial flow is usually smaller than the opposite lung and is supplied by a profusion of bronchial collateral vessels that can be derived from any of the systemic arteries in the chest (Wood and Miller, 1938; Liebow et al., 1950b; Fishman, 1961; Tabakin et al., 1960).

It appears that these vessels can function in gas exchange. In a number of studies using bronchospirometry, the lung without pulmonary arterial flow can participate in carbon dioxide elimination (Tabakin et al., 1960; Bloomer et al., 1949). Some studies were not able to demonstrate participation in oxygen exchange, other studies showed this capability, particularly when the good lung is challenged by hypoxia. One case report described a 21-year-old man who underwent pulmonary artery ligation during surgery for tetralogy of Fallot (Viola and Abbate, 1973). At 8 years after ligation, the occluded lung did not appear to participate in oxygen uptake when breathing hyperoxic gas but did participate when the good lung was exposed to hypoxia. During this 8 year period, the calculated bronchial circulation to the occluded lung greatly increased. Thus, in the absence of a pulmonary artery from birth, the bronchial collateral circulation is able to assume nutritive and gas-exchange functions.

Agenesis is unusual, however, and may not necessarily be analogous to acquired pulmonary artery obstruction in adult disease because of differences in the neonatal pulmonary vasculature. A number of conditions causing obstruction of the pulmonary arteries in adults cause a similar increase in bronchial collateral flow and new bronchial vessel formation. It appears that any cause of chronic pulmonary artery obstruction results in these changes.

Chronic organized thromboembolic obstruction of the central pulmonary arteries is associated with an extensive increase in the bronchial collateral flow to the obstructed regions of lung (Castleman and Bland, 1946; Carroll, 1950; Moser et al., 1965, 1983). These collateral vessels can also arise from any of the systemic vessels in the chest. The profusion of bronchial vessels, which involve the pleura as well, is the reason that surgical correction of this condition is best approached through a sternotomy incision and with the use of cardiopulmonary bypass to avoid incision through the vascular pleura and to provide a bloodless field for dissection of the organized thrombus (Daily et al., 1987).

Other causes of chronic pulmonary artery obstruction are also associated with an expansion of the bronchial collateral circulation. Bronchogenic carcinomas are largely supplied by bronchial collateral vessels (Liebow et al., 1950b; Wood and Miller, 1938; Cudkowicz, 1967; Cudkowicz and Armstrong, 1953; Ryan and Abelmann, 1961; Wagenvoort and Wagenvoort, 1965). In one study, bronchial flow in this setting was estimated as almost 7% of cardiac output as opposed to the normal flow of close to 1% (Cudkowicz, 1967). It is not certain, however, that the bronchial flow to primary bronchogenic carcinomas is related to pulmonary arterial obstruction. Most such tumors cause obstruction of at least small pulmonary arteries by compression or invasion, but they also appear to produce growth factors that stimulate new vessel formation. It is not known if the bronchial collateral supply to bronchogenic carcinomas occurs in the absence of pulmonary arterial obstruction. This issue remains an interesting unanswered question.

Fibrosing mediastinitis may also be associated with an increase in bronchial flow associated with enlarged mediastinal nodes compressing central pulmonary arteries. Angiographically, these cases may simulate chronic thromboembolic pulmonary arterial obstruction (Berry et al., 1986).

All these conditions causing obstruction of major pulmonary arteries are associated with the formation of bronchial collateral vessels and extensive precapillary bronchopulmonary anastomoses, but sickle cell disease, which is associated with diffuse pulmonary microvascular obstruction, does not appear to cause an increase in bronchial collateral vessels. Large-vessel embolization can occur in sickle cell disease, but the predominant pathology is occlusion of small vessels by either thrombi in situ or by sludging of abnormal cells. Only one study examined bronchial vessels in this condition, and they found no evidence for an augmentation in the bronchial arterial circulation (Heath and Thompson, 1969). This finding again raises the question of different responses to large- and small-vessel occlusion.

Regardless of the universality of the response of the bronchial circulation to pulmonary artery occlusion, in the many situations in which the collateral circulation increases, it appears to have a significant physiological effect. The magnitude of the increase in the bronchial circulation in clinical settings is uncertain because of the difficulty in accurately measuring bronchial flow in humans. Bronchopulmonary anastomotic flow can be accurately measured during surgery involving cardiopulmonary bypass by the left ventricular vent flow (Baile et al., 1985), but no data are yet available using this technique in relevant disease states (see Chap. 5). Calculations using simultaneous left and right heart output measurements are the only available data in disease (Cudkowicz et al., 1959, 1960). Although the method is unreliable in conditions of normal flow because of a significant error in each output measurement (Deffebach et al., 1987), it provides an estimate of bronchial collateral flow when the flow is greatly expanded, and, therefore, large enough for the error to be less significant. In one such study, the magnitude of the bronchial flow was 11% of cardiac output in conditions involving either tissue proliferation or obstruction (Ryan and Abelmann, 1961) as opposed to normal flow of 1–3% of cardiac output.

Anastomoses between the bronchial collateral vessels and the pulmonary arterial bed occur in the precapillary zone. This finding was confirmed by histology (Ellis et al., 1952; Liebow et al., 1950b), postmortem angiograms (Liebow et al., 1950b; Marchand et al., 1950; Ellis et al., 1952; Orell and Hultgren, 1966), and vascular casts (Marchand et al., 1950; Liebow et al., 1949). In some settings, elevated pulmonary pressures (Roosenburg and Deenstra, 1954; Williams and Towbin, 1955; Cudkowicz, 1958) and systemic waveforms (Roosenburg and Deenstra, 1954) were recorded in areas of expanded bronchial collateral circulation, although others did not confirm all these findings (Cudkowicz, 1958).

B. Experimental Findings

A number of animal studies focused on the response of the bronchial circulation to chronic pulmonary artery obstruction. In a situation analogous to pulmonary artery agenesis, Haworth et al. (1981) studied the effect of left pulmonary artery ligation on the lung of neonatal pigs. The response of the bronchial circulation is identical to that seen in pulmonary artery agenesis: a great expansion in the bronchial collateral flow to the obstructed lung.

A number of investigators have examined the response of the adult dog lung to left pulmonary artery ligation (Liebow et al., 1950a; Williams and Towbin, 1955; Bloomer et al., 1949; Goetz et al., 1965; Alley et al., 1961). It also appears to be the same as the human response to central pulmonary artery obstruction, such as that seen in chronic thromboembolic disease. In experimental settings, however, additional data are available regarding the nature, magnitude, and time course of the expansion in collateral circulation.

Liebow et al. (1950a) demonstrated the presence of extensive precapillary anastomoses by exquisite vascular casts of dog lungs after ligation of the left pulmonary artery for 4 weeks to 1 year. They noted that the collateral vessels formed from the aorta, intercostal arteries, internal mammaries, and subclavian arteries. In fact, the collaterals can form from any systemic vessel in the chest, including the coronary arteries. This diverse origin has been noted in humans as well.

The magnitude of the increase in collateral flow with chronic pulmonary artery obstruction has been studied by Bloomer et al. (1949) using the left minus right ventricular output method. They found bronchial flow was one-third of the cardiac output by 4 months after ligation in dogs. Williams and Towbin (1955), using the canine left pulmonary artery ligation model with cannulation of the pulmonary arteries to directly measure bronchial collateral flow, found flow increased from baseline values of 4–10 ml/min (1% of cardiac output) to 300–400 ml/min (25–30% of cardiac output) by 1 year after ligation. As mentioned previously, flow initially decreased in the first 4 h after ligation but increased steadily from days to 1 year later. Data are not available in this study beyond the 1 year point, but others found morphological evidence of an increase in collateral vessel formation 2 years after ligation (Alley et al., 1961).

Weibel (1960) examined the time course of the development of bronchial collateral vessels after left pulmonary artery ligation in the rat using light and electron microscopy. In this study, collateral formation began by 2 weeks after ligation. The evidence suggested that new vessel formation occurred, not merely the opening of existing collaterals. Primitive vessel cords with mitoses were seen. In addition, endothelial and smooth muscle cell proliferation occurred first, followed by collagen and elastin deposition. These findings are consistent with earlier studies in rats using postmortem barium sulfate injections (Ellis et al., 1952). The time course for collateral development was the same (2 weeks), and both studies demonstrated significant precapillary bronchopulmonary anastomoses.

IV. Relation of Bronchial Collateral Vessel Formation to Pulmonary Vascular Remodeling

A. Clinical Evidence

One of the earliest reports of chronic pulmonary emboli was a case report of a woman who died from cor pulmonale after repeated episodes clinically consistent with pulmonary emboli (Castleman and Bland, 1946). Autopsy findings were those of chronic organized emboli occluding multiple tertiary vessels. Although the plmonary artery distal to each obstruction appeared grossly thin in contrast to the hypertrophied arteries in the patent areas of the lung, these distal arteries showed true medial hypertrophy on microscopic examination despite the low intravascular pressure likely to have been present. More recently, similar unexpected findings were described in a series of patients who underwent biopsy of the lung distal to chronic pulmonary emboli, as well as biopsy of the lung in patent areas, at the time of thromboendarterectomy for surgical removal of chronic emboli (Spragg et al., 1982). In these patients, both the obstructed and the patent beds showed changes consistent with grades III and IV pulmonary hypertension according to the Heath and Edwards classification. The lesions included medial hypertrophy, intimal proliferation, and plexiform lesions.

A similar pulmonary vascular remodeling was also observed in the lungs of patients with primary bronchogenic carcinoma (Wagenvoort and Wagenvoort, 1965). These workers found medial hypertrophy most marked in the region of the tumor but also present in the remainder of the lobe and, to a lesser extent, in the lung on the side of the tumor. The contralateral lung vasculature was normal.

Both chronic thromboembolic disease and bronchogenic carcinoma are characterized by an increase in bronchial collateral flow. In contrast, sickle cell disease, which causes small-vessel occlusion without an increase in bronchial flow, does not appear to be associated with distal vascular remodeling (Heath and Thompson, 1969). These findings together suggest a possible relationship between collateral formation and vascular remodeling.

B. Experimental Evidence

Using a canine model of hyperkinetic pulmonary flow induced by anastomosis of the aorta to the left lower lobe pulmonary artery, Downing et al. found plexiform lesions at points of high turbulent flow and found that such lesions consisted of bronchial arterial recanalization of pulmonary vessels obstructed by thrombi (Downing et al., 1963). A supporting piece of data for a role of systemic to pulmonary anastomoses in plexogenic remodeling is the finding of plexiform lesions in pulmonary sequestrations (Wagenvoort, 1984). This could reflect high pressure in the sequestration. However, since sequestrations are supplied by systemic vessels, only the presence of a plexiform lesion in a non-sequestrated lung may indicate the equivalent of a systemic bronchopulmonary anastomosis. No hemodynamic data are available to answer this question.

Because of the interesting findings of pulmonary vascular remodeling distal to obstructed pulmonary arteries in humans with chronic thromboemboli, the canine ligation model was reexamined to focus on the effect of ligation on the pulmonary arterial bed rather than the bronchial circulation as in previous studies. Shure et al. (1984) found that changes consistent with pulmonary arterial hypertension occurred distal to a chronically ligated pulmonary artery in adult dogs. The changes observed consisted of medial hypertrophy, intimal proliferation, and plexiform lesions (Fig. 1). Medial hypertrophy was assessed by the medial muscle area ratio: the ratio of the medial area to the total vessel determined by planimetry (Harker et al., 1981). The pathological changes occurred only in the ligated left lung, not on the patent right side (Shure et al., 1984, 1985).

Physiological studies showed that these changes occurred without high pressure or high flow (Shure et al., 1985). The pressure in the obstructed pulmonary artery dropped initially after ligation but was comparable to the patent pulmonary artery pressure at 3 weeks or longer after ligation (12 mmHg in the obstructed artery versus 16 mmHg in the patent artery). Thus, the changes were not due to transmission of systemic pressure through precapillary bronchopulmonary anastomoses.

Another interesting observation was the temporal relation between bronchial collateral formation and remodeling in the pulmonary bed (Shure et al., 1986, 1987). Postobstructive changes occur only at 3 weeks or longer after ligation, coincident with the formation of significant bronchial collateral vessels. The pulmonary changes are not seen at 1 or 2 weeks when bronchial

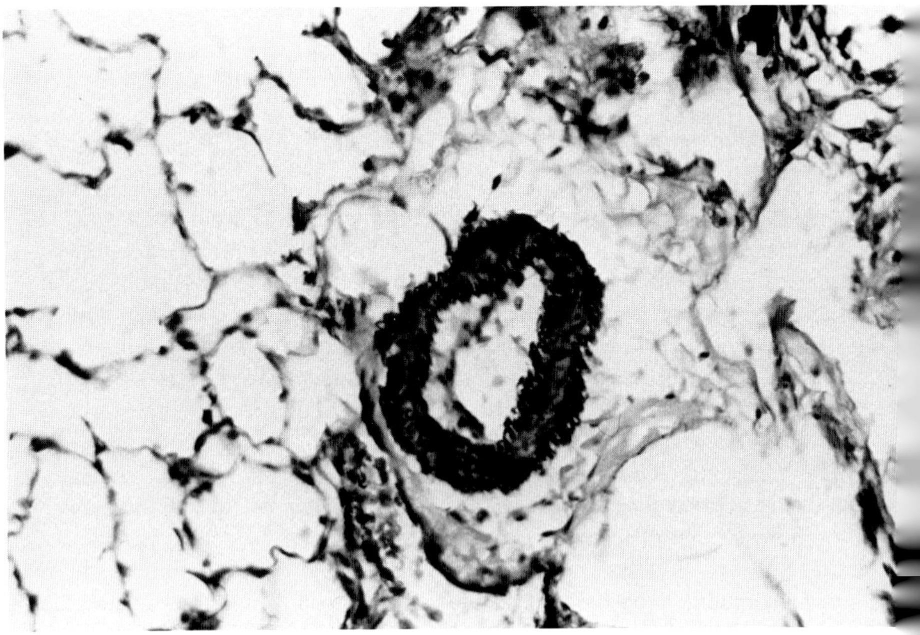

Figure 1 Medial hypertrophy of a small pulmonary artery from the left (chronically obstructed) lung of a dog.

collaterals are not established (Shure et al., 1987). This temporal relationship suggests a possible role for growth factors affecting both bronchial collateral development and the established pulmonary arterial bed. This possibility remains to be investigated.

One animal study provides evidence contrary to a role of the bronchial circulation in pulmonary vascular remodeling (Rabinovitch et al., 1983). Rabinovitch et al. studied rats with pulmonary arteries banded to reduce pulmonary arterial flow to one lung to 20% of normal. Reduced flow (as opposed to complete obstruction) was not a stimulus to bronchial collateral flow. Despite the absence of an increase in collateral flow, remodeling was noted in the banded lungs. The changes consisted of the extension of muscularization into peripheral pulmonary arteries. This study does not disprove a relation between collateral formation and pulmonary vascular remodeling, since the changes with banding may occur by a different mechanism, but it does suggest that the relationship found in dogs and people could be coincidental. Further studies of this area are needed.

V. Role of the Bronchial Circulation in Reperfusion Edema

An interesting form of pulmonary edema has been described in patients who have undergone pulmonary thromboendarterectomy for the relief of chronic pulmonary emboli (Levinson et al., 1986). In these patients, edema develops in regions of the lung that have been chronically obstructed by organized thromboemboli. The edema develops within 24–72 h after surgery only in the regions from which chronic emboli have been removed (Fig. 2). Because of the obvious increase in bronchial collateral flow to these regions, it is tempting to assume a role for the bronchial circulation in the genesis of this edema, perhaps by disruption of bronchopulmonary anastomotic connections during the surgery with subsequent pulmonary vascular leakage.

There are, however, many other candidates as etiological factors in reperfusion edema. Surgical endarterectomy disrupts the intimal surface of the involved pulmonary artery, which could result in the release of a variety of vasoactive factors, both vascoconstrictive and vasodilatory. The roughened endothelial surface remaining after surgery may well be a focus for platelet aggregation despite the postoperative use of heparin. These platelets may in turn be a source of vasoactive factors.

In addition, some preliminary data suggest that the pulmonary arterial bed may be injured early after obstruction, long before the formation of bronchial collateral vessels. Evan's blue dye staining of pulmonary arterial intima distal to a central ligation revealed injury as early as 48 h after ligation in dogs

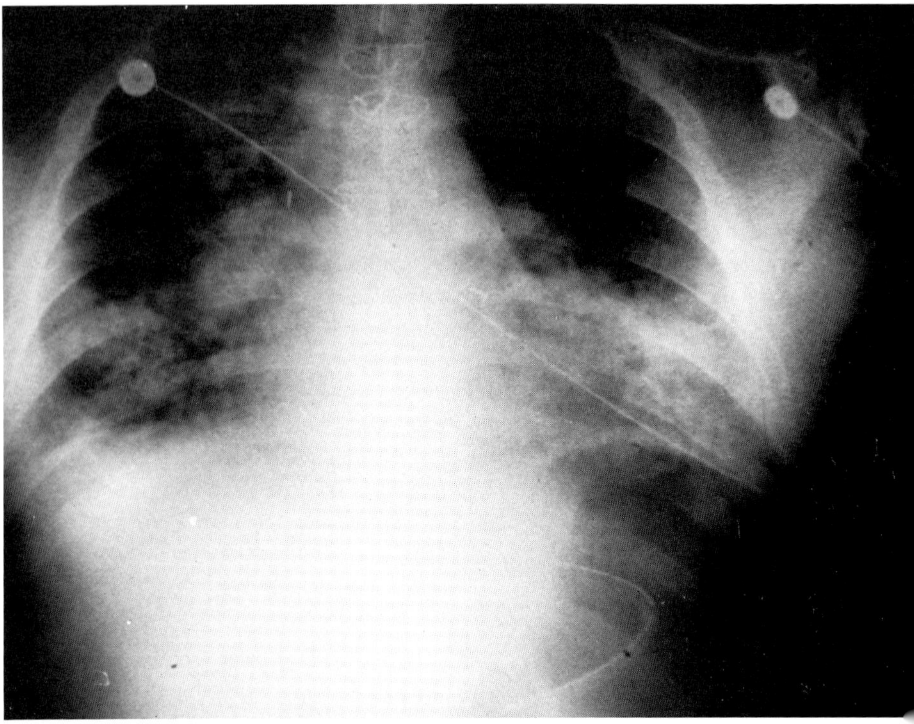

Figure 2 Reperfusion edema. Patches of pulmonary edema in areas from which chronic organized thrombi were surgically removed.

(Shure and Jacobs, 1989); collateral formation does not occur for 3 weeks after ligation (Shure et al., 1986, 1987). In a study of edema formation with reperfusion in rabbits, edema was found after 24 h of pulmonary arterial obstruction—again, long before formation of collateral vessels (Bishop et al., 1989). Thus, early reperfusion edema may result from injury to the pulmonary arterial bed unrelated to the bronchial collateral circulation, although it is possible that the collateral circulation plays a facilitatory role in some late settings, perhaps by being a source of inflammatory mediators during the period of pulmonary vascular obstruction.

VI. What Is the Stimulus to Bronchial Collateral Formation After Pulmonary Artery Obstruction?

A common assumption is that the bronchial circulation increases in response to a drop in pressure in the pulmonary arterial bed. Evidence exists to demonstrate an inverse relation between pulmonary arterial pressure and bronchial flow in a some settings (State et al., 1957; Jindal et al., 1984, 1985), but the bulk of the evidence suggests that the acute response to complete pulmonary arterial obstruction (with a drop in distal pressure to close to zero) is a drop in bronchial flow (Malik and Tracy, 1980; Williams and Towbin, 1955; Agostoni et al., 1987; Kowalski et al., 1989). Flow increases only slowly over days to months. The initial increase in flow is apparently due to dilatation of existing vessels followed by formation of new vessels (Weibel, 1960). With time, the pressure in the obstructed pulmonary artery increases (Williams, and Towbin, 1955; Shure et al., 1985; Cudkowicz, 1958). Despite this increase in pulmonary artery pressure, bronchial collateral formation continues over a period of months (Shure et al., 1985), possibly years (Liebow et al., 1950a; Williams and Towbin, 1955), in the face of prolonged pulmonary artery obstruction.

The stimulus to bronchial collateral formation is currently unknown and presents one of the challenges in the study of the bronchial circulation. The release of growth factors is a possibility to be considered and needs to be investigated in an appropriate model. The stimulus to the release of growth factors is an additional question to be addressed. There is evidence of early metabolic dysfunction of the obstructed lung in the form of a surfactant deficit, although this defect is transient (Baritussio and Clements, 1981). To account for prolonged bronchial collateral formation over months, one needs to find a continuing stimulus. Early data from Evan's blue dye studies of chronically ligated canine pulmonary arteries suggest that intimal injury is present for at least 8 weeks after ligation (Shure and Jacobs, 1989). This finding may make endothelial injury a candidate for the continuing stimulus that may evoke the formation of bronchial collateral vessels, perhaps in a response similar to that of acute inflammation. This area is an interesting source of future studies.

VII. Summary

Acute obstruction of the pulmonary artery appears to result in a decrease (but not a cessation) in bronchial arterial flow. This decrease lasts for minutes to hours and is followed by a gradual increase in bronchial flow, at first by dilation and increased flow through existing vessels. This decrease in flow with acute obstruction calls into question the assumption that infarction is rare after pulmonary embolization because bronchial flow increases immediately as a result of the drop in pulmonary artery pressure.

With chronic obstruction (weeks to months), bronchial flow increases by the formation of new collateral vessels with extensive precapillary bronchopulmonary anastomoses to the obstructed bed. Chronic obstruction is also associated with remodeling of the obstructed pulmonary bed with changes identical to those of pulmonary hypertension. Although these pulmonary vascular changes are temporally related to the formation of bronchial collateral vessels in an animal model, a causal relationship to the formation of bronchial vessels has not been established. Some data from animal studies suggest that ongoing endothelial cell injury in the obstructed pulmonary bed may be a cause of pulmonary remodeling. It may also be a stimulus to collateral formation, but both these hypotheses require additional study.

Many interesting questions remained unanswered about the role of the bronchial circulation in pulmonary artery obstruction, but even less is known about the role of the bronchial circulation in other diseases involving the pulmonary vasculature such as primary pulmonary hypertension, interstitial pulmonary fibrosis, and pulmonary emphysema. Basic observations remain to be made in these conditions before more involved issues can be addressed.

References

Agostoni, P. G., Deffebach, M. E., Kirk, W., Mendenhall, J. M., Albert, R. K., and Butler, J. (1987). Temperature alters the bronchial blood flow response to pulmonary artery obstruction. *J. Appl. Physiol.* **62**:1907–1911.

Alley, R. D., van Mierhop, L. H. S., Peck, A. S., Kausel, H. W., and Stranahan, A. (1961). Bronchial arterial collateral circulation. *Am. Rev. Respir. Dis.* **83**:31–37.

Baile, E. M., Ling, H., Heyworth, J. R., Hogg, J. C., and Pare, P. D. (1985). Bronchopulmonary anastomotic and noncoronary collateral blood flow in humans during cardiopulmonary bypass. *Chest* **87**:749–754.

Baritussio, A., and Clements, J. A. (1981). Acute effects of pulmonary artery occlusion on the pool of alveolar surfactant. *Respir. Physiol.* **45**:323–331.

Berry, D. F., Bacigrossi, D., Peabody, J., Peterson, K. L., and Moser, K. M. (1986). Pulmonary vascular occlusion and fibrosing mediastinitis. *Chest* **89**:296–300.

Bishop, M. J., Albert, R. K., Lamm, W., and Guidotti, S. M. (1989). Pulmonary ischemia increases vascular permeability even without reperfusion. *Am. Rev. Respir. Dis.* **139**:A414.

Bloomer, W. E., Harrison, W., Lindskog, G. E., and Liebow, A. A. (1949). Respiratory function and blood flow in the bronchial artery after ligation of the pulmonary artery. *Am. J. Physiol.* **157**:317–328.

Carlens, E., Hanson, H. E., and Nordenstrom, B. (1951). Temporary unilateral occlusion of the pulmonary artery. *J. Thorac. Surg.* **22**:527–536.

Carroll, D. (1950). Chronic obstruction of major pulmonary arteries. *Am. J. Med.* **9**:175–185.

Castleman, B., and Bland, E. F. (1946). Organized emboli of the tertiary pulmonary arteries. An unusual cause of cor pulmonale. *Arch. Pathol.* **42**:581–589.

Charan, N. B., Turk, G. M., and Ripley, R. (1985). Measurement of bronchial arterial blood flow and bronchovascular resistance in sheep. *J. Appl. Physiol.* **59**:305–308.

Chernick, V., Hodson, W. A., and Greenfield, L. J. (1966). Effect of chronic pulmonary artery ligation on pulmonary mechanics and surfactant. *J. Appl. Physiol.* **21**:1315–1320.

Cudkowicz, L. (1952). Some observations of the bronchial arteries in lobar pneumonia and pulmonary infarction. *Br. J. Tuberc.* **46**:99–102.

Cudkowicz, L. (1958). Pressure and oxygen content measurements distal to temporary and permanent unilateral occlusion of a pulmonary artery in dogs. *Circ. Res.* **6**:728–734.

Cudkowicz, L. (1967). Cardio-respiratory studies in patients with lung tumors. *Dis. Chest* **51**:427–432.

Cudkowicz, L. and Armstrong, J. B. (1953). The blood supply of malignant pulmonary neoplasms. *Thorax* **8**:152–156.

Cudkowicz, L., Calabresi, M., Nims, R. G., and Gray, F. D., Jr. (1959). The simultaneous estimation of right and left ventricular outputs applied to a study of the bronchial circulation in dogs. *Am. Heart J.* **58**:732–742.

Cudkowicz, L., Abelmann, W. H., Levinson, G. E., Katznelson, G., and Jreissaty, R. M. (1960). Bronchial arterial blood flow. *Clin. Sci.* **19**:1–15.

Daily, P. O., Dembitsky, W. P., Peterson, K. L., and Moser, K. M. (1987). Modifications of techniques and early results of pulmonary thromboendarterectomy for chronic pulmonary embolism. *J. Thorac. Cardiovasc. Surg.* **93**:221–233.

Deffebach, M. E., Charan, N. B., Lakshminarayan, S., and Butler, J. (1987). The bronchial circulation. Small, but a vital attribute of the lung. *Am. Rev. Respir. Dis.* **135**:463–481.

Downing, S. E., Vidone, R. A., Brandt, H. M., and Liebow, A. A. (1963). The pathogenesis of vascular lesions in experimental hyperkinetic pulmonary hypertension. *Am. J. Pathol.* **43**:739–765.

Ellis, J. H., Jr., Grindlay, J. H., and Edwards, J. E. (1952). The bronchial arteries. III. Structural changes after division of the rat's left pulmonary artery. *Am. J. Pathol.* **28**:89–103.

Fisher, A. B., Kollmeier, H., Brody, J. S., Hyde, R. W., Hansell, J., Friedman, J. N., and Waldhausen, J. A. (1970). Restoration of systemic blood flow to the lung after division of bronchial arteries. *J. Appl. Physiol.* **29**:839–846.

Fishman, A. P. (1961). The clinical significance of the pulmonary collateral circulation. *Circulation* **24**:677–690.

Goetz, R. H., Rohman, M., and State, D. (1965). The hemodynamics of bronchopulmonary anastomoses. *Surg. Gynecol. Obstet.* **120**:517–529.

Harker, L. C., Kirkpatrick, S. E., Friedman, W. F., and Bloor, C. M. (1981). Effects of indomethacin on fetal rat lungs: A possible cause of persistent fetal circulation (PFC). *Pediatr. Res.* **15**:147–151.

Haworth, S. G., de Leval, M., and Macartney, F. J. (1981). How the left lung is perfused after ligating the left pulmonary artery in the pig at birth: Clinical implications for the hypoperfused lung. *Cardiovas. Res.* **15**:214–226.

Heath, D., and Thompson, I. M. (1969). Bronchopulmonary anastomoses in sickle-cell anaemia. *Thorax* **24**:232–238.

Huber, G. L., and Edmunds, L. H., Jr. (1967). Pulmonary artery occlusion. II. Morphologic studies. *J. Appl. Physiol.* **22**:1002–1011.

Isawa, T., Taplin, G. V., Beazell, J., and Criley, J. M. (1972). Experimental unilateral pulmonary artery occlusion. *Radiology* **102**:101–109.

Jindal, S. K., Lakshminarayan, S., Kirk, W., and Butler, J. (1984). Acute increase in anastomotic bronchial blood flow after pulmonary artery obstruction. *J. Appl. Physiol.* **57**:424–428.

Jindal, S. K., Lakshminarayan, S., Kirk, W., and Butler, J. (1985). Regulation of increase in anastomotic blood flow following pulmonary arterial occlusion. *J. Appl. Physiol.* **59**:180–182.

Julian, D. G., Travis, D. M., Robin, E. D., and Crump, C. H. (1960). Effect of pulmonary artery occlusion upon end-tidal CO_2 tension. *J. Appl. Physiol.* **15**:87–91.

Kowalski, T. F., Guidotti, S. M., Deffebach, M. E., and Bishop, M. J. (1989). The bronchial circulation in pulmonary artery occlusion and reperfusion. *Am. Rev. Respir. Dis.* **139**:A414.

Levinson, R. M., Shure, D., and Moser, K. M. (1986). Reperfusion pulmonary edema after pulmonary artery thromboendarterectomy. *Am. Rev. Respir. Dis.* **134**:1241–1245.

Liebow, A. A., Hales, M. R., and Lindskog, G. E. (1949). Enlargement of the bronchial arteries and their anastomoses with the pulmonary arteries in bronchiectasis. *Am. J. Pathol.* **25**:211–231.

Liebow, A. A., Hales, M. R., Bloomer, W. E., Harrison, W., and Lindskog, G. E. (1950a). Studies on the lung after ligation of the pulmonary artery. II. Anatomical changes. *Am. J. Pathol.* **26**:177–195.

Liebow, A. A., Hales, M. R., Harrison, W., Bloomer, W. E., and Lindskog, G. E. (1950b). The genesis and functional implications of collateral circulation of the lungs. *Yale J. Biol. Med.* **22**:19–49.

Malik, A. B., and Tracy, S. E. (1980). Bronchovascular adjustments after pulmonary embolism. *J. Appl. Physiol.* **49**:476–481.

Malmstrom, G., Michas, P., and Nordenstrom, B. (1954). A comparison between the oxygen and carbon dioxide tensions in blood from occluded branches of the pulmonary artery and vein. *Acta Med. Scand.* **154**:431–436.

Marchand, P., Gilroy, J. C., and Wilson, E. H. (1950). An antomical study of the bronchial vascular system and its variations in disease. *Thorax* **5**:207–221.

Mathes, M. E., Holman, E., and Reichert, F. L. (1932). A study of the bronchial, pulmonary, and lympathic circulations of the lung under various pathologic conditions experimentally produced. *J. Thorac. Surg.* **1**:339–362.

Moser, K. M., Rhodes, P. G., and Hufnagel, C. A. (1965). Chronic unilateral pulmonary artery thrombosis: Successful thromboendarterectomy with thirty-month follow-up. *N. Engl. J. Med.* **272**:1195–1199.

Moser, K. M., Spragg, R. G., Utley, J., and Daily, P. O. (1983). Chronic thrombotic obstruction of major pulmonary arteries: Results of thromboendarterectomy in 15 patients. *Ann. Intern. Med.* **99**:299–304.

Naimark, A. (1966). Pulmonary blood flow and the incorporation of palmitate-I-C^{14} by dog lung in vivo. *J. Appl. Physiol.* **21**:1292–1298.

Nordenstrom, B., Norden, I., and Norhagen, A. (1966). Oxygen tension distally to a temporary occlusion of the pulmonary artery during oxygen breathing. *Acta Radiol.* **4**:385–393.

Orell, S. R., and Hultgren, S. (1966). Anastomoses between bronchial and pulmonary arteries in pulmonary thromboembolic disease. *Acta Pathol. Microbiol. Scand.* **67**:322–338.

Rabinovitch, M., Konstam, M. A., Gamble, W. J., Papanicolaou, N., Aronovitz, M. J., Treves, S., and Reid, L. (1983). Changes in pulmonary blood flow affect vascular response to chronic hypoxia in rats. *Circ. Res.* **52**:432–441.

Roosenburg, J. G., and Deenstra, H. (1954). Bronchial-pulmonary vascular shunts in chronic pulmonary affections. *Dis. Chest* **26**:664–671.

Ryan, T. J., and Abelmann, W. H. (1961). Response of bronchial blood flow to tissue proliferation in the human lung (abstract). *J. Clin. Invest.* **40**:1077.

Said, S. I., Harlan, W. R., Jr., Burke, G. W., and Elliott, C. M. (1968). Surface tension, metabolic activity, and lipid composition of alveolar cells in washings from normal dog lungs and after pulmonary artery ligation. *J. Clin. Invest.* **47**:336–343.

Severinghaus, J. W., Swenson, E. W., Finley, T. N., Lategola, M. T., and Williams, J. (1961). Unilateral hypoventilation produced in dogs by occluding one pulmonary artery. *J. Appl. Physiol.* **16**:53–60.

Shepard, J. W., Jr., Hauer, D., Miyai, K., and Moser, K. M. (1980). Lamellar body depletion in dogs undergoing pulmonary artery occlusion. *J. Clin. Invest.* **66**:36–42.

Shepard, J. W., Jr., Witzum, K. F., Fletcher, J. W., and Dolan, G. F. (1981). Pulmonary venous pathway for substrate delivery to the lung in the absence of arterial blood flow (abstract). *Am. rev. Respir. Dis.* **123**:246A.

Shure, D., and Jacobs, K. (1989). Endothelial injury consequent to prolonged pulmonary artery obstruction. *Am. Rev. Respir. Dis.* **139**:A174.

Shure, D., Swain, J. A., Abraham, J. L., and Moser, K. M. (1984). Pulmonary arterial hypertensive changes distal to a central vascular obstruction in the dog (abstract). *Am. Rev. Respir. Dis.* **129**:331.

Shure, D., Dockweiler, D. W., and Peters, R. M. (1985). Post-obstructive pulmonary arteriopathy occurs without elevation of distal (obstructed) pulmonary artery pressure (abstract). *Am. Rev. Respir. Dis.* **131**:402.

Shure, D., Lammers, R. J., Dockweiler, D. W., and Bloor, C. M. (1986). The role of the bronchial circulation in post-obstructive pulmonary arteriopathy (abstract). *Clin. Res.* **34**:80A.

Shure, D., Dockweiler, D. W., and Bloor, C. M. (1987). Post-obstructive pulmonary arteriopathy does not precede significant bronchial collateral formation in an animal model (abstract). *Am. Rev. Respir. Dis.* **135**:A514.

Spragg, R. G., Moser, K. M., Utley, J., Long, W., and Abraham, J. (1982). Reperfusion of the pulmonary vasculature following removal of chronic thrombotic obstruction. *Am. Rev. Respir. Dis.* **125**:122A.

State, D., Salisbury, P. F., and Weil, P. (1957). Physiologic and pharmacologic studies of collateral pulmonary flow. *J. Thorac. Surg.* **34**:599–608.

Stunick, A. I., and Soloff, L. A. (1967). Pulmonary arterial occlusion and surfactant production in humans. *Ann. Intern. Med.* **67**:549–555.

Tabakin, B. S., Hanson, J. S., Adhikari, P. K., and Miller, D. B. (1960). Physiologic studies in congenital absence of the left main pulmonary artery. *Circulation* **22**:1107–1111.

Viola, A. R., and Abbate, E. H. (1973). Respiratory function and effective collateral flow 8 years after ligation of the left pulmonary artery. *Am. Rev. Respir. Dis.* **108**:1216–1220.

Virchow, R. (1847). Uber die standpunkte in den wissenschaftlichen medizin. *Virchows Arch.* **1**:1.

Wagenvoort, C. A. (1984). In *Pulmonary Hypertension.* Edited by E. K. Weir and J. T. Reeves. Mount Kisco, NY, Futura, pp. 393–437.

Wagenvoort, C. A., and Wagenvoórt, N. (1965). Pulmonary arteries in bronchial carcinoma. *Arch. Pathol.* **79**:529–533.

Weibel, E. R. (1960). Early stages in the development of collateral circulation to the lung in the rat. *Circ. Res.* **8**:353–376.

Williams, M. H., and Towbin, E. J. (1955). Magnitude and time of development of the collateral circulation to the lung after occlusion of the left pulmonary artery. *Circ. Res.* **3**:422–424.

Wood, D. A., and Miller, M. (1938). The role of the dual pulmonary circulation in various pathologic conditions of the lung. *J. Thorac. Surg.* **7**:649–670.

21

The Bronchial Arteries and Anomalous Systemic Arteries to the Lungs in Congenital Heart and Lung Disease

KENT ELLIS

Columbia Presbyterian Medical Center
New York, New York

I. Introduction

The bronchial arteries are the normal systemic arterial supply to the lungs (Huntington, 1919; Cauldwell et al., 1951; Liebow, 1965; Cudkowicz, 1979; Deffebach et al., 1988), but in congenital heart and lung disease, the anatomical bronchial arteries may not be the only systemic arterial supply. Other pathways, such as a patent ductus arteriosus, major aortopulmonary collateral arteries, right or left pulmonary arteries taking origin from the aorta, and other systemic connections, may occur. In this chapter the various forms of systemic artery supply to the lungs are reviewed, and the most important congenital cardiovascular and pulmonary conditions associated with anomalous or abnormal arterial supply to the lungs are discussed.

Systemic arterial supply to lungs can be classified as follows (exclusive of truncus arteriosus and aorticopulmonary septal defect):

1. Bronchial arteries and associated regional arteries
2. Patent ductus arteriosus (PDA; abnormal after neonatal period)
3. Major aortopulmonary collateral arteries (MAPCA)

4. Right or left pulmonary arteries arising from the ascending aorta
5. Other systemic connections

II. The Bronchial Arteries

The bronchial arteries are the only normal systemic arterial supply to the lungs after the neonatal period (Cauldwell et al., 1951; Liebow, 1965; Cudkowicz, 1979; Deffebach et al., 1987). As is well known, these vessels may greatly enlarge and proliferate after birth, especially in cyanotic congenital heart disease and some types of chronic pulmonary inflammatory disease. Even in these conditions, however, the bronchial arteries are apparently normal at birth.

Formerly, the bronchial arteries were considered to derive from the common "splanchnic plexus" or "postbranchial plexus" that surrounded the developing lung buds, trachea, and esophagus and was supplied by a series of arteries arising from the ventral aspects of the paired dorsal aortae (Huntington, 1919; Liebow, 1965; Cudkowitz, 1979; Deffebach et al., 1987; Congdon, 1922). Boyden's more recent work (Boyden, 1970a,b), however, showed that the development of the bronchial arteries occurs later. Instead of developing in the fourth to sixth weeks of fetal life from the aortic branches of the primitive pulmonary plexus, they arise de novo from the aorta at about the ninth to twelfth weeks.

When the bronchial circulation is stimulated to enlarge and provide collateral flow to the pulmonary arteries, any actual or potential connections with other systemic arteries may contribute to the bronchial blood flow: esophageal, intercostal, phrenic, internal mammary, coronary, and so on. Transpleural adhesions can also provide a rich source of collateral arterial connections, not only directly to the small peripheral pulmonary arteries and capillaries but also apparently to the peripheral bronchial arteries.

Pertinent to these considerations is the site (or sites) of anastomosis between the bronchial and pulmonary circulations. According to many authorities, direct connections between the bronchial and pulmonary circulations do not normally occur proximal to the capillary level (Cauldwell et al., 1951; Liebow, 1965; Cudkowitz, 1979; Berry, 1935). Some studies in the human using injection techniques have shown numerous direct anastomosis of up to 0.5 mm diameter between bronchial and pulmonary arteries (Tobin, 1952; Pump, 1963). The issue is not fully settled.

In chronic inflammation, such as bronchiectasis, interarterial connections become numerous and occur as far proximal as the fourth-order of bronchial branching in arteries that may have developed in granulation tissue replacing damaged bronchial wall (Liebow et al., 1949). Classic experimental studies following pulmonary artery ligation in the dog (Liebow et al., 1950) and in the rat (Weibel, 1960) showed a prompt increase in bronchial artery size and numbers as well as the development of multiple connections to the pulmonary arteries of up to 50 μm diameter. Weibel (1960) also showed the development of transpleural collateral in postoperative adhesions between the intercostal arteries and the small pulmonary and bronchial arteries as well as with adjacent alveolar capillaries.

III. Patent Ductus Arteriosus (PDA)

Persistence of a patent ductus after the neonatal period is a well-known congenital abnormality, usually with left-to-right shunting and, sometimes, with pulmonary hypertension. Persistent patent ductus also commonly complicates other forms of congenital cardiovascular disease (Cassels et al., 1975; Lenox et al., 1977). In the presence of lesions causing obstruction to pulmonary blood flow, a patent ductus may serve a useful function in augmentation of the pulmonary blood flow.

A right patent ductus normally regresses and disappears in early fetal life, but it may persist in congenital heart or lung disease (Edwards and McGoon, 1973; Ellis et al., 1967). When a right PDA persists in the presence of a normal left aortic arch, it arises from structures originally part of the primitive right arch: ventrally, from the proximal right subclavian or innominate artery (Fig. 1A), or dorsally, from an aberrant right subclavian artery or an aortic diverticulum. When a right arch is present the left PDA arises in mirror image fashion from the left subclavian or innominate artery or from the proximal portion of a left aberrant subclavian artery. For example, when a PDA is present in tetralogy of Fallot with right aortic arch, it usually arises from the proximal left subclavian or left innominate artery (Fig. 1B and C).

IV. Major Aortopulmonary Collateral Arteries (MAPCA)

These relatively large arteries coursing from the aorta and its branches to the lung are generally thought to represent persistence of primitive "splanchnic plexus" or "postbranchial plexus" arteries that supply the early lung bud and normally regress by the seventh fetal week after the definitive pulmonary arteries have developed (Fig. 2) (Huntington, 1919; Cudkowitz, 1979; Rabinovitch et al., 1981). These arteries are particularly characteristic of pulmonary atresia with ventricular septal defect (Fig. 3) but may occasionally occur in

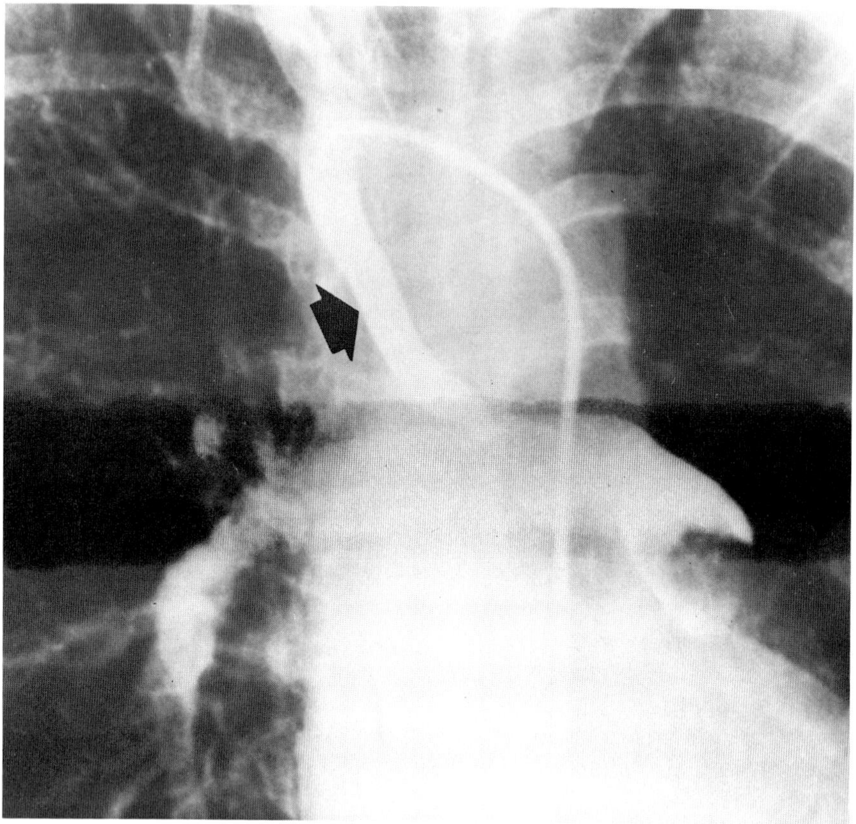

(A)

Figure 1 Patent ductus arteriosus (PDA) supplying lung on side opposite aortic arch. (A) Selective injection of rare right PDA (black arrow) arising from bifurcation of right innominate artery in patient with tetralogy of Fallot and left aortic arch. The proximal left pulmonary artery is absent. The distal left pulmonary artery was probably supplied by a left PDA during fetal life that closed after birth. (B) Severe tetralogy of Fallot at 3 months with right aortic arch. Angiocardiogram showing left PDA (white arrow) from left innominate artery to left pulmonary artery, almost closed on pulmonary end. (From Ellis, 1991, with permission.) (C) Same child 7 years later with left Blalock anastomosis (left subclavian artery to left pulmonary artery, end to side; white arrow) paralleling the smaller, still patent left PDA (small black arrow).

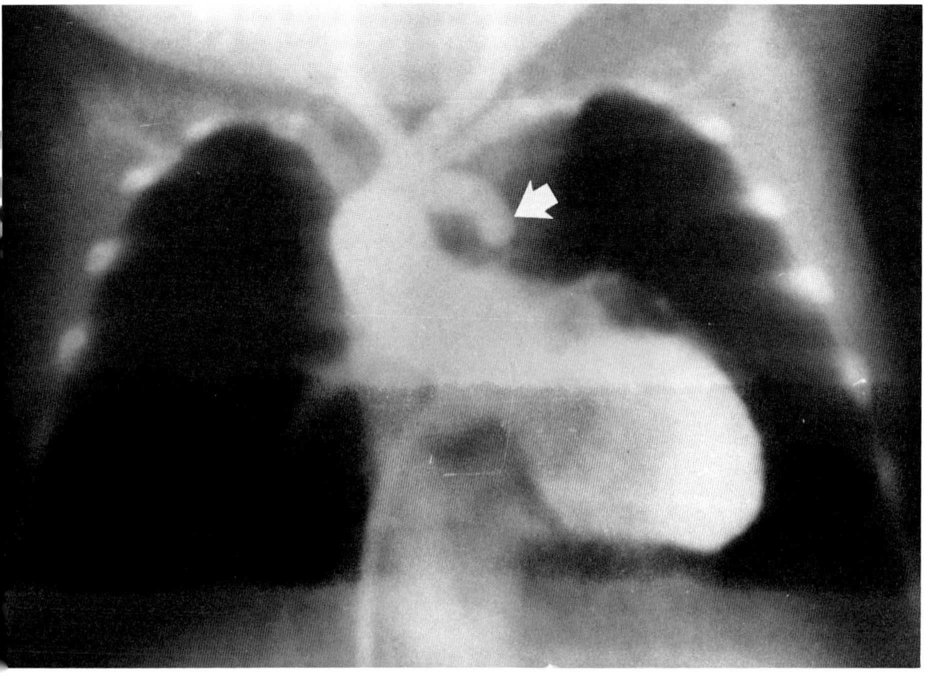

(B)

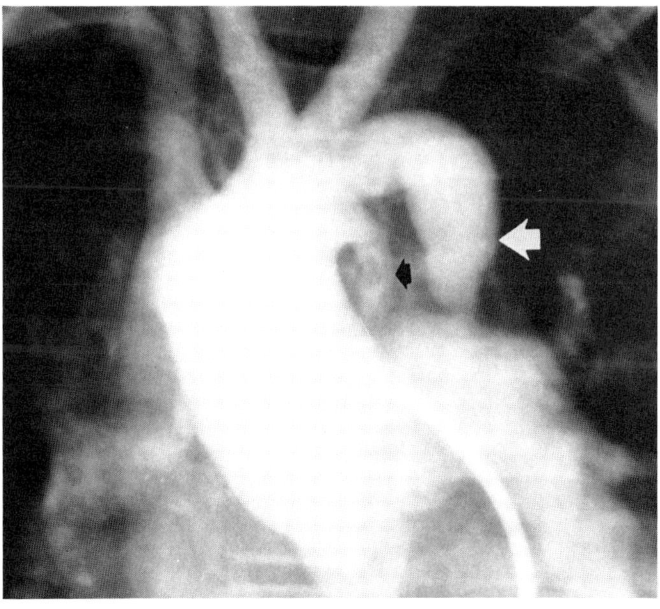

(C)

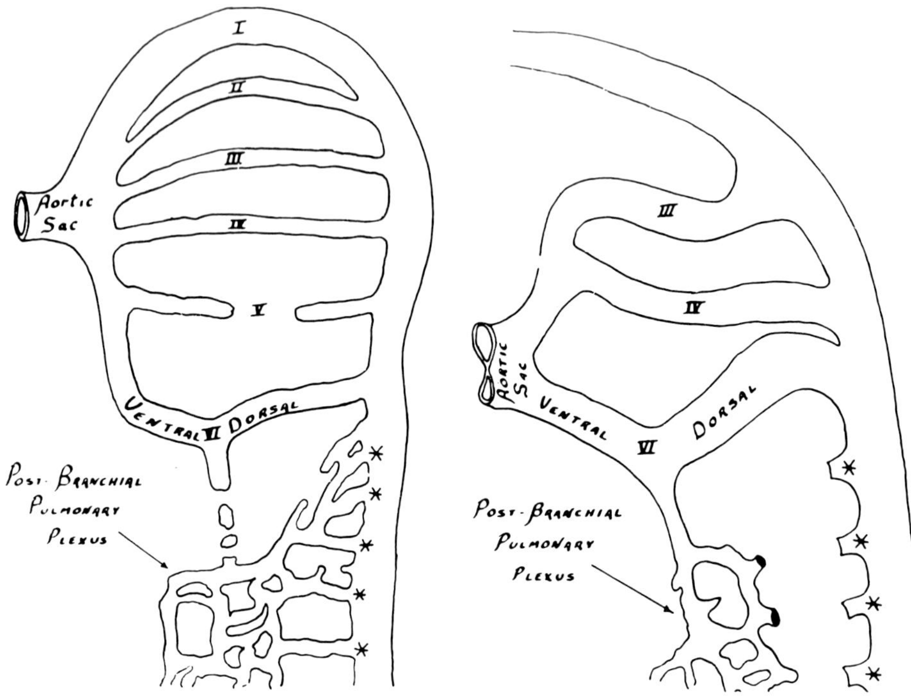

Figure 2 Genesis of major aorticopulmonary collateral arteries (MAPCA). One side of paired arch system. (From Pool et al., 1962, with permission.) (Left) After Huntington (1919), showing the pulmonary post-branchial plexus associated with lung bud being supplied by descending aortic branches (*). (Right) After Congdon (1922), showing postbranchial pulmonary plexus now connected to central pulmonary artery at junction with sixth dorsal arch (PDA). The earlier direct branches from the descending aorta normally atrophy and disappear. Persistence of some of these primitive arteries is thought to be the source of major aortopulmonary collateral arteries.

other congenital heart disease, especially tetralogy of Fallot. They probably also account for the anomalous systemic arteries found in various congenital abnormalities of the lungs, such as pulmonary sequestration and hypogenetic lung syndrome (scimitar syndrome).

V. Anomalous Right or Left Pulmonary Artery Origin from the Aorta

The origin of these arteries from the aorta or its branches instead of from the main pulmonary artery can usually be regarded as the consequence of failure of the proper development of the normal proximal connections to the main pulmonary artery.

VI. Other Systemic Connections

An apparently isolated systemic artery may at times supply normal lung. Other systemic arterial supplies to the lung (excluding truncus arteriosus and aorticopulmonary septal defect) include coronary artery to bronchial artery collateral arterial flow, anomalous left coronary artery arising from the pulmonary artery with retrograde flow, and congenital fistula between various regional systemic arteries and the pulmonary arteries (e.g., coronary artery to pulmonary artery fistula).

The bronchial circulation and other forms of systemic arterial supply to the lungs in congenital cardiovascular and congenital lung disease can be conveniently considered as follows.

A. Systemic Blood Supply to the Lung in Congenital Cardiovascular Disease

Pulmonary Atresia with Ventricular Septal Defect

This relatively common form of congenital heart disease (Figs. 3 through 8), often regarded as an extreme tetralogy of Fallot, has the most variable pulmonary blood supply (Allanby et al., 1950; Thiene and Anderson, 1983; Diethelm et al., 1985; Liao et al., 1985) probably implying that the pulmonary atresia was present in early fetal life. At birth either major aortopulmonary collateral arteries (Fig. 3) or a patent ductus arteriosus provide the pulmonary blood flow. A ductus may supply both lungs (Fig. 4) or part or all of one lung. Very rarely both right and left ductus persist and supply separate lung regions. Virtually never, however, do MAPCAs supply a region of lung that is or was at birth supplied by a PDA (Thiene and Anderson, 1983; Bharati et al., 1975; Thiene et al., 1981; Frescura et al., 1984). The observation suggests that MAPCAs persist for regions that otherwise would have no source of pulmonary blood supply in early fetal life (before the eighth fetal week).

Characteristically, the lung supplied in utero by a PDA is normally developed at birth. After birth the PDA tends to narrow or to close, which may leave the bronchial arteries, which are generally small and not developed as collateral arteries at birth, as the only source of pulmonary blood flow. In subsequent months or years, however, the bronchial arteries may greatly enlarge; some believe 5 or 6 years is required for substantial bronchial collateral development (Somerville, 1988).

Major aortopulmonary collateral arteries (Macartney and Haworth, 1983) are the major source of pulmonary blood supply in many cases of pul-

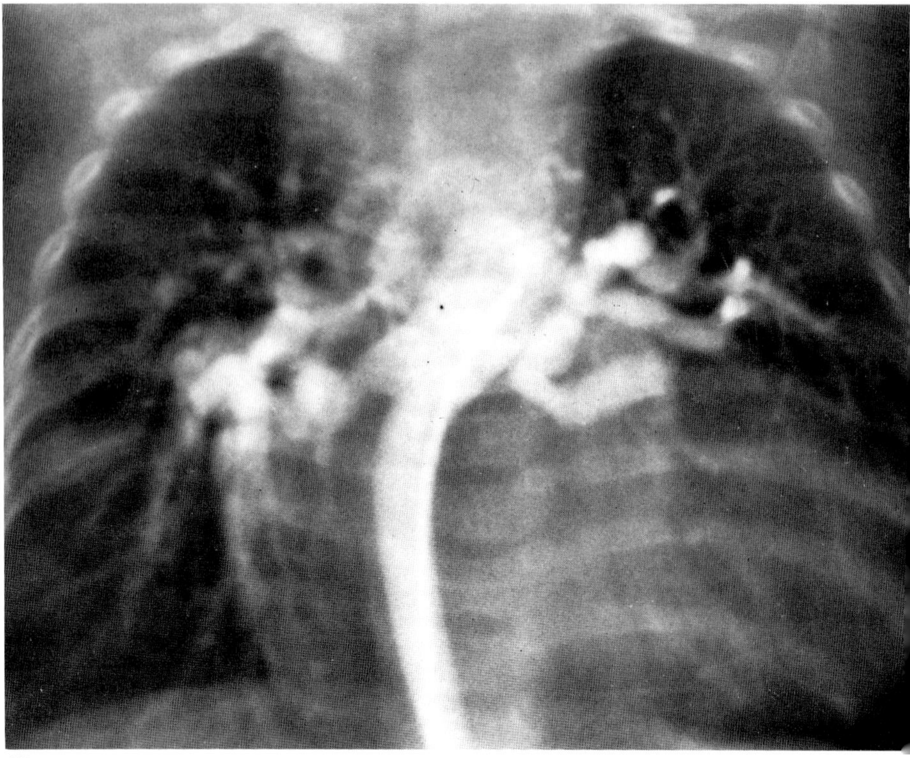

(A)

Figure 3 Major aortopulmonary collateral arteries. (A) Aortogram showing large arteries (MAPCAs) from the descending aorta supplying both lungs in infant with pulmonary atresia and ventricular septal defect (PA and VSD). At necropsy the main and proximal right and left pulmonary arteries were represented by fibrous cords.

monary atresia (PA) with ventral septal defect (VSD). These arteries are present at birth and are regarded by most authorities as persistent primitive arteries of the splanchnic plexus, not as bronchial arteries. Synonyms for MAPCA are systemic collateral arteries, direct aortic collateral arteries (Rabinovitch et al., 1981), large systemic-pulmonary collateral arteries, major collateral arteries (Allanby et al., 1950), persistent intersegmental arteries, primitive arteries of the splanchnic plexus, and others. MAPCA have been described as differing from bronchial arteries in a number of ways:

1. They present as large collateral arteries at birth.
2. Anastomoses with the intrapulmonary arteries are typically at or near the lung hilum instead of in the periphery.

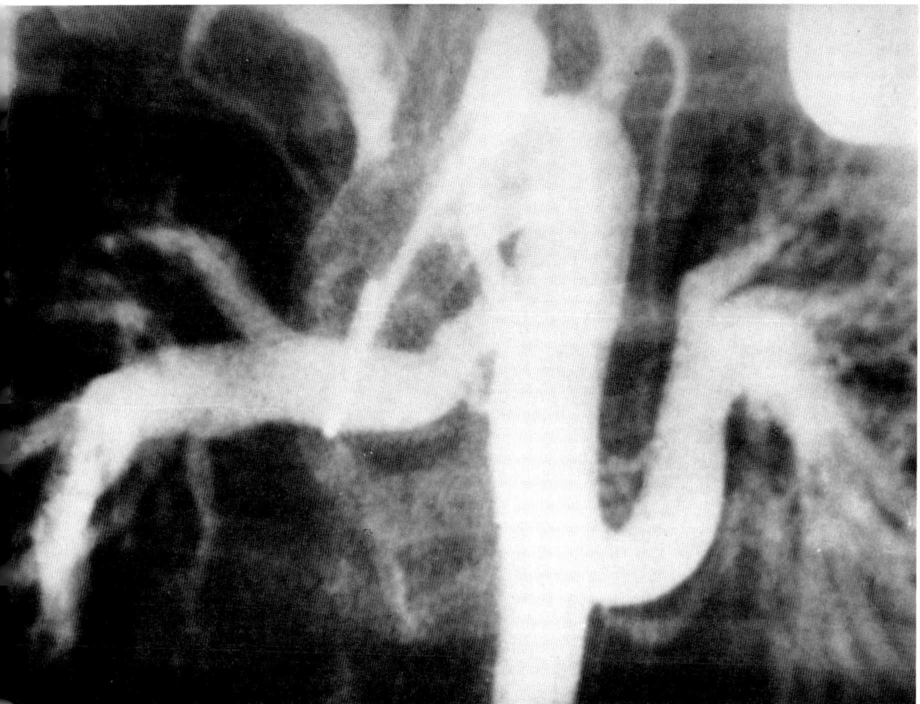

(B)

(B) Aortogram in an 8 year old also with pulmonary atresia and ventricular septal defect. The flow to the left lung is by an unobstructed major aortopulmonary collateral artery arising from the middle of the descending aorta. Another more proximally arising large artery, which is proximally stenotic, supplies the right lung. It is not certain whether this artery is a MAPCA or a PDA. (From Ellis, 1991, with permission.)

3. They may accompany bronchi but do not form nutritive plexus around bronchi (Macartney and Haworth, 1973).
4. Unlike bronchial arteries, MAPCA are virtually never connected with intercostal arteries (Macartney and Haworth, 1973).
5. Intimal stenosis of varying degree is usually present adjacent to anastomosis with an intrapulmonary artery and often also more proximal in the MAPCA.
6. Most MAPCAs have an elastic wall structure resembling the pulmonary artery or aorta rather than bronchial arteries.
7. MAPCAs tend to maintain the same relative caliber throughout life instead of progressively increasing in size as is typical of bronchial arteries.

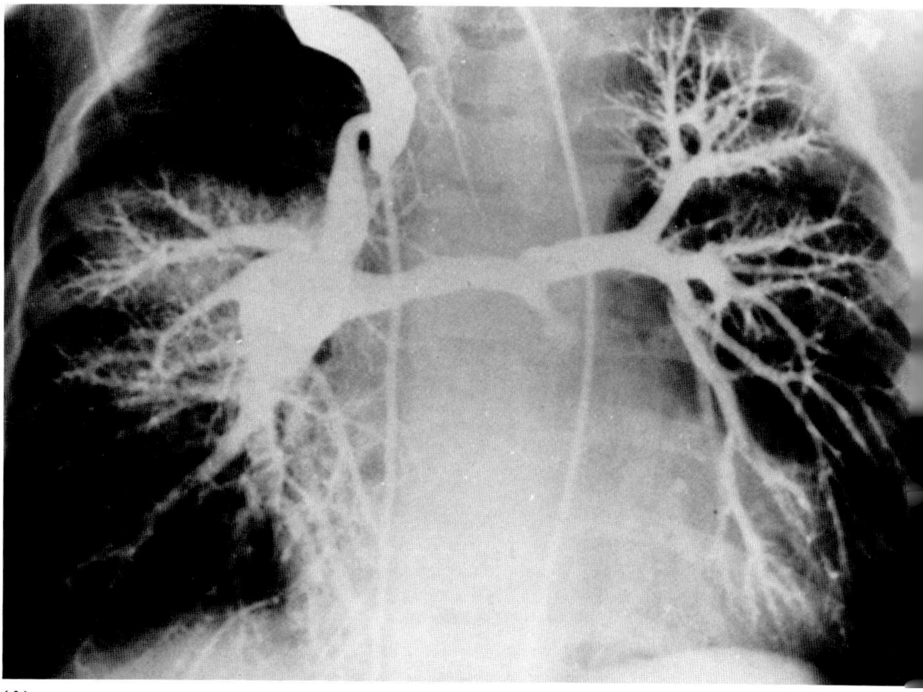

(A)

Figure 4 Pulmonary atresia and ventricular septal defect. (A) MAPCA (possibly interpreted as a patent ductus arteriosus) from right internal mammary artery supplies most of the right lung, the central pulmonary artery confluence, and most of the left lung. Note filling of small proximally occluded main pulmonary artery. (From Ellis,

8. MAPCAs apparently do not usually connect with the "normal" bronchial arteries.

The number of major aortopulmonary collateral arteries usually ranges from one to six, with two to four most representative. They may branch to supply parts of both lungs and most typically anastomose with the parenchymal pulmonary arteries (which are usually intrinsically normal) near the hilum. They may also connect directly with lobar or segmental peripheral pulmonary arteries (Fig. 5). Stenosis (Macartney et al., 1973) at the anastomosis due to intimal fibrous thickening or along the course of the collateral artery is characteristic but not always present. Multiple sources of supply to individual pulmonary arteries imply numerous connections between pulmonary arteries (Faller et al., 1981) and angiography may show dilution of the radiopaque contrast material at arterial junctions or intermittent arterial filling, implying

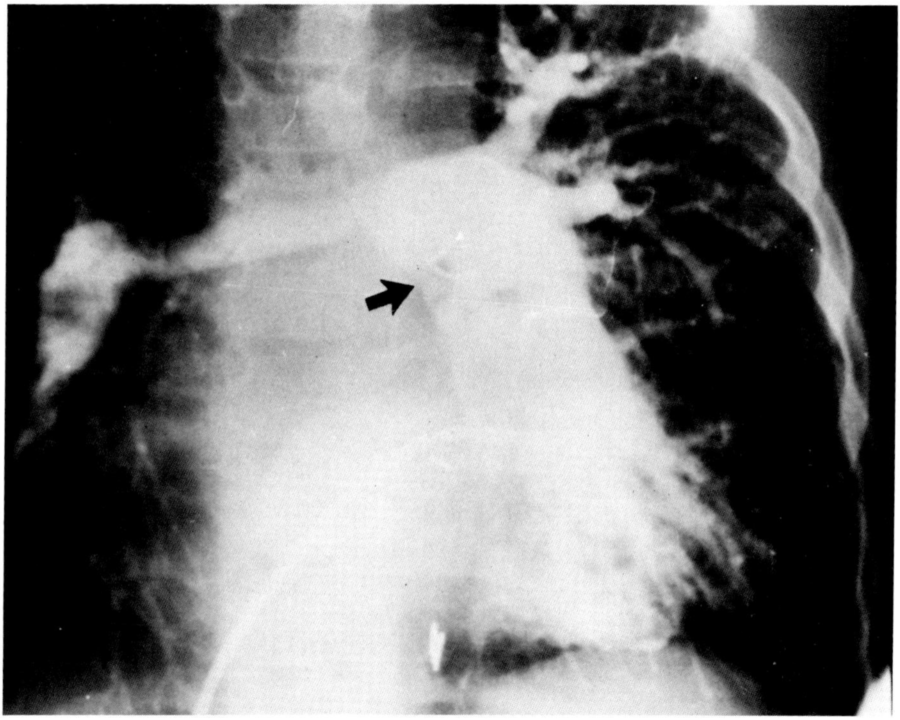

(B)

1991, with permission.) (B) A conduit was surgically placed between the right ventricle and pulmonary artery confluence; the ventricular septal defect and the MAPCA were closed. This right ventriculogram shows filling of the pulmonary arteries via the conduit (black arrow).

interarterial connections. Some MAPCA, however, seem to be the only supply to certain regions of the lung. MAPCAs usually arise from the aorta but may arise from brachiocephalic branches (Brown and Fellows, 1988), especially the subclavian and internal mammary arteries and more rarely from other vessels, such as the coronary arteries, the carotid arteries, or the subdiaphragmatic vessels.

In pulmonary atresia (pulmonary valve atresia) with ventricular septal defect the main pulmonary artery may be present, atretic, or absent. Continuity between the right and left pulmonary arteries is present in 70–90% of cases (Davis et al., 1978), but these central arteries are often small, their size being related to local blood flow. Complete absence or atresia of the central pulmonary arteries occasionally occurs and has been attributed to the absence of the sixth aortic arches (Manhoff and Howe, 1949; Stuckey et al., 1968).

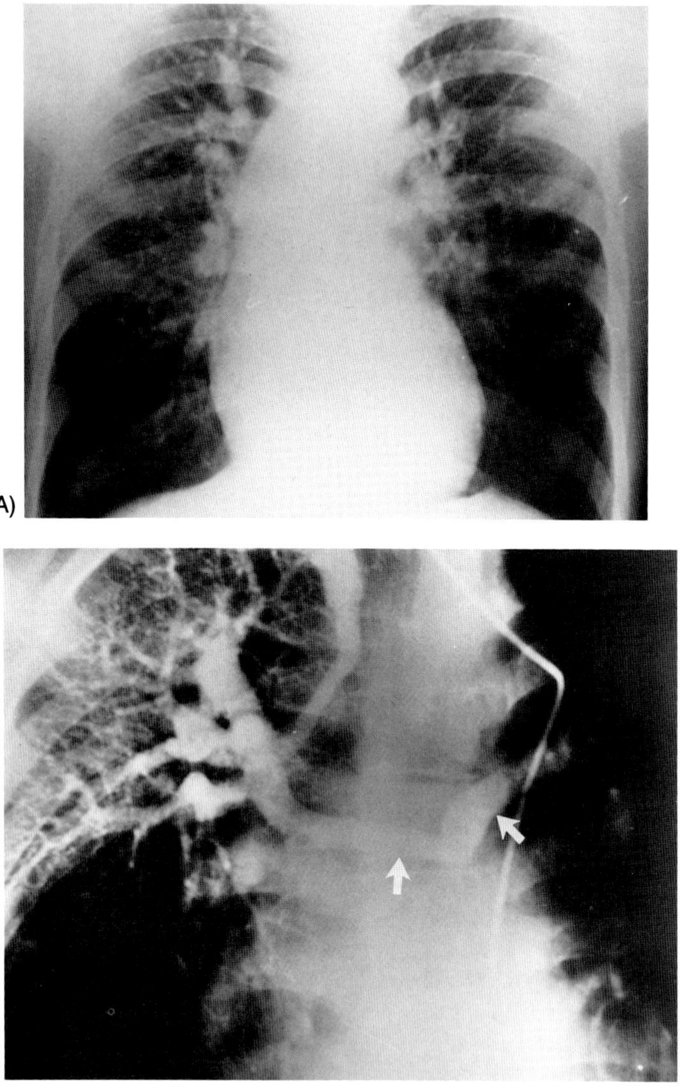

(A)

(B)

Figure 5 Pulmonary atresia with ventricular septal defect and major aortopulmonary collateral arteries. (A) Plain frontal chest roentgenogram showing abnormal appearance of hilar vasculature. (B) Selective arteriogram of large artery arising from right subclavian artery with a left aortic arch. The artery supplies right upper lung vessels and fills by collateral flow the "seagull" confluence of right and left pulmonary arteries

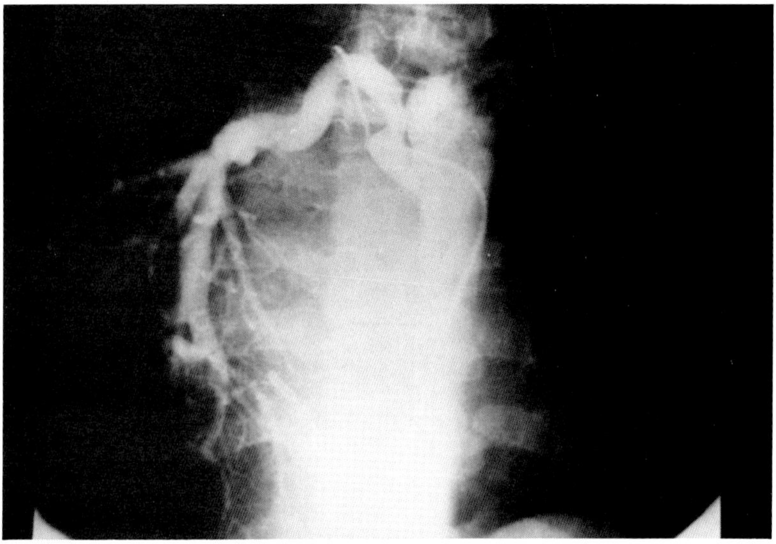

(C)

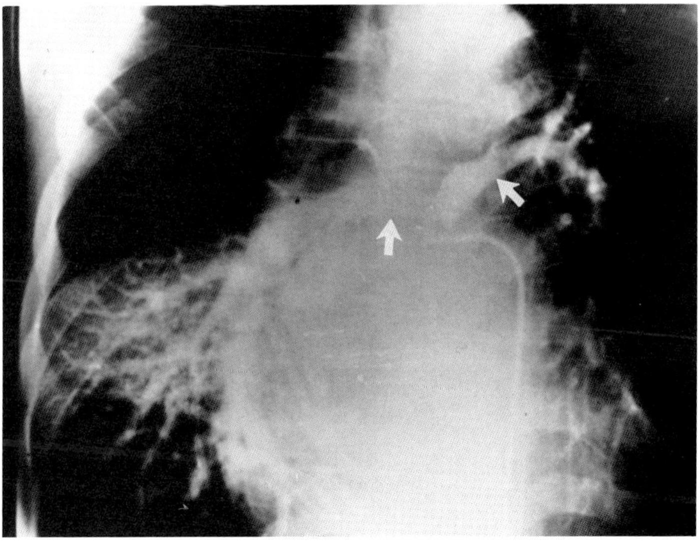

(D)

(arrows). (From Ellis, 1991, with permission.) (C) Selective injection of large descending aortic branch (MAPCA) that has a proximal stenosis but supplies much of the right lower lung. (D) The same seagull confluence (arrows) of the central pulmonary arteries is again opacified 1 s later, implying multiple communications between MAPCA and the native pulmonary arteries.

Angiographic demonstration of central pulmonary artery continuity may require a large bolus of contrast material selectively injected into a particular collateral artery (Figs. 5 and 6A) (Rees et al., 1987). Magnetic resonance imaging can be helpful (Rees et al., 1987; Kersting-Sommerhoff et al., 1988) in demonstrating this central pulmonary artery confluence, which is hypoplastic in about 82% and tends to have a "seagull" configuration (Figs. 5 and 6) (Somerville, 1988). The structure of the more distal intrapulmonary (Jefferson et al., 1972; Johnson et al., 1985) and intracinar arteries depends mainly upon the pressure and amount of blood flow (Haworth et al., 1981; Haworth and

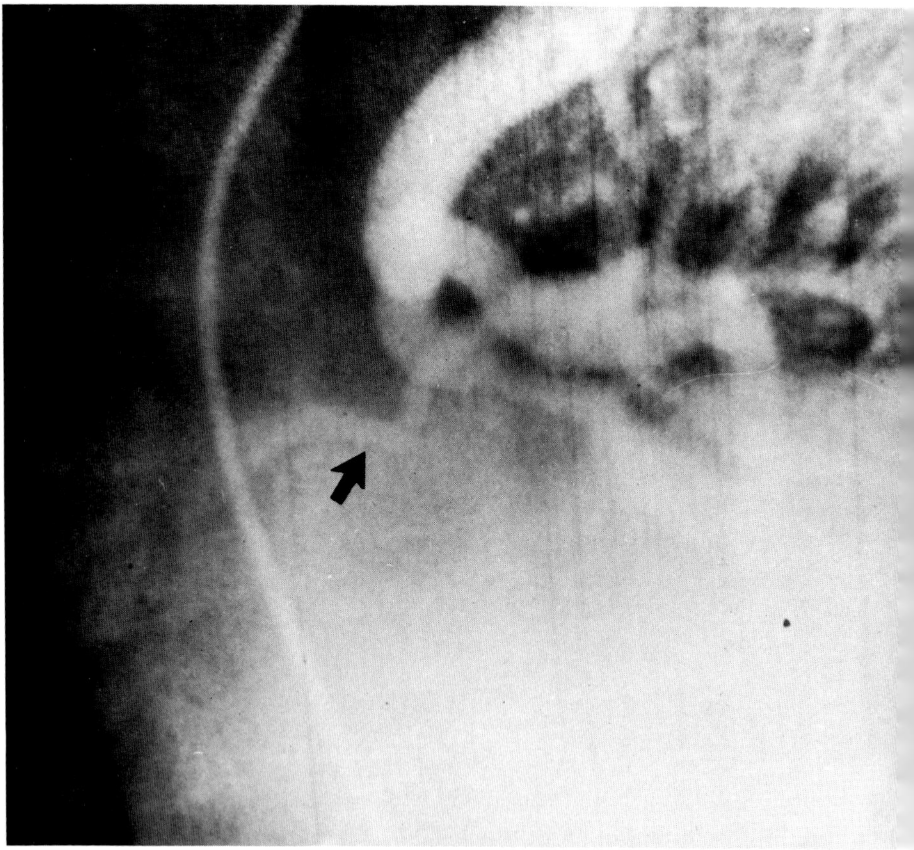

(A)

Figure 6 Pulmonary atresia and ventricular septal defect. (A) Selective injection of major aortopulmonary collateral artery fills many left lung arteries and a very small seagull (black arrow), the confluence of the central right and left pulmonary arteries.

Macartney, 1983; Rabinovitch, 1988) irrespective of whether the source is a central pulmonary artery or a collateral artery.

Surgical treatment of PA with VSD requires clear demonstration of virtually the entire complex pulmonary blood supply, with hemodynamic measurements when possible (Macartney and Haworth, 1983; Davis et al., 1978; Chesler et al., 1974; McGoon et al., 1977). Selective injections of contrast material into each of the major aortopulmonary collateral arteries is usually required (Macartney et al., 1973; Faller et al., 1981; Davis et al., 1978; Chesler et al., 1970; Levin et al., 1974). In addition, selective balloon occlu-

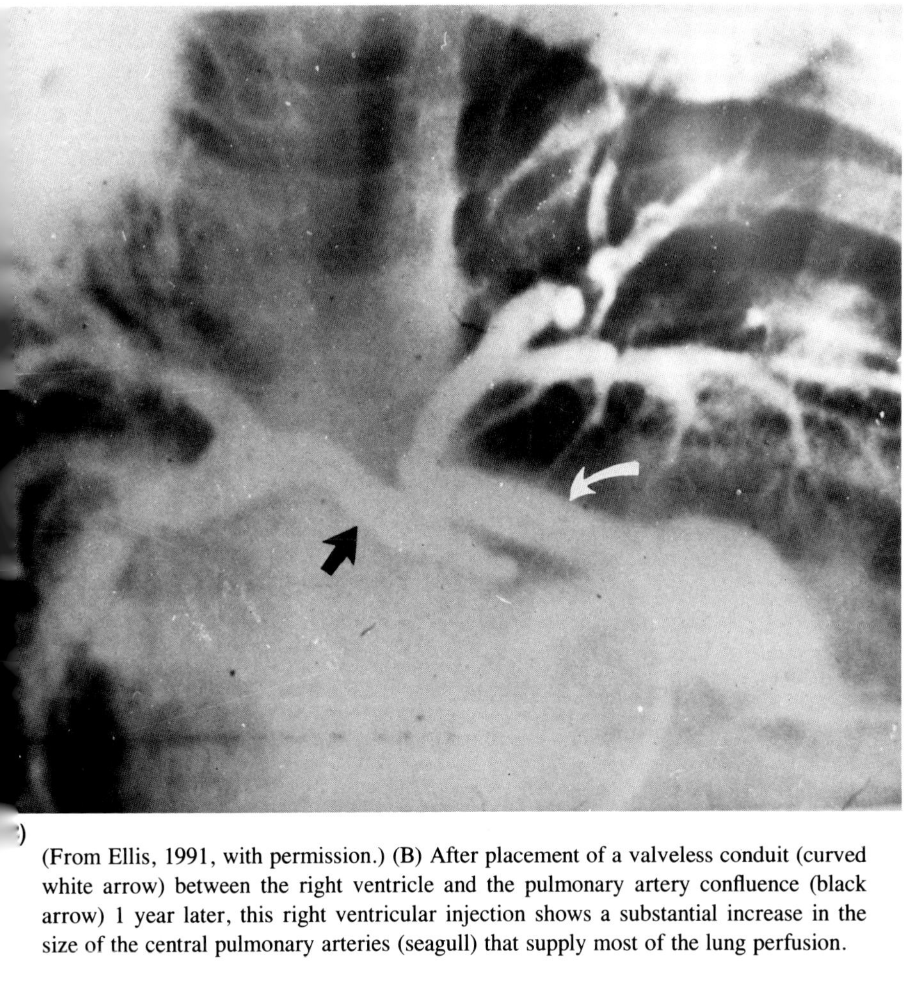

(From Ellis, 1991, with permission.) (B) After placement of a valveless conduit (curved white arrow) between the right ventricle and the pulmonary artery confluence (black arrow) 1 year later, this right ventricular injection shows a substantial increase in the size of the central pulmonary arteries (seagull) that supply most of the lung perfusion.

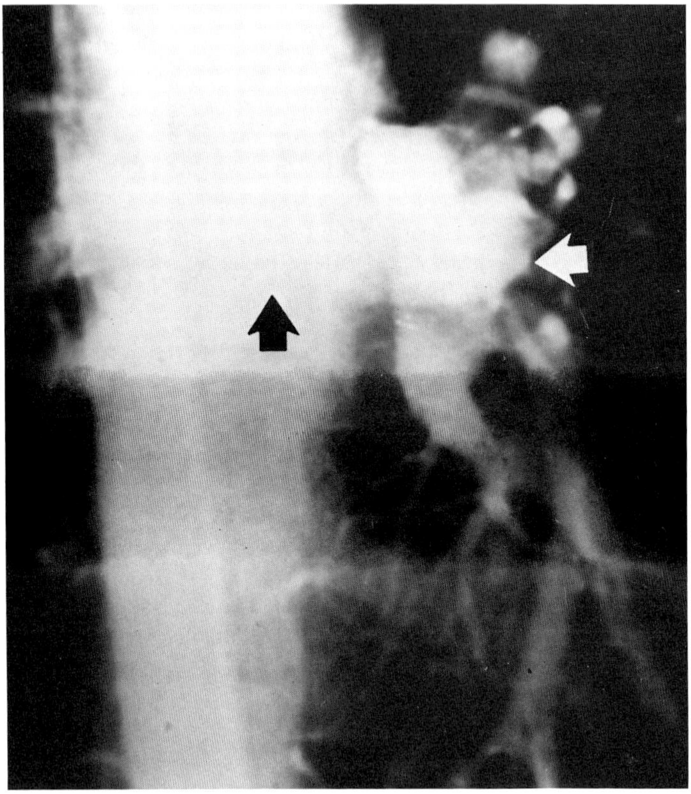

(A)

Figure 7 Pulmonary atresia and ventricular septal defect. (A) Following an aortogram the central pulmonary arteries (black and white arrows) have filled by collateral blood flow. These central arteries are quite unusual in being of about normal size despite pulmonary atresia, which is usually associated with small central pulmonary arteries. (B and C) Frontal and lateral views of right ventriculogram after a conduit was placed surgically between the right ventricle and the central pulmonary artery confluence and the ventricular septal defect and MAPCA were closed. The patient is asymptomatic. The right ventriculogram shows filling of the pulmonary arteries via the conduit. An aortic homograft is preferred today for long-range function instead of the fabric conduit with a porcine valve supported by a metallic ring that was used in this patient.

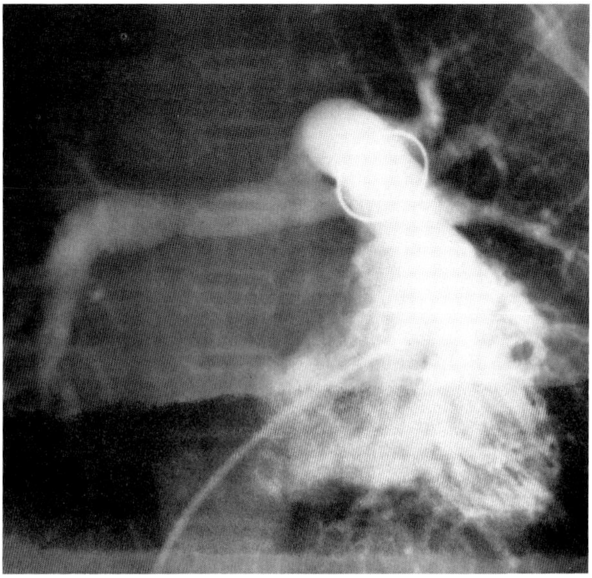

(B)

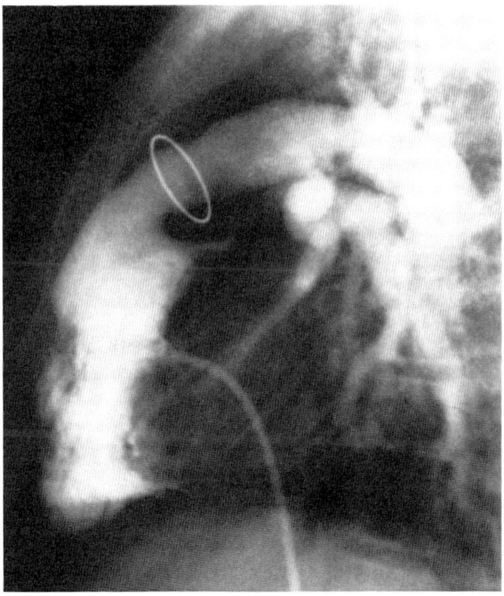

(C)

sion of one MAPCA together with selective contrast material injection into another MAPCA may be very helpful in showing the presence as well as the anatomy of anastomotic connections between major aortopulmonary collateral arteries and/or pulmonary arteries (Diethelm et al., 1985; Hruda and Julsvud, 1989). Such detailed information is necessary for planning an optimal surgical repair (Blackstone et al., 1988; Milikan et al., 1986; Shimazaki et al., 1988), and each patient must be considered individually. When the central pulmonary arteries are large (about 8%) (Somerville, 1988) and well connected to the intrapulmonary arteries without serious obstruction, a conduit between the right ventricle and central pulmonary arteries can be very successful (Fig. 7) (Ross and Somerville, 1966). The great majority of patients, however, require more complex connections (Fig. 8) or staged procedures or may not be surgically reparable. Several techniques have been advocated for predicting whether the central pulmonary arteries or any available set of vessels is capable of accepting the postsurgical right ventricular output without excessive pressure (Blackstone et al., 1988; Wallace et al., 1969). A 50% reduction in the pulmonary vascular bed does not normally produce pulmonary hypertension in the adult, but it may do so in the immature lung. Numerous thoughtful surgical procedures have been tried with varying results (Ross and Somerville, 1966; Wallace et al., 1969; Kirklin et al., 1977, 1988; McGoon et al., 1975). A frequently advised technique of staged treatment is to connect the right ventricle or a systemic artery to the hypoplastic central pulmonary arteries in early life, postponing definitive repair in expectation that increased blood flow may substantially enlarge these central pulmonary arteries and thus make them suitable for more complete surgical correction (Fig. 6B).

Most cases of pulmonary atresia and ventricular septal defect with pulmonary blood supply by MAPCA are not in severe distress in the first months of life and have arterial oxygen saturations of over 70%, implying considerable pulmonary blood flow (Somerville, 1988). Some survive many years without severe symptoms. A few cases (2–5%) have such large MAPCA connections and so little resistance to flow that they present in the first months of life with congestive heart failure because of excessive pulmonary blood flow. Percutaneous pre- or postoperative embolization of major collateral arteries has become increasingly useful in such situations (Lois et al., 1988; Perry et al., 1989). We have seen two cases in whom large tortuous anomalous collateral arteries caused serious airway obstruction with stridor, relieved in one case by surgical repositioning of the anomalous artery.

Pulmonary Stenosis (PS) and Ventricular Septal Defect; Tetralogy of Fallot

In tetralogy of Fallot in contrast to pulmonary atresia, a portion of the right ventricular output goes to the lungs via the stenotic pulmonary outflow tract.

The residual output is shunted via ventricular septal defect to left ventricle and aorta. Occasionally a partially closed but patent ductus supplies some additional blood flow to the lungs. In striking contrast to PA with VSD, major aortopulmonary collateral arteries (Ramsay et al., 1985; Lintermans et al., 1966) are seldom found. Later in postnatal life enlarged bronchial and acquired transpleural arteries may substantially contribute to pulmonary blood flow (Hales and Liebow, 1948). The transpleural collateral development is facilitated by any process causing transpleural adhesions, such as thoracotomy for performing a Blalock anastomosis between a subclavian artery and a pulmonary artery. Therapeutic procedures designed to create transpleural adhesions were used in the early years of heart surgery (Barrett and Daley, 1949).

Such collateral connections are responsible for the visualization of the macroscopic pulmonary arteries during aortography in many clinical cases of severe pulmonary stenosis or atresia. Similar systemic arterial connections to the pulmonary arteries may occur across the mediastinal pleura as well as via the hilum or pulmonary ligaments.

In tetralogy of Fallot the bronchial collateral circulation increases with time and often produces a profusion of small, irregular vessels in the lung that can be recognized on the chest radiograph (Fig. 9) (Campbell and Gardner, 1950). The lung findings, of course, are typically accompanied by other radiographic features: a "cour en sabot" configuration of the heart, a concave main pulmonary artery segment and small hilar vessels. Occasionally in adults with severe pulmonary obstruction apical lung densities develop that resemble tuberculosis but that are due to rich collateral vasculature and scarring subsequent to small-vessel thrombosis and hemorrhage (pulmonary pseudofibrosis) (Haroutunian and Neill, 1972).

Other Congenital Heart Diseases With or Without Pulmonary Stenosis or Atresia

Any form of congenital heart disease with pulmonary stenosis, especially with cyanosis, tends to have enlargement of the bronchial arteries and other routes of acquired blood flow to the lungs.

Commonly, considerable acquired bronchial collateral circulation is found in transposition of the great arteries (Aziz et al., 1977) even without associated pulmonary stenosis. This is especially evident when the interventricular septum is intact. Somewhat surprisingly, when pulmonary atresia is part of more complicated congenital heart disease, such as transposition of the great arteries, single ventricle, double-outlet right ventricle, or atrioventricular canal, a patent ductus arteriosus is usually the major source of pulmonary blood flow. In a group of 40 such cases (Marino et al., 1987), only 2 had MAPCA, both with nonconfluent central pulmonary arteries; the other 38 cases had confluent central arteries and a PDA.

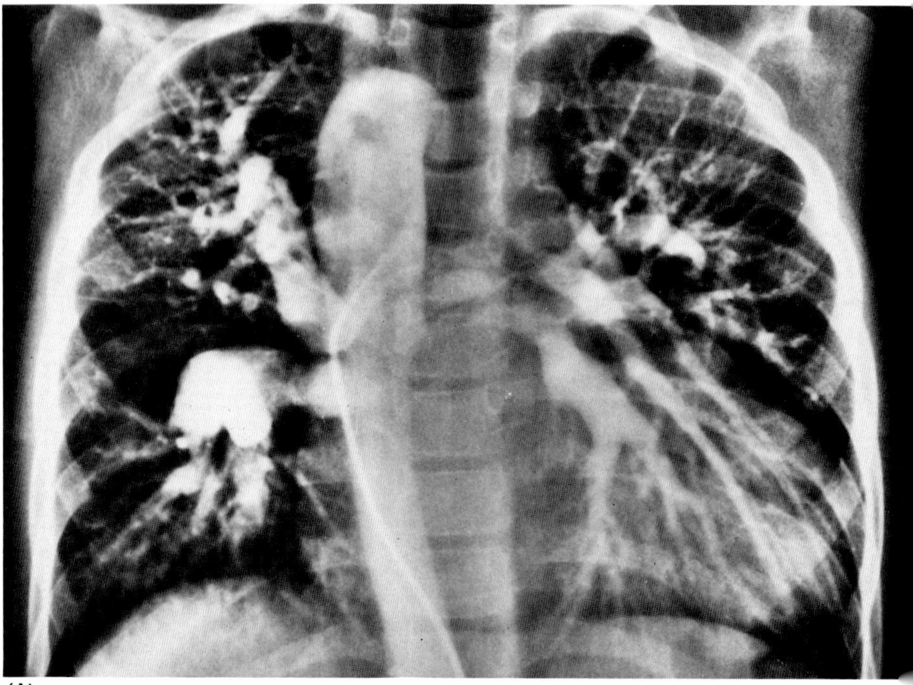

(A)

Figure 8 Pulmonary atresia and ventricular septal defect. (A) Descending aortogram shows right-sided aorta with two MAPCAs to each lung, those on the left with severe proximal stenoses. (B) A conduit was surgically placed between the right ventricle and the surgically isolated descending aortic segment giving origin to the four MAPCAs. This right ventriculogram shows filling of the distal end of the conduit and the MAP-

Absence of Proximal Right or Left Pulmonary Artery

When a right or left pulmonary artery is not normally connected to the main pulmonary artery, several anatomic arrangements may occur (Pool et al., 1962; Sherrick et al., 1962). The entire artery including the intrapulmonary vessels may be missing, which usually translates to agenesis of the lung. Since in the great majority of cases lung parenchymal development is normal at birth, however, intrauterine perfusion must have been adequate for lung growth. Thus although the central or proximal arterial connection is missing, the more peripheral circulation is (or was) provided by an alternate route (Sotomora and Edwards, 1978; Presbitero et al., 1984; Pfefferkorn et al., 1982; Anderson et al., 1958; Freedom et al., 1984). The major possibilities for alternative supply are:

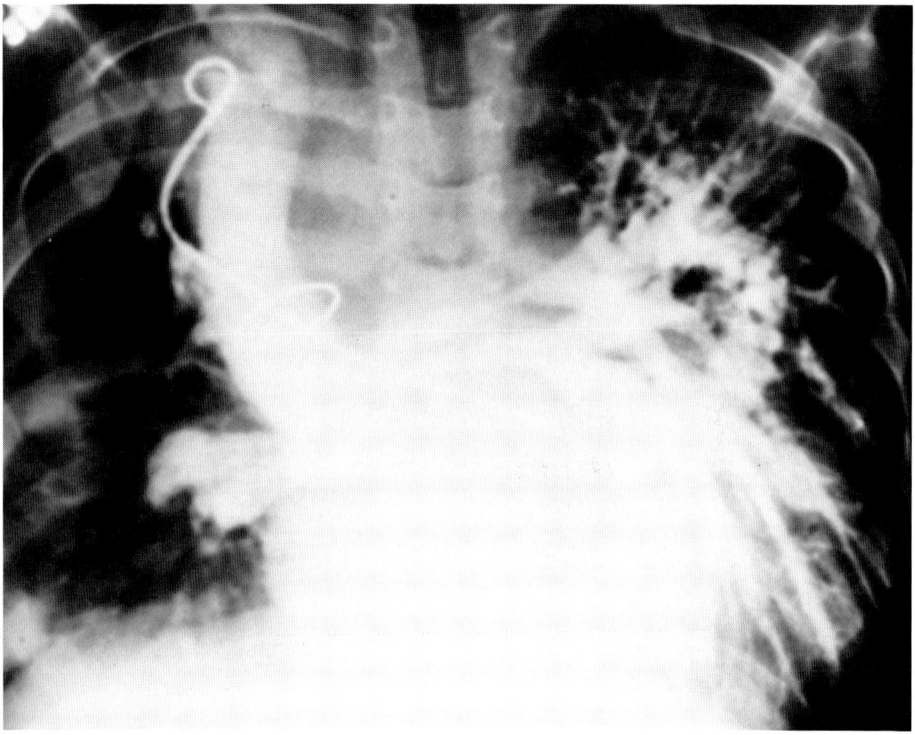

(B)
CAs. The ventricular septal defect was closed, and a bypass aortic graft was placed between the aorta proximal and that distal to the isolated aortic segment. The slow flow in large right-sided vessels is due to high peripheral vascular resistance. (A and B from Ellis, 1991, with permission.)

1. Patent ductus arteriosus
2. Acquired bronchial and other collateral circulation
3. Direct origin of pulmonary artery from aorta
4. Major aortopulmonary collateral artery (theoretical possibility)

Absent Proximal Right Pulmonary Artery with Peripheral Right Arteries Supplied by PDA and/or Bronchial Collateral

Right PDA supply to the hilum of the right lung is probably the most common association with absent right pulmonary artery (AbRPA) at birth (Fig. 10), but since the infant is typically asymptomatic very few cases have been documented to have an open ductus to the right lung. The ductus referred to is an

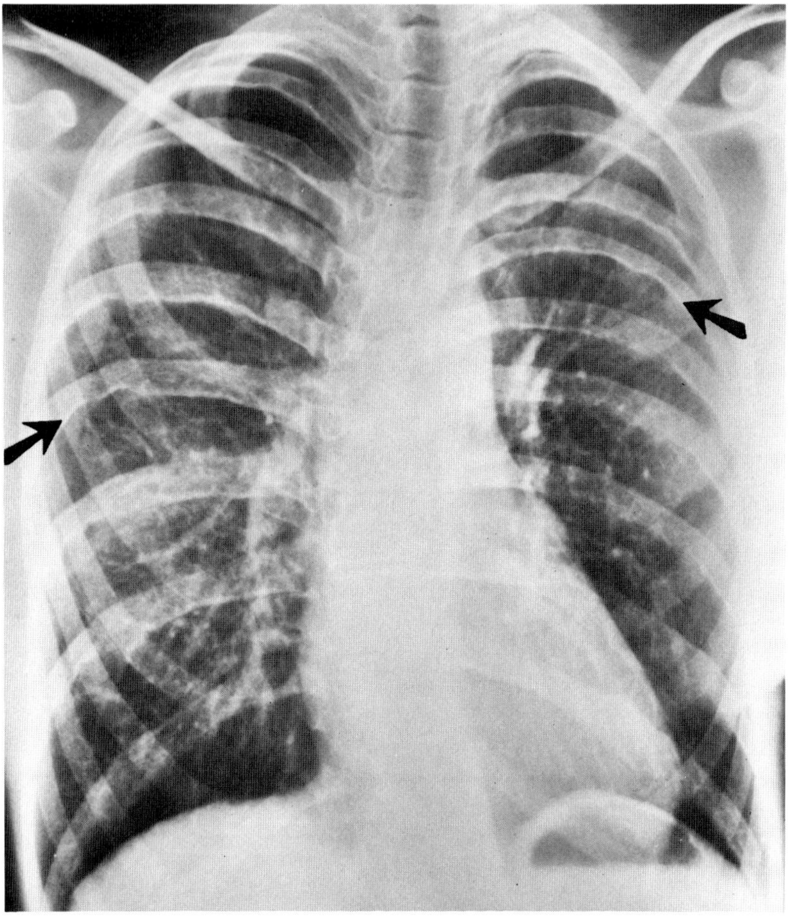

Figure 9 Tetralogy of Fallot. This chest roentgenogram shows small bilateral hilar pulmonary vasculature and some peripheral small curvilinear densities typical of bronchial collateral circulation. Rib notching (arrows) is seen on several ribs bilaterally secondary to erosions by large tortuous intercostal arteries supplying blood to the lungs via collateral arteries connecting to the lung by pleural adhesions. The intercostal arteries also supply collateral blood flow to the arm because of subclavian artery interruption by prior bilateral Blalock anastomoses of proximal subclavian artery to the ipsilateral pulmonary artery.

abnormally persistent in utero right ductus arteriosus arising from the region of the right innominate artery (Pfefferkorn et al., 1982). It usually closes shortly after birth. Nearly all these patients have a left aortic arch and also the usual left ductus arteriosus open at least until the neonatal period.

During childhood, collateral circulation is acquired through bronchial and associated arteries. The right lung generally grows less than the left, may be slightly more opaque than the left, and develops parenchymal roentgenographic features that may suggest bronchial collateral circulation. The left hilar vascular structures enlarge; those on the right appear smaller than usual or absent. Transpleural collateral development may be so marked as to cause visible pleural thickeinig, and rib notching may occur as a result of enlarged intercostal arteries. Angiocardiography is the mainstay of radiological diagnosis (Madoff et al., 1952; Wyman, 1954), but echocardiography, magnetic resonance imaging (MRI), computed tomography (CT), and nuclear medicine studies have been increasingly used. Chronic thromboembolic occlusion of a right or left pulmonary artery in the adult can mimic the proximal absence of a pulmonary artery on angiography (Moser et al., 1989).

Bronchograms have been near normal in most cases (Pool et al., 1962), although some show abnormal bronchial development (Pool et al., 1962; Hislop et al., 1973) and/or bronchiectasis. Hemoptysis (Pool et al., 1962) from the abnormal lung occurs in up to 16% of cases and may require pulmonary resection or selective arterial embolization. A variable number (16–40%) have a history of repeated respiratory infections (Pool et al., 1962; Shakibi et al., 1978).

In 1978, Shakibi et al. reviewed the world literature after the landmark paper of Pool et al. (1962) and discussed guidelines for surgical repair. Only three patients (Shakibi et al., 1978; Kieffer et al., 1965; Winship et al., 1967) had surgical connection of the right hilar pulmonary artery to the main pulmonary artery. One died soon after operation (Winship et al., 1967), one graft closed (Kieffer et al., 1965), and the other died 1 month later with severe pulmonary hypertension and apparent diffuse arteriovenous fistulas in the right lung (Shakibi et al., 1978). (In 1963, however, Green et al. reported successful direct anastomosis of a *left* hilar pulmonary artery to the main pulmonary artery.) Since 1976 a number of successful grafts to the right hilar pulmonary artery have been accomplished (Presbitero et al., 1984; Kucera et al., 1982; Toews and Pappas, 1983; Cobanoglu et al., 1984; Grillo et al., 1986; Sosa et al., 1987).

Patients with congenital absent right pulmonary artery can be conveniently divided into several groups (Pool et al., 1962; Bahler et al., 1969):

1. Isolated AbRPA without pulmonary hypertension. These patients are typically asymptomatic, and the diagnosis is often clinical and radio-

(A)

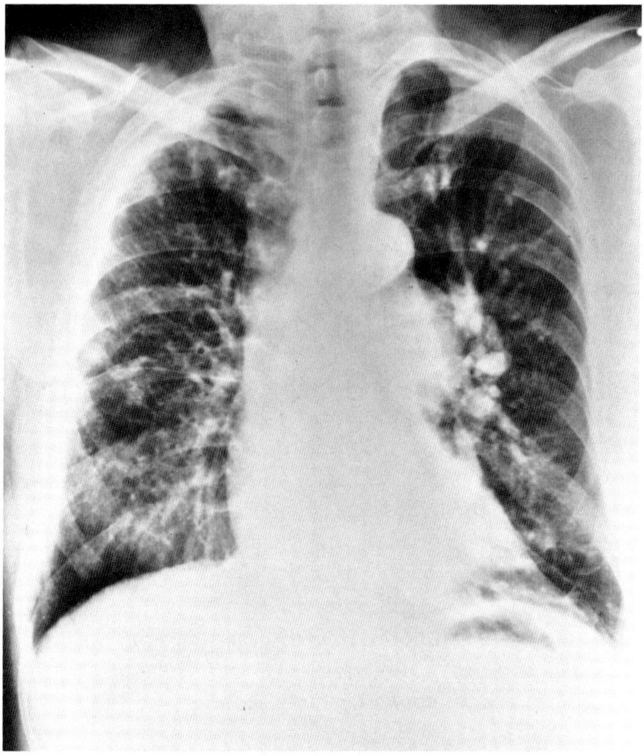

Figure 10 Absent proximal right pulmonary artery in an 80-year-old man. (A) Plain film showing a very large left pulmonary artery system and a small or absent central right pulmonary artery. The right lung is smaller than usual. Note the many small peripheral curvilinear densities in the right lung due to collateral circulation and also the apparent pleural thickening and increased density over the right apex. The patient had some pulmonary hypertension but was active and asymptomatic and had been followed medically for more than 50 years. (B) Pulmonary arteriogram shows huge left pulmonary arteries and no evidence of a proximal right pulmonary artery. (From Ellis, 1991, with permission.) (C) Late film from an aortogram showing filling of numerous "bronchial" collateral arteries, particularly evident over the apex of the right lung. Transpleural collateral connections developed secondary to adhesions, perhaps secondary to microinfarctions in the lung apex (Haroutunian and Neill, 1972). The intercostal arteries are much enlarged.

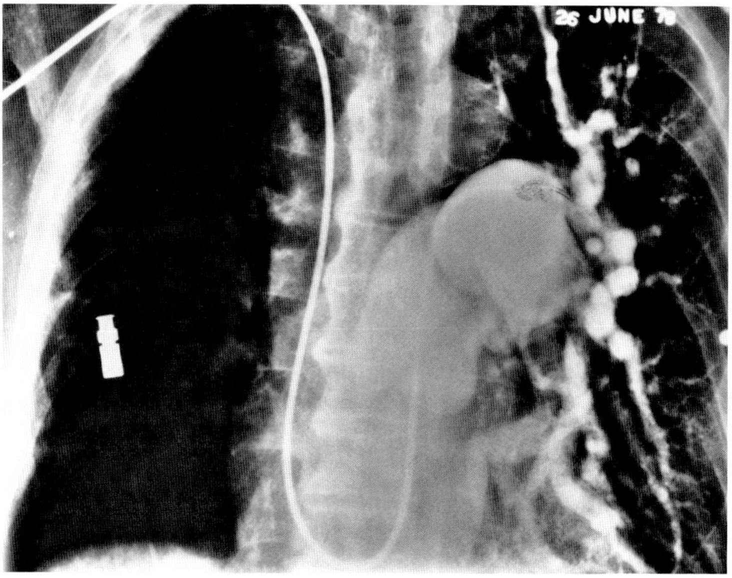

(B)

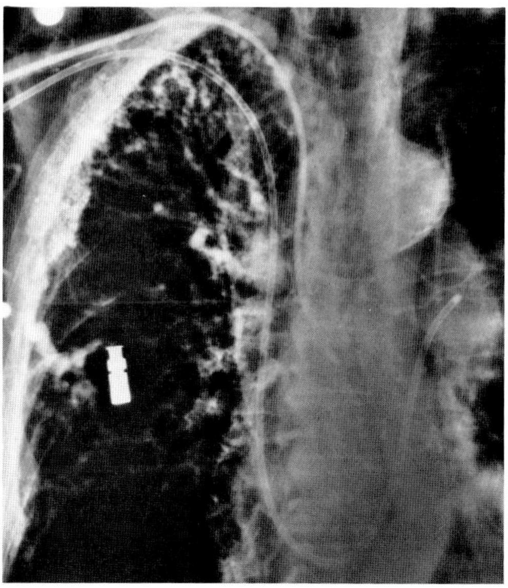

(C)

graphic without surgical or pathological confirmation. Some of these patients eventually develop pulmonary hypertension (Pool et al., 1962; Ferguson et al., 1969; Hubsch et al., 1987), but the prognosis is too uncertain for a definite recommendation for surgical connection of the hilar pulmonary artery to the main pulmonary artery unless pulmonary hypertension is present. Pulmonary hypertension is occult in an uncertain portion of these patients, and they are remarkably vulnerable to development of high-altitude pulmonary hypertension and pulmonary edema (Pool et al., 1962; Vogel et al., 1967; Hackett et al., 1980).

2. Isolated AbRPA with pulmonary hypertension. Patients are seen at all ages but infants and young children are most common. Surgical connection of the right hilar artery to the main pulmonary artery can be lifesaving (Toews and Pappas, 1983; Sosa et al., 1987) and perhaps should be done prophylactically.
3. Isolated AbRPA with intractable pulmonary infection or hemoptysis from right lung. Some of these lungs are congenitally malformed. Resection or bronchial artery embolization may be required.
4. AbRPA with left PDA or other congenital heart disease (Vasquez-Sanchez et al., 1983; Buchler et al., 1986). All these patients have pulmonary hypertension (Pool et al., 1962; Vasquez-Sanchez et al., 1983) and are usually much benefited by closure of the left PDA (Pool et al., 1962). The same is true for closure of other congenital defects, permitting a left-to-right shunt (Kumar et al., 1984).

Fortunately, the majority are in the first group (Werber et al., 1983). Exercise tolerance is usually good, and survival may be long (Fig. 10) despite the eventual development of pulmonary hypertension in some patients.

Absent Proximal Left Pulmonary Artery with Peripheral Left Arteries Supplied by PDA and/or Bronchial Collateral

Absence of the left pulmonary artery is usually associated with significant congenital heart disease, especially tetralogy of Fallot, and frequently a right aortic arch is present (Figs. 11 and 12). Because of this angiocardiography may be performed, and in some infants a patent ductus supplying the left lung has been documented (Fig. 11). In these cases, after the ductus has closed the bronchial and associated arteries provide the only arterial supply to the lung. The radiographic findings on chest films are most typically those of tetralogy of Fallot with unusually small left hilar vessels. Diagnosis usually requires angiography.

Absent proximal left pulmonary artery can usefully be considered in two groups depending upon whether the aortic arch is right or left. In 1954,

McKim and Wiglesworth added three proven cases of absent left pulmonary artery to the three previously recorded. All their cases had a *right aortic arch* and a cord representing an obliterated ductus arteriosus between the left innominate artery and the peripheral (hilar) left pulmonary artery. They suggested that the most likely mechanism producing this anomaly was disappearance (i.e., resorption) of the primitive left pulmonary artery proximal to its junction with the sixth left aortic arch. These authors (McKim and Wiglesworth, 1954), supported by the later report of Sotomora and Edwards (1978) and others, confirmed radiologically (Nordenström, 1963; Freedom et al., 1983) that the distal pulmonary artery at the hilum of the lung and the intrapulmonary vessels persisted even though the more central artery was lost.

In 1984, Presbitero et al. reported the results of surgical exploration in nine clinical cases of congenital heart disease with absent left pulmonary artery. Four of these nine cases had a *right aortic arch,* and in them no intrapericardial remnant of the pulmonary artery was found. Like the cases of McKim and Wiglesworth (1954) each had a ligamentum arteriosum connecting the left innominate artery to the left hilar pulmonary artery. The authors suggested early embryological involution of the proximal left pulmonary artery had occurred, leaving the left ductus arteriosus to supply the left lung. Such a ductus usually closes after birth. Absence of the left pulmonary artery with right aortic arch may or may not be associated with other congenital heart disease (Pfefferkorn et al., 1982), but it was present in these cases (Presbitero et al., 1984).

The other five cases (Presbitero et al., 1984) with absent left pulmonary artery had a *left aortic arch,* and all of them had an "intrapericardial left pulmonary artery in continuity with the (left) hilar vessels," even though the artery was proximally occluded. All five cases had severe right ventricular outflow tract obstruction and also had a left ductus that descended vertically from under the aortic arch, as is characteristic of anomalies dependent upon reversed ductal flow in utero (i.e., flow from aorta to pulmonary artery), such as pulmonary atresia with ventricular septal defect (Santos et al., 1980; Heymann and Rudolph, 1972; Cassels et al., 1975). The authors postulated that this type of absent left pulmonary artery may be acquired after birth secondary to narrowing or closure of the left ductus arteriosus.

Nearly all of this second group of cases of absent left pulmonary artery (LPA) with left aortic arch occurred in conjunction with pulmonary atresia or severe stenosis and ventricular septal defect. In 1986, Elzenga and Gittenberger-de Groot in a large pathological study of obstructions of the pulmonary arteries in pulmonary atresia, including 20 cases with left aortic arch and left ductus, found that stenosis (or atresia) of the left pulmonary artery occurred exclusively in relation to a ductus and was located in the segment of the left pulmonary artery between the main pulmonary trunk and the ductus.

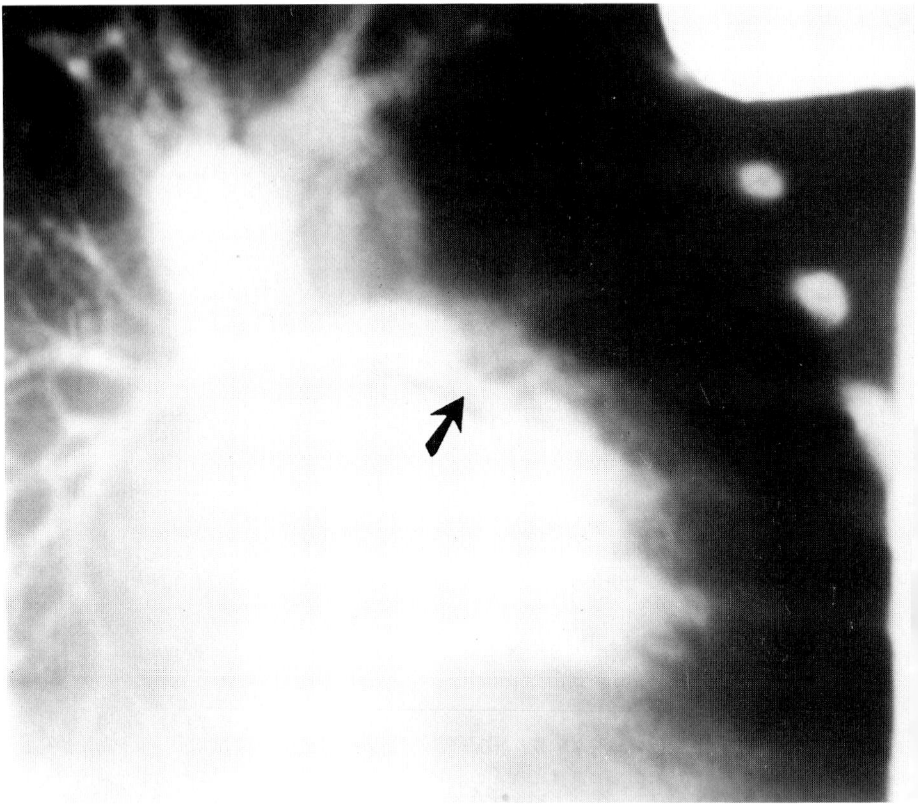

(A)

Figure 11 Absent proximal left pulmonary artery in tetralogy of Fallot. (A) Right venticulogram in a newborn shows severe infundibular stenosis (black arrow) with filling of the right pulmonary artery but no definite visualization of a proximal left pulmonary artery. Most of the contrast material flows through a ventricular septal defect into the large right-sided aortic arch. This right-to-left shunt causes a severe clinical

The majority of cases with a stenotic or occluded pulmonary artery exhibited a ridge on the interior wall of the pulmonary artery opposite the site of ductal entry (analogous to the aortic shelf found opposite the entry of the ductus in coarctation of the aorta (Hutchins, 1971). In addition, ductal tissue was noted histologically in the wall of the affected pulmonary artery in more than half these cases. The authors imply that the ductal tissue in the pulmonary artery wall may be responsible for the pulmonary artery narrowing.

In 1986, Mommo et al. reported a series of 21 unoperated cases of pulmonary atresia (with left aortic arch implied, ages 11 days to 21 years; median

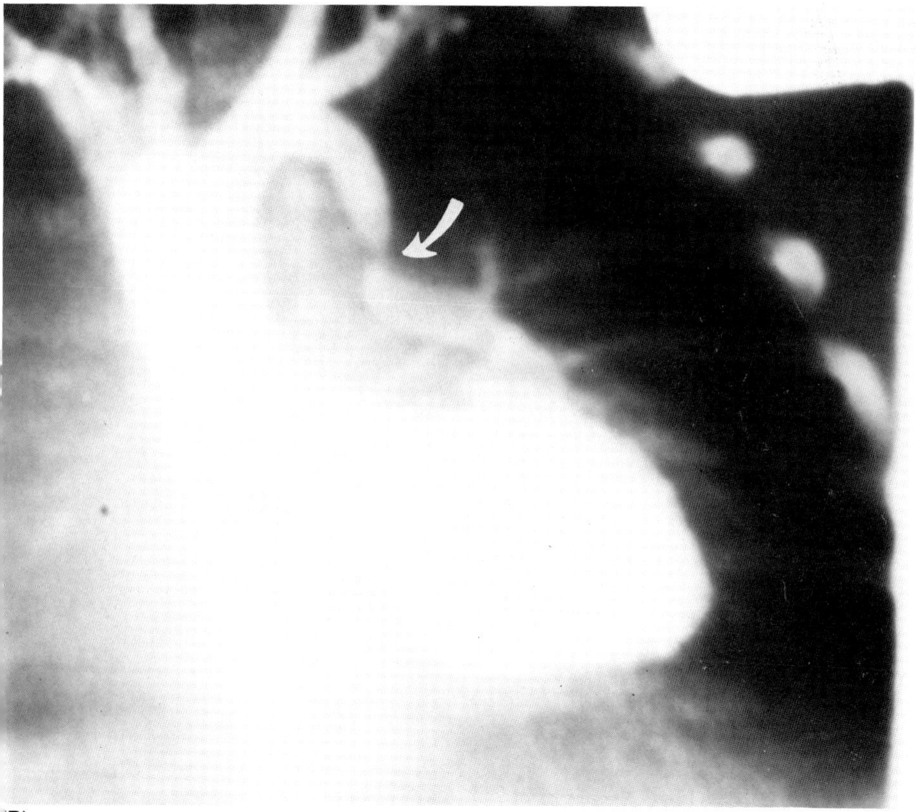

B)

cyanosis. The left lung is of normal size at birth. (B) Left ventriculogram on same day again shows filling of aorta and clearly shows a left PDA from the distal left innominate artery to the peripheral left pulmonary artery, which appears to be closing at the distal end (white arrow). This ductus had closed spontaneously 3 months later. (A and B from Ellis, 1991, with permission.)

age 4 years) in whom the central pulmonary artery originally gave rise to both right and left pulmonary arteries. Of these cases 5 developed proximal left pulmonary artery atresia; another 9 developed juxtaductal stenosis of the left pulmonary artery. The left pulmonary artery atresia was considered to have developed as a consequence of ductal contracture, augmented in some cases by local intimal fibrosis and thrombosis. No right pulmonary artery obstructions were found. A subsequent paper (Mommo et al., 1987) by this group showed that left pulmonary artery atresia was even more common and its site more variable after palliative shunt operations.

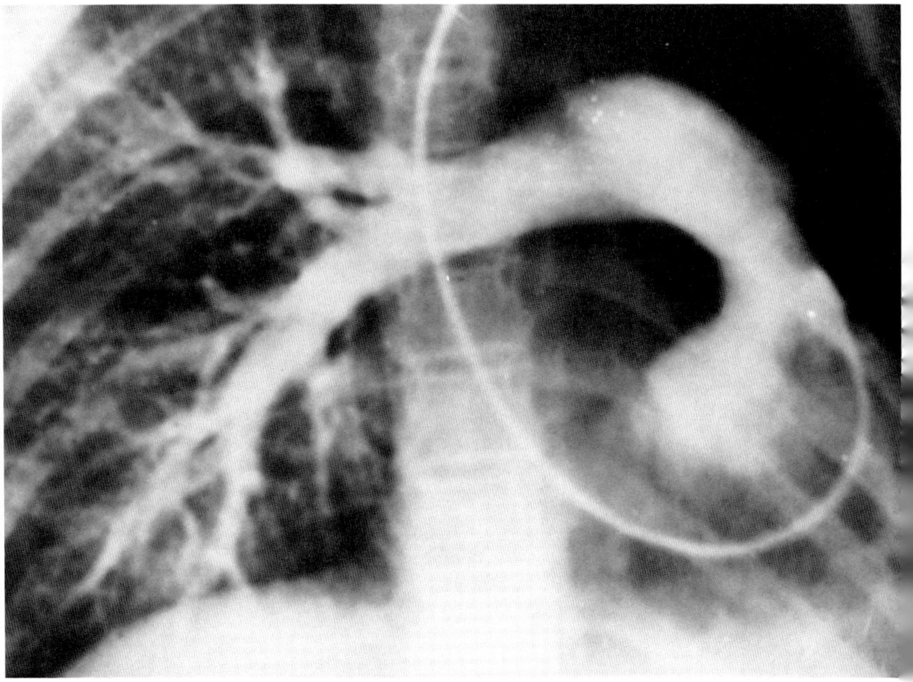

(A)

Figure 12 Absent proximal left pulmonary artery in a 12-year-old child with right aortic arch. (A) Right ventriculogram showing filling of right pulmonary arteries but no filling of a left pulmonary artery. The left lung was relatively small (hypoplastic), and

Thus the absence of the proximal left pulmonary artery *with right aortic arch* appears to develop before birth. The distal left pulmonary artery is supplied by a left ductus arteriosus arising from the region of the innominate artery, and the intrapericardial proximal left pulmonary artery may be absent. On the other hand, with a *left aortic arch* atresia of the proximal left pulmonary artery may develop after birth, with ductal closure almost always in the presence of pulmonary atresia or severe pulmonary stenosis with ventricular septal defect.

In the typical clinically cyanotic patient with pulmonary obstruction and absent proximal left pulmonary artery, early shunting, for example, anastomosis of the left subclavian artery by a graft to the hilar left pulmonary artery, is desirable (Presbitero et al., 1984). When successful the operation (Presbitero et al., 1984) provides more pulmonary blood flow and may keep the peripheral left pulmonary artery large and available for future procedures and may result in more normal maturation of the left lung.

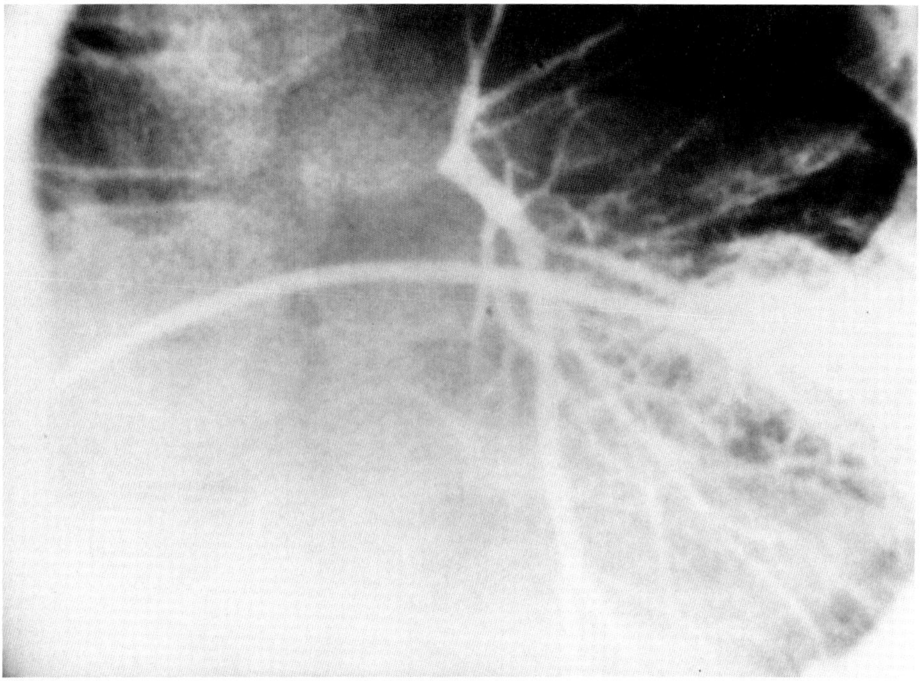

(B)

the heart is secondarily shifted toward the left. A right aortic arch was present. (B) Wedge pulmonary vein angiogram showing retrograde filling of the small but normally formed left pulmonary arteries back to the region of left hilum despite the absence of a proximal left pulmonary artery. (From Ellis, 1991, with permission.)

Absent Proximal Right Pulmonary Artery with Origin of the Right Pulmonary Artery from the Ascending Aorta

Anomalous origin of a pulmonary artery from the ascending aorta (Fig. 13) was beautifully studied by Kutsche and Van Mierop (1988). They were able to analyze 99 cases from the literature and 9 of their own. In 89 cases the artery was on the right and in 19 cases on the left. In 76 of the 89 right-sided cases the artery arose on the posterior wall or left posterior wall of the ascending aorta near the aortic valve; in the other 13 cases it arise from the distal ascending aorta near the origin of the innominate artery. The authors believe, as did others, that the two sites of origin imply different embryologies, the more common proximal type due to incomplete or delayed leftward migration of the fetal right pulmonary artery (Fig. 14); origin from the distal ascending aorta is attributed to persistence of the right fifth aortic arch. Other developmental possibilities were also discussed. All these patients had a left aortic arch, and over

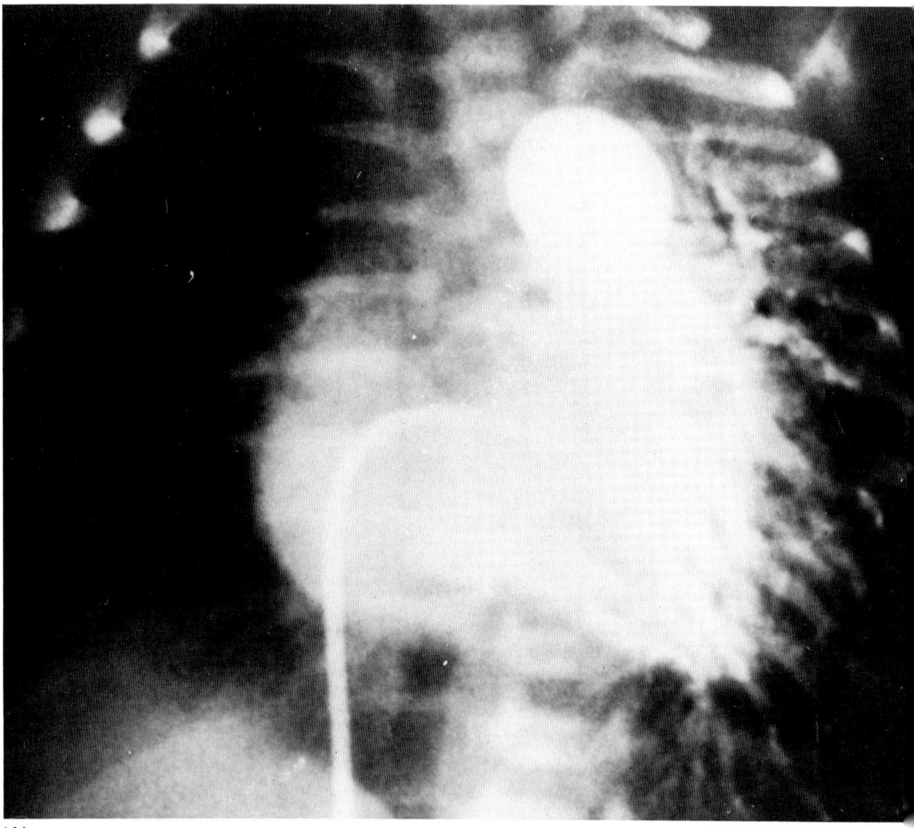

(A)

Figure 13 Right pulmonary artery directly from ascending aorta with congestive heart failure in the first week of life. (A) Right ventriculogram showing filling of the right heart and a large main pulmonary artery with only left branches. No filling of the

two-thirds had a patent ductus arteriosus on the left side. Aorticopulmonary septal defect was present in 12 patients. Interrupted aortic arch or coarctation of the aorta was present in 11 cases, and 8 of these also had an aorticopulmonary septal defect. Kutsche and Van Mierop (1988) rejected a large group of cases with the right pulmonary artery arising more peripherally from the innominate artery or its subclavian branch, all of whom were regarded as persistent right-sided patent ductus arteriosus.

For nearly all of this group pulmonary arterial hypertension rapidly ensues, and death from congestive heart failure is usual before the first year even if no other anomalies are present (Griffiths et al., 1962; Odell and Smith, 1963; Kauffman et al., 1967; Long et al., 1985). Plain chest films show car-

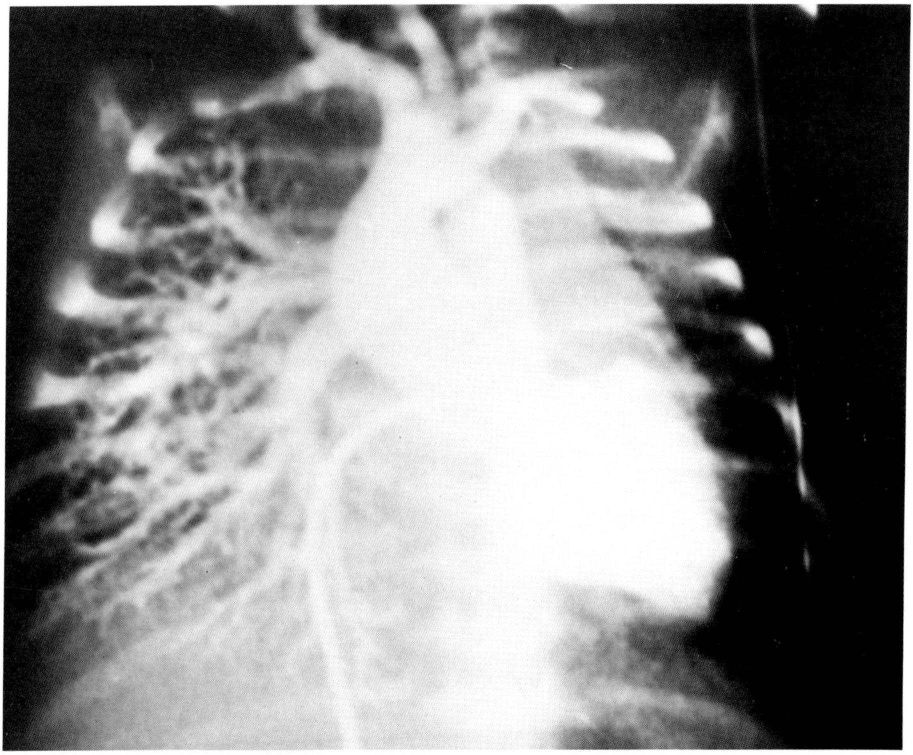

(B)

right pulmonary arteries is seen. (B) Left ventriculogram shows the left ventricle and a large aorta with left arch and filling of the large right pulmonary aterial vasculature. The right pulmonary artery arose from the posterior wall of the proximal ascending aorta. Prompt surgical transfer of the right pulmonary artery origin to the main pulmonary artery was lifesaving. (From Ellis, 1991, with permission.)

diomegaly and increasing vascular engorgement. Surgery in early infancy with transfer of the origin of the right pulmonary artery from the aorta to the main pulmonary artery is quite regularly a curative procedure (Fig. 13) (Cumming et al., 1972; Penkoske et al., 1983; Nashef et al., 1987; Benatar et al., 1987). The operation becomes more hazardous as the evolving high pulmonary vascular resistance worsens.

Untreated, very few of these patients have reached the age of 2 years. Right ventricular endocardial fibroelastosis (Pahlajani et al., 1985) may be recognized as a consequence of the severe pulmonary hypertension. The oldest survivor is 23 years. Clearly, early recognition and surgical treatment provide the only chance for long survival.

A

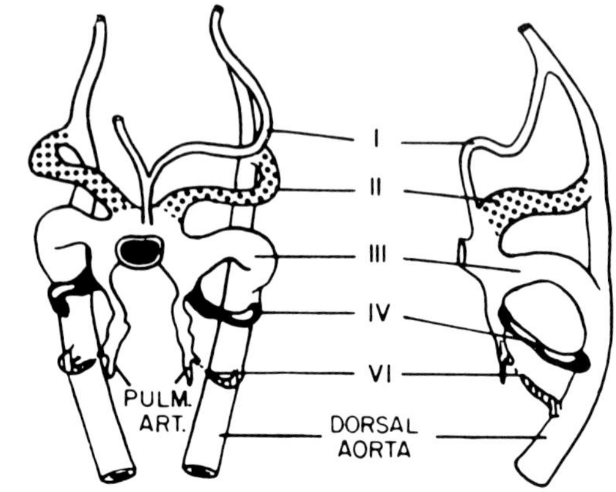

Figure 14 Successive early stages of development of the aortic arch system. (From Kutsche and Van Mierop, 1988, with permission.) (B) The asterick indicates the proximal right and left pulmonary arteries, which are usually but erroneously considered derived from the ventral parts of the sixth arches (Congdon, 1922; Kutsche and Van Mierop, 1988). These arteries are earlier primary extensions (A) from the truncoaortic sac. The right and left sixth arches (cross-hatched) account only for the respective right and left ductus arteriosus. (C) The right pulmonary artery origin has migrated to the left and fused with the left pulmonary artery to create the distal pulmonary trunk. Incomplete (or delayed?) leftward migration of the origin of the right pulmonary artery is almost certainly the mechanism for the anomalous origin of the right pulmonary artery from the posterior aspect of the proximal ascending aorta (Kutsche and Van Mierop, 1988). ART = artery; ARTER = arteriosus; ASC = ascending; PULM = pulmonary artery. (Redrawn after Congdon, 1922.) A = 4 mm; B = 5 mm; C = 11 mm embryo.

Absent Proximal Left Pulmonary Artery with Origin of the Left Pulmonary Artery from the Ascending Aorta

Much less common than right pulmonary artery from ascending aorta (Fig. 15) (Kutsche and Van Mierop, 1988; Robida and Fetlich, 1985) only 19 cases were in the Kutsche and Van Mierop (1988) series. All cases had either tetralogy of Fallot or a right aortic arch, or both: 14 (75%) had tetralogy of Fallot and 12 (63%) had a right aortic arch. Half had anomalous origin of a subclavian artery; 3 had a PDA, all on the right side, and 4 had no trace of a ductus or a ligamentum arteriosum. No patient had arch interruption, coarctation, or aorticopulmonary window. The authors believe that the genesis of this anomaly is failure of development of the left sixth arch. These authors believe that neither of these forms of origin of the pulmonary arteries from the ascending

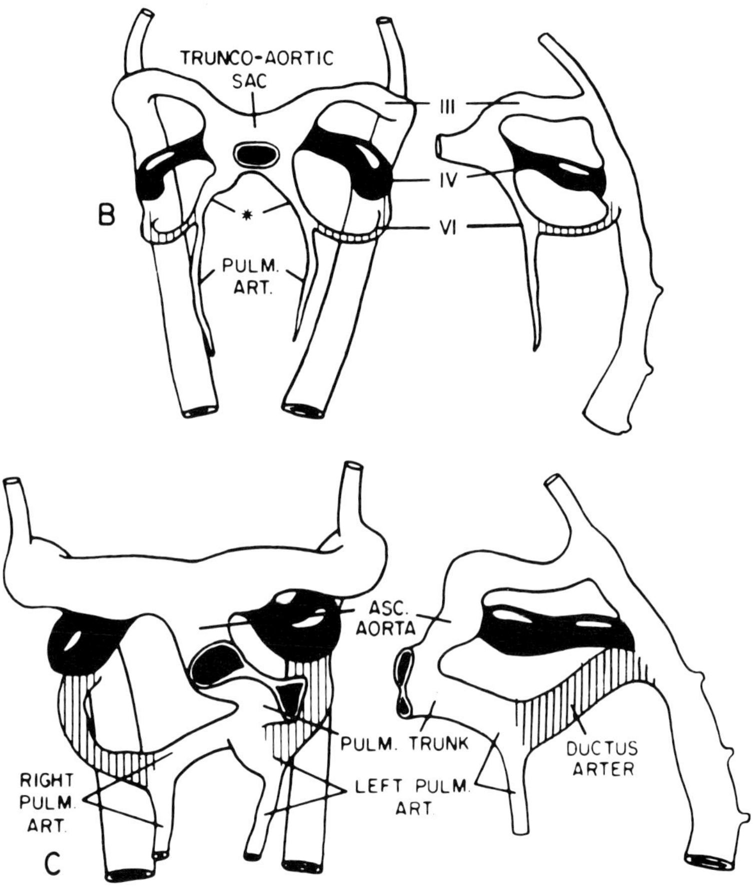

aorta should be considered partial types of persistent truncus arteriosus (Kutsche and Van Mierop, 1988).

These patients with tetralogy of Fallot and aortic origin of the left pulmonary artery survive longer than those with aortic origin of the right pulmonary artery. In two personal cases when the tetralogy was repaired in childhood and the left pulmonary artery was reanastomosed to the main pulmonary artery the patients survived but flow via the left lung was small, presumably because of acquired high peripheral vascular resistance. The diagnosis can be made by angiocardiography, magnetic resonance imaging, or echocardiography. The plain chest film shows an unusually large left pulmonary artery, often with unusually small peripheral vessels (Fig. 15).

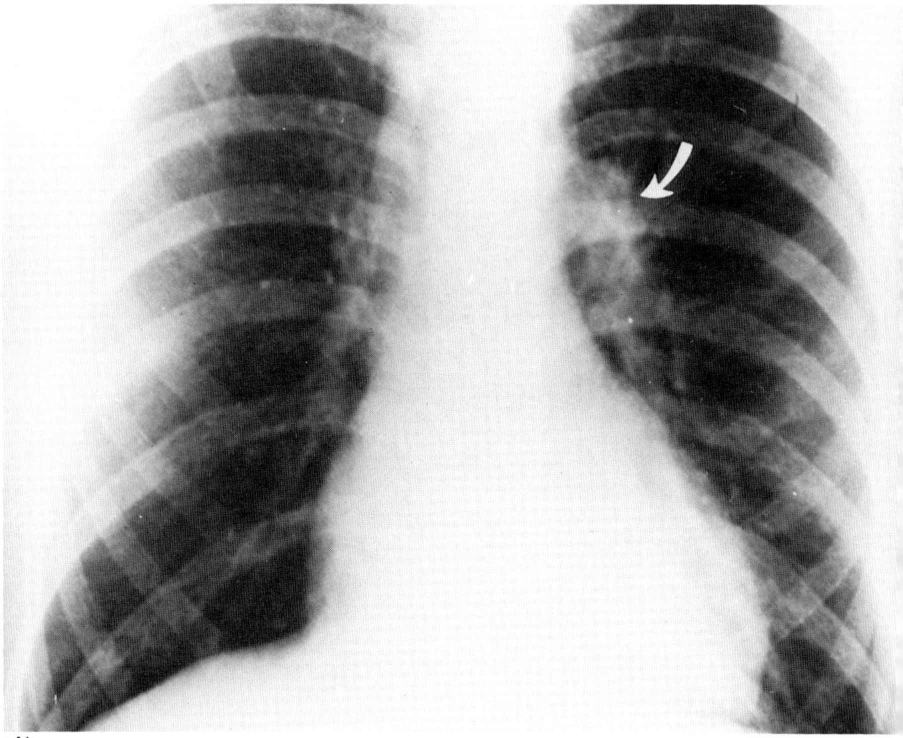

(A)

Figure 15 Anomalous origin of the left pulmonary from the ascending aorta in tetralogy of Fallot. (A) Plain chest film at age 8 showing a small right hilum and exceptionally small vessels in the right lung; the central left pulmonary artery (arrow) is large. The peripheral pulmonary resistance on the left was high, as suggested by the disproportionally small peripheral vessels. (B) Right ventriculogram showing filling of

Collateral Flow via the Coronary Arteries

The coronary arteries frequently contribute to collateral pulmonary blood flow in the presence of congenital heart disease with pulmonary obstruction. Tiny anastomoses between the coronary arteries and mediastinal branches of the bronchial arteries are evidently present at all ages (Berry, 1935; Tobin, 1952; Moberg, 1968). These connections may enlarge under conditions stimulating increased bronchial artery flow or in certain cases of coronary artery obstruction. Bjork (1966) demonstrated by aortography flow between the coronary arteries and the bronchial arteries in 12 of 67 cases with tetralogy of Fallot or pulmonary atresia with ventricular septal defect. By selective coronary

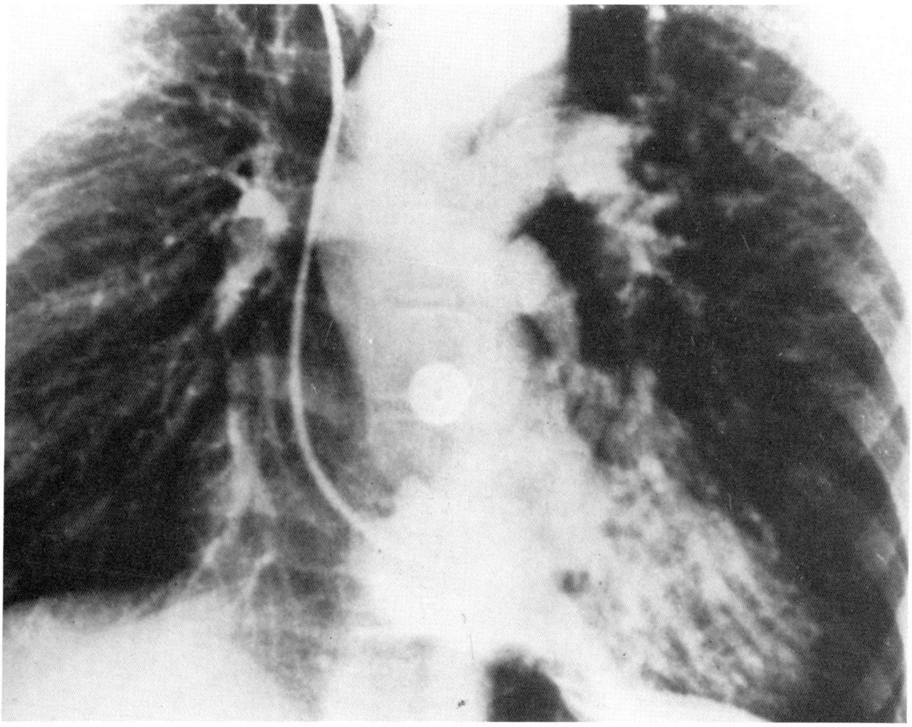

(B)

the stenotic pulmonary outflow tract as well as the ascending aorta. The right pulmonary arteries are relatively small. The left pulmonary artery is larger and arises directly from the ascending aorta, not from the main pulmonary artery, although this is not easily recognized on this angiocardiogram. (From Ellis, 1991, with permission.)

arteriography (Zureikat, 1980), 5 of 23 patients with cyanotic congenital heart disease had demonstrable collateral flow into the bronchial arteries; none was seen in 44 patients with noncyanotic congenital heart disease. A case has been reported in whom a large branch from the right coronary artery contributed most of the flow to a left lung with absent proximal left pulmonary artery (Thompson et al., 1986).

A few cases were reported in whom a proximal congenital connection or fistula between a major coronary artery, usually the left coronary, and the main or proximal right or left pulmonary artery is the supplier of a major portion of the pulmonary blood flow (Krongrad et al., 1972; Krongrad et al., 1973; Dark and Pollock, 1985; Pahl et al., 1989). Nearly all such patients have had pulmonary atresia with ventricular septal defect. They can be diagnosed by aortic root angiography. Preoperative recognition is crucial to planning an optimal surgical approach to these potentially correctable lesions.

In congenital origin of the left or the right coronary artery from the main pulmonary artery instead of from the aorta, coronary blood flow after infancy is characteristically retrograde into the pulmonary artery (Fig. 16). Small coronary vascular malformations that empty into the main pulmonary artery are occasionally encountered in routine coronary arteriography (Baim et al., 1982).

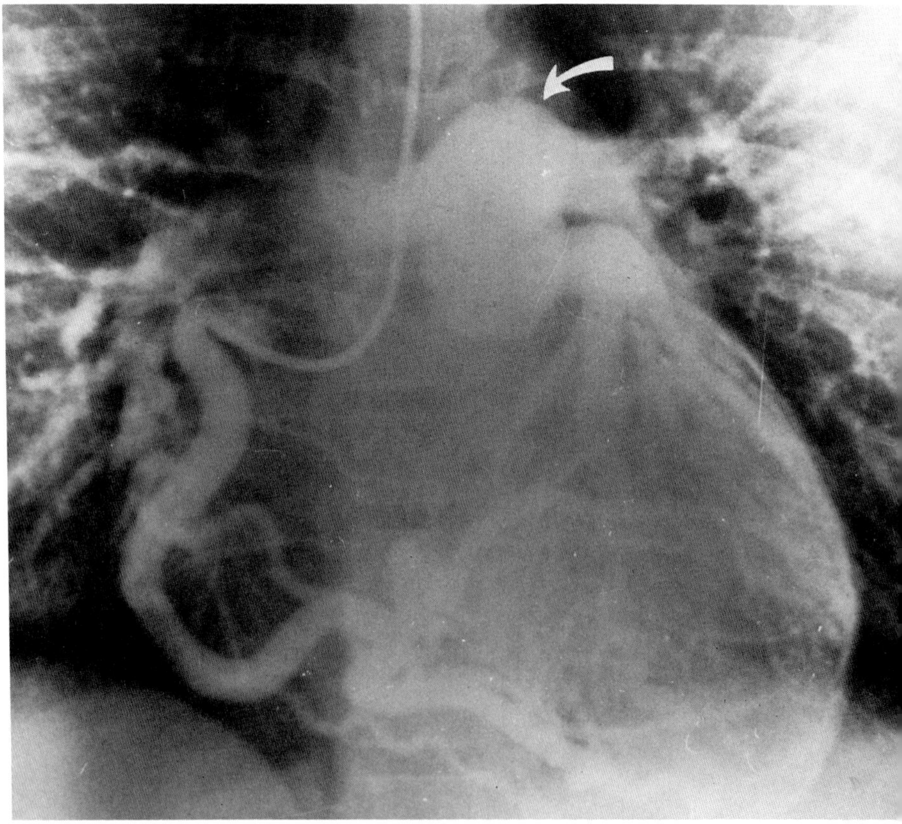

Figure 16 Anomalous origin of left coronary artery from pulmonary artery with large retrograde flow into the pulmonary artery at age 12 years. This selective right coronary arteriogram shows filling of the left coronary artery by collateral intercoronary flow. Retrograde opacification of the pulmonary artery (curved arrow) occurs via the anomalous origin of the left main coronary artery.

The mediastinal branches of the bronchial artery normally also have small connections with the esophageal, internal mammary, phrenic, and other regional vessels. Thus collateral flow via these sources can be expected under suitable conditions.

Other Systemic Arterial Connections to the Lung in Congenital Cardiovascular Disease

Unique cases continue to be reported. Both right and left pulmonary arteries may arise directly from the ascending aorta, with the main pulmonary artery supplying only the ductus (Beitzke and Shinebourne, 1980). A heart was encountered with three arterial trunks, an extra one arising from the left ventricle and supplying the right lung (Diaz-Gongora et al., 1982). It is not possible to encompass all the variations found in nature. In this review the focus is on anomalous systemic arterial supply to the lung in situs solitus (normal visceroatrial situs). Analogous connections may be observed in situs inversus or situs ambiguous.

The possibility of a prior surgical intervention being responsible for alterations in pulmonary blood supply, of course, can be an important consideration in many clinical cases. Anastomoses directly (or by graft) between a subclavian artery and the ipsilateral pulmonary artery (Blalock anastomoses), between descending aorta and left pulmonary artery (Potts), and between the proximal ascending aorta and the right pulmonary artery (Waterston) are the most well known anastomoses performed to increase pulmonary blood flow. There are many other surgical maneuvers, however, so an accurate history is invaluable when prior operations have been performed.

B. Systemic Blood Supply in Congenital Anomalies of the Lung

Agenesis, aplasia, and hypoplasia, as well as dysplasia of the lung, may be classified as developmental anomalies (Boyden, 1955; Ferencz, 1961; Felson, 1972; Currarino and Williams, 1985). By definition agenesis and aplasia have no substantial blood supply (Boyden, 1955), and failure of development of such a blood supply could be etiological. Congenital hypoplasia of one lung is of two main types (Currarino and Williams, 1985): (1) that caused by diaphragmatic hernia or other conditions limiting space available for the developing fetal lung, and (2) and that due to a primary embryological defect. Hypoplasia of a lung can be associated with an abnormal systemic blood supply, most notably in congenital absence of the right or left pulmonary artery (see earlier) and in the hypogenetic lung syndrome (scimitar syndrome). It should not be surprising that certain lung dysplasias dating from early fetal life (third to seventh weeks) may retain primitive aortopulmonary connections (MAPCA) prevailing at the time of developmental arrest.

In recent years experts in the field of congenital pulmonary anomalies have tended to regard the major clinical pulmonary anomalies as a spectrum (Gerle et al., 1968; Sade et al., 1974; Heifhoff et al., 1976; Haller et al., 1979; Thilenius et al., 1983; Rodgers et al., 1986; Clements and Warner, 1987; Panicek et al., 1987; Felson, 1988). For example, Panicek et al. (1987) defined a continuum of pulmonary developmental anomalies that included

1. Congenital lobar emphysema
2. Bronchogenic cyst
3. Congenital cystic adenomatoid malformation
4. Bronchopulmonary sequestration
5. Hypogenetic lung syndrome
6. Pulmonary arteriovenous malformation

Major aortopulmonary collateral arteries are characteristic of bronchopulmonary sequestration, are often present in the hypogenetic lung syndrome, and have been reported in a few cases of cystic adenomatoid malformation of the lung. Large systemic arteries supplying apparently normal lung parenchyma have also been documented in a number of cases (Felson, 1988). These entities follow, presented with focus upon their abnormal systemic arteries (Findlay and Maier, 1951; Rees, 1981).

Bronchopulmonary Sequestration

In 1946 and 1947, D. M. Pyrce masterfully described and named intralobar sequestration of lung, the most common of the clinically significant lung anomalies (Figs. 17, 18, and 19). He presented seven cases and found only three had been previously reported. The abnormality was twofold:

1. A large anomalous systemic artery arising from the aorta near the diaphragm, supplying a
2. Congenital bronchopulmonary dislocation (sequestration or ectopia)

The large artery, not related to any cardiac malformation, typically enters the lung via the pulmonary ligament and has an elastic wall resembling a pulmonary artery rather than a bronchial artery. The arterial distribution may be confined to the sequestered lung or may also supply adjacent lung. In addition it was recognized that such arteries sometimes supply normally connected lung without a definite bronchopulmonary sequestration (see the next section). The anomalous arteries were considered to be persistent primitive

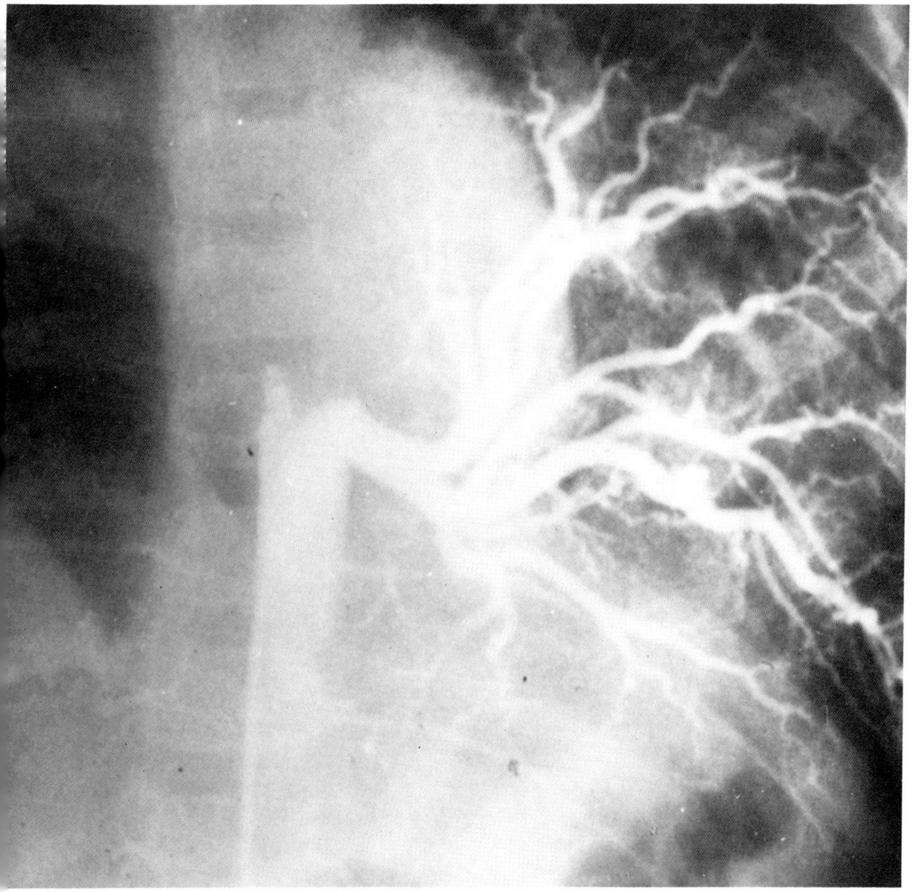

Figure 17 A major aortopulmonary collateral artery supplies a large bronchopulmonary sequestration in the left lower lobe. The contrast material is being injected into the distal discending aorta in this aortogram.

aortic branches that earlier supplied the vascular plexus surrounding the developing lung bud. Atheromatous changes are commonly noted in these arteries after infancy. The venous return is nearly always via the pulmonary veins.

A congenital bronchopulmonary sequestration is dissociated from the normal bronchial tree and is located almost always in the posterior medial lung base (posterior basal segment) somewhat more often on the left. The lung

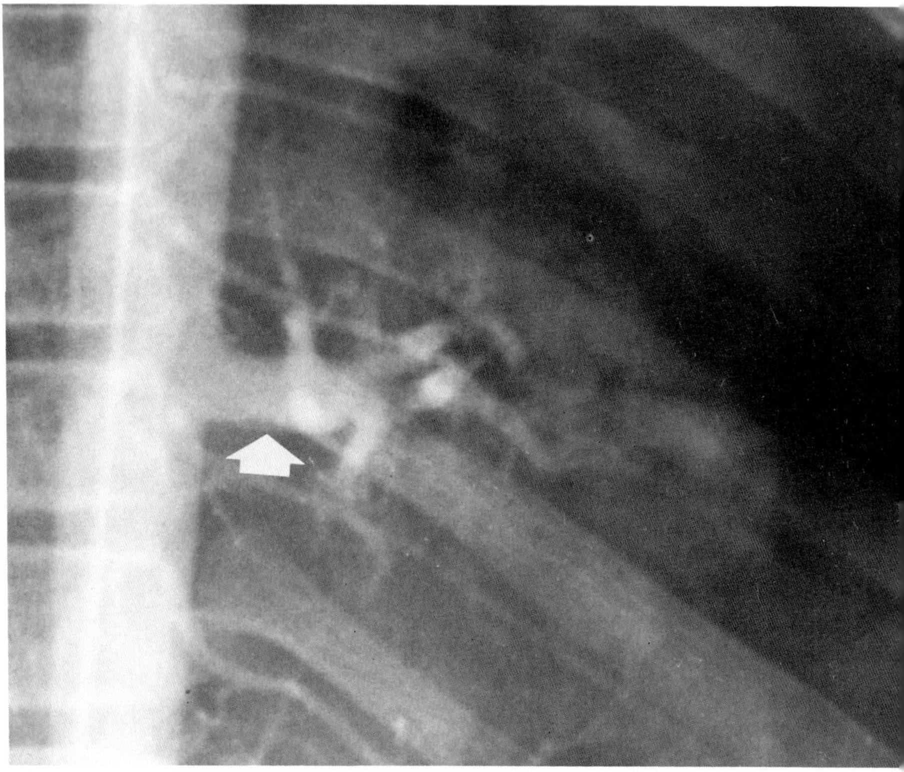

Figure 18 Retrocardiac intralobar sequestration. Aortogram showing a large systemic artery (MAPCA; arrow) arising on the left margin of the distal descending aorta to supply the sequestered lung. Several episodes of pneumonia involved the left lung base.

parenchyma of nearly all sequestrations has some cystic regions (Boyden, 1958). Sometimes single or multiple cysts predominate. Often the sequestered and therefore occluded bronchi are distended by mucus plugs. Inflammatory changes are common since infection spreading from adjacent lung tends to become chronic in these poorly draining regions. Rarely, sequestration of large regions or an entire lung may occur.

Pryce also recognized extralobar sequestrations, lung tissue separate from the normal lungs, usually comprising a mass between the lungs and the liver and often associated with diaphragmatic hernias. These anomalies were called lower accessory lungs. He noted that 40 of 43 reported cases were on the left. These extralobar sequestrations are also supplied by anomalous aortic branches and nearly always drain into the azygos system or inferior vena cava.

Pryce proposed that abnormal tension by the aberrant artery on the developing lung buds resulted in both the detachment (sequestration) and the aberrant arterial supply. Over 40 hypotheses have been proposed without widely accepted concordance on the mechanism of sequestration development, but most authrities agree that the aberrant systemic arteries represent the persistence of primitive aortic branches to the lung buds (i.e., MAPCAs).

Since 1947, many additional examples of sequestration anomalies have been reported. Fistulous connections between foregut derivatives, the stomach and the esophagus, and the sequestered lung have been documented (Gerle et al., 1968; Heithoff et al., 1976; Halasz et al., 1962). A spectrum of sequestration anomalies as well as associations with other developmental anomalies have been described.

By 1979, Savic et al. were able to review 540 reported cases, 400 of whom were intrapulmonary sequestrations. Six cases of simultaneous intra- and extrapulmonary sequestration were recorded (Pendse et al., 1972). Another six involved a whole lung, and two were bilateral. Four sequestrations were located in the right upper lobe; two others were in the left upper lobe. Of the intralobar sequestrations 4% had venous drainage to systemic instead of pulmonary veins. By 1986 (Hoeffel and Bernard, 1986), 16 upper lobe sequestrations were recorded.

In 74% of cases the aberrant artery arises from the thoracic aorta, most of the others coming from the upper abdominal aorta or its branches (Pedersen et al., 1988). The artery averages more than 6 mm in diameter (range 1–15 mm) in the intralobar sequestration and is similar in extralobar sequestrations. In 15% of cases more than one large anomalous systemic artery is present. Savic et al. showed in 1971 that the sequestered pulmonary parenchyma is not supplied by the bronchial arteries.

The first radiographic sign of a sequestration is usually a lower lung field paraspinal mass or air- or fluid-filled cavity or cyst. Aortography is the most definitive technique for establishing the presence and position of the large systemic artery. Computed tomography (Fig. 19B) (Wimbash et al., 1983) Doppler sonography, and magnetic resonance imaging have each been shown to be useful in demonstration of the abnormal artery as well as the sequestration itself. Bronchography is occasionally helpful in showing the lack of bronchial communication with a sequestration. Sequestrations, as mentioned can be bilateral (Felson, 1988; Wimbash et al., 1983; Roe et al., 1980).

Surgical treatment, usually resection, is required for most clinical complications of sequestration. Intractable infection, hemoptysis, and occasionally congestive heart failure (Ransom et al., 1978) are the most important reasons

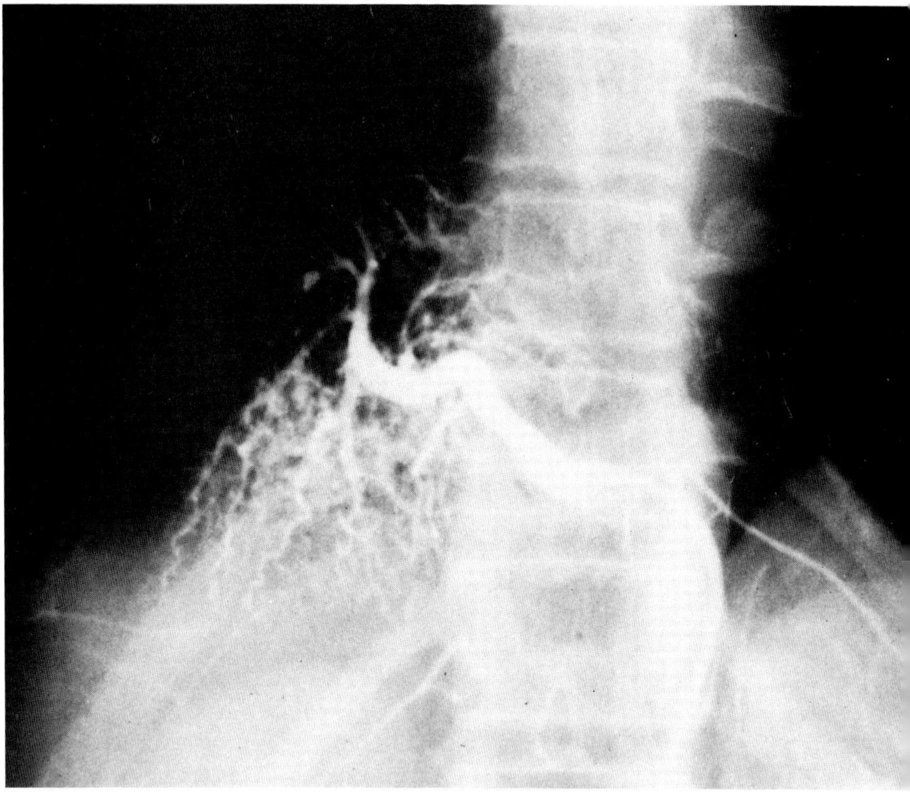

(A)

Figure 19 Right lower lobe intralobar sequestration. (A) Selective arteriogram showing a large systemic artery (MAPCA) arising from the distal descending aorta to supply

for intervention. Symptoms occur before age 10 in 37% of patients. In 4% pleural effusions are conspicuous. It is most important that the diagnosis be considered preoperatively so that the surgeon is alert to the presence of a large abnormal artery, particularly when the surgical field is likely to be obscured by extensive inflammatory changes.

Remarkably, large systemic collateral arteries have been proven to be acquired (Gebauer and Mason, 1959; Fraser and Pare, 1977; Laffey et al., 1985; Livingston et al., 1986) mainly reaching the lungs via the pulmonary ligaments, which normally carry small arteries from the aorta to the pleura (Stocker & Malczak, 1984). Large aortic branches connected to regions of chronic pulmonary infection (Webb and Jacobs, 1977), bronchiectasis, or other inflammation or to the site of a prior surgical procedure, especially in the pres-

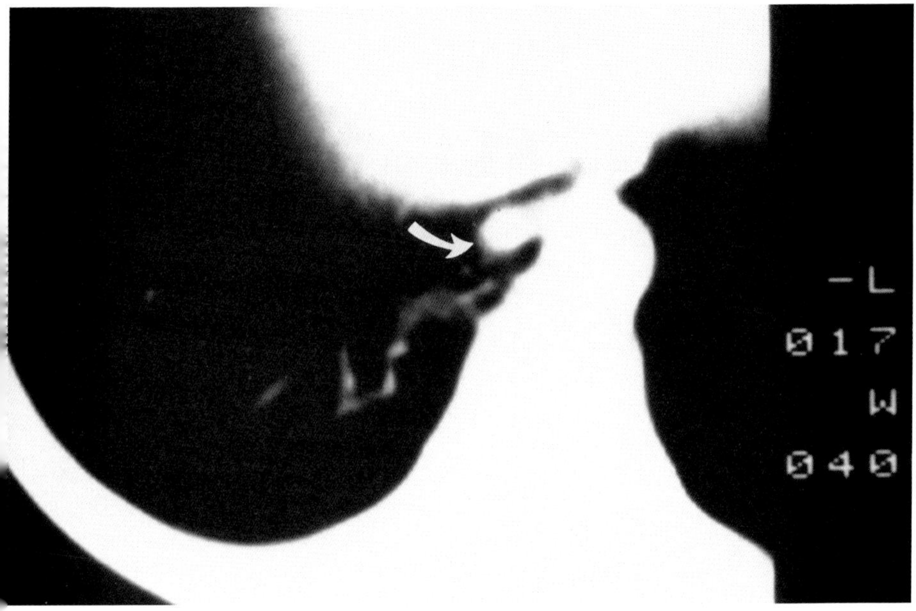

(B)

an intralobar sequestration at the right medial lung base. (B) Transaxial scan by computer tomography showing the origin of the large artery (arrow) from the distal descending aorta.

ence of cyanotic congenital heart disease, can be acquired rather than of congenital origin. These observations, together with an observed very low incidence of intralobar (compared to extralobar) sequestration in the newborn at necropsy (Stocker, 1986), have raised the question of whether intralobar sequestration is truly a developmental anomaly (Gebauer and Mason, 1959; Livingston et al., 1986; Stocker and Malczak, 1984; Webb and Jacobs, 1977). Thus, not every case in which a large aortic collateral artery is demonstrated is a congenital sequestration, especially if bronchial sequestration from the adjacent lung cannot be proven. Confusion is most likely when an acquired chronic inflammatory process is located at the posterior medial lung base, especially if abscess with air-fluid level is present. Webb and Jacobs (1977) noted that arterial collateral acquired secondary to chronic pulmonary inflammation tends to derive from enlarged inferior phrenic arteries and become a tangle of small vessels at the pleural surface instead of entering the lungs as large arteries via the pulmonary ligaments as in most sequestrations. In some instances it may be impossible to prove whether a large collateral artery is either congenital or acquired, so that the diagnosis becomes a matter of opinion. These considerations led Felson to concede that in rare cases "sequestration" is acquired (Felson, 1988).

Some such large acquired arteries have been shown to have regressed somewhat after successful treatment of the inflammatory disease (Botenga, 1968). Whether the large artery is a component of congenital sequestration or acquired pathology, surgical precautions are warranted. Aortography should be considered before surgical exploration of suspect lesions.

Anomalous Systemic Arterial Supply to Apparently Normal Lung

A number of cases, about 50, have been reported in whom a large systemic artery arising from the descending thoracic or upper abdominal aorta or branches, such as celiac or inferior phrenic, supplied apparently normal lung parenchyma (Fig. 20) (Hessel et al., 1970; Litwin et al., 1970; Currarino et al., 1975; Clarke et al., 1976; Kirks et al., 1976; Hofschire et al., 1976; Macpherson and Whytehead, 1977; Yabek et al., 1981; Flisak et al., 1982; Gay et al., 1983; Pernot et al., 1988; Levine et al., 1982). In some cases the arterial supply was accessory since the normal pulmonary arteries were present and functional. In other cases the systemic artery was exclusively supplied the pulmonary arteries of a region of lung. The venous drainage in virtually all cases was via the pulmonary veins to the left atrium. Currarino et al. (1975) distinguish cases with and without congenital fistulas between the aberrant systemic artery and the pulmonary veins. A fistula is strongly suggested by the rapid flow in certain patients. Little detailed anatomic study, however, of these rare cases has been possible for the demonstration of the partially semantic difference between a fistulous malformation and an unusually dilated compliant regional pulmonary vascular bed.

Most patients are asymptomatic, but flow can be large enough to precipitate congestive heart failure. Continuous or systolic-diastolic machinery-type murmurs are common. The basal regions of the lower lobes are most often involved, but any part of the lung can apparently be affected. For example, a 4-year-old girl had a large accessory systemic artery supplying the right upper lobe (Hofschire et al., 1976). The artery was excised from its origin on the right side of the middescending aorta to its branching in the parenchyma of the lung and was found histologically to be a normal elastic artery. Most authors have considered these large systemic arteries as equivalent to the major aorto-pulmonary collateral arteries that have persisted from the time of the primitive splanchnic plexus supply to the lung in early fetal life.

In some patients the anomalous systemic arteries (MAPCA) are the only pulmonary arterial supply to the involved lung region. Treatment of these cases can be either by transfer of the arterial origin to the central pulmonary

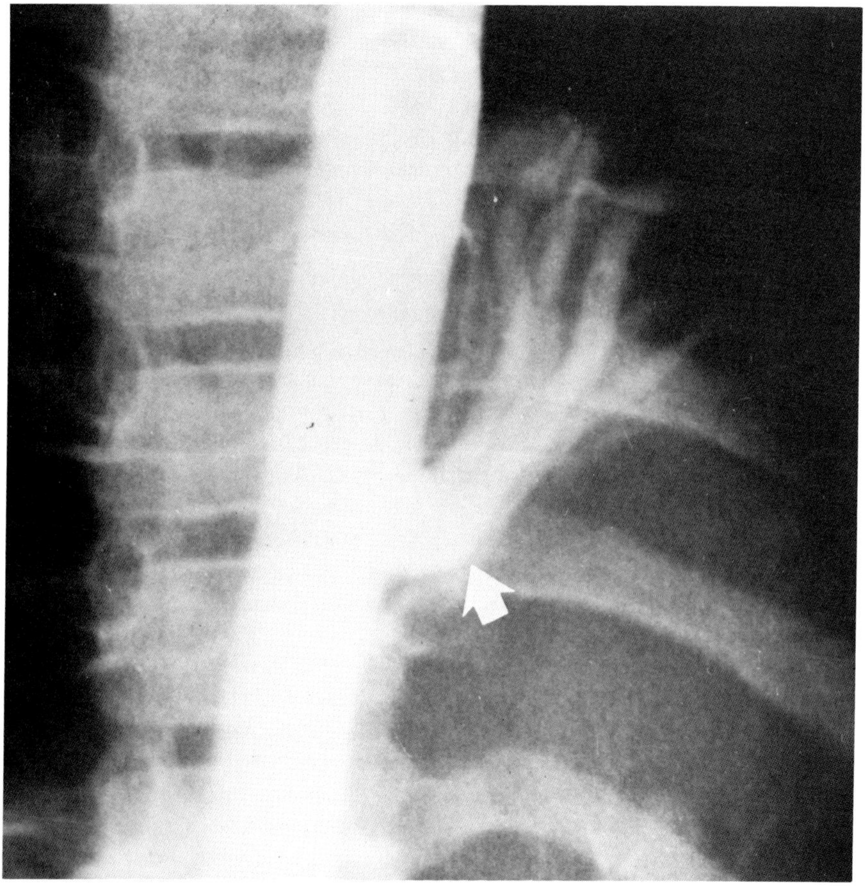

Figure 20 Anomalous major aortopulmonary collateral artery (arrow) to apparently normal lung. Asymptomatic. Bronchogram and pulmonary pressures and oxygen saturations were all normal.

artery or by resection. A 6-year-old boy had the origin of a large systemic artery supplying the basal segments of the left lower lobe successfully transferred to the native left pulmonary artery (Hessel et al., 1970). On the other hand, congestive heart failure in a 6-month-old girl with large MAPCA supplying the left lower lobe was successfully treated by lobectomy (Yabek et al., 1981). In another example, right lower lobectomy was required for treatment of a 10 mm diameter branch of the celiac axis that profusely supplied the basilar segments in a 26-year-old woman with hemoptysis and dyspnea on exertion (Flisak et al., 1982). Bilateral anomalous arteries with congestive heart failure have been reported (Gay et al., 1983).

The cause for the persistence of these remnants of the apparent embryonic arterial circulation is not known. These rare cases are probably best regarded as a mild form of the process that, when more severe, can cause sequestration of both bronchial and arterial supplies to the lung.

Hypogenetic Lung Syndrome (Scimitar Syndrome)

The "scimitar" image (Figs. 21, 22, and 23) (Neill et al., 1960), resembling a Turkish sword, is produced on the frontal chest radiography by an anomalous pulmonary vein draining all or part of the right lung into the inferior vena cava just above or below the diaphragm (Fig. 21) (Halasz et al., 1956; Neill et al., 1960; Kiely et al., 1967; Folger, 1976). A large anomalous systemic artery (MAPCA) arising from the lower thoracic or upper abdominal aorta often supplies at least the basal part of the maldeveloped right lung (Figs. 21 and 22). The right lung is to a variable degree malformed and hypoplastic, most commonly with only two lobes and a hyparterial bronchus thus resembling an anatomic left lung. Other anomalies, such as bronchial cysts or diverticula, hemivertebrae, horseshoe lung (Kiely et al., 1967; Folger, 1976; Dische et al., 1974), accessory diaphragm, and diaphragm hernia, are associated. Dextrocardia secondary to the hypoplastic right lung may be marked (Alivizatos et al., 1985). About a quarter of the patients have congenital heart disease, most often an atrial septal defect (Kiely et al., 1967). The right pulmonary artery is usually smaller than normal, and the pulmonary blood flow is smaller than expected so that symptoms due to the abnormal pulmonary venous connection are uncommon. Symptoms due to acute or chronic right lung infection are not unusual. A spectrum of variations occur with each feature of the scimitar syn-

There seems to be wide agreement that the large systemic artery arising from the lower descending aorta represents persistence of one of the primitive aortic branches supplying the postbranchial plexus about the developing lung bud. If surgery is required for the anomalous vein or associated heart or lung disease, an aortogram is desirable to search for an anomalous artery. Several cases have been shown to have a bronchopulmonary sequestration in association with the scimitar syndrome (Thilenius et al., 1983; Panicek et al., 1987; Halasz et al., 1962; Alivizatos et al., 1985), although the definition of sequestration has not been uniform. Total right lung ectoplasia (Masaoka et al., 1979) or sequestration with systemic arterial supply and venous drainage into the azygos system may represent an extreme form of hypogenetic lung syndrome.

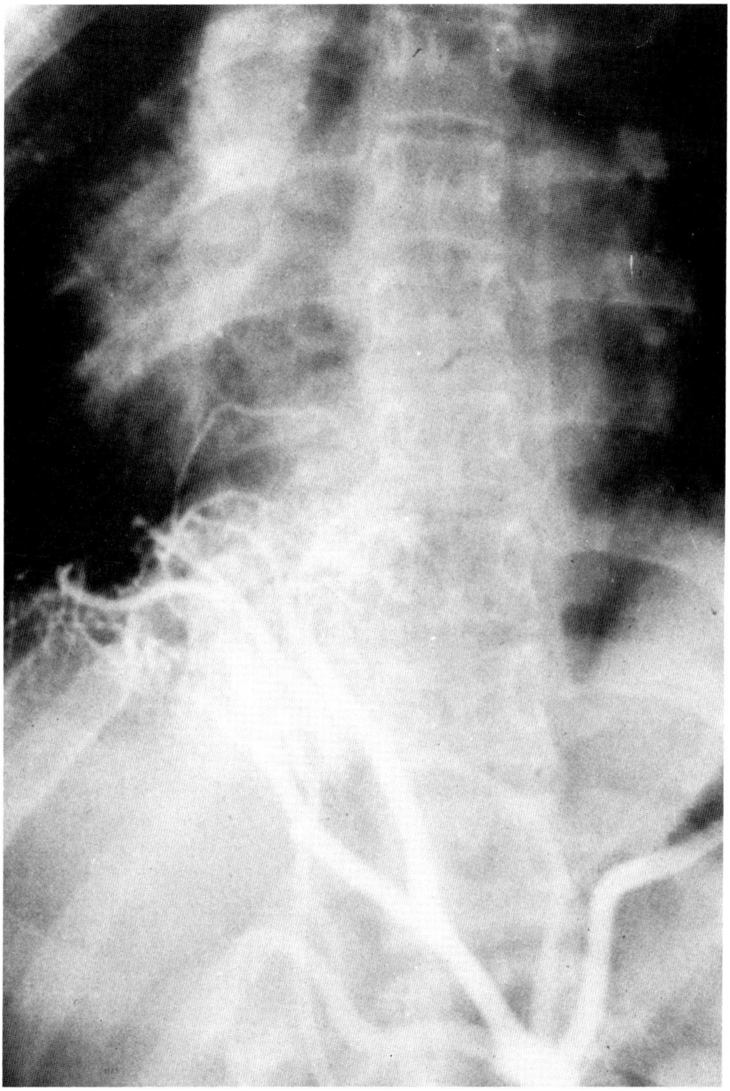

Figure 21 Scimitar syndrome, hypogenetic lung syndrome. Selective arteriogram showing a large major aortopulmonary collateral artery arising from the upper abdominal aorta and supplying the lower right lung. Note the dextrocardia secondary to the small right lung. The venous drainage was into the pulmonary veins. (From Ellis, 1991, with permission.)

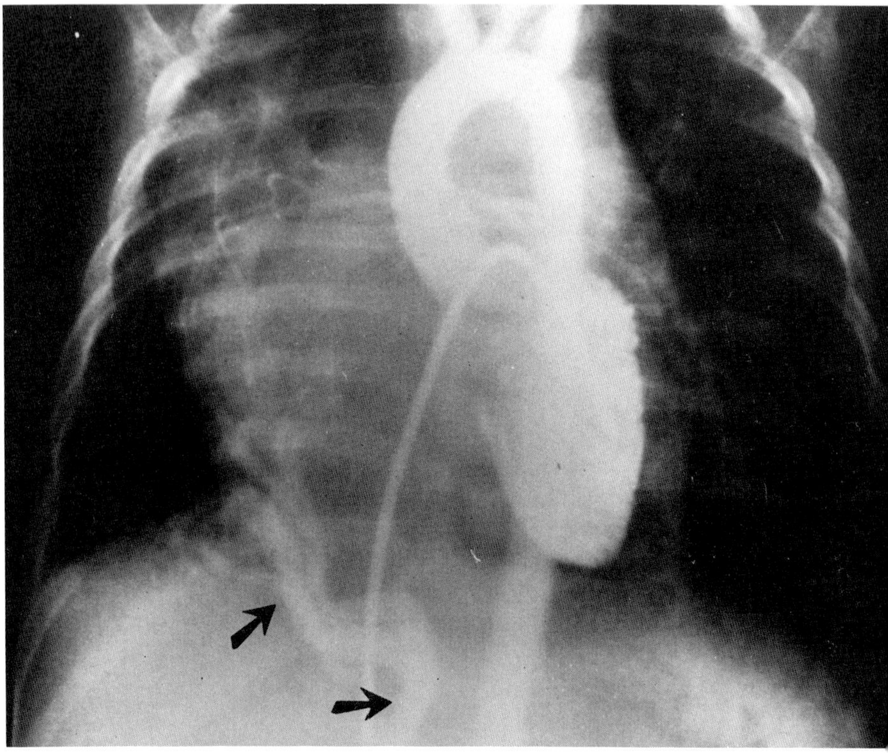

Figure 22 Scimitar syndrome, hypogenetic lung syndrome. This left ventricular angiocardiogram shows an opacified left ventricle and aorta with large arterial branch from below the diaphragm supplying the lower right lung (arrows).

Congenital Cystic Adenomatoid Malformation of the Lung

A few cases of cystic congenital adenomatoid malformations have been descrbed in which an associated large aortic branch (MAPCA) contributed to the blood supply of the malformation (Panicek et al., 1987; Hutchin et al., 1971). Apparently three examples have been noted in well over 200 reported cases. An additional case had a bronchopulmonary sequestration in the other lung. Typically, part or all of a lobe is involved; occasionally multiple lobes or a whole lung is affected. Two cases with bilateral disease are reported.

Described in 1949, the main histological feature is overgrowth of the terminal respiratory structures with development of varying sizes of cystic spaces lined with "adenomatoid" proliferation of cuboidal or ciliated columnar

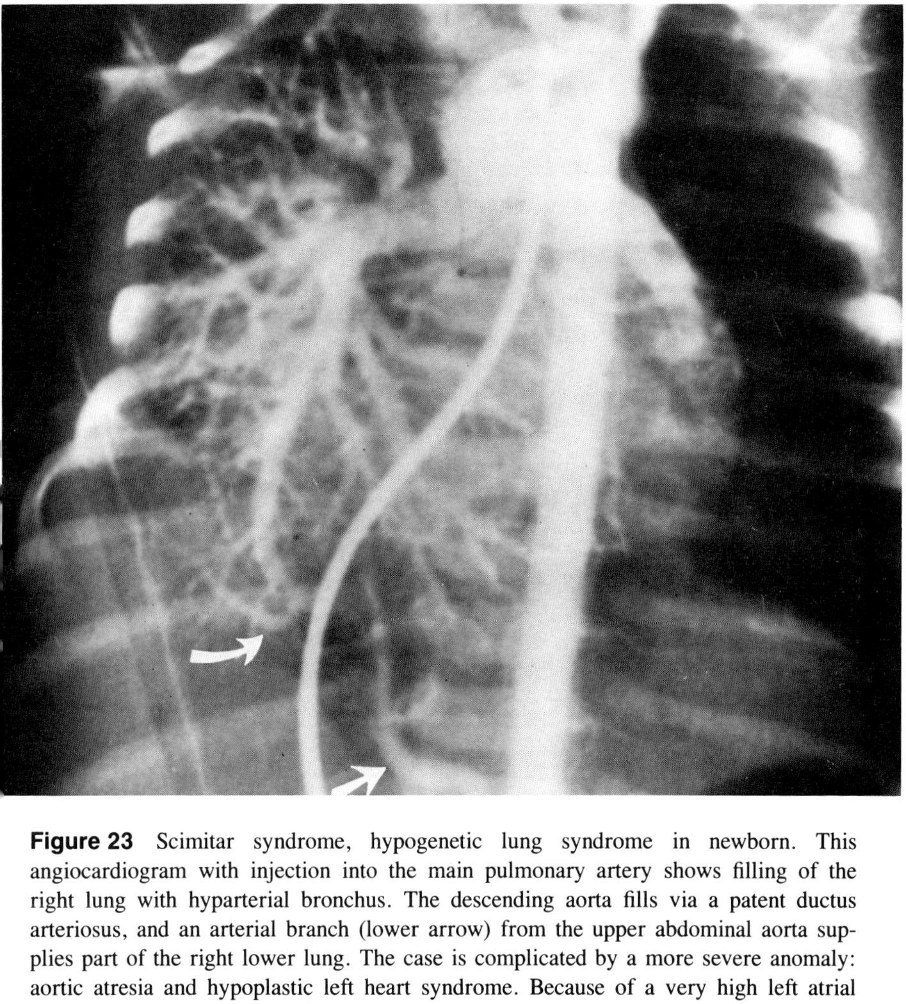

Figure 23 Scimitar syndrome, hypogenetic lung syndrome in newborn. This angiocardiogram with injection into the main pulmonary artery shows filling of the right lung with hyparterial bronchus. The descending aorta fills via a patent ductus arteriosus, and an arterial branch (lower arrow) from the upper abdominal aorta supplies part of the right lower lung. The case is complicated by a more severe anomaly: aortic atresia and hypoplastic left heart syndrome. Because of a very high left atrial pressure there is very slow flow in the left lung, but the right lung draining into the inferior vena cava (not shown) does not have venous obstruction and thus flow via the right lung is relatively large. The sharp turn of the branch pulmonary artery (curved arrow) in the right lower lung is a consequence of lung deformity caused by an accessory diaphragm.

epithelium (Madewell et al., 1975; Miller et al., 1980). Cartilage does not develop in the cystic parenchyma. The majority of lesions are cystic with either single or multiple gross cysts; a few are mostly solid, with the others intermediate.

Clinically the disease usually presents in a child with cough, fever, and recurrent respiratory infections or in a newborn with respiratory distress. Only rarely is the diagnosis first made in an adult. Radiographically, multicystic spaces, some with air-fluid levels, compressing adjacent lung and shifting the mediastinum suggest the diagnosis. In the newborn the cystic spaces may be filled with fluid and appear as large or multiple masses. Angiography of the pulmonary arteries and aorta is advocated by some, especially when the preoperative differential diagnosis includes pulmonary sequestration.

Other Abnormal Systemic Arterial Connections in Congenital Lung Disease

A number of very unusual vascular connections to the pulmonary arteries have been reported (Brain and Kauntze, 1960; Good, 1961; Syme, 1973; Dines et al., 1974; Burke et al., 1986). Congenital pulmonary arteriovenous fistulas with a systemic arterial supply from the chest wall are extremely rare.

References

Alivizatos, P., Cheatle, T., DeLaval, M., and Stark, J. (1985). Pulmonary sequestration complicated by anomalies of venous return. *J. Pediatr. Surg.* **20**:76–79.

Allanby, R. D., Brinton, W. D., Campbell, M., and Gardner, F. (1950). Pulmonary atresia and the collateral circulation to the lungs. *Guy's Hosp. Rep.* **99**:110–152.

Anderson, R. C., Char, F., and Adams, P. Jr. (1958). Proximal interruption of a pulmonary arch (absence of one pulmonary artery). Case report and a new embryologic interpretation. *Dis. Chest* **34**:73–86.

Aziz, K. U., Paul, M. H., and Rowe, R. D. (1977). Bronchopulmonary circulation in d-transposition of the great arteries: Possible role in genesis of accelerated pulmonary vascular disease. *Am. J. Cardiol.* **39**:432–438.

Bahler, R. C., Carson, P., Traks, E., Levine, A., and Gillepsie, D. (1969). Absent right pulmonary artery. *Am. J. Med.* **46**:64–71.

Baim, D. S., Kline, H., and Silverman, J. F. (1982). Bilateral coronary artery-pulmonary artery fistulas. Report of five cases and review of the literature. *Circulation* **65**:810–815.

Barrett, W. R., and Daley, R. (1949). A method of increasing the lung blood supply in cyanotic congenital heart disease. *Br. Med. J.* **1**:699–702.

Beitzke, R., and Shinebourne, E. A. (1980). Single origin of right and left pulmonary arteries from ascending aorta, with main pulmonary artery from right ventricle. *Br. Heart J.* **43**:363–365.

Benatar, A., Kinsley, R. H., Milner, S., Dansky, R., Hummel, D. A., and

Levin, S. E. (1987). Surgical correction for one pulmonary artery arising from ascending aorta—report of five cases. *Int. J. Cardiol.* **16**:249–255.

Berry, J. L. (1935). The relation between bronchial and pulmonary circulations in the human lung, investigated by radiopague injections. *Q. J. Exp. Physiol.* **24**:305–315.

Bharati, S., Paul, M. H., Idriss, F. S., Potkin, R. T., and Lev, M. (1975). The surgical anatomy of pulmonary atresia with ventricular septal defect: Pseudotruncus. *J. Thorac. Cardiovasc. Surg.* **69**:713–721.

Bjork, L. (1966). Anastomoses between the coronary and the bronchial arteries. *Acta Radiol. (Diagn.)* **4**:93–96.

Blackstone, E. H., Shimazaki, Y., Machara, T., Kirklin, J. W., and Bargeron, L. M., Jr. (1988). Prediction of severe obstruction to the right ventricular outflow after repair of tetralogy of Fallot and pulmonary atresia. *J. Thorac. Cardiovasc. Surg.* **96**:288–293.

Botenga, A. S. J. (1968). The role of bronchopulmonary anastomoses in chronic inflammatory processes in the lung. *AJR* **104**:829–839.

Boyden, E. A. (1955). Developmental anomalies of the lungs. *Am. J. Surg.* **89**:79–89.

Boyden, E. A. (1958). Bronchogenic cysts and the theory of intralobar sequestration: New embryologic data. *J. Thorac. Surg.* **35**:604–616.

Boyden, E. A. (1970a). The developing bronchial arteries in a fetus of the twelfth week. *Am. J. Anat.* **129**:357–368.

Boyden, E. A. (1970b). Time lag in the development of bronchial arteries. *Anat. Rec.* **166**:611–614.

Brain, R., and Kauntze, ? (1960). Systemic-pulmonary arteriovenous aneurysm of chest wall and lung. *Guy's Hosp. Rep.* **109**:110–115.

Brown, R. T., and Fellows, K. E. (1988). Cervical collateral arteries in pulmonary atresia with ventricular septal defet. *Am. J. Cardiol.* **62**:1310–1311.

Buchler, J. R., Jatene, A. D., and deAndrade, J. (1986). Congenital unilateral absence of the right pulmonary artery and complex of Fallot. A rare association. *Jpn. Heart J.* **27**:885–892.

Burke, C. M., Safai, C., Nelson, D. P., and Raffin, T. A. (1986). Pulmonary arteriovenous malformations: A critical update. *Am. Rev. Respir. Dis.* **134**:334–339.

Campbell, M., and Gardner, F. (1950). Radiological features of enlarged bronchial arteries. *Br. Heart J.* **12**:183–200.

Cassels, D., Bharati, S., and Lev, M. (1975). The natural history of the ductus arteriosus in association with other congenital cardiac defects. *Perspect. Biol. Med.* **Summer**:541–572.

Cauldwell, E. W., Siekert, R. G., Lininger, R. E., and Anson, B. J. (1951).

The bronchial arteries—an anatomic study of 150 human cadavers. *Surg. Gynecol. Obstet.* **86**:395–412.

Chesler, E., Beck, W., and Schrire, V. (1970). Selective catheterization of pulmonary or bronchial arteries in the preoperative assessment of pseudotruncus arteriosus and truncus arteriosus type IV. *Am. J. Cardiol.* **26**:20–24.

Chesler, E., Matisonn, R., and Beck, W. (1974). The assessment of the arterial supply to the lungs in pseudotruncus arteriosus and truncus arteriosus type IV in relation to surgical repair. *Am. Heart J.* **88**:542–552.

Clarke, C. P., Goh, T. A., Blackwood, A., and Venables, A. W. (1976). Massive pulmonary arteriovenous fistula in the newborn. *Br. Heart J.* **38**:1092–1095.

Clements, B. S., and Warner, J. P. (1987). Pulmonary sequestration and related congenital bronchopulmonary-vascular malformations: Nomenclature and classification based on anatomical and embryological considerations. *Thorax* **42**:401–408.

Cobanoglu, A., Abbtuzzese, P., Brauner, B., Ferre, B., Issenberg, H., and Starr, A. (1984). Therapeutic considerations in congenital absence of right pulmonary artery. Use of internal mammary as a preparatory shunt. *J. Cardiovasc. Surg. (Torino)* **25**:241–245.

Congdon, E. D. (1922). Transformation of the aortic-arch system during development of the human embryo. *Carnegie Inst. Contrib. Embryol.* **14**:47–110.

Cudkowitz, L. (1979). Bronchial arterial circulation in man. Normal anatomy and responses to disease. In *Pulmonary Vascular Disease.* Edited by K. M. Moser. New York, Marcel Dekker, Chap. 2, pp. 111–232.

Cumming, G. R., Ferguson, C. C., and Sanchez, J. (1972). Aortic origin of the right pulmonary artery. *Am. J. Cardiol.* **30**:674–679.

Currarino, G., and Williams, B. (1985). Causes of congenital unilateral pulmonary hypoplasia: A study of 33 cases. *Pediatr. Radiol.* **15**:15–24.

Currarino, G., Willis, K., and Miller, W. (1975). Congenital fistula between aberrant systemic artery and a pulmonary vein without sequestration. *J. Pediatr.* **87**:554–557.

Dark, J. H., and Pollock, J. C. S. (1985). Coronary artery-pulmonary artery fistula in tetralogy of Fallot with pulmonary atresia. *Eur. Heart J.* **6**:714–716.

Davis, G. D., Fulton, R. E., Ritter, D. G., Mair, D. D., and McGoon, D. W. (1978). Congenital pulmonary atresia with ventricular septal defect: Angiographic and surgical correlates. *Radiology* **128**:133–144.

Deffebach, M. E., Charan, N. B., Lakshminarayam, S., and Butler, J. (1987). The bronchial circulation. *Am. Rev. Respir. Dis.* **135**:463–481.

Diaz-Gongora, G., Quero-Jiminez, M., Espino-Vela, J., Arteaga, M., and Bargeron, L. M., Jr. (1982). A heart with three arterial trunks (tritruncal heart). Report of a case. *Pediatr. Cardiol.* **3**:293–299.

Diethelm, E., Soto, B., Nath, P. H., Bargeron, L. M., Jr., and Kirlkin, J. K. (1985). The pulmonary vascularity in patients with pulmonary atresia and ventricular septal defect. *Radiographics* **5**:243–254.

Dines, D. E., Arms, R. A., Bernatz, P. E., and Gomes, M. R. (1974). Pulmonary arteriovenous fistulas. *Mayo Clin. Proc.* **49**:460–465.

Dische, M. R., Teixeira, M. L., Winchester, P. H., and Engle, M. A. (1974). Horseshoe lung associated with a variant of the "scimitar" syndrome. *Br. Heart J.* **36**:617.

Edwards, J. E., and McGoon, D. C. (1973). Absence of anatomic origin from heart of pulmonary arterial supply. *Circulation* **47**:393–398.

Ellis, K. (1991). Fleischner Lecture: Developmental abnormalities in the systemic blood supply to the lungs. *AJR* **156**:669–679.

Ellis, K., Seaman, W. B., Griffiths, S. P., Berdon, W. F., and Baker, D. H. (1967). Some congenital anomalies of the pulmonary arteries. *Semin. Roentgenol.* **2**:325–341.

Elzenga, N. J., and Gittenberger-de Groot, A. C. (1986). The ductus arteriosus and stenoses of the pulmonary arteries in pulmonary atresia. *Int. J. Cardiol.* **11**:195–208.

Faller, K., Haworth, S. G., Taylor, J. F. W., and Mccartney, F. J. (1981). Duplicate sources of pulmonary blood supply in pulmonary atresia with ventricular septal defect. *Br. Heart J.* **46**;263–268.

Felson, B. (1972). Pulmonary agenesis and related anomalies. *Semin. Roentgenol.* **7**:17–30.

Felson, B. (1988). Pulmonary sequestration revisited. *Med. Radiogr. Photogr.* **64**:1–27.

Ferencz, C. (1961). Congenital anomalies of the pulmonary vessels and their relationship to malformations of the lung. *Pediatrics* **28**:993–1010.

Ferguson, A., Belleau, R., and Gaensler, E. A. (1969). Congenital absence of one pulmonary artery. *Respiration* **26**:300–312.

Findlay, C. W., Jr., and Maier, H. C. (1951). Anomalies of the pulmonary vessels and their surgical significance, with a review of the literature. *Surgery* **29**:604–641.

Flisak, M. E., Chandrasekar, A. J., Marsan, R. E., and Ali, M. M. (1982). Systemic arterialization of lung without sequestration. *AJR* **138**:751–753.

Folger, G. M. (1976). The scimitar syndrome: Anatomic, physiologic, developmental and therapeutic considerations. *Angiology* **27**:373–407.

Fraser, R. G., and Pare, J. A. P. (1977). *Diagnosis of Diseases of the Chest,* Vol. I, 2nd Ed. Philadelphia, W. B. Saunders, p. 649.

Freedom, R. M., Williams, W. G., Trusler, G. A., Moss, C. A., and Rowe, R. D. (1983). Pulmonary vein wedge angiography: Indication, results and surgical correlates in 25 patients. *Am. J. Cardiol.* **51**:936–941.

Freedom, R. M., Moes, C. A. F., Pelech, A., Smallhorn, J., Rabinovitch, M., Olley, P. M., Williams, W. G., Trusler, G. A., and Rowe, R. D. (1984). Bilateral ductus arteriosis (or remnant): An analysis of 27 patients. *Am. J. Cardiol.* **53**:884–891.

Frescura, C., Talenti, E., Pellegraino, P. A., Mazzuco, A., Faggian, G., and Thiene, G. (1984). Coexistence of ductal and systemic pulmonary arterial supply in pulmonary atresia with ventricular septal defect. *Am. J. Cardiol.* **53**:348–349.

Gay, B B., Jr., Atkinson, G. O., Jr., Ball, T. I., Edwards, K., and Vandersalm, D. (1983). Systemic arterial supply to normal pulmonary parenchyma. Pediatric case of the day. *AJR* **140**:1016–1018.

Gebauer, P. W., and Mason, C. B. (1959). Intralobar pulmonary sequestration associated with anomalous pulmonary vessels: A nonentity. *Chest* **345**:282–288.

Gerle, R. D., Jaretzki, A., III, Ashley, C. A., and Berne, A. S. (1968). Congenital bronchopulmonary-foregut malformation. *N. Engl. J. Med.* **278**:1413–1419.

Goldstein, J. D., Rabinovitch, M., Van Praagh, R., and Reid, L. (1979). Unusual vascular anomalies causing persistent pulmonary hypertension in a newborn. *Am. J. Cardiol.* **43**:962–968.

Good, C. A. (1961). Certain vascular abnormalities of the lungs. Hickey Lecture 1961. *AJR* **85**:1009–1024.

Green, G. E., Reppert, E. H., Cohlan, S. Q., and Spencer, F. C. (1963). Surgical correction of absence of proximal segment of left pulmonary artery. *Circulation* **37**:62–end.

Griffiths, S. P., Levine, O. R., and Anderson, D. H. (1962). Aortic origin of the right pulmonary artery. *Circulation* **25**:73–84.

Grillo, R., Pipstone, S., Piero, D., Spataro, G., Basile, G., and Sperandeo, V. (1986). Clinical and angiocardiographic observations on the so-called absence of a branch of the pulmonary artery. *G. Ital. Cardiol.* **16**:1027–1031.

Hackett, P., Creagh, C. E., Grover, R. F., Honigman, B., Houston, C. S., Reeves, J. T., Sophocles, P. M., and Van Hardenboeck, M. (1980). High altitude pulmonary edema in patients without the right pulmonary artery. *N. Engl. J. Med.* **302**:1070–1073.

Halasz, N. A., Halloran, K. H., and Liebow, A. A. (1956). Bronchial and arterial anomalies with drainage of the right lung into the inferior vena cava. *Circulation* **14**:826–846.

Halasz, N. A., Lindskog, G. E., and Liebow, A. A. (1962). Esophagobronchial fistula and bronchopulmonary sequestration. *Ann. Surg.* **155**:215–220.

Hales, M. R., and Liebow, A. A. (1948). Collateral circulation to the lungs in congenital pulmonary stenosis. *Bull. Int. Assoc. Med. Museums* **28**:1–22.

Haller, J. A., Golladay, E. S., Pickard, L. R., Tepas, J. J., III, Shorter, N. A., and Shermeta, D. W. (1979). Surgical management of lung bud anomalies: Lobar emphysema, bronchogenic cyst, cystic adenomatoid malformation and intralobar pulmonary sequestration. *Ann. Thorac. Surg.* **28**:33–43.

Haroutunian, L. M., and Neill, C. A. (1972). Pulmonary pseudofibrosis in cyanotic heart disease: A clinical syndrome mimicking tuberculosis in patients with extreme pulmonary stenosis. *Chest* **62**:587–592.

Haworth, S. G., and Macartney, F. J. (1983). In *Pediatric Cardiology*. Edited by R. H. Anderson, F. J. Macartney, E. A. Shinebourne, and M. Tynan. New York, Churchill Livingston, Chap. 10, pp. 102–110.

Haworth, S. G., DeLaval, M., and Macartney, F. J. (1981). Hypoperfusion and hyperperfusion in the immature lung. *J. Thorac. Cardiovasc. Surg.* **82**:281–292.

Heithoff, K. B., Sane, S. M., Williams, H. J., Jarvis, C. J., Carter, J., Kane, P., and Brennom, W. (1976). Bronchopulmonary foregut malformations: A unifying etiological concept. *AJR* **126**:46.

Hessel, E. A., II, Boyden, E. A., Stamm, S. J., and Sauvagc, L. R. (1970). High systemic origin of the sole artery to the basal segments of the left lung: Findings, surgical treatment, and embryologic interpretation. *Surgery* **67**:624–632.

Heymann, M. A., and Rudolph, A. M. (1972). Effects of congenital heart disease on fetal and neonatal circulation. In *Neonatal Heart Disease*. Edited by W. F. Friedman, M. Leach, and E. M. Sonnenblick. New York, Grune and Stratton, p. 70.

Hislop, A., Sanderson, M., and Reid, L. (1973). Unilateral congenital dysplasia of lung associated with vascular anomalies. *Thorax* **28**:435–441.

Hoeffel, J., and Bernard, C. (1986). Pulmonary sequestration of the upper lobe in children. *Radiology* **160**:513–514.

Hofschire, P. J., Todd, E. P., Varro, R. L., Kaplan, E. L., and Edwards, J. E. (1976). Anomalous double blood supply to the lung. *Chest* **69**:439–441.

Hruda, J., and Julsrud, P. R. (1989). Diagnostic selective balloon occlusion technique in pulmonic valve atresia and ventricular septal defect. *Am. J. Cardiol.* **63**:1408–1409.

Hubsch, P., Pichler, W., Lang, I., and Miczoch, J. (1987). Isolated agenesis of the right pulmonary artery with late manifestation of pulmonary artery hypertension. *Roentgenblatler* **40**:23–25.

Huntington, G. S. (1919). The morphology of the pulmonary artery in the mammalia. *Anat. Rec.* **17**:165–201.

Hutchin, P., Friedman, P. J., and Saltstein, S. L. (1971). Congenital cystic adenomatoid malformation with anomalous blood supply. *J. Thorac. Cardiovasc. Surg.* **62**:220–225.

Hutchins, G. M. (1971). Coarctation of the aorta explained as a branch-point of the ductus arteriosus. *Am. J. Pathol.* **63**:203–214.

Jefferson, K., Rees, S., and Somerville, J. (1972). Systemic arterial supply to the lungs in pulmonary atresia and its relation to pulmonary artery development. *Br. Heart J.* **34**:418–427.

Johnson, R. J., Sauer, U., Buhlmeyer, K., and Haworth, S. G. (1985). Hypoplasia of the intrapulmonary arteries in children with right ventricular outflow tract obstruction, ventricular septal defect and major aortopulmonary collateral arteries. *Pediatr. Cardiol.* **6**:137–143.

Kauffman, S. L., Yao, A. C., Webber, C. B., and Lynfield, J. (1967). Origin of right pulmonary artery from the aorta. *Am. J. Cardiol.* **19**:741–748.

Kersting-Sommerhoff, B. A., Sechtein, V. P., and Higgins, C. B. (1988). Evaluation of pulmonary blood supply by nuclear magnetic resonance imaging in patients with pulmonary atresia. *J. Am. Coll. Cardiol.* **11**:166–171.

Kieffer, S. A., Amplatz, K., Anderson, R. C., and Lillehei, C. W. (1965). Proximal interruption of a pulmonary artery. *AJR* **95**:592–597.

Kiely, B., Filler, J., Stone, S., and Doyle, E. F. (1967). Syndrome of anomalous venous drainage of the right lung to the inferior vena cava. *Am. J. Cardiol.* **20**:102–116.

Kirklin, J. W., Bargeron, L. M., Jr., and Pacifico, A. D. (1977). The enlargement of small pulmonary arteries by preliminary palliative procedures. *Circulation* **56**:612–617.

Kirklin, J. W., Blackstone, E. H., Shimazaki, Y., Machara, T., Pacifico, A. D., Kirklin, J. K., and Bargeron, L. M. (1988). Survival, functional status, and reoperation after repair of tetralogy of Fallot with pulmonary atresia. *J. Thorac. Cardiovasc. Surg.* **96**:102–116.

Kirks, D. R., Kane, P. E., Free, E. A., and Taybi, H. (1976). Systemic arterial supply to normal basilar segments of left lower lobe. *AJR* **126**:817–821.

Krongrad, E., Ritter, D. G., Hawe, A., Kincaid, O. W., and McGoon, D. C. (1972). Pulmonary atresia or severe stenosis and coronary to pulmonary artery fistula. *Circulation* **46**:1005–1012.

Krongrad, E., Ritter, D. G., and Kincaid, O. W. (1973). Aorticopulmonary tunnel: Angiographic recognition of pulmonary atresia and coronary artery-to-pulmonary artery fistula. *AJR* **119**:498–502.

Kucera, V., Fiser, B., Tuma, B., and Hucin, B. (1982). Unilateral absence of pulmonary artery: A report of 19 selected clinical cases. *Thorac. Cardiovasc. Surg.* **30**:152–158.

Kumar, A., Sharma, S., Desai, A., and Hansoti, R. C. (1984). Absent right pulmonary artery with atrial septal defect. *Am. Heart J.* **108**:1037–1038.

Kutsche, L. M., and Van Mierop, L. H. S. (1988). Anomalous origin of a pulmonary artery from the ascending aorta: Associated anomalies and pathogenesis. *Am. J. Cardiol.* **61**:850–856.

Laffey, K. J., Thomashow, B., Jaretzki, A., III, and Martin, E. C. (1985). Systemic supply to pulmonary arteriovenous malformation: A relative contraindication to surgery. *AJR* **145**:720–722.

Lenox, C. C., Neches, W. H., Zuberbuhler, J. K., Park, S. C., Mathews, R. A., Siewers, R. D., Lerberg, D. B., and Bahnson, H. T. (1977). Management of bilateral ductus arteriosus in complex congenital heart disease. *J. Thorac. Cardiovasc. Surg.* **74**:607–613.

Levin, D. C., Baltaxe, H. A., Goldberg, H. P., Engle, M. A., Ebert, P. A., Sos, T. A., and Levin, A. R. (1974). The importance of selective angiography of the systemic arterial to the lungs in planning surgical correction of pseudotruncus arteriosus. *Am. J. Roentgenol.* **121**:606–613.

Levine, M., Nudel, D. B., Gootman, N., Wolpowitz, A., and Wisoff, B. G. (1982). Pulmonary sequestration causing failure in infancy: A report of two cases and review of the literature. *Ann. Thorac. Surg.* **34**:581–585.

Liao, P., Edwards, W. D., Julsrud, P. R., Puga, F. J., Danielson, G. K., and Feldt, R. H. (1985). Pulmonary blood supply in patients with pulmonary atresia and ventricular septal defect. *J. Am. Coll. Cardiol.* **6**:1343–1415.

Liebow, A. A. (1965). Patterns of origin and distribution of the major bronchial arteries in man. *Am. J. Anat.* **117**:19–32.

Liebow, A. A., Hales, M. R., and Lindskog, G. E. (1949). Enlargement of the bronchial arteries and their anastomoses with the pulmonary arteries in bronchiectasis. *Am. J. Pathol.* **25**:211–232.

Liebow, A. A., Hales, M. R., Bloomer, W. E., Harrison, W., and Lindskog, G. E. (1950). Studies of the lung after ligation of the pulmonary artery II anatomical changes. *Am. J. Pathol.* **26**:177–195.

Lintermans, J. P., Guntheroth, W. G., and Figley, M. M. (1966). Extensive accessory pulmonary arteries in the presence of relatively normal primary pulmonary arteries. *Am. Heart J.* **71:**527–532.

Litwin, S. B., Plauth, W. H., and Nadas, A. S. (1970). Anomalous systemic arterial supply to lung causing pulmonary hypertension. *N. Engl. J. Med.* **283**:1098–1099.

Livingston, D. R., Mehtra, A. C., O'Donovan, P. B., and Cordasco, E. M. (1986). An angiographic dilemma: Bronchopulmonary sequestration versus pseudosequestration: Case reports. *Angiology* 37:896–904.

Lois, J. F., Gomes, A. S., Smith, D. C., and Laks, H. (1988). Systemic-to-pulmonary collateral vessels and shunts: Treatment with embolization. *Radiology* **169**:671–676.

Long, W. A., Perry, J. R., and Henry, G. W. (1985). Radionuclide diagnosis of anomalous origin of the right pulmonary artery from the ascending aorta (so-called hemitruncus). *Int. J. Cardiol.* **8**:492–496.

Macartney, F., and Haworth, S. G. (1983). Pulmonary atresia with VSD. Investigation of pulmonary atresia with ventricular septal defect. In *Paediatric Cardiology,* Vol. 5. Edited by R. H. Anderson, F. J. Macartney, E. A. Shinebourne, and M. Tynan. New York, Churchill Livingstone, pp. 111–125.

Macartney, F., Deverall, P., and Scott, O. (1973). Haemodynamic characteristics of systemic arterial blood supply to lungs. *Br. Heart J.* **35**:28–37.

Macpherson, R. I., and Whytehead, L. (1977). Pseudosequestration. *J. Can. Assoc. Radiologists* **28**:17–25.

Madewell, J. E., Stocker, J. T., and Korsower, J. M. (1975). Cystic adenomatoid malformation of the lung—morphologic analysis. *AJR* **124**:436–448.

Madoff, I. M., Gaensler, E. A., and Strieder, J. W. (1952). Congenital absence of the right pulmonary artery. *N. Engl. J. Med.* **247**:147–157.

Manhoff, L. J., Jr., and Howe, J. S. (1949). Absence of the pulmonary artery: A new classification for the pulmonary arteries of anomalous origin. *Arch. Pathol.* **48**:155–170.

Marino, B., Calabro, R., Gagliardi, M. G., Bevilacqua, M., Ballerini, L., and Marcelletti, C. (1987). Patterns of pulmonary arterial anatomy and blood supply in complex congenital heart disease with pulmonary atresia. *J. Thorac. Cardiovasc. Surg.* **94**:518–520.

Masaoka, A., Masazumi, M., Monden, Y., Nakahara, K., and Tani, Y. (1979). Total lung ectoplasia with systemic arterial supply. *Ann. Thorac. Surg.* **27**:76–79.

McGoon, D. C., Baird, D. K., and Davis, G. D. (1975). Surgical management of large bronchial collateral arteries with pulmonary stenosis or atresia. *Circulation* **52**:109–118.

McGoon, M. D., Fulton, R. E., Davis, G. D., Ritter, D. G., Neill, C. A., and White, R. I., Jr. (1977). Systemic collateral and pulmonary artery stenosis in patients with congenital pulmonary valve atresia and ventricular septal defect. *Circulation* **56**:473–479.

McKim, J. S., and Wiglesworth, F. W. (1954). Absence of the left pulmonary artery. *Am. Heart J.* **47**:845–859.

Milikan, J. S., Puga, F. J., Danielson, G. K., Schaff, H. V., Julsrud, P. R., and Mair, D. D. (1986). Staged surgical repair of pulmonary atresia, ventricular septal defect, and hypoplastic confluent pulmonary arteries. *J. Thorac. Cardiovasc. Surg.* **91**:919–925.

Miller, R. K., Sieber, W. K., and Yonis, E. J. (1980). Congenital adenomatoid malformation of the lung: A report of 17 cases and review of the literature. *Pathol. Annu.* **15**:387–407.

Moberg, A. (1968). Anastomoses between extracardiac vessels and the coronary arteries. *Acta Med. Scand. Suppl.* **485**:5–26.

Mommo, K., Takao, A., Ando, M., Nakazawa, M., Satomi, G., Imai, Y., Takanash, Y., and Kurosawa, H. (1986). Juxtaductal pulmonary artery obstruction in pulmonary atresia. *Br. Heart J.* **55**:39–44.

Mommo, K., Takao, A., Imai, Y., and Kurosawa, H. (1987). Obstruction of the central pulmonary artery after shunt operations in patients with pulmonary atresia. *Br. Heart J.* **57**:534–542.

Moser, K. M., Olson, L. K., Schlusselberg, M., Daly, P. O., and Dembitsky, S. P. (1989). Chronic thromboembolic occlusion in adult can mimic pulmonary artery agenesis. *Chest* **95**:503–608.

Nashef, S. A. M., Jamieson, M. P. G., Pollock, J. C. S., and Houston, A. B. (1987). Aortic origin of right pulmonary artery: Successful surgical correction of three consecutive patients. *Ann. Thorac. Surg.* **44**:536–538.

Neill, C. A., Ferenz, C., Sabiston, D. C., and Sheldon, H. (1960). The familial occurrence of hypoplastic right lung with systemic arterial supply and venous drainage "scimitar syndrome." *Bull. Johns Hopkins Hosp.* **107**:1–21.

Nordenstrom, B. (1963). Methods of altering circulatory dynamics to improve roentgen examination of the cardiovascular system. *AJR* **89**:233–253.

Odell, J. E., and Smith, J. C., II (1963). Right pulmonary artery aising from ascending aorta. *Am. J. Dis. Child.* **105**:53–62.

Pahl, E., Fong, L., Anderson, R. A., Park, S. C., and Zuberbuhler, J. R. (1989). Fistulous communications between a solitary coronary atery and the pulmonary arteries as a primary source of pulmonary blood supply in tetralogy of Fallot with pulmonary atresia. *Am. J. Cardiol.* **63**:140–143.

Pahlajani, D. B., Pantvaidya, S. H., Pandit, S., Patwardhan, A. M., and Chaukar, A. P. (1985). Anomalous origin of right pulmonary atery from ascending aorta with right ventricular endocardial fibroelastosis. *Pediatr. Cardiol.* **6**:47–50.

Panicek, D. M., Heitzman, E. R., Randall, P. A., Groskin, S. A., Chew, F. S., Lane, E. J., Jr., and Markarian, B. (1987). The continuum of pulmonary developmental anomalies. *Radiographics* **7**:747–772.

Pedersen, M. L., LeQuire, M. H., Spies, J. B., and Ladd, W. A. (1988). Computed tomography of intralobar bronchopulmonary sequestration supplied from the renal artery. *J. Comput. Assist. Tomogr.* **12**:874–875.

Pendse, P., Alexander, J., Khademi, M., and Groff, D. B. (1972). Pulmonary sequestration: Coexisting classic intralobar and extralobar types in a child. *J. Thorac. Cardiovasc. Surg.* **64**:127–131.

Penkoske, P. A., Castaneda, A. R., Fyler, D. C., and Van Praagh, R. (1983). Origin of pulmonary artery branch from ascending aorta: Primary surgical repair in infancy. *J. Thorac. Cardiovasc. Surg.* **85**:537–545.

Pernot, C., Simon, P., Hoeffel, J. C., Worms, A. M., Marcon, F., and Prevot, J. (1988). Systemic artery to pulmonary vein fistula. *J. Radiol.* **69**:437–441.

Perry, S. B., Radtke, W., Fellows, K. E., Keane, J. F., and Lock, J. E. (1989). Coil embolization to occlude aortopulmonary collateral vessels and shunts in patients with congenital heart disease. *J. Am. Coll. Cardiol.* **13**:100–108.

Pfefferkorn, J. R., Loser, H., Pech, G., Toussaint, R., and Hilgenberg, F. (1982). Absent pulmonary artery—a hint to its embryogenesis. *Pediatr. Cardiol.* **3**:283–286.

Pool, P. E., Vogel, J. H. K., and Blount, S. G. (1962). Congenital unilateral absence of a pulmonary artery. *Am. J. Cardiol.* 706–732.

Presbitero, P., Bull, C., Haworth, S. G., and deLeval, M. R. (1984). Absent or occult pulmonary artery. *Br. Heart J.* **52**:178–185.

Pryce, D. M. (1946). Lower accessory pulmonary artery with intralobar sequestration of lung: A report of seven cases. *J. Pathol. Bacteriol.* **58**:457–467.

Pryce, D. M., Sellors, T. H., and Blair, L. G. (1947). Intralobar sequestration of lung associated with an abnormal pulmonary artery. *Br. J. Surg.* **35**:18–29.

Pump, K. K. (1963). The bronchial arteries and their anastomoses in the human lung. *Dis. Chest* **43**:245–255.

Rabinovitch, M. (1988). Intrapulmonary connections and nonconnections in tetralogy of Fallot with pulmonary atresia. In *Perspectives in Pediatric Cardiology,* Vol. I. Edited by R. H. Anderson, W. H. Neches, S. C. Park, and J. R. Zuberbuhler. Mount Kisco, New York, Futura, Chap. 33, pp. 169–182.

Rabinovitch, M., Herrera-DeLeon, V., Casteneda, A. R., and Reid, L. (1981). Growth and development of the pulmonary vascular bed in patients with tetralogy of Fallot with or without pulmonary atresia. *Circulation* **64**:1234–1248.

Ramsay, J. M., Macartney, F. J., and Haworth, S. G. (1985). Tetralogy of Fallot with major aortopulmonary collateral arteries. *Br. Heart J.* **53**:167–172.

Ransom, J. M., Worton, J. B., and Williams, S. G. (1978). Pulmonary sequestration presenting as congestive heart failure. *J. Thorac. Cardiovasc. Surg.* **76**:378–380.

Rees, R. S. O., Somerville, J., Underwood, S. R., Wright, J., Firmin, D. N., Klipstein, R. H., and Longmore, D. B. (1987). Magnetic resonance imaging of the pulmonary arteries and their systemic connections in pulmonary atresia; comparison with angiographic and surgical findings. *Br. Heart J.* **58**:621-626.

Rees, S. (1981). Arterial connections of the lung: The inaugural Keith Jefferson Lecture. *Clin. Radiol.* **32**:1-15.

Robida, A., and Fetlich, D. (1985). Tetralogy of Fallot with origin of the left pulmonary artery from the ascending aorta. *Pediatr. Radiol.* **15**:422-423.

Rodgers, B. M., Harman, P. K., and Johnson, A. M. (1986). Bronchopulmonary foregut malformations—spectrum of anomalies. *Ann. Surg.* **213**:517-524.

Roe, J. P., Mack, J. W., and Shirley, J. H. (1980). Bilateral pulmonary sequestrations. *J. Thorac. Cardiovasc. Surg.* **80**:8-10.

Ross, D. N., and Somerville, J. (1966). Correction of pulmonary atresia with a homograft aortic valve. *Lancet* **2**:1446-1447.

Sade, R. M., Clouse, M., and Ellis, F. H., Jr. (1974). The spectrum of pulmonary sequestration—collective review. *Ann. Thorac. Surg.* **18**:644-658.

Santos, M. A., Moll, J. N., Drumond, C., Araujo, W. B., Roma, O., and Reis, N. B. (1980). Development of the ductus arteriosus in right ventricular outflow tract obstruction. *Circulation* **62**:818.

Savic, B., Birtel, F. J., Tholen, W., Funke, H. D., and Knoche, R. (1979). Lung sequestration: Report of seven cases and review of 540 published cases. *Thorax* **34**:96-101.

Shakibi, J. G., Rastan, H., Mazarian, I., Paydar, M., Aryanpour, I., and Siassi, B. (1978). Isolated unilateral absence of the pulmonary artery. *Jpn. Heart J.* **19**:439-451.

Sherrick, D. W., Kincaid, O. W., and DuShane, J. W. (1962). Agenesis of a main branch of the pulmonary artery. *AJR* **87**:917-928.

Shimazaki, Y., Machara, T., Blackstone, E. H., Kirklin, J. W., and Bargeron, L. M., Jr. (1988). The structure of the pulmonary circulation in tetralogy of Fallot with pulmonary atresia. *J. Thorac. Cardiovasc. Surg.* **95**:1048-1058.

Somerville, J. (1988). Clinical identification of the pulmonary blood supply in pulmonary atresia. In *Perspectives in Pediatric Cardiology,* Vol. I. Edited by R. H. Anderson, W. H. Neches, S. C. Park and J. R. Zuberbuhler. Mount Kisco, New York, Futura, Chap. 32, pp. 155-168.

Sosa, E. S., Kratz, C., Spier, S., Gauthier-Chouinard, M., Stanley, P., and Chartrand, C. (1987). Congenital unilateral absence of a pulmonary artery. *Chir. Pediatr.* **28**:204-208.

Sotomora, R. F., and Edwards, J. E. (1978). Anatomic identification of so-called absent pulmonary artery. *Circulation* **57**:624-633.

Stocker, J. T. (1986). Sequestrations of the lung. *Semin. Diagn. Pathol.* **3**:106–121.

Stocker, J. T., and Malczak, M. T. (1984). A study of pulmonary ligament arteries: Relationship to intralobar pulmonary sequestration. *Chest* **86**:611–615.

Stuckey, D., Bowdler, J. D., and Reye, R. D. K. (1968). Absent sixth aortic arch: A form of pulmonary atresia. *Br. Heart J.* **30**:258–264.

Syme, J. (1973). Systemic to pulmonary arterial fistula of the chest wall and lung following lobectomy. *Australas. Radiol.* **19**:326–333.

Thiene, G., and Anderson, R. H. (1983). Pulmonary atresia with VSD. In *Paediatric Cardiology,* Vol. 5. Edited by R. H. Anderson, F. J. Macartney, E. A. Shinebourne, and M. Tynan. New York, Churchill-Livingston, pp. 80–101.

Thiene, G., Frescura, C., Bortolotto, U., Del Maschio, A., and Valente, M. (1981). The systemic pulmonary circulation in pulmonary atresia with ventricular septal defect: Concept of reciprocal development of the fourth and sixth arches. *Am. Heart J.* **101**:339–344.

Thilenius, A. G., Ruschhaupt, D. G., Replogle, R. L., Bharati, S., Herman, T., and Arcilla, R. A. (1983). Spectrum of pulmonary sequestration: Association with anomalous pulmonary venous drainage in infants. *Pediatr. Cardiol.* **4**:97–103.

Thompson, J. A., Lewis, S. A., and Mauck, H. P. (1986). Absence of left pulmonary artery: Anomalous collateral from coronary artery to affected lung. *Am. Heart J.* **111**:418–420.

Tobin, C. E. (1952). The bronchial arteries and their connections with other vessels in the human lung. *Surg. Gynecol. Obstet.* **95**:741–750.

Toews, W. H., and Pappas, G. (1983). Surgical management of absent right pulmonary artery with associated pulmonary hypertension. *Chest* **84**:497–499.

Vasquez-Sanchez, J., Pinto-Tortolero, P., Testelli, M. R., and Herrera, E. L. (1983). Unilateral agenesis of main branch of pulmonary artery. *Arch. Inst. Cardiol. Mex.* **53**:381–386.

Vogel, J. H. K., McNamara, D. G., Hallman, G., Rosenberg, H., Jamieson, G., and McCrady, J. D. (1967). Effects of mild chronic hypoxia on the pulmonary circulation in calves with reactive pulmonary hypertension. *Circ. Res.* **21**:661–669.

Wallace, R. B., Rastelli, G. C., Ongley, P. A., Titus, J. H., and McGoon, D. C. (1969). Complete repair of truncus arteriosus defects. *J. Thorac. Cardiovasc. Surg.* **57**:95–107.

Webb, W. R., and Jacobs, R. P. (1977). Transpleural abdominal systemic artery—pulmonary artery anastomosis in patients with chronic pulmonary infection. *AJR* **129**:233–236.

Weibel, E. R. (1960). Early stages in the development of collateral circulation to the lung in the rat. *Circ. Res.* **8**:353–376.

Werber, J., Ramilo, J. L., London, R., and Harris, V. J. (1983). Unilteral absence of a pulmonary artery. *Chest* **84**:729–732.

Wimbash, K. H., Agha, F. P., and Brady, T. M. (1983). Bilateral pulmonary sequestration: Computed tomographic appearance. *AJR* **140**:689–690.

Winship, W. S., Beck, W., and Schrire, V. (1967). Congenital absence and anomalous origin of the main pulmonary arteries. *Br. Heart J.* **29**:34–42.

Wyman, S. M. (1954). Congenital absence of the pulmonary artery; its demonstration by roentgenography. *Radiology* **62**:321–327.

Yabek, S. M., Burstein, J., Berman, W., Jr., and Dillon, T. (1981). Aberrant systemic arterial supply to left lung with congestive heart failure. *Chest* **80**:636–637.

Zureikat, H. Y. (1980). Collateral vessels between the coronary and bronchial arteries in patients with cyanotic congenital heart disease. *Am. J. Cardiol.* **45**:599–603.

Part VII

THERAPY

22

Endovascular Management of Bronchial Bleeding

JACQUES RÉMY, MARTINE RÉMY-JARDIN, and CYR VOISIN

Hôpital Albert Calmette
Lille, France

I. Introduction

Until recent years the pathophysiological mechanisms underlying bronchial bleeding have been incompletely understood. Before the advent of angiography it was believed the pulmonary arteries were the principal source of bleeding, and when tuberculosis was more common, Rasmussen's aneurysm was often indicted. With the beginning of bronchial arteriography about 1965, bleeding from bronchial arteries was demonstrated and Rasmussen's aneurysm was all but forgotten. As experience has accumulated, other systemic arteries contributing to the blood supply of pulmonary lesions through transpleural collateral circulation have been recognized. Thus, we now understand that pulmonary, bronchial, and nonbronchial systemic arteries may be involved in complex arrangements in congenital, inflammatory, and neoplastic processes in the lung. If cessation of bleeding after arterial embolization is used to identify the responsible blood vessel, our experience indicates bronchial arteries are the immediate source of blood in 88% of cases, nonbronchial arteries in 7%, and pulmonary arteries in 5%.

In this chapter we take up the pathogenesis of bleeding, discuss the most common clinical circumstances for bleeding, and consider the contribution endoscopy may make to its management. This is followed by indications and contraindications to endovascular treatment and a description of our technique. We conclude with a resume of complications and the results of embolotherapy in our hands.

II. Pathophysiology of Bronchial Bleeding

Angiography explains the genesis of bronchial bleeding when contrast material is seen to enter a bronchus from a blood vessel or when obstruction of a blood vessel stops the bleeding. The second is the more frequent experience, but it does not precisely delineate the bronchoarterial communication. As is briefly reviewed here, many thoracic arteries may be the source of bronchial bleeding.

A. Bronchial Arteries

The bronchial arteries are the source of bleeding in about 90% of clinical cases. Nevertheless, experience has revealed some paradoxes. Cessation of bleeding by bronchial arterial embolization does not prove the communication to the bronchus involves the bronchial artery. It may derive from a pulmonary artery with which the bronchial artery has anastomosed. Nor is there any correlation between the extent of bronchial artery hypervascularization and the extent of bronchial bleeding. Even angiographically normal bronchial arteries may bleed with no apparent abnormality although huge hypervascularization may not. Further, demonstration of a communication between a bronchial artery and a bronchus is very exceptional. We have seen it only twice in 260 patients treated by embolization (Fig. 1). Nevertheless, the majority of bronchial bleeding relates to bronchial hypervascularization, which in itself is a nonspecific response to several stimuli: reduced pulmonary artery flow, hypoxemia, alveolar hypoxia, fibrosis, inflammation, and chronic suppuration. Clinical conditions in which bronchial artery hypervascularization relates to bronchial bleeding are taken up in detail later. Figure 2 illustrates bronchial hypervascularization developing in response to hypoxemia in congenital tricuspid valve atresia.

B. Pulmonary Arteries

Fistulas between the pulmonary arteries and the bronchi arise by erosive processes, primarily in either the lung or the artery, where the artery and bronchus are in close contiguity. This is illustrated by neoplastic bronchial and arterial necrosis (Fig. 3). Arterial necrosis may also result in formation of aneurysm. Bartter et al. (1988) proposed a classification of pulmonary artery aneurysms based on their etiology and pathogenesis (Table 1). From a thera-

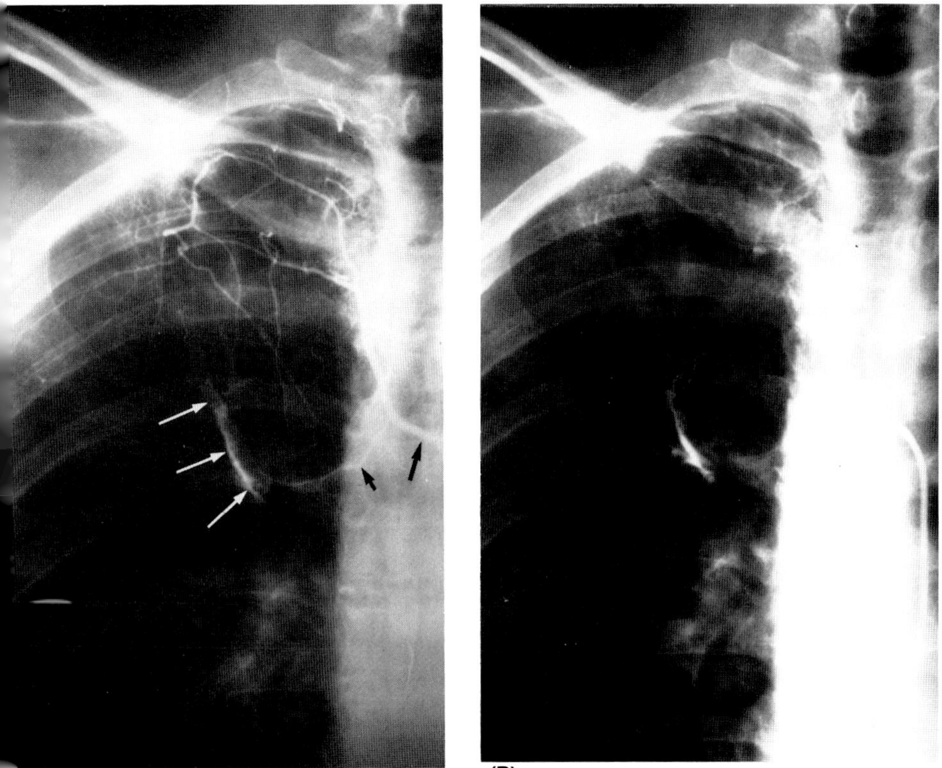

(B)

Figure 1 Demonstrable bronchoarterial fistula. Endoscopy demonstrated bleeding from the right upper lobe. (A) Angiography of the intercostobronchial trunk (long black arrow) shows a small right bronchial artery (short black arrow) and contrast material in a segmental bronchus (white arrows). (B) A second film shows this is not interstitial extravasation but a direct communication as the contrast moves rapidly in the bronchial lumen.

peutic point of view, pulmonary artery aneurysms are more usefully classified as central, requiring surgical treatment, and peripheral, amenable to vasoocclusive control. A further important consideration is whether they involve the full circumference of the wall or simply a segment, thereby allowing a saccular cavity to develop. In either case, the rule of Laplace applies, namely, the stress in the vessel wall is directly proportional to the intravascular pressure and the diameter of the vessel and inversely proportional to the wall thickness (Butto et al., 1987). This means that the risk of rupture increases as aneurysms enlarge. Bleeding from pulmonary artery aneurysms is not frequent. Remy et al. (1977) treated 184 patients for bronchial bleeding of whom 6% had a pulmonary arterial cause. In 306 patients with bleeding, Rabkin et al. (1987)

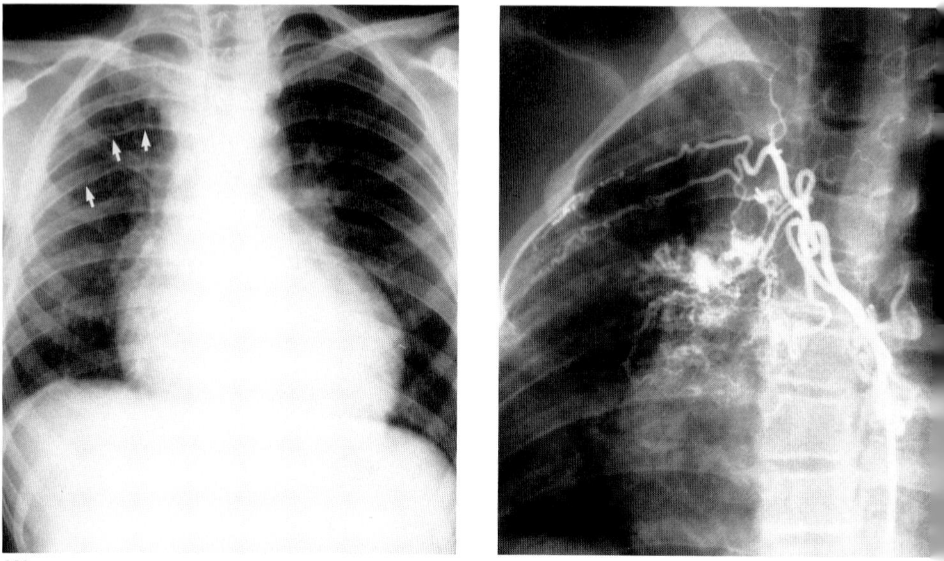

(A) (B)

Figure 2 Bronchial hypervascularization after Glenn anastomosis for tricuspid atresia (superior caval-right pulmonary artery anastomosis). (A) Standard radiograph shows rib notching on the right side indicating dilated intercostal arteries (arrows). (B) Massive bronchial bleeding from the right upper lobe prompted arteriography of the intercostobronchial trunk, which shows hypervascularization in the right lung hilum and tortuous intercostal arteries supplying transpleural collaterals. Embolization with fragments of Gelfoam arrested the bleeding until a fatal recurrence 1 year later.

found a pulmonary arterial cause in 10%. Both groups found the most frequent underlying diseases were tuberculosis and abscess of the lung.

Rasmussen's aneurysm has long been familiar (Rasmussen, 1868; Auerbach, 1939; Plessinger and Jolly, 1949). It takes on new significance now that it can be treated. The aneurysm develops in tuberculous cavities as the granulation tissue destroys the elastic fibers of the arterial media. The vessel wall, then only intima, herniates into the cavity. This intracavitary protrusion explains the episodic character of bleeding when the aneurysm ruptures. If the cavity is poorly drained, an intracavitary clot tamponades the bleeding. With retraction of the clot, bleeding may recur. Fragile Rasmussen's aneurysms may vary from a few millimeters to several centimeters in diameter and may not be discovered until a clot is removed from the cavity (Fig. 4).

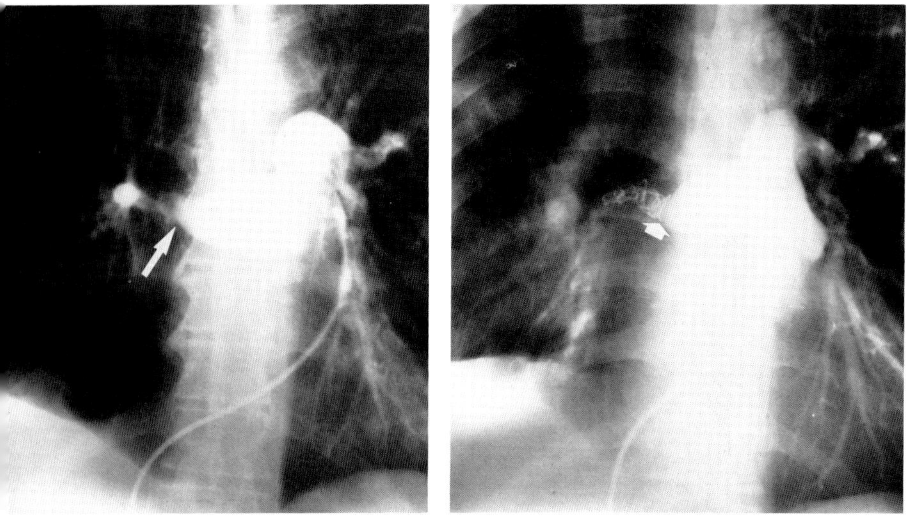

(B)

Figure 3 Epidermoid bronchial cancer eroding the right pulmonary artery. Endoscopic examination for bleeding showed an ulcer in the right main bronchus at the base of which the pulsating right pulmonary artery could be seen. (A) Pulmonary angiography shows the artery is stenosed (arrow). (B) Thrombosis of the artery was attempted with metal coils (arrow). Bleeding was arrested, but at subsequent endoscopy some of the metal coils were visible. A third endoscopy 3 weeks later showed more extraarterial coils, indicating progressive erosion of the artery. Death occurred by bronchial bleeding.

Rasmussen's aneurysm may be suspected when bleeding complicates a necrotizing process in the lung, such as tuberculosis and other infections, notably mycoses. Vascular erosions have been observed with invasive aspergillosis and sarcoidosis (Edelman et al., 1985).

Mycotic aneurysms of pulmonary arteries may complicate peripheral thrombophlebitis as in drug addicts or right heart endocarditis (Choyke et al., 1982). The mechanism is either septic embolism to a small-vessel lumen or to the vasavasorum of larger arteries.

Pulmonary arterial aneurysms may develop in certain diffuse vascular diseases and syndromes. Behçet's disease is perhaps the most common cause of bronchial bleeding with high mortality (Park et al., 1984; Raz et al., 1989). The vasculitis affects large and small arteries, capillaries, and veins, with resulting thombosis, hemorrhage, and infarction. Inflammatory destruction of elastic tissue and occlusion of the vasavasorum may be followed by aneurysm,

Table 1 Aneurysms of the Pulmonary Arteries

Aneurysms of the Pulmonary Arteries
Infection (mycotic aneurysm)
Tuberculosis (Rasmussen's aneurysm)
Syphilis
Other bacteria and fungi
Cardiovascular
Congenital
Patent ductus arteriosus
Atrial septal defect
Others
Acquired
Mitral stenosis, pulmonary stenosis
Tricuspid incompetence, pulmonary incompetence
Vasculopathies
Congenital
Cystic medial necrosis
Acquired (atheroma)
Marfan's syndrome
Vasculitides
Behçet's disease
Takayasu's disease
Kawasaki disease
Pulmonary hypertension
Idiopathic
Hughes-Stovin syndrome
Others
Traumatic
Diverse

Source: After Bartter et al. (1988).

which may then develop a fistula into a bronchus. Hughes-Stovin syndrome, considered by some to be related to Behçet's disease, includes peripheral thrombophlebitis, fever, cough, and a high proclivity to bronchial bleeding (Roberts et al., 1982). Proximal artery aneurysms need to be treated individually, whether by surgery (Salamon et al., 1988) or endovascular occlusion (Lacombe et al., 1985). Such aneurysms may be overlooked at conventional angiography if they are thrombosed or have a very small neck. Digital angiography may be more sensitive in their detection.

Pulmonary arteriovenous fistulas and aneurysms are associated with bronchial bleeding in 10–30% of two large series of patients (Prager et al., 1983; White et al., 1988). Bleeding may be expected more frequently with these thin-walled sacs.

C. Aorta and Systemic Arteries

Fistulas between the aorta, brachiocephalic arteries, and tracheobronchial tree may occasionally develop as a result of aneurysms or trauma. The aneurysms may be atherosclerotic, mycotic, and congenital. Surprisingly, initial bronchial bleeding is not always fatal. A "sentinel" bleed may occur to be followed by exsanguination days or weeks later. Bronchoscopy must be done very carefully; better to begin with computed tomography (CT) or angiography when the possibility of aortobronchial fistula is suspected (Hampson and Pepper, 1987). Tracheostomy, tracheal reconstruction, and prolonged tracheal intubation may occasionally result in fistulas between the innominate artery and trachea as a result of pressure necrosis, postoperative infection, or direct surgical injury (Conrad et al., 1977). These fistulas may also have minor prodromal bleeding. Angiography in the latent interval with oblique projections may delineate the fistula.

Unfortunately, many of these fistulas between large arteries and the bronchi are revealed only at autopsy. Often simple radiography gives no clue. If prodromal sentinel bleeding is investigated with angiography, however, computed tomography or magnetic resonance imaging (MRI), rare entities may be revealed. Palliative treatment is not possible except to the extent that balloons of a Swan-Ganz or Fogarty catheter may temporarily stop cataclysmic bleeding.

III. Bronchial Bleeding Amenable to Endovascular Treatment

As of this writing (1989), we have treated 260 patients for bronchial bleeding by embolization or vasoocclusion (Table 2). The causes reflect the socioeconomic conditions in northern France, where there are 8000 active and 28,000 retired coal miners. In this respect, our experience differs from that reported elsewhere (Ferris, 1981).

A. Tuberculosis

Tuberculosis causes about 2000 deaths annually in the United States, some by bronchial bleeding. Davis et al. (1985) estimates this at 10%, Muthuswamy et al. (1987) at 1–5%. We found tuberculosis the most frequent indication for

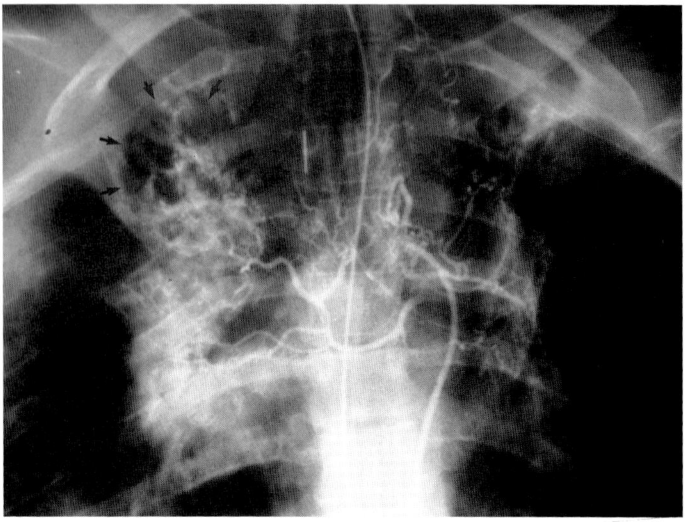

(A)

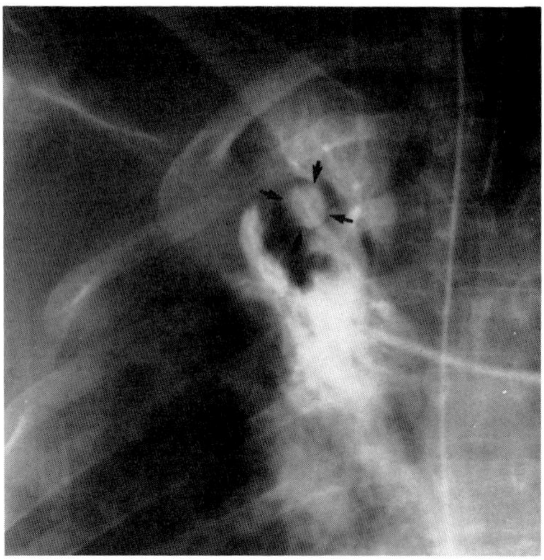

(B)

Figure 4 Bleeding Rasmussen's aneurysm in tuberculous cavity. (A) Bronchial arteriography shows moderate hypervascularization of the cavity (arrows). Bronchial embolization did not stop the bleeding. (B) Pulmonary angiography suggests an aneurysm in the superior aspect of the cavity (arrows). (C) Selective pulmonary angiography confirms the aneurysm (arrows). (D) The bronchial bleeding was controlled by three coils in segmental artery branches. The first two (single and double arrows) were ineffective, but the third (triple arrow) was successful.

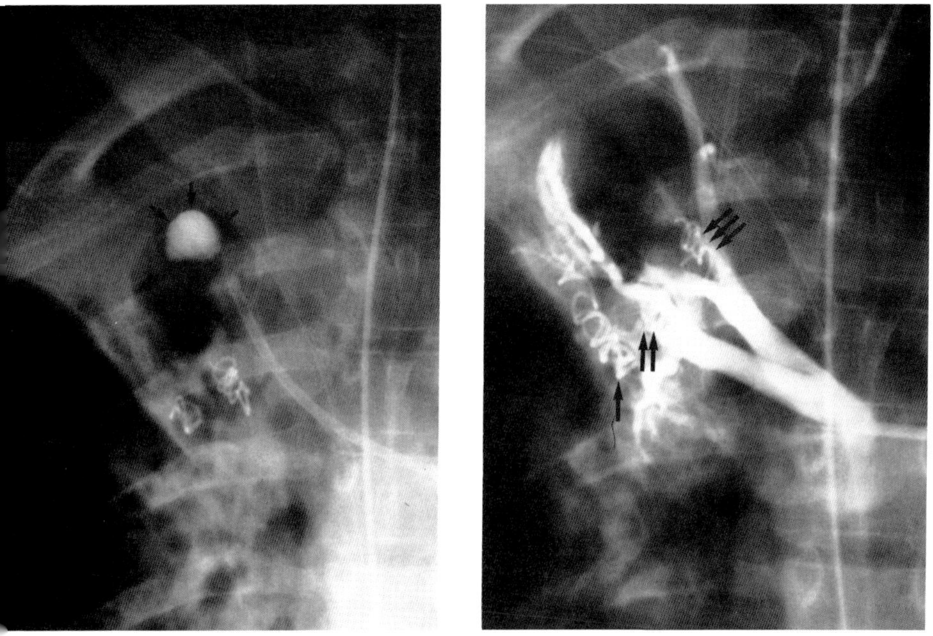

) (D)

Table 2 Author's Experience with Endovascular Treatment of Bronchial Bleeding (to 1989)

Tuberculosis	64
Coal miner's pneumoconiosis	49
Bronchiectasis	33
Mycoses	29
Tumors	23
Chronic obstructive bronchial disease	16
Cardiovascular causes	12
Lung abscess	7
Cystic fibrosis	1
Miscellaneous	26
Total	260

endovascular treatment, approximately 25% of our patients. Bleeding episodes are said to be fatal in 20%. The majority of massive bleeding occurs in cavitary disease (Teklu and Felleke, 1982). We believe bronchial bleeding in tuberculosis patients warrants computed tomography to search for cavities. If cavities are demonstrated, we further believe that angiographic exploration of both the bronchial and pulmonary circulations is indicated (Bookstein et al., 1977; Remy et al., 1988). Surgical resection is seldom used nowadays, and only when postoperative specimens are carefully injected is the source of bleeding precisely established. It may be bronchial hypervascularization or erosion of vessels by cavities or lymph nodes, and it may relate to bronchiectasis.

B. Pneumoncoiosis

About 5% of patients with pneumonoconiosis experience bleeding; it made up 20% of our experience. It complicates both black lung disease and progressive massive fibrosis.

C. Bronchiectasis

The bronchial hypervascularization in bronchiectasis is characterized by large sinuous arteries with spindle-shaped and saccular microaneurysms (Delarue et al., 1953; Cockett and Vass, 1951). The anastomotic connections between the bronchial and pulmonary circulations may range from 50 μm to 1 mm in diameter. Whereas there is no correlation between the type of bronchiectasis—cylindrical, or saccular—and the extent of hypervascularization, drainage of infection appears to be important, as well-drained bronchi have less vascularization.

The angiographic features of bronchiectasis reflect the vascular pathology, sinuous corkscrewlike arteries, saccular aneurysms, and contrast blushing of bronchial walls (hyperemia). Bronchopulmonary anastomoses are numerous, sometimes affecting distal pulmonary arteries, which are approximately normal (Fig. 5). Aneurysms in the proximal bronchial arteries may rupture into a bronchus, the esophagus, the mediastinum, and even into a regional pulmonary artery with resulting bronchopulmonary shunt. The large flow in the dilated vasculature may divert contrast material such that more normal territories are not perfused during pulmonary angiography (Botenga, 1968).

D. Pulmonary Mycoses

Intracavitary aspergilloma is a relatively frequent cause of bleeding, 10% in our experience. Others report bleeding in 70% of intracavitary aspergillomas with a mortality of 2–26% (Jewkes et al., 1983). As in other conditions, premortal episodic bleeding occurs. The definitive treatment is, preferably, surgery, and 5 year survival after massive bleeding is 85%. However, surgery for resection and cavernostomy has a high morbidity, 25%, and mortality of 8% due to hemorrhage and bronchopleural fistula (Jewkes et al., 1983). Percutaneous drainage of cavities containing fungus balls can also be complicated by hemorrhage requiring endocavitary instillation of aminocaproic acid to enhance coagulation (Fernandez, 1984). Presurgical embolization may be useful to lessen the risks of hemorrhage when surgical interventions on aspergillomas are planned (Fig. 6).

Invasive aspergillosis is also associated with bleeding due to fungal invasion of vessel walls with resulting rupture and thrombosis. Orr et al. (1978) describe the mechanisms in Table 3. Massive bleeding in invasive aspergillosis was formerly unfamiliar (Pittokopitis et al., 1983), but fungal pneumonia, especially in hematological malignancies, is now more frequently recognized as a cause of fatal bleeding. Albelda et al. (1985) state bleeding occurs in 26% of leukemic patients with invasive aspergillosis during recovery from drug-induced marrow suppression. Among 26 patients with leukemia and invasive aspergillosis, he has seen 4 with massive bleeding, 1 fatal and 3 requiring lobectomy. In 3 of these cases, cavitation developed 1–2 days before the bleeding and 2 had minor prodromal bleeding. The quasi-synchronization of cavitation, bleeding, and recovery of granulocytes suggests that a proteolytic enzyme from the leukocytes may contribute to vessel wall destruction.

Kibbler et al. (1988) describe 38 patients with invasive aspergillosis, 6 dying of massive bleeding. They recommended CT search for cavities when immunocompromised patients develop focal opacities and begin to bleed. According to some authors, an intracavitary nodule is an indication for prophylactic surgery. Embolotherapy must now be considered for those with bleeding and opacities suspected or shown to be invasive aspergillosis.

Mucormycosis is another fungus associated with bleeding. In leukemia and lymphoma and in diabetic patients with central bronchial obstruction, endobronchial mucormycosis may result in invasion of adjacent pulmonary arteries with fatal bleeding (Reich and Renzetti, 1970; Donohue, 1983).

E. Pulmonary Neoplasm

Several mechanisms may be operative when bleeding complicates bronchial neoplasm: tumoral hypervascularization, invasion of blood vessels, obstruction of pulmonary venous return, obstruction of pulmonary arteries with infarction and hemorrhage, and as a complication of surgical biopsy or laser therapy. Necrotic squamous carcinomas invading central large arteries and veins are the usual culprits (Panos et al., 1988).

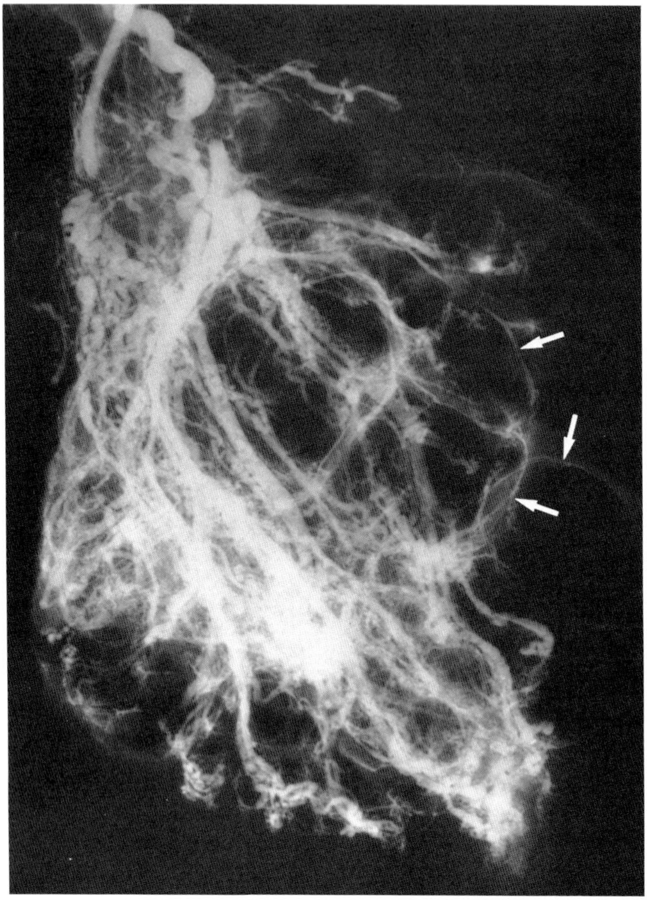

(A)

Figure 5 Bronchiectasis with profuse systemic hypervascularization and diversion of pulmonary blood flow. (A) Bronchial artery injection in the surgically resected left lower lobe shows massive hypervascularization and encirclement of bronchial cysts by small aterial bronches (arrows). (B) Presurgical bronchial arteriography demonstrates retrograde flow in the small-caliber left inferior pulmonary artery (arrows) but normal antegrade flow in other pulmonary artery branches (large curved arrow). (C) Preoperative injection in the intercostobronchial trunk (long arrow) shows large-caliber bronchial arteries supplying the bronchiectatic lobe (short arrows).

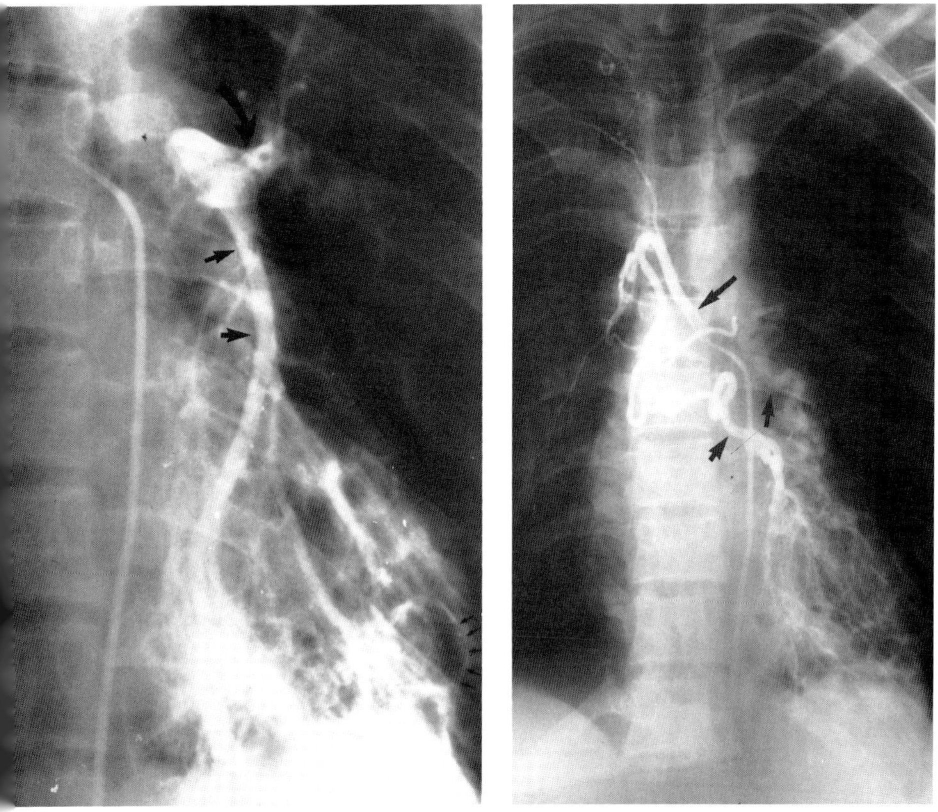

(B) (C)

Bronchial adenomas are very vascular tumors and notable bleeders, both spontaneously and on endoscopic biopsy (Mojab et al., 1974). Endobronchial and pulmonary metastases may also bleed as they have both pulmonary and bronchial artery supply (Milne et al., 1969). The very vascular metastases from hypernephroma may be treated by intraarterial chemotherapy (Kakizoe et al., 1984).

F. Obstructive Pulmonary Disease

We encountered 16 patients with bleeding from chronic obstructive pulmonary disease. They had hyperaeration and thick bronchial walls by radiography, obstructive physiology by functional tests, normal or hyperemic bronchial mucosa by endoscopy, and control of bleeding without recurrence by bronchial artery embolization. When present, bronchial hyperemia was moderate and

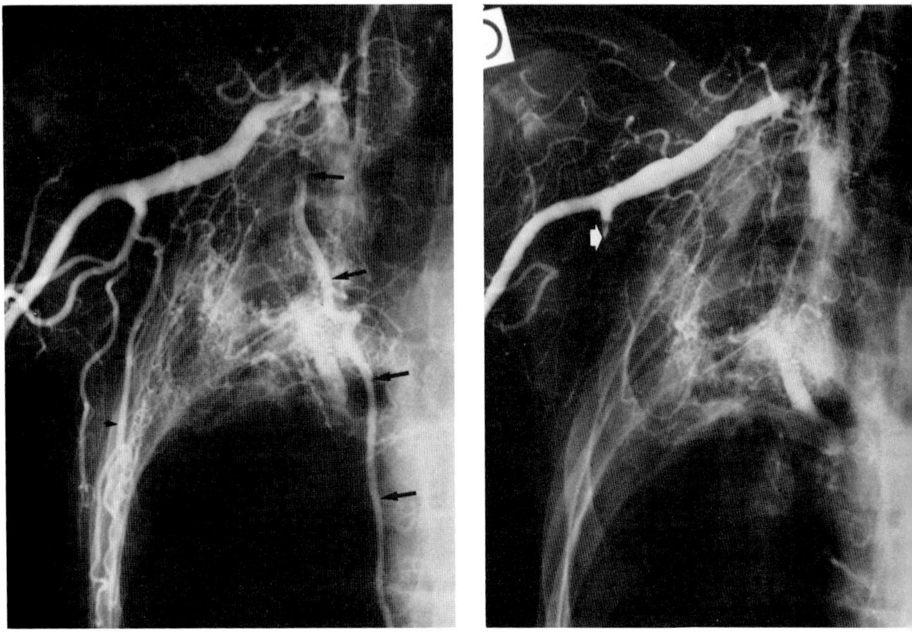

(A) (B)

Figure 6 Intracavitary aspergilloma with massive bleeding. (A) Axillary and right subclavian arteriography show hypervascularization of the cavity supplied by the internal mammary artery (large arrows) and a branch of the external mammary artery (small arrows). Atheromata of the right subclavian artery prevented selective embolization of these feeding arteries. (B) They were explored under local anesthesia and ligated (white arrow). This treatment, together with embolization of the right bronchial artery, arrested bronchial bleeding for 2 years. (Reproduced from *Radiology* 1988; **168**:377–383, with permission.)

symmetrical (Fig. 7). Bleeding in chronic obstructive pulmonary disease has been recognized but not recently studied (Boushy et al., 1969; Berry and Ochsner, 1972).

G. Cardiovascular Abnormalities

Reduction in pulmonary blood flow is regularly followed by augmentation of systemic artery collateral flow, which may be profoundly developed. This is notably true in congenital heart disease with pulmonary stenosis and atresia. Occasionally it is complicated by bronchial bleeding.

In congenital pulmonary artery atresia, the ductus arteriosus may remain patent and three types of collateral circulation may develop to provide blood to

Table 3 Mechanism of Bleeding in Bronchial Aspergillosis

Endobronchial and transbronchial proliferation

∅	∅
Lobar and segmental bronchi	Peripheral bronchi
∅	∅
Contiguous arteries in lobar and segmental arteries	Contiguous arteries in peripheral bronchi
∅	∅
Hemorrhagic infarction (5–10 cm diameter)	Nodules 1–3 cm. Ischemic necrosis and excavation

∅

Hemoptysis

Source: After Orr et al. (1978).

the lungs. The bronchial arteries anastomose with the pulmonary arteries in the lung, the sites of anastomosis being marked by stenosing, eccentric, intimal hyperplasia. Nonbronchial systemic arteries from the descending aorta (also called direct aortopulmonary collaterals) anastomose with the pulmonary arteries in the hila (Burrows et al., 1985). These may also have anastomotic stenoses. Further systemic collaterals arise in the subclavian, internal mammary, intercostal, coronary, and splanchnic arteries. They anastomose with central pulmonary and subpleural intrapulmonary arteries (Figs. 8 and 9).

Bronchial bleeding can complicate the development of anastomotic collateral circulation by atheromata or aneurysms that rupture (Haroutunian and Neill, 1972). Sometimes transpleural collateral vessels can be so large in the lung apices as to suggest pulmonary tuberculosis—pseudofibrosis of the apex (Haroutunian and Neill, 1972). These transpleural collaterals may offer difficulties in control of bleeding when the chest is open for cardiac repair (Matsuda et al., 1985). Postoperatively these collaterals can lead to left heart failure. If they are not closed at the time of complete surgical repair, the resulting condition is physiologically similar to intralobar pulmonary sequestration.

Another anomaly, absent pulmonary artery, is also complicated by bleeding in 5–10% of patients according to Pool et al. (1962) and Kucera et al.

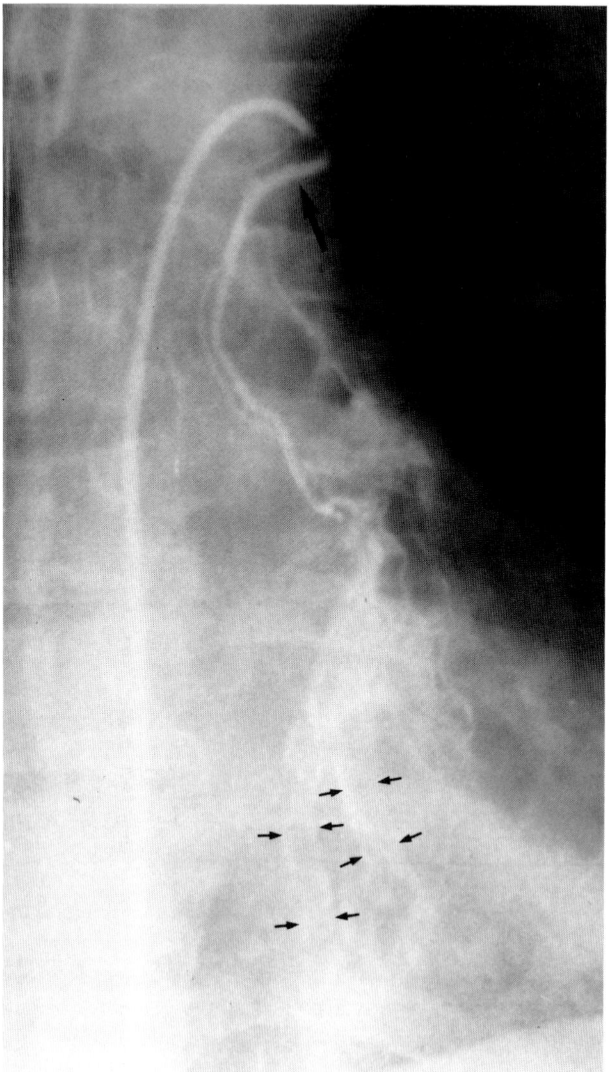

Figure 7 Chronic obstructive pulmonary disease with bronchial bleeding. Left bronchial arteriography (large arrow) shows opacification of the walls of cylindrically dilated bronchi in the left lower lobe (small arrows). Bleeding was controlled by embolization. No recurrence after 4 years.

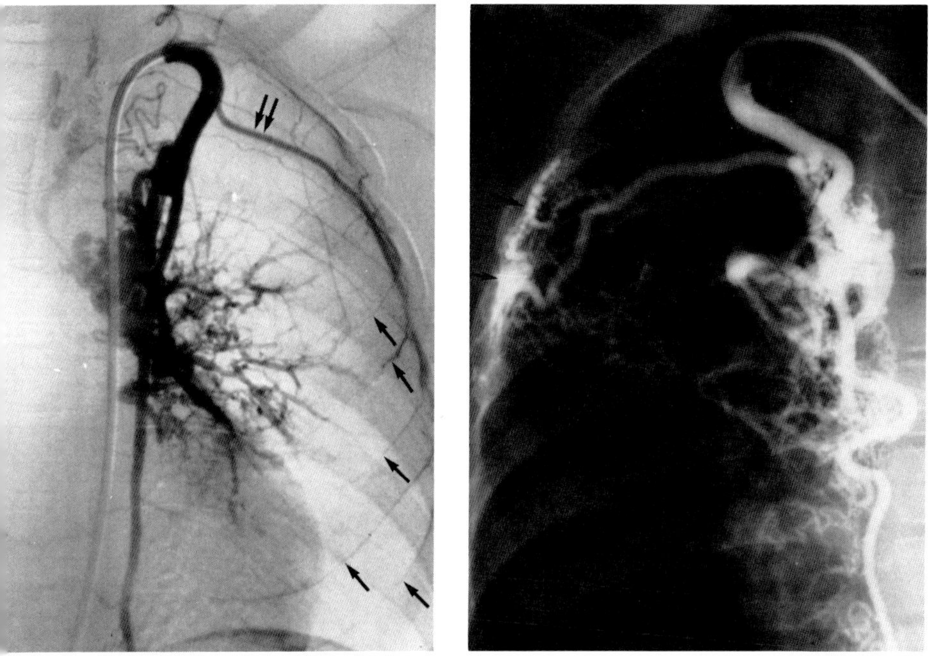

(B)

Figure 8 Pulmonary atresia with collateral circulation from internal mammary arteries. (A) Selective injection in the left internal mammary artery shows it is very large with extensive central communication with the pulmonary arteries in which there is antegrade flow. An accessory internal mammary artery (double arrows) supplies numerous small intercostal arteries (single arrows). (B) Angiography of the right internal mammary artery shows these same features with a somewhat larger accessory mammary artery and transpleural collateral circulation (arrows).

(1982). Pneumonectomy has been required (Byrne and Bloom, 1970; Taguchi et al., 1987). Transpleural collateral flow in this anomaly is facilitated by the development of pleural adhesions after surgery or infection (Kleinman, 1979). Sometimes bronchial angiography reveals a hidden hilar or intrapericardial pulmonary artery, in which case surgical repair may be considered.

Pulmonary hypertension complicating congenital heart disease and the obliterative modifications of the peripheral arteries accompanying it can lead to the development of precapillary bronchopulmonary anastomoses (Reid, 1986). These "dilatation lesions" with thin fragile walls may rupture (Charan et al., 1985). Pulmonary venous obstruction and hypertension may also be associated with bronchial bleeding. Whereas these are rare congenital and

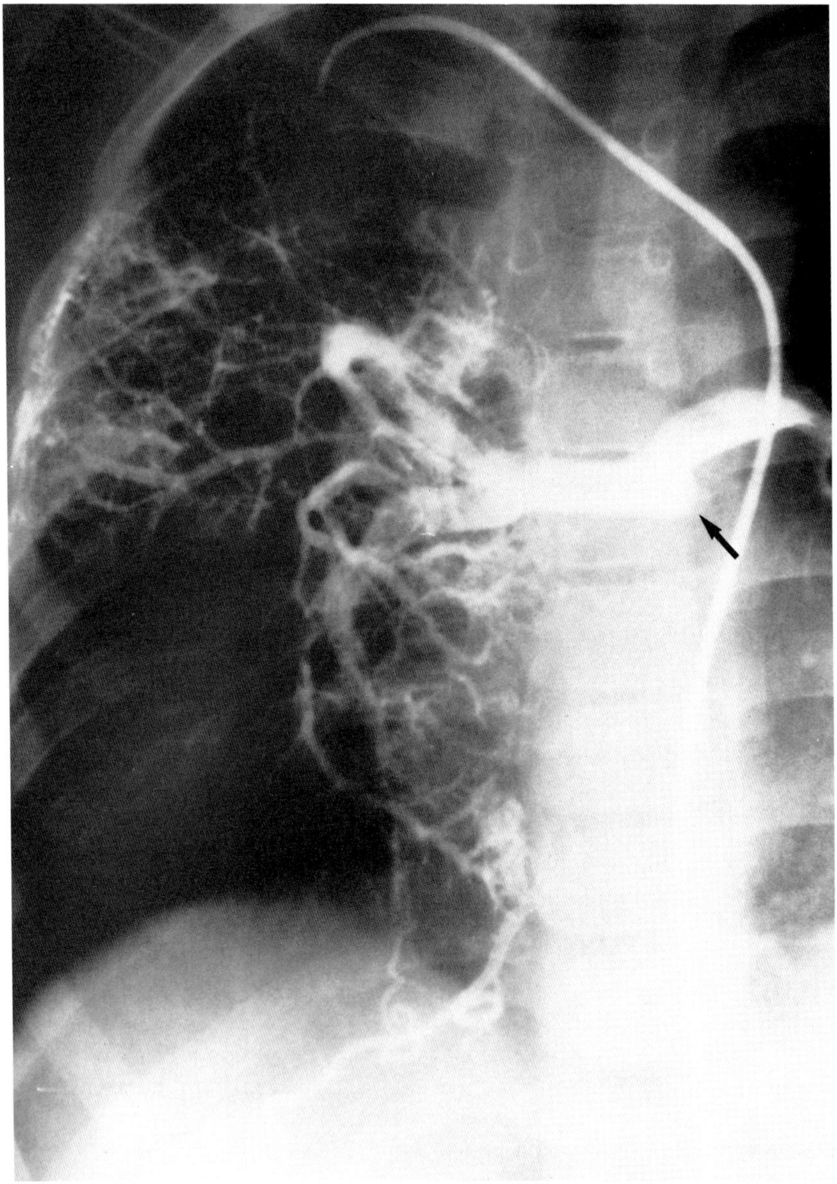

Figure 9 Systemic collateral circulation in pulmonary atresia. Injection of the right internal mammary artery provides central pulmonary artery opacification (arrow) via transpleural anastomoses in the superior right thorax.

acquired causes of obstruction of the pulmonary veins, venous hypertension with bleeding is probably most commonly due to mitral valve disease. It is said as many as 10–15% of patients experience it (Jouve et al., 1965).

H. Lung Abscess

Life-threatening bleeding in lung abscess is said to occur in 11–15% of patients (Thoms et al., 1972; Spencer, 1985). The mechanism is either erosion through the wall of a large artery in the abscess cavity or capillaries in the granulation tissue of the wall, which is supplied by highly developed bronchial arteries (Charan et al., 1985). Thus, both pulmonary and systemic circulations must be examined in bleeding lung abscess (Fig. 10).

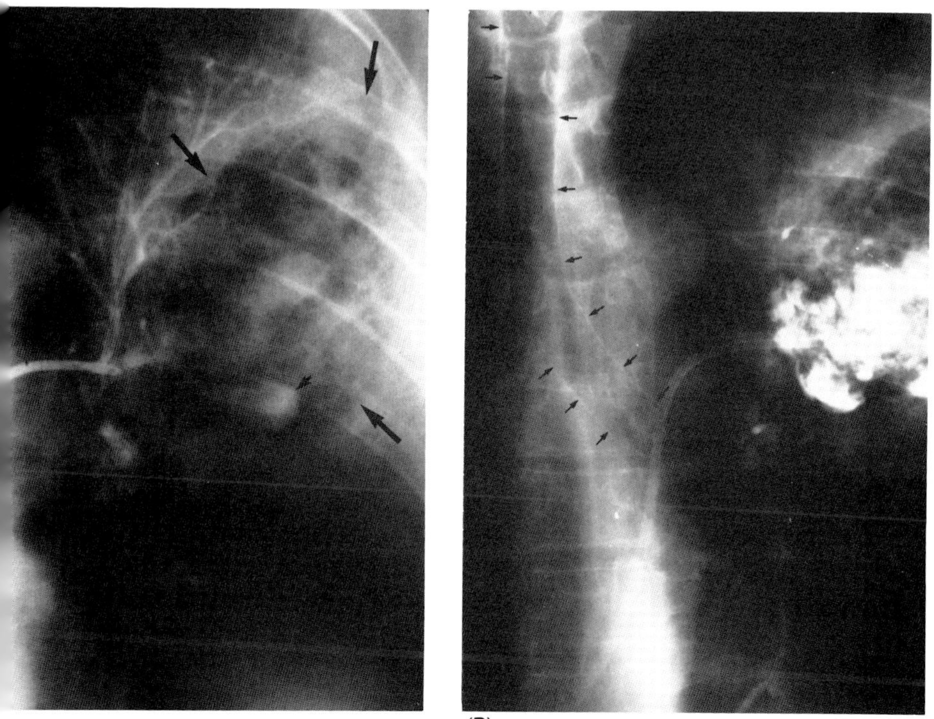

(B)

Figure 10 Lung abscess with pulmonary artery aneurysm ruptured during angiography. (A) Selective left pulmonary angiography with a side-hole catheter shows hypervascularization of the abscess wall (large arrows) and an aneurysmal sac (small arrow). (B) A second injection, manual and slow, with an end-opening catheter ruptured the aneurysmal sac with flooding of the tracheobronchial tree with contrast material (arrows). The bleeding was controlled with two metal coils.

Two clinical feature are notable. Larger abscesses have more complications (Harber and Terry, 1981), and positive-pressure ventilation in the presence of a bleeding abscess can lead to fatal gas embolism (Cholankeril et al., 1982). Bleeding may complicate the percutaneous drainage of abscesses (Snow et al., 1985; Mengoli, 1985; Rice et al., 1987) and occur in necrotizing pneumonia or pulmonary gangrene (Murthy et al., 1981).

I. Cystic Fibrosis

It can be expected that, as more patients survive to adulthood, the frequency of bronchial bleeding in cystic fibrosis may increase, for bronchial hypervascularization is very well developed in this disease. According to Stern et al. (1978), massive bleeding occurred in 38 (5%) of 728 patients, both children and adults. It was recurrent in 45%. Fink et al. (1978) reported bleeding in 9 of 40 patients, or about 20%, and Porter et al. (1983) observed it to be fatal in 11%. Holsclaw et al. (1970) observed bleeding to be even more serious, 6 of 19 patients dying within 2 days of its onset. Emergency surgery in this condition carries a high mortality, 18% according to Porter et al. (1983), indicating a role for treatment by embolization. The best results are obtained when all bronchial arteries are embolized, because of numerous interarterial anastomoses (Fellows et al., 1979).

J. Miscellaneous Causes

Endoscopic biopsy may occasionally be complicated by serious bleeding (Flick et al., 1975). We successfully saved a patient with postbiopsy bleeding by embolization (Fig. 11). Transthoracic needle biopsy for diagnosis and transbronchial laser therapy for bronchial cancer can occasionally be complicated by bleeding. In one case, preoperative CT was preventative, as it showed bronchial cancer invading the pulmonary artery (Personne et al., 1976). Bronchial telangiectasia in Rendu-Weber-Osler syndrome may occasionally bleed (Lincoln and Shigeoka, 1988), and rarely, seemingly normal bronchial arteries may spontaneously rupture as a result of local defects in their media (Sheffield et al., 1988).

IV. Endoscopy for Bronchial Bleeding

The indications for endoscopy in bronchial bleeding depend basically on whether the need is for diagnosis or treatment (Selecky, 1978). Repeated chronic low-volume hemoptysis in which bronchial cancer is a primary consideration is primarily investigated endoscopically, usually with a fiberoptic instrument. In massive hemoptysis for which embolotherapy may eventually be necessary, endoscopy can be useful by clearing bronchi of clots, identifying the bleeding territory, protecting other lung regions from aspiration, and applying local hemostasis. In this circumstance, the rigid bronchoscope is usually used. Bronchial cancer frequently presents with bleeding, in 40% of cases in fact (Weaver et al., 1979). Often the chest radiograph is abnormal, but if it is not, the incidence of cancer discovered by endoscopy is low. Jackson et al. (1985) report 3% and Poe et al. (1988) report 6%. Thus, with a normal radiograph, bleeding is predominantly of nonneoplastic or indeterminate origin.

The value of endoscopy in localizing active bleeding is variably assessed. Smiddy and Elliott (1973) report that localization was correct in 93% of cases, whereas Gonz and Salvatierra (1981) state that localization was not possible in as many as 60% of patients undergoing fiberoptic bronchoscopy during or within 48 h of the cessation of bleeding. Table 4 shows our experience in 141 cases. Neither site nor cause of bleeding was established in 55 patients, or 39%. Conversely, endoscopy provided useful information in 61%. If there are no radiographic or endoscopic clues to the site of bleeding, proper angiography requires exploration not only of the bronchial arteries but the intercostal, subclavian, and axillary arteries as well. If the bleeding lobe or segment is known beforehand, however, angiography may be more limited. In our embolized patients, about 80% of bleeding came from the upper lobes.

V. Indications and Contraindications for Endovascular Treatment of Bronchial Bleeding

A. Indications

The prime indication for vasoocclusion or embolization is severe bronchial bleeding that resists medical treatment in a patient who cannot be surgically managed. Authors vary in their use of adjectives for bleeding. For instance, "massive bleeding" is said to be more than 1 L in 24 h (Muthuswamy, 1987) or 600 ml in 24 h (Garzon, 1982). "Exsanguinating bleeding" is the loss of a liter of blood at a flow rate of 150 ml/h. "Especially massive bleeding" is 600 ml in 16 h or 200 ml every 24 h (Middleton et al., 1977). "Severe bleeding" is less than 200 ml in 24 h (Poe et al., 1988). The initial quantity of blood may be deceptive, however. Premonitory or sentinel bleeding may be followed by a grace period of hours to days before massive and even fatal bleeding occurs. Such sentinel bleeding has been described in intracavitary aspergilloma (Fernandez, 1984), invasive aspergillosis (Albelda et al., 1985; Panos et al., 1988), mucormycosis (Reich and Renzetti, 1970), necrotizing pneumonia (Murthy et

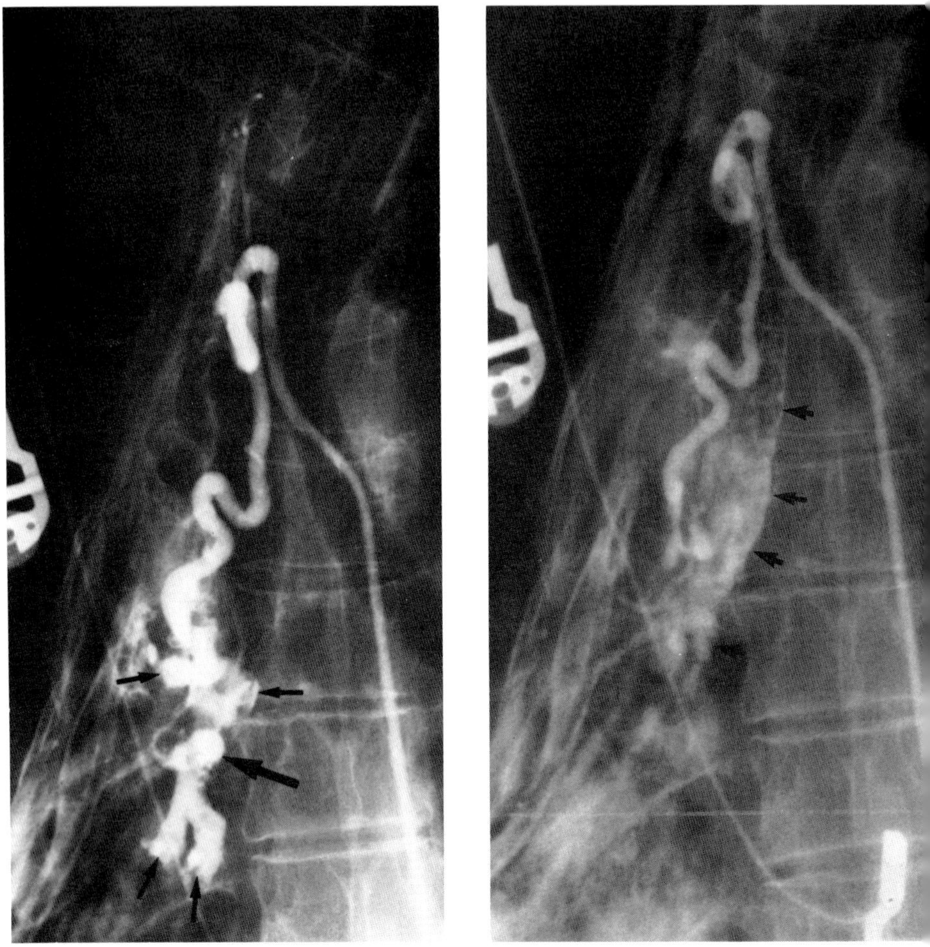

(A) (B)

Figure 11 Postbronchoscopic biopsy bleeding controlled by endovascular embolization. Previous thoracoplasty for tuberculosis. Biopsy of a submucosal nodule in the right middle lobe bronchus was followed by cataclysmic bleeding. (A) Selective arteriography of the intercostobronchial trunk shows the right bronchial artery is very dilated and sinuous (small arrows). A bronchoarterial fistula is shown (large arrow). (B) Bleeding into a bronchus is shown (arrows). Embolization of the artery with large fragments of Gelfoam was ineffective, the fragments being retrieved from aspirated blood. (C) A bronchial balloon was used to isolate the bleeding site. (D) Proximal embolization of the right bronchial artery (arrows) with isobutyl-2-cyanoacrylate effectively controlled the bleeding. No recurrence in 6 years.

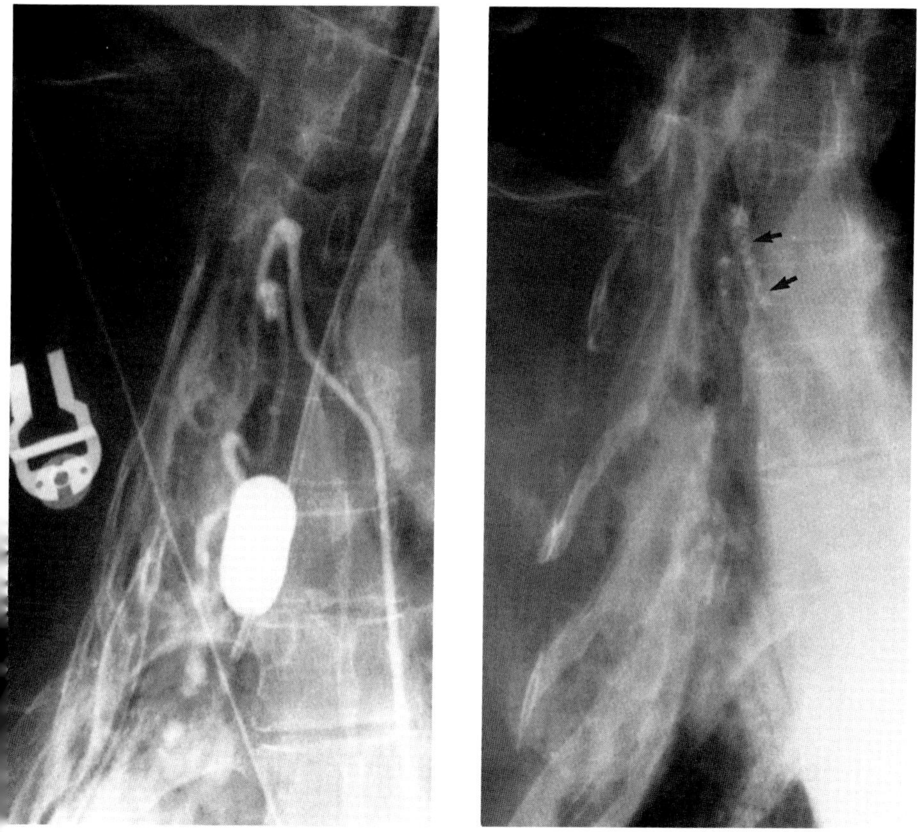

(C) (D)

al., 1981), tuberculosis (Middleton et al., 1977), lung abscess (Remy et al., 1984), and Swan-Ganz catheter trauma (Martin et al., 1982; Davis et al., 1987).

Besides the quantity of blood, other considerations before undertaking embolotherapy are respiratory function, the extent of the lesions, the adequacy of equipment, the competence of personnel, and the general prognosis for the patient. Most of the causes of severe bronchial bleeding are primarily medical rather than surgical problems (Conlan et al., 1983). In 123 patients who expectorated more than 600 ml blood in 24 h, Conlan et al. (1983) found the causes to be as follows: tuberculosis in 47, bronchiectasis in 37, chronic necrotizing pneumonia in 11, lung abscess in 6, cancer in 6, bronchovascular fistulas in 5, fungal infection in 4, and others in 7. Also according to Conlan et al. (1983),

Table 4 Location of Bronchial Bleeding by Endoscopy (Author's Experience)

Location	Number of patients
Right or left lung	13
Lobar bronchus	39
Segmental bronchus	33
Subsegmental bronchus	1
No bleeding, no lesion	28
Bilateral bleeding	15
Endoscopy incomplete	12
Total	141

emergency surgery in this circumstance carries a high mortality (17%). According to Garzon et al. (1982), surgical mortality is 25%. Embolotherapy does not carry this high risk, and since it is often effective, at least temporarily, it allows a period for medical treatment or the proper preparation of the patient for definitive surgery.

Although it is difficult to predict the future behavior of minor bleeding, when it occurs in necrotizing lung disease, we believe it justifies angiographic exploration and prophylactic embolization of the blood supply to the necrotic region. Angiographic exploration and preventive embolotherapy are also indicated when surgery carrying a high risk of bleeding is planned. This is true in the resection of vascular tumors, thoracoplasty, and cavernostomy (Hughes et al., 1986).

Occasionally, clues to the risk of bleeding are provided by CT, MRI, and angiography, such as the discovery of aneurysms of the pulmonary artery, pulmonary arteriovenous malformations, vessels in close proximity to a cavity, extravasation of contrast material during angiographic exploration, and arterial injuries from Swan-Ganz catheters. Contrast-enhanced CT is particularly useful in noninvasively identifying circumstances in which preventive treatment may be considered (Furuse et al., 1987).

B. Contraindications

The single most important contraindication to endovascular occlusion is the risk of spinal cord injury as determined at the time of angiography. This is taken up later. Chronic pulmonary embolism seems to be a relative contraindication. Recurrent hemoptysis is a symptom or a complication of chronic pulmonary thromboembolism (Mills et al., 1980; Cabrol et al., 1978; Chitwood et al., 1985). The mechanisms of bleeding are either oozing from a hyperemic, friable bronchial mucosa due to proliferation of bronchial arteries or the development of hypertensive lesions in the nonoccluded pulmonary arterial branches. If the hemoptysis is due to the first mechanism, bronchial arteries can be embolized for its management, but there is a danger of causing infarction from interruption of a systemic collateral supply (see Fig. 22).

VI. Techniques of Angiography and Embolization

A. Bronchial Arteriography and Embolization

The anatomy of the bronchial arteries varies with the method of examination. Cudkowicz's (1968) description is based on nonperfused arteries. Botenga (1969) dealt with diseased lungs and pathological arteries. During angiography in a patient, the arteries may appear to be different depending on the technique: global aortography versus selective ostial injection or conventional versus digital imaging. Notably lacking in most anatomic descriptions are the interarterial anastomoses that are so prominent in the pathological lung and probably preexist in the normal lung.

The location of the arterial ostia is an important technical point. The bronchial arteries emerge at right angles from the anterior, the right anterior, and the left anterior aspects of the descending aorta over a few centimeters extending above, at, and below the crossing of the left mainstem bronchus. In many cases (80%), the right bronchial arteries are branches of the intercostobronchial artery, which has an axis of about 130° to the axis of the aorta and is easily catheterized with a catheter of proper shape. With advancing age, tortuosity of the iliac arteries and aorta make catheterization more difficult, even though the ostium is 1.5–2.0 mm in diameter. Changing the catheter insertion to the other femoral artery is sometimes helpful.

With precurved 5–7F catheters for the left or right arteries, injection is first made in the aorta above the arteries to define their location and size. We prefer not to catheterize an ostium immediately lest it be injured and other bronchial arteries overlooked. Further, it is desirable to know the size and flow in large arteries to determine the contrast volume for selective injection.

The first injection is made in the first centimeter of the artery. Ultraselective catheterization must not be attempted in the first instance for two reasons: the risk of trauma to the endothelium and the risk of injecting beyond a strategic bronchial branch.

Embolization must not be carried out too close to the ostium as interarterial anastomoses may continue to supply the lesion downstream of the embolus. In the bronchial arteries we do not use metal coils, large emboli, electrocoagulation, or cyanoacrylate tissue glue, nor do we place the emboli too far peripherally lest tissue necrosis result (Naar et al., 1983). Absolute alcohol is hazardous in this respect (Naar et al., 1983). In our hands, Gelfoam particles about 300 μm in diameter have proved the most satisfactory.

It is seldom that angiography displays the bleeding vessel. This is recognized only when the contrast material has entered the bronchus from the injection site. Some normal and noninvolved arteries are necessarily occluded but the bleeding artery(s) is included. As long as there is concordance between the territory fed by the artery, the location of the lesion by radiography, and the site of bleeding by endoscopy, embolization of the artery can proceed.

B. Hemodynamic Consequences of Angiography and Embolization

Selective injection of an artery temporarily augments the distal flow by raising the intraarterial pressure and by reducing the peripheral resistance because of the vasodilating effect of contrast agents (Levin, 1978). This temporary perturbation may modify the direction of flow through anastomoses (Fig. 12), augment the venous return, suggesting an arteriovenous fistula, cause opacification, a blush of the lung lesion or bronchus, and provoke otherwise nonexistent arterial extravasation (Fig. 13). These effects are more pronounced if large volumes of contrast agent are used and the artery is occluded by the catheter.

Embolization also has hemodynamic effects. By redistributing flow, it may allow opacification of arteries not previously seen (Fig. 14), including the anterior spinal artery (Fig. 15), discovery of interarterial anastomoses not previously known, and unexpected extravasation of contrast agent. This last can occur in the aortic wall and must be avoided at all costs as the resulting dissection could compromise spinal cord perfusion and bronchial artery patency. For these reasons, the speed of injection of contrast agent and emboli must be continuously adapted to the speed of flow as seen fluoroscopically (Kerber, 1980; Levin, Beckmann and Hillman, 1980).

Embolus size is important, and discrepancies between the embolus and blood vessel arise under special circumstances. If systemic hypotension from bleeding has required vasoconstrictive drugs, these may reduce bronchial artery caliber during embolization such that the emboli become ineffective or change position after cessation of the drug. If a large number of emboli appear to be necessary to occlude a small artery, the catheterization is probably poor and the emboli may be flowing backward to escape to other vessels. Conversely, if an artery seems to obstruct too rapidly, there may be conglomeration of emboli in a clot at the tip of the catheter rather than being dispersed into the arterial branches. This conglomeration may be broken up with a guide

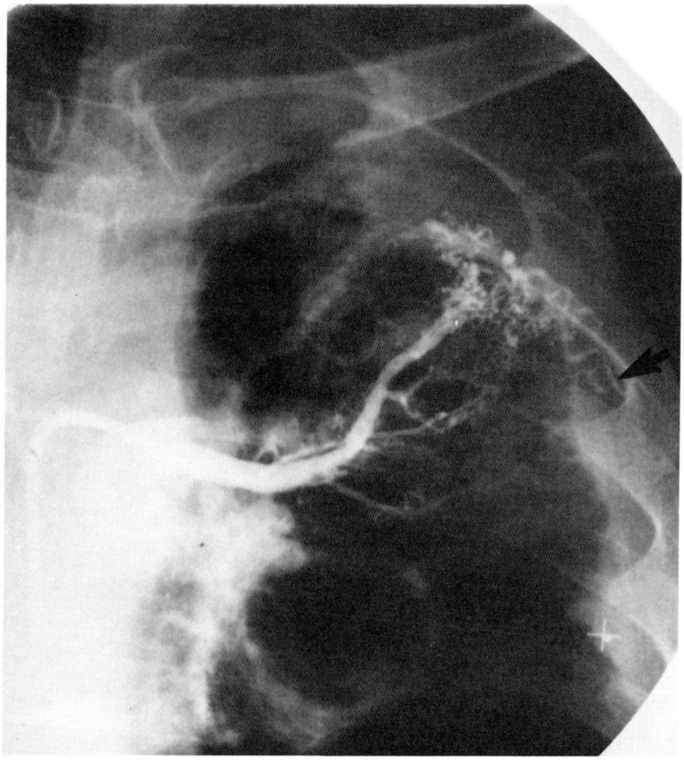

Figure 12 Transpleural intercostal-pulmonary anastomosis demonstrated by reverse flow. A patient with large intracavitary aspergilloma. Selective angiography in a pulmonary arterial branch in the left upper lobe opacifies an aortic intercostal artery (arrow) by transpleural symphysis. The reverse flow presumably reflects momentary elevation of intravascular pressure during injection.

wire. An uncontrollable effect appears to be vasoconstriction of an artery proximal to a distal embolus. This may frustrate further catheterization of the artery.

The choice of embolic material is a large subject that can be dealt with only superficially here. Gelfoam has many advantages: easy use, low cost, preparation at the time of need, and biodegradability. Fragments are sized as appropriate and lead to temporary (7–21 days) occlusion. Sometimes Gelfoam's friability leads to more distal embolization than desired. A Gelfoam slurry of Pantopaque, 50% dextrose solution, a sclerosing agent, and amino-

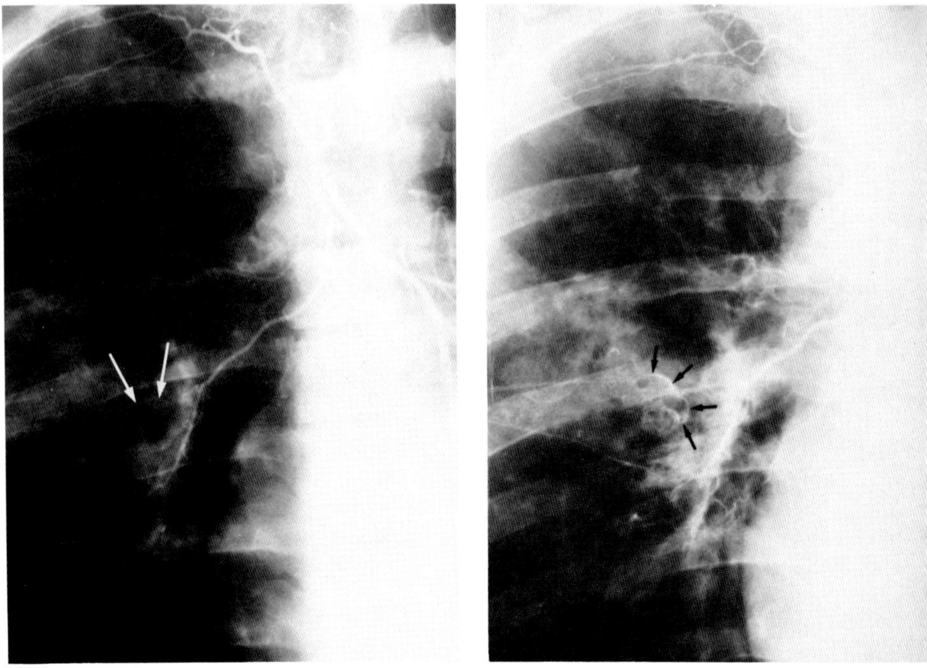

(A) (B)

Figure 13 Extravasation at angiography in cavitary tuberculosis. (A) Bronchial arteriogram shows branches surrounding the cavity (arrows). (B) The catheter was advanced, and a second injection shows more cavitary opacification, suggesting extravasation of contrast material (arrows).

caproic acid (an antifibrinolytic agent) was used by Mauro and Jaques (1987). This preparation has the advantage of x-ray opacity.

The frequency of recanalization after Gelfoam has led to nonresorbable materials, among them isobutyl-2-cyanoacrylate, a tissue glue also known as IBC (Grenier et al., 1983). The injection technique must be mastered as this material rapidly polymerizes in blood. Polymerization can be slowed by mixing with Ethiodol, a radiopaque oil, or by pre- and postinjections of saline into the artery. Preinjection of fragments of lyophilized dura mater prevents the IBC from peripheral distribution where tissue necrosis would result. IBC produces permanent occlusion, the initial inflammatory reaction leading to later obliterative endarteritis (Cromwell et al., 1986). We do not use IBC because it is more difficult to handle than solid emboli and because its viscosity may

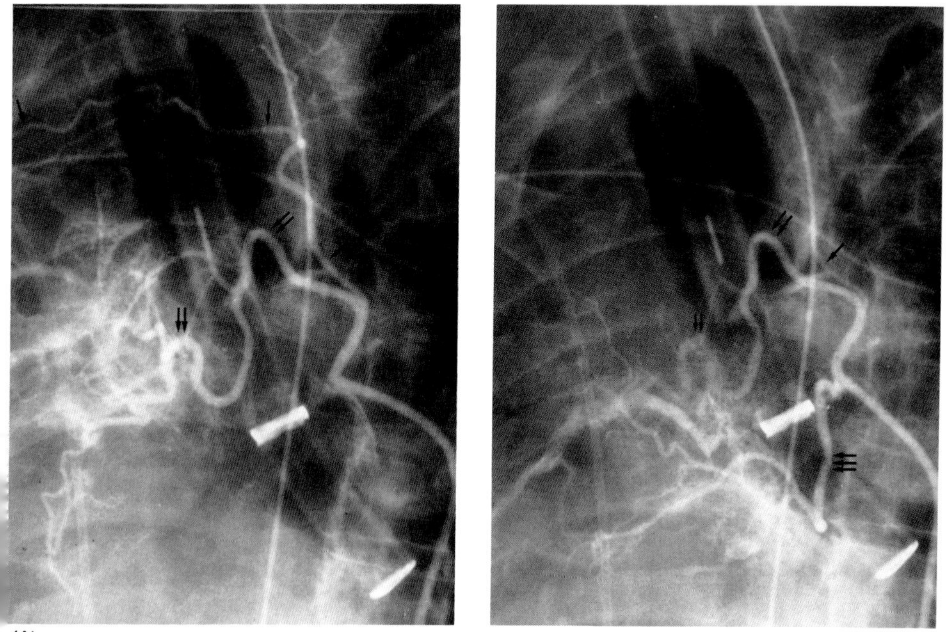

(A) (B)

Figure 14 Redistribution of blood flow after embolization. Intracavity aspergilloma. (A) Injection of the intercostobronchial trunk shows an intercostal artery (single arrows) and a right bronchial artery (double arrows). The intercostobronchial trunk was embolized with fragments of dura mater. (B) Subsequent arteriography shows occlusion of the intercostal artery (single arrow) and right bronchial artery (double arrows) and new opacification of a second bronchial artery (triple arrow).

cause undesirable proximal occlusion. Further, since occlusion is permanent, subsequent entry into the vessel is impossible should the situation require a second embolization.

Polyvinyl alcohol (Ivalon) is also used in bronchial arteries. Subsequent histological study showed the particles in vessels and in peribronchial connective tissue. The vessels are destroyed and fibrosed. Absolute alcohol has also been used (Naar et al., 1983), but we do not use it because it causes vascular damage down to the capillary level that could lead to tissue necrosis (Cromwell et al., 1986).

Lyophilized dura mater is easy to use. We use it when arterial catheterization is selective and stable. In subsequent histological study at 2 years we

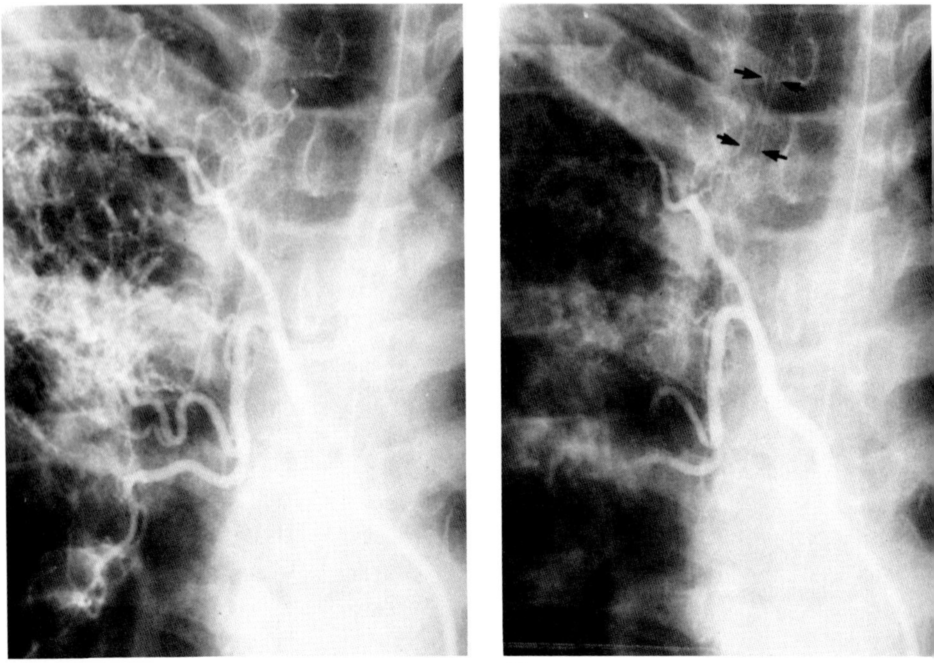

(A) (B)

Figure 15 Demonstration of spinal arteries requiring cessation of embolization. (A) Bronchial arteriography and embolization were undertaken for bronchial bleeding due to tuberculosis. Extensive hypervascularization in the lung apex was demonstrated. (B) Repeat angiography after embolization shows tiny, rather straight arteries near the midline arising from the intercostal artery (arrows). These are spinal afferent arteries, and their demonstration requires cessation of further embolization in the intercostobronchial trunk.

observed this material was not biodegraded and did not incite inflammatory reaction or thombus. Apparently the particles alone stopped the flow.

Endovascular treatment of bronchial bleeding may be combined with surgical, medical, and endobronchial methods. Most often it is used after unsuccessful medical treatment and before or instead of surgical treatment. As a generalization, surgery carries a mortality of about 18% (Gourin and Garzon, 1975), and preoperative embolization can reduce this by half (Vujic et al., 1982).

Medical treatment with indomethacin has been tried, analogous to its use in newborns with patent ductus arteriosus. It is given by suppository and inhibits the production of vasodilating prostaglandins derived from arachidonic acid (Deffebach et al., 1987). However, indomethacin also inhibits platelet aggregation and prolongs bleeding time. We have no experience with it.

Endobronchial treatment usually involves cautery of the bleeding site or isolation of the bleeding territory and protection of the normal lung from aspiration with endobronchial tubes (Martin et al., 1982; Shivaram et al., 1987). Double-lumen plastic tubes, easier to use than Carlen's tubes, allow protection of normal lung and fiberoptic inspection of the affected lung. A Fogarty catheter passed under television (TV) guidance can also be used to isolate the bleeding bronchus.

C. Spinal Injury Complications

The anatomy of the blood supply of the spinal cord explains the occurrence of injury to it during bronchial arteriography. Adamkiewicz's artery, which supplies the anterior spinal artery, arises from intercostal arteries and enters the spinal canal at the level of the fifth to eighth dorsal vertebrae in about 8–15% of individuals (Beg et al., 1987). Thus, manipulations within the intercostal arteries or the bronchointercostal artery may risk spinal cord injury.

The mechanisms responsible are not entirely clear. Possibilities include ischemia by direct or indirect occlusion of spinal cord blood flow, endothelial toxicity of the contrast material, and direct neurotoxicity of the contrast agent (Schrodt et al., 1987). The recording of somatosensory evoked potentials has been useful in detecting anterior spinal ischemia during aortic surgery, in myelopathies, and during spinal angiography (Wadouh et al., 1986; Drummond et al., 1987; Laschinger et al., 1987). Such recordings may be advantageous during bronchial arteriography (Schrodt et al., 1987).

The risk of spinal injury is greater on the right than left because of the common origin of spinal and bronchial arteries from the intercostobronchial trunk. On the left side there is no intercostobronchial trunk. The intercostals and bronchials have separate orifices from the aorta, the former from the posterior aspect and the latter on the anterior aspect. Still, they may be confused unless multiplane TV viewing is used.

Schrodt et al. (1987) describe using evoked sematosensory potentials to guide catheterization. When the intercostobronchial artery was entered, a test injection of Amytal Sodium (amobarbital) caused painful evoked potentials. The catheter was advanced into the bronchial branch, where evoked potentials were painless and uncomplicated embolization was carried out. Still there is a possibility of cord injury if in superselective catheterization the intercostobronchial artery is occluded or if during injection contrast agent or emboli flow back from it. Drugs have been used to protect the cord: Amytal and lidocaine (Horton, 1986) and papavarine to dilate the anterior spinal artery (Svensson et al., 1988).

Ultimately, however, safety requires observing basic precautions. Any intercostal artery should be searched for spinal branches, and special care should be used in the right intercostobronchial trunk. An adequately large field of view and high-quality images are essential as spinal arteries may be very narrow. Prolonged entry of intercostal arteries should be avoided, and contrast material of low neurotoxicity and endothelial toxicity should be used. Injection that produces backflow toward the aorta must be avoided. Frequent testing of neurological responses during the procedure is mandatory. With respect for these essentials, we believe that recognition of spinal branches of the intercostobronchial artery is not an absolute contraindication to embolization. However, other angiographers disagree (Miller and Mineau, 1983).

D. Angiography of Other Systemic Arteries

In addition to the bronchial arteries and the pulmonary arteries, a third group of vessels can contribute to bronchial bleeding. These systemic arteries become functional only in disease states and may be very numerous. Principally the internal mammary, intercostal, and diaphragmatic arteries supply the lung by anastomoses across the pleural space (Remy et al., 1977; Keller et al., 1987; Hickey et al., 1988).

The internal mammary artery is the most important. Its branches, which can take part in transpleural vascularization of the lung, are the pericardiophrenic and the anterior intercostals (Fig. 16). The former can terminate in musculophrenic and diaphragmatic arteries deriving from the celiac trunk and aorta. The anterior intercostals anastomose with the posterior intercostals from the axillary arteries and aorta to encircle the chest (Fig. 17). Sternal, paracardiac, and mediastinal branches may join with bronchial arteries to create a mediastinal plexus. An accessory internal mammary artery is found in 16% of subjects (Nathan et al., 1982). Because of rich anastomoses with vessels below the diaphragm, including the ascending trunk of the deep iliac circumflex artery and the superior epigastric branch of the inferior epigastric artery, blood flow may be reversed in the internal mammary artery should the artery be occluded near its origin (Chait, 1976; Cohen et al., 1988). Bleeding both in the chest wall and from the lung can be controlled by embolization of the internal mammary artery. To be effective, the occlusion must be close to the vessels supplying the hemorrhage, or the generous anastomoses of the artery continue to allow the bleeding.

The posterior intercostal arteries from the aorta may supply the lung via pleural adhesions that at times may be profusely vascularized (Baile et al.,

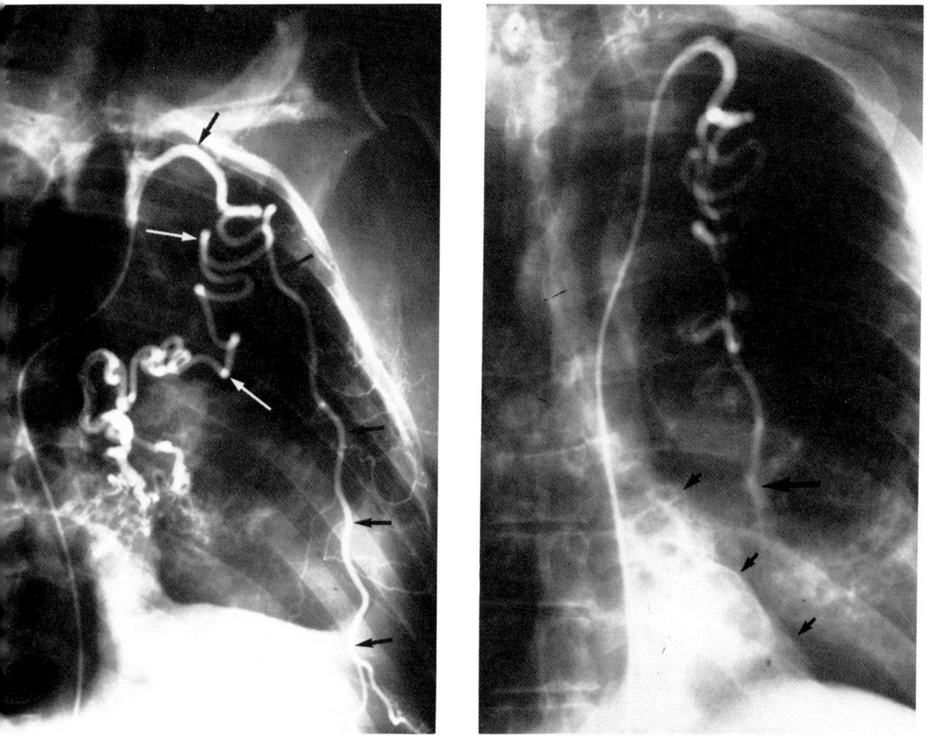

(A) (B)

Figure 16 Pericardiophrenic artery as the source of bronchial bleeding. The left lower lobe was retracted and bronchiectatic. (A) Angiography of the left internal mammary artery in the left posterior oblique projection shows that artery (black arrows) with a very large pericardiophrenic branch (white arrows) directed toward massive hypervascularization in the lower lobe. The pericardiophrenic artery was embolized with more than 100 fragments of lyophilized dura. (B) Repeat angiography in the frontal projection shows that the internal mammary artery is occluded (large arrow), and much of the hypervascularization in the left lower lobe is suppressed (small arrows). No recurrence of bleeding for 4 months until left lower lobe lobectomy.

1985). Their embolization has been effective in controlling bronchial bleeding (Prioleau et al., 1980; Vujic et al., 1980). The left intercostals emerge from the posterior aspect of the aorta, but the more superior right intercostals exit from the lateral aspect of the vessel. As discussed earlier, angiography and embolization of intercostal arteries must be undertaken very carefully because of the risk to small spinal cord branches. Even prolonged catheterization of a small intercostal ostium could lead to endothelial injury and thrombosis. A too

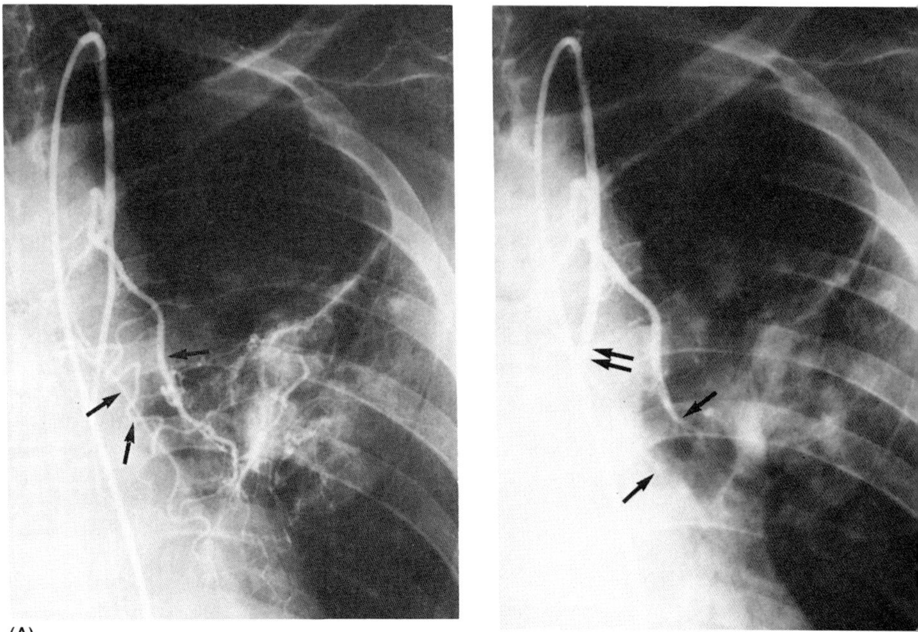

(A) (B)

Figure 17 Bleeding from intracavitary aspergilloma controlled by internal mammary artery embolization. Bronchial artery embolization failed to control serious bleeding. (A) Arteriography of the left internal mammary artery shows a hypervascularization network, probably fed by the pericardiophrenic artery (arrows). (B) Embolization with fragments of Gelfoam occludes the hypervascularization, the mammary artery (double arrow), and the pericardiophrenic artery (single arrows). (C) Upon recurrence of bleeding, the external mammary artery was injected. Its hypervascular network, including anterior intercostal arteries (arrows), was effectively obliterated by embolization (D), stopping bronchial bleeding for 2 years.

vigorous injection, especially after embolization, may lead to dissection and ostial occlusion.

At times, the thyrocervical and costocervical branches of the subclavian arteries can contribute collateral circulation (Moore et al., 1986), but caution must be used in embolizing these vessels because of their spinal branches and the proximity of the vertebral artery (Fig. 18).

Other systemic arteries that may supply the lung are pulmonary ligament arteries (Fig. 19) (Stocker and Malczak, 1984), inferior phrenic arteries (Figs. 20 and 21), and rarely branches of the subclavian and vertebral arteries (Darrason et al., 1986).

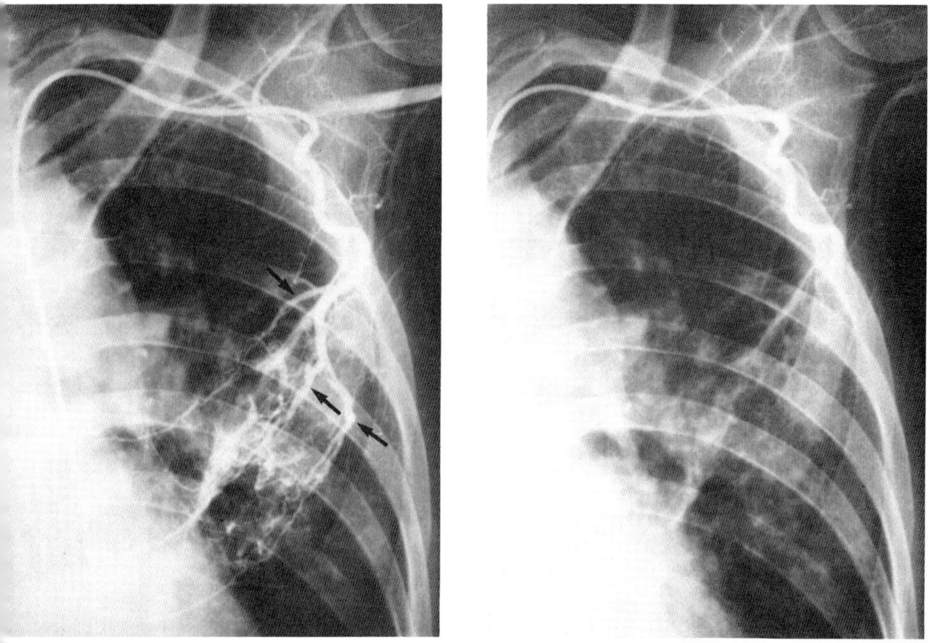

(D)

The hemodynamic effects of systemic hypervascularization of the lung are interesting and important. Hypervascularization allows a territory of the lung to be perfused at systemic pressure and high flow rates with as much as 6–20% of the cardiac output when it is grossly developed. Pulmonary venous return is augmented, and pulmonary artery perfusion is diverted away from the hypervascularized territory. To some extent, this diversion is desirable in the sense that pulmonary arterial blood does not perfuse hypoventilated lung. Yet, the systemic blood perfusing the diseased lung may return to the left heart somewhat desaturated. Both ventricles may be stressed, the left by the augmented pulmonary venous return and the right by pulmonary hypertension.

Systemic-pulmonary shunts are of two basic types depending on the direction of blood flow in the peripheral pulmonary arteries (Table 5). Retrograde flow from peripheral to more proximal pulmonary arteries is usually seen in disease of the parenchyma. Peripheral pulmonary vascular resistance is high, and blood flows centrally until it reaches branches that serve lung territories with lesser resistance where antegrade flow resumes. Figure 5 illustrates retrograde flow in bronchiectasis. Antegrade flow in the arteries from the hila to the periphery usually reflects central pulmonary artery obstruction of either congenital or acquired origin. Chronic pulmonary thromboembolism can be

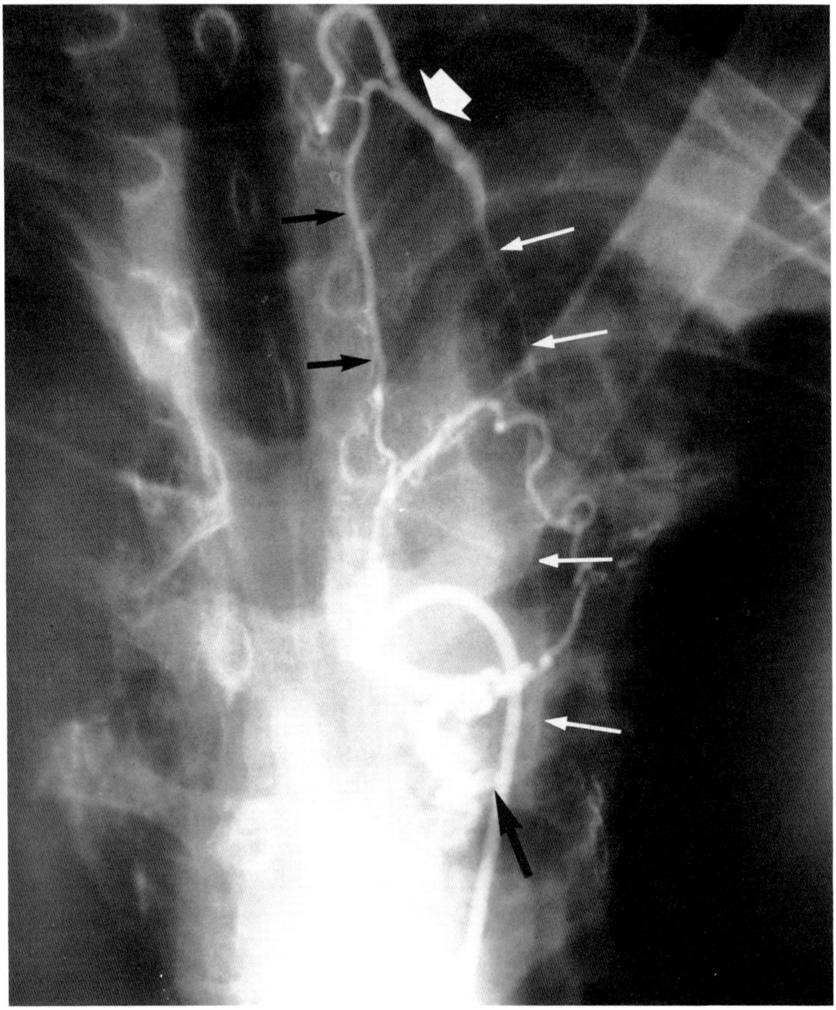

Figure 18 Anastomoses between thyrocervical trunk, internal mammary, and bronchial arteries. Bronchial bleeding due to intracavitary aspergilloma in the apical segment of the left lower lobe was treated by embolization of the left bronchial artery (large black arrow). Injection in the partially occluded bronchial artery demonstrates anastomosis between the thyrocervical trunk (large white arrow) and bronchial artery (small black arrows) and the internal mammary artery (small white arrows).

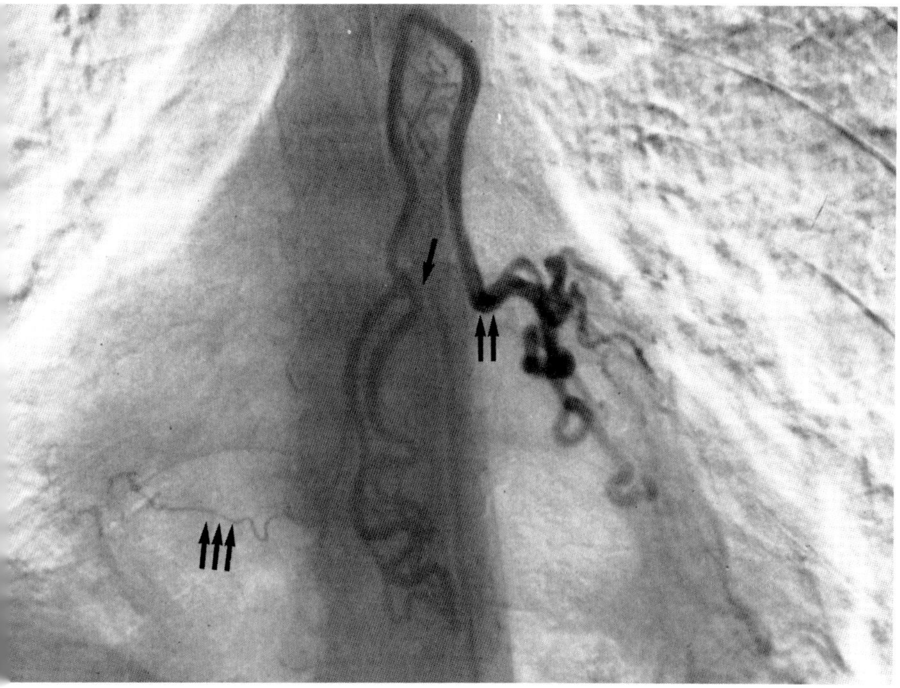

Figure 19 Mediastinal artery with blood supply to both lungs. Exploration of bleeding from the left lower lobe revealed an artery (single arrow) arising from the descending aorta, ascending and then descending to give origin to a large left inferior bronchial artery (double arrow) and a smaller right inferior bronchial artery (triple arrow). The arteries probably penetrate the lower lobes via the pulmonary ligaments. Embolization of the unnamed artery controlled the bleeding.

suspected when bronchial arteriography reveals large arteries providing antegrade flow in distal pulmonary arteries (Fig. 22). In this circumstance, lung perfusion by systemic arteries can contribute to gas exchange.

E. Angiography and Vasoocclusion of the Pulmonary Circulation

Bleeding from the pulmonary circulation can be temporarily stemmed with a Swan-Ganz balloon catheter, but more permanent occlusion is obtained with detachable balloons (White et al., 1979; Renie et al., 1982; Grinnell et al., 1982) or metal coils (Gianturco et al., 1975; Wallace et al., 1976; Chuang et al., 1980). Our experience is with the latter (Remy et al., 1988).

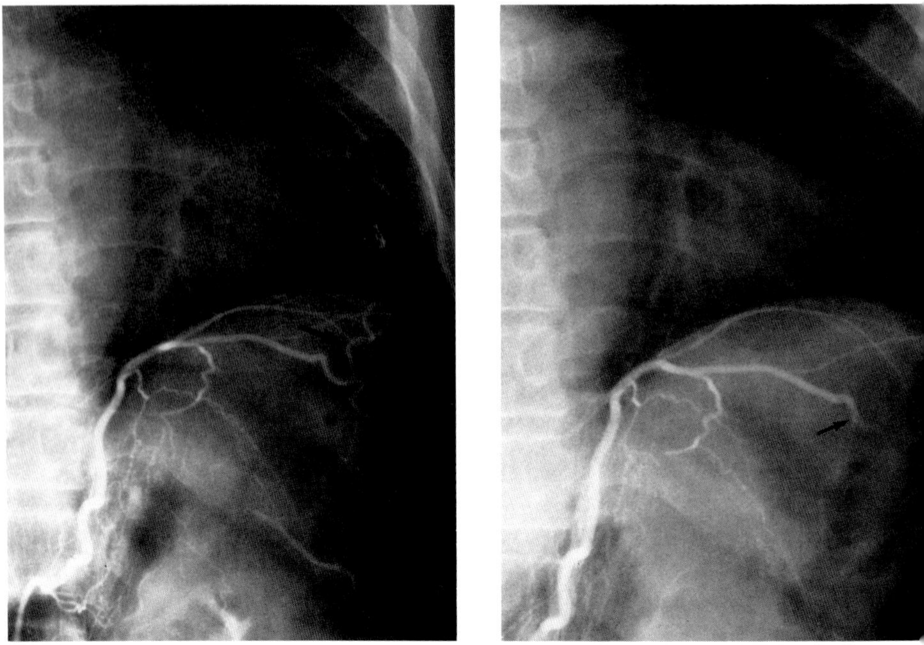

(A) (B)

Figure 20 Bronchial bleeding supplied by inferior phrenic artery. (A) In exploring bleeding from the lingula in a patient with chronic obstructive bronchial disease, the left inferior phrenic artery was catheterized. It has a transpleural branch (large black arrows) and phrenicopulmonary anastomoses (small arrows). (B) Release of emboli in the inferior phrenic artery (small black arrow) provoked no diaphragmatic complication and controlled bleeding for 4 years.

The metal coils are introduced in the uncoiled configuration by catheter and resume their shape when expelled into the vessel. They carry thrombogenic Dacron fibers. Considerable experience is needed in choosing the proper coil size and placing it properly (Chuang et al., 1980; Anderson, 1979). In general, a coil 15–25% larger than the diameter of the vessel provides optimal coiling and stability of position. Selective catheterization of the bleeding artery can be difficult because the heartbeat moves the catheter tip. Preferably coils are cast off when the catheter tip is still (Fig. 23).

The first coils carried wool fibers, which caused a pyogranulomatous reaction that destroyed the vessel wall. Silk, Ivalon, and Dacron are more histocompatible. With these, the occlusion is limited to thrombosis within the coil. Systemic-to-pulmonary hypervascularization distal to the coil may allow

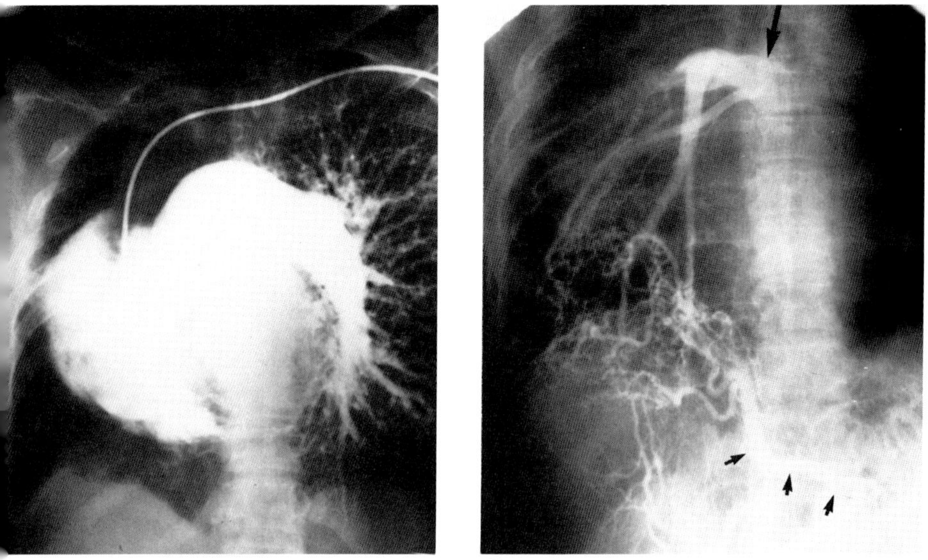

(A) (B)

Figure 21 Collateral circulation to the right lung from the inferior phrenic artery. Dyspnea and dextrocardia led to the discovery of unilateral agenesis of the right pulmonary veins. (A) Pulmonary angiography with injection in the right ventricle shows no filling of the right pulmonary artery. (B) Arteriography in the celiac trunk reveals extensive transdiaphragmatic and transpleural hypervascularization fed by the right inferior phrenic artery (small arrows) with retrograde flow in a small right pulmonary artery up to its origin (large arrow). (Courtesy of Dr. Personne.)

bleeding to continue. Also, coagulopathies, such as those after multiple transfusions, can frustrate control of bleeding as thrombogenesis is required (McLean et al., 1986). In the case of Rasmussen's aneurysms, the aneurysmal sac may be filled with coils (Fig. 24). At times it becomes necessary to occlude both systemic and pulmonary arteries to a bleeding region. This can be anticipated if blood samples from the pulmonary artery indicate a systemic shunt into more distal branches.

VII. Complications of Endovascular Control of Bronchial Bleeding

Several general reviews of selective angiography and endovascular occlusion are available (Miller and Mineau, 1983; Feldman et al., 1983; White and Lun-

Table 5 Classification of Systemic-to-Pulmonary Shunts (Numerous Sources)

I. Retrograde flow in pulmonary arteries
  Pleural or pulmonary disease
    Trauma: postlobectomy, abscess drainage, pneumothorax
    Inflammatory
    Neoplastic
    Congenital
    Idiopathic
  Mediastinal disease
  Bronchopulmonary disease
  Obstruction of pulmonary venous return
  Idiopathic

II. Antegrade flow in pulmonary arteries
  Congenital heart disease with pulmonary stenosis or atresia
  Palliative anastomoses: Blalock, Waterston, Potts
  Unilateral absence or atresia of pulmonary artery
  Peripheral pulmonary stenosis
    Congenital
      Rubeola, Williams and Beuren syndrome, Keutel syndrome,
  Conradi's syndrome, arteriohepatic dysplasia
    Acquired
      Chronic thromboembolism, mediastinitis, Takayasu's disease
    Pulmonary hypertension

dell, 1984; Hemingway and Allison, 1988). Our own experience through 1989 is shown in Table 6. This includes 350 patients undergoing systemic arteriography without embolism in 1967–1973 and 260 patients with systemic or pulmonary angiography and embolization in 1973–1989. Several complications warrant special consideration.

Bronchial arteries are necessary for the nutrition of the central bronchi and lobar branches. In 1951, Ellis et al. experimentally demonstrated that interruption of the arteries resulted in ulceration of proximal bronchial walls and the middle third of the esophagus. Hilar lymph nodes were infarcted. Subsequently, Fisher et al. (1970) demonstrated that the bronchial circulation was restored within a month of complete interruption. In practice, bronchial injury after bronchial artery embolization is uncommon but has been described: focal necrosis of the right main bronchus with subsequent nonstenotic scarring (Remy et al., 1977), bronchoesophageal fistula (Helenon et al., 1977), bronchial mucosal infarction (Baile et al., 1985), bronchial stenosis requiring pneu-

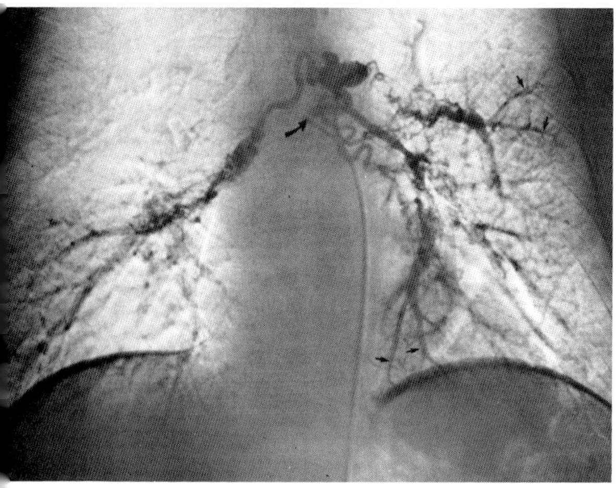

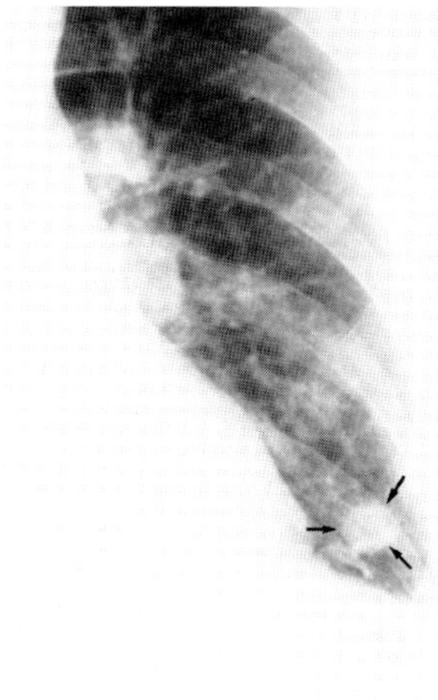

(B)

Figure 22 Chronic pulmonary embolism with recurrent bronchial bleeding. (A) Bronchial arteriography shows a common trunk with dilated sinuous, proximal right and left branches (curved arrow). These anastomose near the hila with pulmonary artery branches in which there is antegrade pulmonary flow (small arrows). Central pulmonary artery emboli were suspected. The common trunk was embolized. (B) A pulmonary nodule (arrows) and some pleural fluid developed 24 h later, suggesting pulmonary infarction; both resolved spontaneously a few days later.

monectomy, and bronchopulmonary artery fistula (Ivanick et al., 1983). Generalizations are difficult from these reports, in which differing sites and differing embolic materials were used.

Myocardial ischemia is also a potential complication of bronchial embolization inasmuch as the bronchial circulation anastomoses with the coronary circulation, providing the possibility of collateral flow between the two (Baile et al., 1985; Bolling et al., 1984; Lajos, 1985). At coronary angiography anastomoses are found in 22% of normal subjects and 48% of those with stenosing coronary lesions. The communications may be as large as 2 mm in diameter (Bjork, 1966). Other collateral vessels to the coronary arteries may derive from various mediastinal branches, the pericardiophrenic, inferior phrenic, and esophageal arteries (Smith et al., 1972). Whereas the bronchial arteries may supply the coronaries, they may also steal from the coronaries when profuse systemic-to-pulmonary collateralization develops as in Fallot's tetralogy and pulmonary atresia. This raises the possibility of bronchial steal in older individuals with acquired systemic collateralization. It also emphasizes the need for care during bronchial embolization in such persons as emboli may escape to the coronary circulation (Durand-Gasselin et al., 1988).

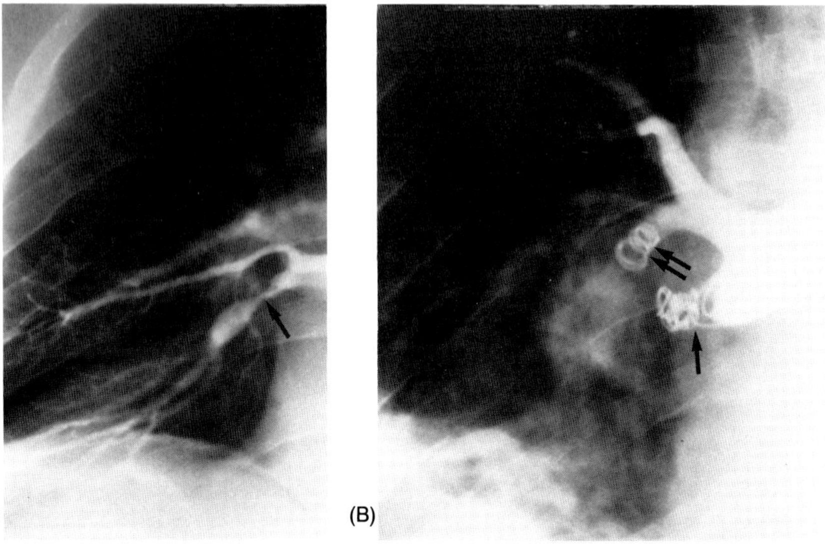

(A) (B)

Figure 23 Bronchial cancer invading the right inferior pulmonary vein and left atrium treated with coils. (A) Pulmonary angiography shows a serrated stenosis of the right middle lobe artery (arrow) and nonopacification of the right inferior pulmonary vein. There was a mass in the left atrium. The bleeding was controlled by placing metal coils in the artery. (B) Repeat angiography at 7 weeks for recurrent bleeding. A second coil was placed (double arrow) and controlled the bleeding again. Neoplastic venoatrial invasion was demonstrated at autopsy.

Aside from the spinal complications previously discussed, other rare complications of bronchial embolization are intercostal and paraspinal muscle infarction (Doppman and Di Chiro, 1976) and pulmonary necrosis with erosion of the pulmonary artery (Rabkin et al., 1987).

VIII. Results of Endovascular Treatment

Our cumulative experience in 260 patients with endovascular management of bronchial bleeding is summarized in Table 7. Hemoptysis was immediately arrested in 182, or 70%. Although 70% immediate control of bleeding is helpful, this control is not always permanent. Recurrent hemorrhage occurs in about 15% of patients within a month of embolization (Table 8) and even more frequently the longer the posttreatment interval (Table 9). When bleeding

Table 6 Complications of Angiographic Techniques in the Treatment of Bronchial Bleeding

Cerebrovascular injury: 4
Hemiplegia: 2 (1 reversible, 1 irreverisble)
Diffuse injury to the cerebral trunk: 1 fatal
Blindness, transitory: 1
Spinal cord injury: 2
(1 reversible, 1 irreversible)
Extravasation, aortic or mediastinal:
8 without complications
Ischemic incidents in the territory of embolization
Bronchial: 2
bronchus intermedius injury, spontaneously resolved
Pulmonary infarction: 2
(1 spontaneous resolution, 1 evolved into necrosis and secondary infection)
Esophageal: 8
painful dysphagia clearing after several hours
Ischemic incidents remote from the territory of embolization
Splanchnic: 2
epigastric pain spontaneously resolved
Digital: 2
ischemia of digital pulp
Complications of Seldinger technique
Thrombosis of femoral artery: 1
Thrombosis of axillary artery: 1
Cardiovascular collapse by anaphylaxis: 1
recovery without sequelae

recurs, it is of the same amount in about one-half of patients, less voluminous in 35%, and more in 15%.

These results compare favorably with other methods of treatment of massive bronchial bleeding in which the mortality of surgery is 13% and the mortality of medical treatment 22% (Bobrowitz et al., 1983). The primary risk of embolization is spinal cord injury, which occurs in 0.5–1.0%.

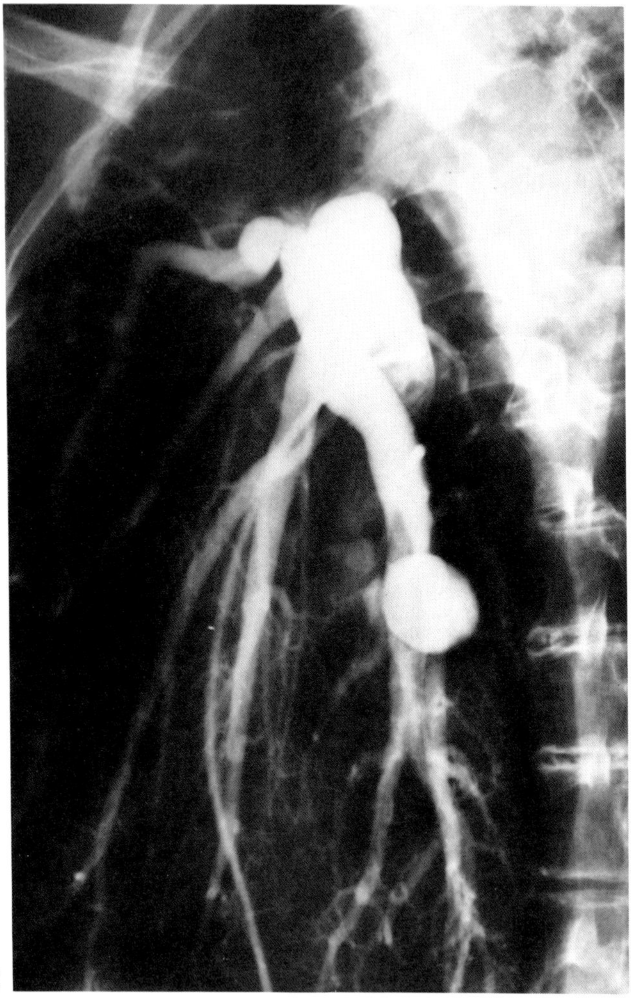

(A)

Figure 24 Rasmussen's aneurysm treated with coils. (A) Pulmonary angiography in right posterior oblique projection revealed an unsuspected aneurysm in the lower lobe. We believe this is properly considered Rasmussen's aneurysm because a tuberculous cavity at the site was demonstrated earlier. (B) Profile angiography showed the eccentric origin of the aneurysm from the segmental artery (large arrows). (C) The aneurysm was thrombosed with 12 coils placed in the sac. This was complicated by thrombosis of the segmental artery as well. (Reproduced from *AJR* 1984; **143**:963–969, with permission.)

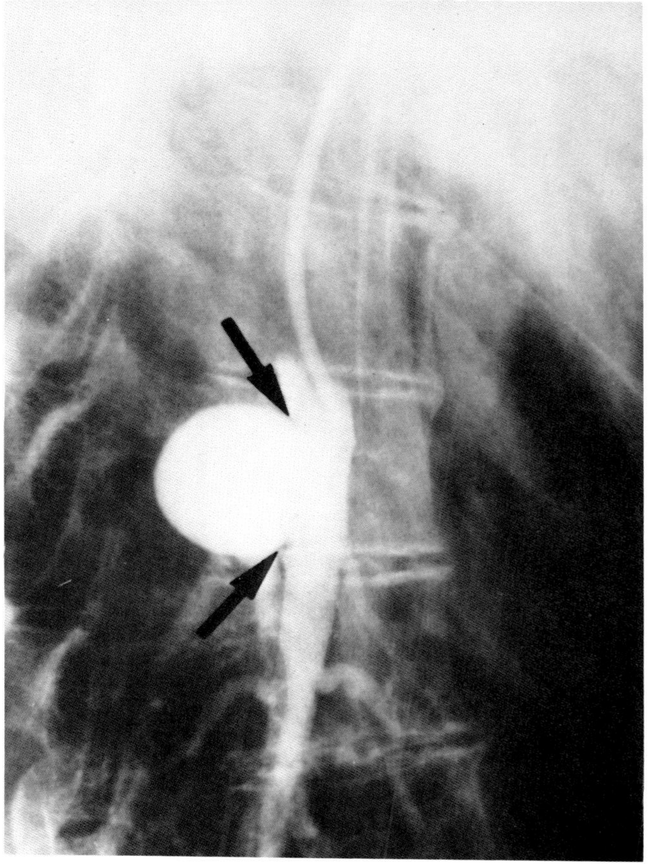

(B)

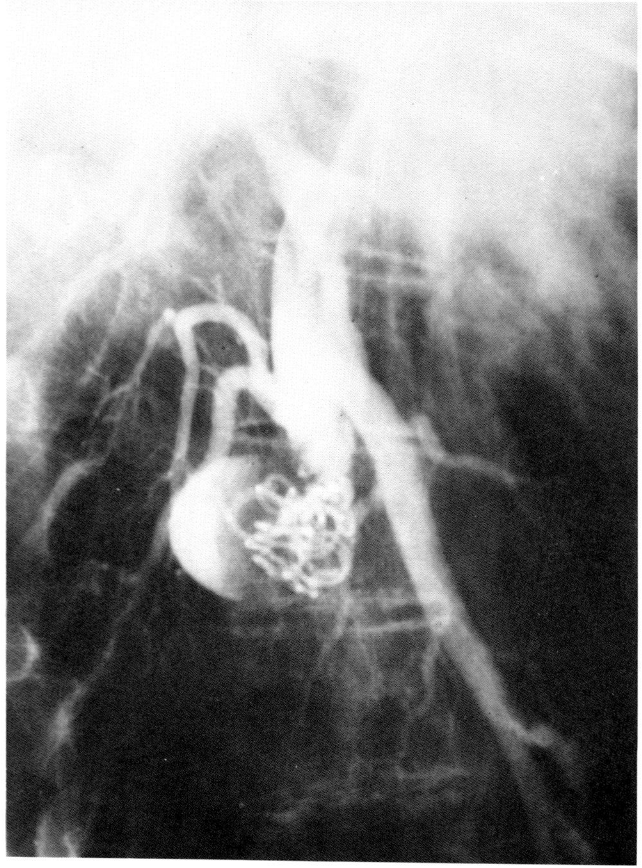

(C)

Figure 24

Table 7 Author's Results in 260 Endovascular Procedures for Control of Bronchial Bleeding

Year of publication	Cumulative number of patients	Immediate arrest of bleeding after embolization
1973	7	6
1976	43	35
1977	49	41
1983	98	68
1989	260	182

Table 8 Frequency of Recurrent Bleeding 1 Month After Embolization

Reference	Frequency of recurrence
Remy et al. (1977)	6/41
Magilligan et al. (1981)	2/7
Barret et al. (1983)	4/18
Uflacker et al. (1983)	6/33
Uflacker et al. (1985)	12/56
Rabkin et al. (1987)	39/278
Fellows et al. (1979)	0/12
Wholey et al. (1976)	0.14
Ferris (1981)	2/16

Table 9 Frequency of Recurrent Bleeding in Different Conditions: Author's Experience, Multiyear Follow-up

Conditions	%
Sequelae of tuberculosis	30
Coal miner's pneumonoconioses	50
Bronchiectasis	60
Intracavitary aspergilloma	100

IX. Conclusions

Despite the contribution that endovascular treatment can make, this management of bronchial bleeding has not yet been fully exploited. Lacking full understanding of the mechanism of bleeding when it begins, it is still difficult to choose the least harmful and most quickly effective method. The problem arises with sentinel bleeding. If it were definitely known that slight bronchial bleeding would be followed by massive hemorrhage, aggressive preventive treatment could be confidently undertaken. Not all slight bleeding justifies extensive angiographic effort, however, and although generally effective, endovascular treatment is costly and carries a small risk. Only by stopping the bleeding can we be sure that endovascular treatment is warranted, yet this may involve exploration of many vessels and the embolization of several. This dilemma requires us to refine our studies of the conditions associated with bronchial bleeding and to publish and share our experiences so that this method of treatment is most knowledgeably applied.

Acknowledgment

We thank Professor Melvin Figley for his enormous work of translation, editing, and rewriting.

References

Albelda, S. M., Talbot, G. H., Gerson, S. L., Miller, W. T., and Cassileth, P. A. (1985). Pulmonary cavitation and massive hemoptysis in invasive pulmonary aspergillosis. *Am. Rev. Respir. Dis.* **131**:115–120.

Anderson, J. H., Wallace, S., Gianturco, C., and Gerson, L. P. (1979). "Mini" Gianturco stainless stell coils for transcatheter vascular occlusion. *Radiology* **132**:301–303.

Auerbach, O. (1939). Pathology and pathogenesis of pulmonary arterial aneurysm in tuberculous cavities. *Am. Rev. Tuberc.* **39**:99–115.

Baile, E. M., Ling, H., Heyworth, J. R., Hogg, J. C., and Pare, P. D. (1985). Bronchopulmonary anastomotic and noncoronary collateral blood flow in humans during cardiopulmonary bypass. *Chest* **87**:749–754.

Barret, F., Mayaud, C., Milleron, B., Carette, M. F., Marsac, J., Akoun, G., Bigot, J. M., and Helenon, C. (1983). Traitement en urgence des hémoptysies graves par embolisation des artères systèmiques. *Presse Med.* **12**:625–629.

Bartter, T., Irwin, R. S., and Nash, G. (1988). Aneurysm of the pulmonary arteries. *Chest* **94**:1065–1075.

Beg, M. H., Ekramullak, Ahmad, S. H., and Rayazuddin, (1987). Paraplegia after ductus ligation accompanied by injury to intercostal artery. *J. Thorac. Cardiovasc. Surg.* **93**:934–935.

Berry, B. E., and Ochsner, A. (1972). Massive hemoptysis associated with localized pulmonary bullae requiring emergency surgery. *J. Thorac. Cardiovasc. Surg.* **63**:94–98.

Bjork, L. (1966). Angiographic demonstration of extracardiac anastomoses to the coronary arteries. *Radiology* **87**:274–277.

Bobrowitz, I. D., Ramakrishna, S., and Shim, Y. S. (1983). Comparison of medical and surgical treatment of major hemoptysis. *Arch. Intern. Med.* **143**:1343–1346.

Bolling, S. F., Kanter, K. R., Flaherty, J. T., Gott, V. L., and Gardner, T. J. (1984). Identification and control of noncoronary collateral blood flow. *Ann. Thorac. Surg.* **38**:232–236.

Bookstein, J. J., Moser, K. M., Kalafer, M. E., Higgins, C. B., Davis, G. B., and James, W. S. (1977). The role of bronchial arteriography and therapeutic embolization in hemoptysis. *Chest* **72**:658–661.

Botenga, A. S. J. (1968). The role of bronchopulmonary anastomoses in chronic inflammatory processes of the lung. *AJR* **104**:829–839.

Botenga, A. S. J. (1969). The significance of broncho-pulmonary anastomoses in pulmonary anomalies: A selective angiographic study. *Radiol. Clin. Biol.* **38**:309–328.

Boushy, S. F., North, L. B., and Trice, J. A. (1969). The bronchial arteries in chronic obstructive pulmonary disease. *Am. J. Med.* **46**:506–515.

Burrows, P. E., Freedom, R. M., Rabinovitch, M., and Moes, C. A. F. (1985). The investigation of abnormal pulmonary arteries in congenital heart disease. *Radiol. Clin. North Am.* **23**:689–717.

Butto, F., Lucas, R. V., and Edwards, J. E. (1987). Pulmonary arterial aneurysm. A pathological study of five cases. *Chest* **91**:237–241.

Byrne, R. J. R., and Bloom, D. L. (1970). Absence of the right pulmonary artery as a cause of hemoptysis. *J. Thorac. Cardiovasc. Surg.* **59**:264–268.

Cabrol, C., Cabrol, A., Acar, J., Gandjbackhch, I., Guiraudon, G., Laughlin, L., Mattei, M. F., and Godeau, P. (1978). Surgical correction of chronic postembolic obstructions of the pulmonary arteries. *J. Thorac. Cardiovasc. Surg.* **76**:620–628.

Chait, A. (1976). The internal mammary artery: An overlooked collateral pathway to the leg. *Radiology* **121**:621–624.

Charan, N. B., Turk, G. M., and Dhand, R. (1985). The role of bronchial circulation in lung abscess. *Am. Rev. Respir. Dis.* **131**:121–124.

Chitwood, W. R., Lyerly, H. K., and Sabiston, D. C. (1985). Surgical management of chronic pulmonary embolism. *Ann. Surg.* **201**:11–26.

Cholankeril, J. V., Johsi, R. R., Cenizal, J. S., Ketyer, S., and O'Connor, W. T. (1982). Massive air embolism from the pulmonary artery. *Radiology* **142**:33–34.

Choyke, P. L., Edmonds, P. R., Markowitz, R. I., Kleinman, C. S., and Laks, H. (1982). Mycotic pulmonary artery aneurysm: Complication of aspergillus endocarditis. *AJR* **138**:1172–1175.

Chuang, V. P., Wallace, S., and Gianturco, C. (1980). A new improved coil for tapered-tip catheter for arterial occlusion. *Radiology* **135**:507–509.

Cockett, F. B., and Vass, C. C. N. (1951). A comparison of the role of the bronchial arteries in bronchiectasis and in experimental ligation of the pulmonary artery. *Thorax* **6**:268–275.

Cohen, A. J., Ameika, J. A., Briggs, R. A., Grishkin, B. A., and Helsel, R. A. (1988). Retrograde flow in the internal mammary artery. *Ann. Thorac. Surg.* **45**:48–49.

Conlan, A. A., Hurwitz, S. S., Krige, L., Nicolaou, N., and Pool, R. (1983). Massive hemoptysis. Review of 123 cases. *J. Thorac. Cardiovasc. Surg.* **83**:120–124.

Conrad, M. R., Cameron, J., and White, R. I. (1977). The role of angiography in the diagnosis of tracheal-innominate artery fistula. *AJR* **128**:35–38.

Cromwell, L. D., Freeny, P. C., Kerber, C. W., Kunz, L. L., Harris, A. B., and Shaw, C. M. (1986). Histologic analysis of tissue response to bucrylate-pantopaque mixture. *AJR* **147**:627–631.

Cudkowicz, L., Editor (1968). *The Human Bronchial Circulation in Health and Disease.* Baltimore, Williams & Wilkins.

Darrason, R., Revert, R., Audebert, M., and Remond, A. (1986). Anastomose artérielle broncho-vertébrale: Une anomalie rare. *Ann Radiol.* **29**:560–562.

Davis, C. E., Carpenter, J. L., MacAllister, C. K., Matthews, J., Bush, B. A., and Ognibene, A. J. (1985). Tuberculosis. Cause of death in antibiotic era. *Chest* **88**:726–729.

Davis, S. D., Neithamer, C. D., Schreiber, T. S., and Sos, T. A. (1987). False pulmonary artery aneurysm induced by Swan-Ganz catheter: Diagnosis and embolotherapy. *Radiology* **164**:741–742.

Deffebach, M. E., Charan, N. B., Lakshminarayan, S., and Butler, J. (1987). The bronchial circulation: Small, but a vital attribute of the lung. *Am. Rev. Respir. Dis.* **135**:463–481.

Delarue, J., Sors, C., and Mignot, J. (1953). Les modifications vasculaires au cours des bronchectasies. *J. Fr. Med. Chir. Thorac.* **7**:225–237.

Donohue, J. F. (1983). Endobronchial mucormycosis. *Chest* **83**:585–585.

Doppman, J. L., and Di Chiro, G. (1976). Paraspinal muscle infarction. *Radiology* **119**:609–613.

Drummond, J. C., Zornow, M. H., and Dembitsky, W. P. (1987). Spurious identification of critical intercostal arteries by evoked responses during aortic resection. *Ann. Thorac. Surg.* **44**:79–81.

Durand-Gasselin, J., Di Stefano, D., Silvestri, M., and Sainty, J. M. (1988). Infarctus du myocarde au cours d'une embolisation artérielle thérapeutique. *Rean. Soins Intens. Med. Urg.* **4**:233–235.

Edelman, R. R., Johnson, T. S., Jhaveri, H. S., Kim, D., Kasdon, E., Frank, H. A., and Simon, M. (1985). Fatal hemoptysis resulting from erosion of a pulmonary artery in cavitary sarcoidosis. *AJR* **145**:37–38.

Ellis, F. H., Grindlay, J. H., and Edwards, J. E. (1951). The bronchial arteries. I. Experimental occlusion. *Surgery* **30**:810–826.

Feldman, L., Greenfield, A. J., Waltman, A. C., Novelline, R. A., Van Breda, A., Luers, P., and Athanasoulis, C. A. (1983). Transcatheter vessel occlusion: Angiographic results versus clinical success. *Radiology* **147**:1–5.

Fellows, K. E., Khaw, K. T., Schuster, S., and Schwachman, H. (1979). Bronchial artery embolization in cystic fibrosis; technique and long-term results. *J. Pediatr.* **95**:959–963.

Fernandez, N. A. (1984). Intracavitary aminocaproic acid for massive pulmonary hemorrhage. *Chest* **85**:839–839.

Ferris, E. J. (1981). Pulmonary hemorrhage. Vascular evaluation and interventional therapy. *Chest* **80**:710–714.

Fink, R. J., Doershuk, C. F., Tucker, A. S., Stern, R. C., Boat, T. F., and Matthews, L. W. (1978). Adult patients with cystic fibrosis. *Chest* **74**:643–647.

Fisher, A. B., Kollmeier, H., Brody, J. S., Hyde, R. W., Hansell, J., Friedman, J. N., and Waldhausen, J. A. (1970). Restoration of systemic blood flow to the lung after division of bronchial arteries. *J. Appl. Physiol.* **29**:839–846.

Flick, M. R., Wasson, K., Dunn, L. J., and Block, A. J. (1975). Fatal pulmonary hemorrhage after transbronchial lung biopsy through the fiberoptic bronchoscope. *Am. Rev. Respir. Dis.* **111**:853–856.

Furuse, M., Saito, K., Kunieda, E., Aihara, T., Touei, H., Ohara, T., and Fukushima, K. (1987). Bronchial arteries: CT demonstration with arteriographic correlation. *Radiology* **162**:393–398.

Garzon, A. A., Cerruti, M. M., and Golding, M. E. (1982). Exsanguinating hemoptysis. *J. Thorac. Cardiovasc. Surg.* **84**:829–833.

Gianturco, C., Anderson, J. H., and Wallace, S. (1975). Mechanical devices for arterial occlusion. *AJR* **124**:428–435.

Gonz, H., and Salvatierra, C. (1981). Clinical efficacy of early and delayed fiberoptic bronchoscopy in patients with hemoptysis. *Am. Rev. Respir. Dis.* **124**:221–225.

Gourin, A., and Garzon, A. A. (1975). Control of hemorrhage in emergency pulmonary resection for massive hemoptysis. *Chest* **68**:120–121.

Grenier, P., Cornud, F., Lacombe, P., Viau, F., and Nahum, H. (1983). Bronchial artery occlusion for severe hemoptysis: Use of Isobutyl-2 cyanoacrylate. *AJR* **140**:467–471.

Grinnell, V. S., Mehringer, C. M., Hieshima, G. B., Stanley, P., and Lurie, P. R. (1982). Transaortic occlusion of collateral arteries to the lung by detachable valved balloons in a patient with tetralogy of Fallot. *Circulation* **65**:1276–1278.

Hampson, S., and Pepper, J. (1987). Aortopulmonary fistula: Role of computer tomography. *Thorax* **42**:395–396.

Harber, P. H., and Terry, P. B. (1981). Fatal lung abscesses: Review of 11 years' experience. *South. Med. J.* **74**:281–283.

Haroutunian, L. M., and Neill, C. A. (1972). Pulmonary complications of congenital heart disease: Hemoptysis. *Am. Heart J.* **84**:540–559.

Harris, P., and Heath, D. (1977). In *The Human Pulmonary Circulation: Its Form and Function in Health and Disease,* 2nd Ed. Edinburgh, Churchill Livingstone, pp. 242–265.

Helenon, C., Chatel, A., Bigot, J. M., and Brocard, H. (1977). Fistule oesophago-bronchique gauche après embolisation bronchique. *Nouv. Presse Med.* **6**:4209.

Hemingway, A. P., and Allison, D. J. (1988). Complications of embolization: Analysis of 410 procedures. *Radiology* **166**:669–672.

Hickey, N. M., Peterson, R. A., Leech, J. A., Chambers, R. J., and Shamji, F. M. (1988). Percutaneous embolotherapy in life-threatening hemoptysis. *Cardiovasc. Intervent. Radiol.* **11**:270–273.

Holsclaw, D. S., Grand, R. J., and Schwachman, H. (1970). Massive hemoptysis in cystic fibrosis. *J. Pediatr.* **76**:829–838.

Horton, J. (1986). Embolization of intramedullary arteriovenous malformations in the spinal cord. *A.J.N.R.* **7**:113–118.

Hughes, C. F., Waugh, R., and Lindsay, D. (1986). Surgery for pulmonary aspergilloma: Preoperative embolization of the bronchial circulation. *Thorax* **41**:324–325.

Isaacs, R. D., Wattie, W. J., Wells, A. U., Rea, H. H., and Bai, T. R. (1987). Massive haemoptysis as a late consequence of pulmonary irradiation. *Thorax* **42**:77–78.

Ivanick, M. J., Thorwarth, W., Donohue, J., Mandell, V., Delany, D., and

Jaques, P. F. (1983). Infarction of the left mainstem bronchus: A complication of bronchial artery embolization. *AJR* **141**:535–537.

Jackson, C. V., Savage, P. J., and Quinn, D. L. (1985). Role of fiberoptic bronchoscopy in patients with hemoptysis and a normal chest roentgenogram. *Chest* **87**:142–144.

Jewkes, J., Kay, P. H., Paneth, M., and Citron, K. M. (1983). Pulmonary aspergilloma: Analysis of prognosis in relation to hemoptysis and survey of treatment. *Thorax* **38**:572–578.

Jouve, A., Gabriel, B., Revelin, J. F., and Colombani, F. (1965). Les hémoptysies graves de l'insuffiscance mitrale pure ou prédominante. *Arch. Mal. Coeur* **9**:1213–1232.

Kakizoe, T., Matsumoto, K., Nishio, Y., Ohtani, M., and Miyazawa, N. (1984). Chemotherapy by bronchial arterial infusion for pulmonary metastases of renal cell carcinoma. *J. Urol.* **131**:1053–1055.

Keller, F. S., Rosch, J., Loflin, T. G., Nath, P. H., and MacElvein, R. B. (1987). Nonbronchial systemic collateral arteries: Significance in percutaneous embolotherapy for hemoptysis. *Radiology* **164**:687–692.

Kerber, C. W. (1980). Flow-controlled therapeutic embolization: A physiologic and safe technique. *AJR* **134**:557–561.

Kibbler, C. C., Milkins, S. R., Bhamra, A., Spiteri, M. A., Noone, P., and Prentice, H. G. (1988). Apparent pulmonary mycetoma following invasive aspergilloma in neutropenic patients. *Thorax* **43**:108–112.

Kleinman, P. K. (1979). Pleural telangiectasia and absence of a pulmonary artery. *Radiology* **132**:281–284.

Kucera, V., Fiser, B., Tuma, S., and Hucin, B. (1982). Unilateral absence of pulmonary artery: A report on 19 selected clinical cases. *Thorac. Cardiovasc. Surg.* **30**:152–158.

Lacombe, P., Frija, G., Parlier, H., Lang, F., Hamza, M., Hamza, R., and Bismuth, V. (1985). Transcatheter embolization of multiple pulmonary artery aneurysms in Behçet's syndrome. *Acta Radiol. Diagn.* **26**:251–253.

Lajos, T. Z. (1985). Noncoronary collateral blood flow. *Am. Thorac. Surg.* **40**:99.

Laschinger, J. C., Izumoto, H., and Kouchoukos, N. T. (1987). Evolving concepts in prevention of spinal cord injury during operations on the descending thoracic and thoracoabdominal aorta. *Ann. Thorac. Surg.* **44**:667–674.

Levin, D. C. (1978). Augmented arterial flow and pressure resulting from selective injections through catheters: Clinical implications. *Radiology* **127**:103–108.

Levin, D. C., Beckmann, C. F., and Hillman, B. (1980). Experimental determination of flow patterns of gelfoam emboli: Safety implications. *AJR* **134**:525–528.

Lincoln, M. J., and Shigeoka, J. W. (1988). Pulmonary telangiectasia without hypoxemia. *Chest* **93**:1097–1098.

Magilligan, D. J., Ravipati, S., Zayat, P., Shetty, P. C., Bower, G., and Kvale, P. (1981). Massive hemoptysis: Control by transcatheter bronchial artery embolization. *Ann. Thorac. Surg.* **32**:392–400.

Martin, C., Saux, P., Auffray, J. P., Aubert, C., and Gouin, F. (1982). Perforation de l'artère pulmonaire au cours d'un catheretisme par sonde a ballonnet. Valeur semioloque d'une hémoptysie mineure. *Nouv. Presse Med.* **11**:1807–1807.

Matsuda, H., Hirose, N., Nakano, S., Shimazaki, Y., Kishimotot, H., Kobayashi, J., Arisawa, J., and Kawashima, Y. (1985). Management of large aortopulmonary collateral arteries in patients with ventricular septal defect and pulmonary atresia: Simultaneous ligation through median sternotomy during intracardiac repair. *Ann. Thorac. Surg.* **40**:595–598.

Mauro, M. A., and Jaques, P. F. (1987). Transcatheter embolisation with a Gelfoam "slurry." *J. Intervent. Radiol.* **2**:157–159.

McLean, G. K., Stein, E. J., Burke, D. R., and Meranze, S. G. (1986). Steel occlusion coils: Pretreatment with thrombin. *Radiology* **158**:549–550.

Mengoli, L. (1985). Giant lung abscess treated by tube thoracostomy. *J. Thorac. Cardiovasc. Surg.* **90**:186–194.

Middleton, J. R., Sen, P., Lange, M., Salaki, J., Kapila, R., and Louria, D. B. (1977). Death-producing hemoptysis in tuberculosis. *Chest* **72**:601–604.

Miller, F. J., and Mineau, D. E. (1983). Transcatheter arterial embolization: Major complications and their prevention. *Cardiovasc. Intervent. Radiol.* **6**:141–149.

Mills, S. R., Jackson, D. C., Sullivan, D. C., Moore, A. V., Heaston, D. K., Wolfe, W. G., and Sabiston, D. C. (1980). Angiographic evaluation of chronic pulmonary embolism. *Radiology* **136**:301–308.

Milne, E. N. C., Noonan, C. D., Margulis, A. R., and Stoughton, J. A. (1969). Vascular supply of pulmonary metastases. *Invest. Radiol.* **4**:215–229.

Mojab, K., Barker, W., Rodriguez, J., and Ramos, M. (1974). Angiographic findings in bronchial adenoma. *AJR* **122**:828–832.

Moore, L. B., McWey, R. E., and Vujic, I. (1986). Massive hemoptysis: Control by embolization of the thyrocervical trunk. *Radiology* **161**:173–174.

Murthy, R., Dosani, A. R., and Zonozi, M. S. (1981). Fatal massive hemoptysis due to pneumonia. *South. Med. J.* **74**:647–648.

Muthuswamy, P. P., Akbik, F., Franklin, C., Spigos, D., and Barker, W. L. (1987). Management of major or massive hemoptysis in active pulmonary tuberculosis by bronchial arterial embolization. *Chest* **92**:77–82.

Naar, C. A., Soong, J., Clore, F., and Hawkins, I. F. (1983). Control of massive hemoptysis by bronchial artery embolization with absolute alcohol. *AJR* **140**:271–272.

Nathan, H., Rubinstein, Z., and Bogart, B. (1982). Accessory internal thoracic artery. *Anat. Clin.* **3**:333–337.

Orr, D. P., Myfrowitz, R. L., and Dubois, P. J. (1978). Patho-radiologic correlation of invasive pulmonary aspergillosis in the compromised host. *Cancer* **41**:2028–2039.

Panos, R. J., Barr, L. F., Walsh, T. J., and Silverman, H. J. (1988). Factors associated with fatal hemoptysis in cancer patients. *Chest* **94**:1008–1013.

Park, J. H., Han, M. C., and Bettmann, M. A. (1984). Arterial manifestations of Behçet disease. *AJR* **143**:821–825.

Personne, C., Colchen, A., Leroy, M., Vourc'h, G., and Toty, L. (1986). Indications and technique for endoscopic laser resections in bronchology. *J. Thorac. Cardiovasc. Surg.* **91**:710–715.

Pittokopitis, K., Herriott, D. T., and Shirey, J. K. (1983). Massive fatal hemoptysis secondary to invasive aspergillosis in a patient with COPD. *Chest* **83**:583–583.

Plessinger, V. A., and Jolly, P. N. (1949). Rasmussen's aneurysms and fatal hemorrhage in pulmonary tuberculosis. *Am. Rev. Respir. Dis.* **60**:589–603.

Poe, R. H., Israel, R. H., Marin, M. G., Ortiz, C. R., Dale, R. C., Wahl, G. W., Kallay, M. C., and Greenblatt, D. G. (1988). Utility of fiberoptic bronchoscopy in patients with hemoptysis and a nonlocalizing chest roentgenogram. *Chest* **92**:70–75.

Pool, P. E., Vogen, J. H. K., and Blount, G. (1962). Congenital unilateral absence of a pulmonary artery. The importance of flow in pulmonary artery. *Am. J. Cardiol.* **10**:706–732.

Porter, D. K., Van Every, M. J., Anthracite, R. F., and Mack, J. W. (1983). Massive hemoptysis in cystic fibrosis. *Arch. Intern. Med.* **143**:287–290.

Prager, R. L., Laws, K. H., and Bender, H. W. (1983). Arteriovenous fistula of the lung. *Ann. Thorac. Surg.* **36**:231–239.

Prioleau, W. H., Vujic, I., Parker, E. F., Voegele, L. D., and Hairston, P. (1980). Control of hemoptysis by bronchial artery embolization. *Chest* **78**:878–880.

Rabkin, J. E., Astafjev, V. I., Gothman, L. N., and Grigorjev, Y. G. (1987). Transcatheter embolization in the management of pulmonary hemorrhage. *Radiology* **163**:361–365.

Rasmussen, V. (1868). On haemoptysis, especially when fatal, in its anatomical and clinical aspects. *Edinburgh Med. J.* **14**:385–401.

Raz, I., Okon, E., and Chajek-Shaul, T. (1989). Pulmonary manifestations in Behçet's syndrome. *Chest* **95**:585–589.

Reich, J., and Renzetti, A. D. (1970). Pulmonary phycomycosis. Report of a case of bronchocutaneous fistula formation and pulmonary arterial mycothrombosis. *Am. Rev. Respir. Dis.* **102**:959–964.

Reid, L. (1986). Structure and function in pulmonary hypertension. New perceptions. The Simon Rodbard Memorial Lecture. *Chest* **89**:279–288.

Remy, J., Arnaud, A., Fardou, J., Giraud, R., and Voisin, C. (1977). Treatment of hemoptysis by embolization of bronchial arteries. *Radiology* **122**:33–37.

Remy, J., Lemaitre, L., Lafitte, J. J., Vilain, M. O., Saint Michel, J., and Steenhouwer, F. (1984). Massive hemoptysis of pulmonary arterial origin: Diagnosis and treatment. *AJR* **143**:963–969.

Remy, J., Remy-Jardin, M., Wallaert, B., and Lafitte, J. J. (1988). La vasoocclusion de l'artère pulmonaire. *Rev. Mal. Respir.* **5**:429–449.

Renie, W. A., Rodeheffer, R. J., Mitchell, S., Balke, W. C., and White, R. I. (1982). Balloon embolization of a mycotic pulmonary artery aneurysm. *Am. Rev. Respir. Dis.* **126**:1107–1110.

Rice, T. W., Ginsberg, R. J., and Todd, T. R. J. (1987). Tube drainage of lung abscesses. *Ann. Thorac. Surg.* **44**:356–359.

Roberts, D. H., Jimenez, J. F., and Golladay, E. S. (1982). Multiple pulmonary artery aneurysms and peripheral venous thromboses. The Hughes-Stovin syndrome. *Pediatr. Radiol.* **12**:214–216.

Salamon, F., Weinberger, A., Nili, M., Avidor, I., Neuman, M., Zelikovsky, A., Levy, M. J., and Pinkhas, J. (1988). Massive hemoptysis complicating Behçet's syndrome: The importance of early pulmonary angiography and operation. *Ann. Thorac. Surg.* **45**:566–567.

Schrodt, J. F., Becker, G. J., Scott, J. A., Warren, C. H., and Benenati, S. V. (1987). Bronchial artery embolization: Monitoring with somatosensory evoked potentials. *Radiology* **164**:135–139.

Selecky, P. A. (1978). Evaluation of hemoptysis through the bronchoscope. *Chest* **73**:741–745.

Sheffield, E. A., Moore-Gillon, J., Murday, A. R., and Addis, B. J. (1988). Massive haemoptysis caused by spontaneous rupture of a bronchial artery. *Thorax* **43**:71–72.

Shivaram, U., Finch, P., and Nowak, P. (1987). Plastic endobronchial tubes in the management of life-threatening hemoptysis. *Chest* **92**:1108–1110.

Smiddy, J. F., and Elliott, R. C. (1973). The evaluation of hemoptysis with fiberoptic bronchoscopy. *Chest* **64**:158–162.

Smith, S. C., Adams, D. F., Herman, M. V., and Paulin, S. (1972). Coronary-to-bronchial anastomoses: An in vivo demonstration by selective coronary arteriography. *Radiology* **104**:289–290.

Snow, N., Lucas, A., and Horrigan, T. P. (1985). Utility of pneumonotomy in the treatment of cavitary lung disease. *Chest* **87**:731–734.

Spencer, H. (1985). *Pathology of the Lung,* 4th Ed, Vol. 1. Elmford, NY, Pergamon Press.

Stern, R. C., Wood, R. E., Boat, T. F., Matthews, L. W., Tucker, A. S., and Doerschuk, C. F. (1978). Treatment and prognosis of massive hemoptysis in cystic fibrosis. *Am. Rev. Respir. Dis.* **117**:825–828.

Stocker, J. T., and Malczak, H. T. (1984). A study of pulmonary ligament arteries. Relationship to intralobar pulmonary sequestration. *Chest* **86**:611–615.

Svensson, L. G., Stewart, R. W., Cosgrove, D. M., Lytle, B. W., Antunes, M. J., Beven, E. G., Furlan, A. J., Gottlieb, A., Grum, D. F., Hinder, R. A., Schoenwald, P., Lewis, B. S., Salgado, A., and Loop, F. D. (1988). Intrathecal papaverine for the prevention of paraplegia after operation on the thoracic or thoracoabdominal aorta. *J. Thorac. Cardiovasc. Surg.* **96**:823–829.

Taguchi, T., Ikeda, K., Kume, K., Nagasaki, A., Goto, S., Matsuo, S., Hasuo, K., and Tamura, S. (1987). Isolated unilateral absence of left pulmonary artery with peribronchial arteriovenous malformation showing recurrent hemoptysis. *Pediatr. Radiol.* **17**:316–318.

Teklu, B., and Felleke, (1982). Massive hemoptysis in tuberculosis. *Tubercle* **63**:213–216.

Thoms, N. W., Wilson, R. F., Puro, H. E., and Arbulu, A. (1972). Life-threatening hemoptysis in primary lung abscess. *Ann. Thorac. Surg.* **14**:347–358.

Trento, A., Estner, S. M., Griffith, B. P., and Hardesty, R. L. (1985). Massive hemoptysis in patients with cystic fibrosis: Three case reports and a protocol for clinical management. *Ann. Thorac. Surg.* **39**:254–256.

Uflacker, R., Kaemmerer, A., Neves, C., and Picon, P. D. (1983). Management of massive hemoptysis by bronchial artery embolization. *Radiology* **146**:627–634.

Uflacker, R., Kaemmerer, A., Picon, P. D., Rizzon, C. F. C., Neves, C. M. C., Oliveira, E. S. B., Oliveira, M. E. M., Azevedo, S. N. B., and Ossanai, R. (1985). Bronchial artery embolization in the management of hemoptysis: Technical aspects and long-term results. *Radiology* **157**:637–644.

Vujic, I., Pyle, R., Parker, E., and Mithoefer, J. (1980). Control of massive hemoptysis by embolization of intercostal arteries. *Radiology* **137**:617–620.

Vujic, I., Pyle, R., Hungerford, G. D., and Griffin, C. N. (1982). Angiography and therapeutic blockage in the control of hemoptysis. *Radiology* **143**:19–23.

Wadouh, F., Arndt, C. F., Oppermann, E., Borst, H. G., and Wadouh, R. (1986). The mechanism of spinal cord injury after simple and double aortic cross-clamping. *J. Thorac. Cardiovasc. Surg.* **92**:121–127.

Wallace, S., Gianturco, C., Anderson, J. H., Goldstein, H. M., Davis, L. J., and Bree, R. L. (1976). Therapeutic vascular occlusion utilizing steel coil technique: Clinical applications. *AJR* **127**:381–387.

Weaver, L. J., Solliday, N., and Cugell, D. W. (1979). Selection of patients with hemoptysis for fiberoptic bronchoscopy. *Chest* **76**:7–10.

White, R. I., and Lundell, C. (1984). Prevention of complications during embolotherapy of the lung. *Ann. Radiol.* **27**:310–315.

White, R. I., Kaufman, S. L., Barth, K. H., De Caprio, V., and Standbert, J. D. (1979). Embolotherapy with detachable silicone balloons. *Radiology* **131**:619–627.

White, R. I., Lynch-Nyhan, A., Terry, P., Buescher, P. C., Farmlett, E. J., Charnas, L., Shuman, K., Kim, W., Kinnison, M., and Mitchell, S. E. (1988). Pulmonary arteriovenous malformations: Techniques and long-term outcome of embolotherapy. *Radiology* **169**:663–669.

Wholey, M. H., Chamorro, H. A., Rao, G., Ford, W. B., and Miller, W. H. (1976). Bronchial artery embolization for massive hemoptysis. *JAMA* **236**:2501–2504.

23

The Human Bronchial Circulation
Anatomy and Lung Transplantation

HANS SCHREINEMAKERS and JOEL D. COOPER

Washington University School of Medicine
St. Louis, Missouri

I. Introduction

More than 25 years following the first human lung allograft transplantation in 1963 by Hardy et al., healing of the airway anastomosis remains a significant problem. With current techniques the systemic arterial supply to the tracheobronchial tree is not reconstructed at the time of transplantation, which makes lung allografts unique among solid organ transplants. The importance of the bronchial artery circulation in human lung transplantation remains controversial. Lima and coworkers at the University of Toronto (1982) used a pedicle of omentum to indirectly revascularize the bronchus in canine lung transplantation and demonstrated improved healing of the bronchial anastomosis. Utilizing this technique, the first successful human lung transplant was performed (Cooper et al., 1986) in 1983. Before this, airway complications were responsible for many of the fatalities following single-lung transplant. Cooper and colleagues also demonstrated successful human double-lung transplantation using the omentopexy for the tracheal anastomosis (Patterson et al., 1988). However, airway healing remained a major concern with this procedure, with 25% of patients dying as a result of airway complication and 20% more having nonfatal airway problems (Patterson et al., 1990).

In human heart-lung transplantation, airway complications are less frequent in comparison to double-lung transplantation. Griffith et al. (1987) described 3 significant airway complications in 33 heart-lung transplantations. Collateral flow from coronary artery to bronchial arteries has been demonstrated radiographically following heart-lung transplantation, and preservation of bronchial artery flow by means of these connections is thought to be responsible for the generally satisfactory airway healing with the combined heart-lung transplant. Nonetheless, airway complications secondary to ischemia have been reported in up to 10% of heart-lung recipients.

It seems apparent that restoration of the bronchial artery circulation at the time of any type of lung transplant would contribute to reduced airway complications. Furthermore, as the period of safe lung preservation is extended, direct revascularization of the airway may assume greater importance in preventing ischemic complications at this vulnerable anastomosis.

II. Anatomy of the Bronchial Circulation

The anatomy of the bronchial arteries has been studied by dissection (Cauldwell et al., 1948; Kasai and Chiba, 1979; Nakamura, 1924; Nathan et al., 1970; Miller, 1925), corrosion casting (Liebow, 1965; Marchand et al., 1950; Pump, 1963, 1972), injections with different techniques and different solutions (Cudkowicz and Armstrong, 1951; Verloop, 1948), and more recently by arteriography (Botenga, 1970; Viamonte et al., 1965; Schreinemakers et al., 1990). Most commonly the bronchial arteries are branches of the descending thoracic aorta. The left bronchial arteries arise from the anterior surface of the aorta between the level of the aortic arch and the level of the third pair of intercostal arteries, and sometimes from the concavity of the aortic arch. In about 30% of cases, they arise from the anterior surface of the thoracic aorta as a common truck with a right bronchial artery. The left bronchial arteries seldom arise in common with an intercostal artery. The left bronchial arteries may be associated with a right intercostal artery. When the lung is supplied by more than one bronchial artery, the upper vessel usually supplies the greater portion of the lung. Additional arteries seldom supply more than the posterior and medial aspects of the lower lobe. The additional bronchial arteries may course in the inferior pulmonary ligament, and the more distal its origin from the aorta, the more limited seems to be its distribution (Marchand et al., 1950). Neither the bronchial artery nor the intercostal arteries leave the aorta at right angles to its axis, but they pass upward, initially forming an acute angle with the aorta. During systole, the effect of the elongation and dilatation of the aorta is to accentuate this angulation. There is never an association with the left intercostal arteries. The right bronchial arteries arise from the right anterolateral, lateral, or posterolateral surface of the thoracic descending aorta. Usually a right bronchial artery is associated with a right intercostal artery, specifically the first intercostal artery. Cauldwell's group described this common trunk from a bronchial artery and a right intercostal artery as the intercostobronchial artery. They studied 150 cadavers and found the right bronchial artery to be related to a right intercostal artery in 89% of cases (Cauldwell et al., 1948). We found this relation present in 90% of 30 autopsy cases. Nakamura (1924), Nathan (1970), Liebow (1965), and Kasai and Chiba (1979) had similar findings. According to Cauldwell's group, the right bronchial artery arises directly from the thoracic aorta in 11% of cases. Rarely, the right bronchial artery may arise from the subclavian, innominate, or internal mammary artery. For the majority of cases, the right and left bronchial arteries arise independently of each other. The pattern encountered in the number and the site of origin of the bronchial arteries may differ considerably. Despite this variation in number and position of origin from the aorta, we found some consistency in the anatomy of the bronchial arteries. At least one left bronchial artery originated from the anterior wall of the thoracic aorta in over 90% of cases. The right bronchial artery arose from the first right intercostobronchial artery in over 80% of cases and, thereby, was the most constant in origin. A major difference in course between the left and right bronchial arteries is that the left bronchial artery usually runs laterally and anteriorly to the esophagus, whereas the right bronchial artery usually runs posterior to the esophagus at the level of the arch of the azygos vein, specifically when related to the first right intercostobronchial artery. This consistency in anatomy of left and right bronchial arteries made it possible to develop techniques for harvesting a lung bloc along with the bronchial arteries and to isoate a left bronchial artery pedicle as well as a right intercostobronchial artery pedicle. Figure 4 shows the relation of the left and right bronchial artery to the mediastinal structures. The course of the left bronchial artery is usually directed to the membranous portion of the left main bronchus close to the bifurcation of the trachea, after originating from the anterior surface of the aorta immediately behind the left main bronchus. The right bronchial artery usually arises at the superior border of the first or second right aortic intercostal artery at a variable distance (0.5–5.0 cm) from the aorta at the level of T5–6. The right bronchial artery then courses obliquely upward and forward toward the right main bronchus. During its course, the right bronchial artery lies initially on the right anterolateral aspect of the vertebral column and then passes anteriorly to the right of the thoracic duct and traverses the right side of the esophagus to terminate at the lower end of the trachea and right main bronchus. During its course, the azygos arch may totally or partially overlap the artery (Nathan et al., 1970). Figure 4 shows the relation of the right inter-

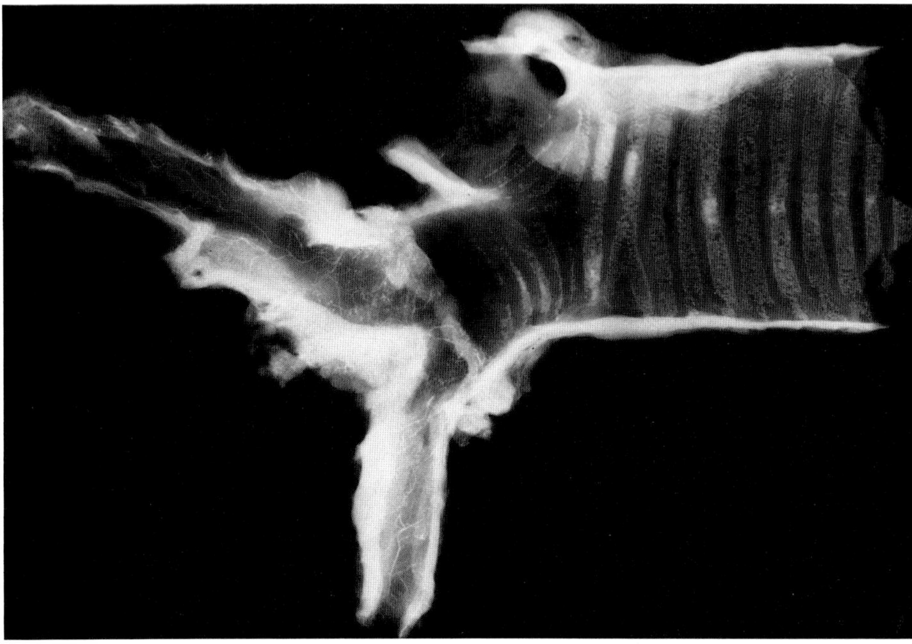

Figure 1 Omental injection study of a dog 4 days after left lung reimplantation with bronchial omentopexy. A network of fine vessels is evident in the anastomosis of the left bronchus (black arrowhead). The distal left bronchial arteris are filled with contrast material (white arrowhead). (From Lima et al., 1982; used by permission.)

costobronchial artery to the spine. It is embedded in the fatty tissue covering the spine. For this reason, we modified our extraction technique to obtain a donor lung bloc along with the bronchial arteries by excision not only of the lungs but also the thoracic aorta, esophagus, and the fatty tissue covering the spine.

After the bronchial arteries reach the main bronchus on each side, having a diameter of 1.5 mm at the hilum in adults (Deffebach et al., 1987), they arborize along the entire intrapulmonary airways. Both left and right main bronchial arteries enter the lung closely applied to the membranous portion of the mainstem bronchus and continue along the posterior aspect of the main bronchus. The mediastinal pleura is prolonged into the lung with the bronchi. The bronchial arteries can be followed into the substance of the lung without coming in contact with the lung parenchyma. They lie between the invaginated pleura and the fibrous layer covering the lung. The invaginated pleura fuses with the outer bronchial coat at the origin of the segmental bronchi. If the

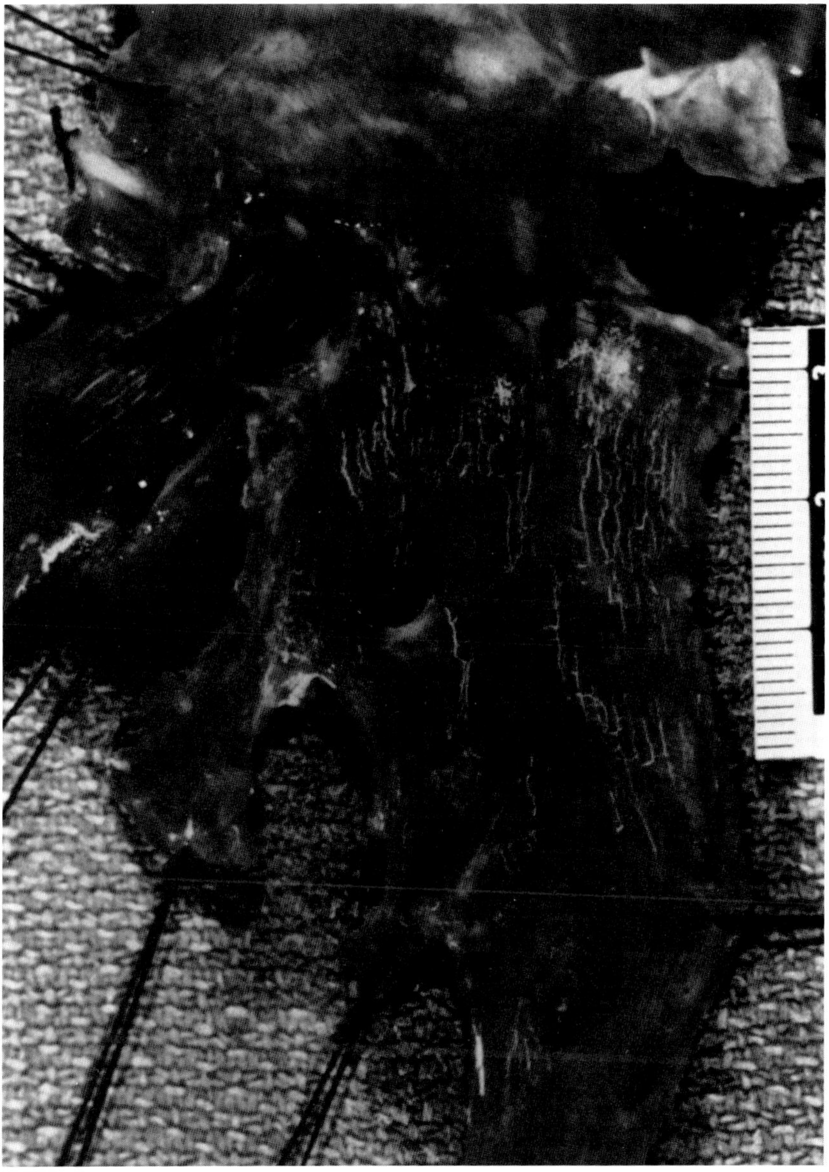

Figure 2 Photograph of specimen described in Figure 1. The bronchial mucosal capillaries distal to the anastomosis are filled with the silicone rubber injected into omental vessels at sacrifice of the animal 4 days after left lung reimplantation with bronchial omentopexy. (From Lima et al., 1982; used by permission.)

bronchial arteries are followed farther than this point, the interstitial tissue of the lung itself must be exposed. The bronchial arteries then become truly intrapulmonary and from there onward branch repeatedly and by renastomosis form an arterial mesh around the bronchi (Marchand et al., 1950).

III. Consistency of Bronchial Artery Anatomy

We undertook an anatomic study to establish the consistency in the anatomy of the bronchial arteries. Table 1 shows the incidence of left and right bronchial arteries. In 30 autopsy cases, we found a total of 41 right bronchial arteries and 65 left bronchial arteries, which implies a mean of 1.3 right bronchial arteries and a mean of 2.2 left bronchial arteries, consistent with the findings of others (Cauldwell et al., 1948; Nakamura, 1924). Differences exist mainly in the method used to count the individual arteries (Kasai and Chiba, 1979). All authors agree that the left bronchial arteries in the vast majority of cases arise from the anterior wall of the descending thoracic aorta. In our findings, at least one left bronchial artery arose from the anterior wall of the descending thoracic aorta in 93% of cases. It was Nathan et al. (1970) who first stressed the consistency in the anatomy of the right bronchial arteries. Table 2 shows

Table 1 Numbers of Left and Right Bronchial Arteries and Their Combination in 30 Autopsy Cases[a]

Number of autopsy cases	Number of right bronchial arteries	Number of left bronchial arteries
1	1	0
4	1	1
9	1	2
4	1	3
1	1	4
1	1	5
1	2	1
6	2	2
1	2	3
1	2	4
1	3	2
Total 30	41	65

[a] Right: mean = 1.3. Left: mean = 2.2.

Table 2 Incidence of a First Right Intercostobronchial Artery

Source	Number	%
Cauldwell et al. (1948)	121/150	80.7
Kasai and Chiba (1979)	32/40	85
Nathan et al. (1970)	60	"Almost all"
Schreinemakers et al. (1990)	25/30	83.3

the presence of the right intercostobronchial artery found by anatomists in autopsy studies. All authors could demonstrate in at least 80% of cases a right bronchial artery related to the first right intercostobronchial artery. We found this relation present in 25 of 30 autopsy studies. Cauldwell et al. (1948), Kasai and Chiba (1979), Liebow (1965), Nakamura (1924), and Nathan et al. (1970) all found in some instances a right bronchial artery related to a second or third right intercostobronchial artery. In our study, we found this relation in 2 of the 30 autopsy studies, bringing the total of right bronchial arteries related to an intercostobronchial artery to 90%. We also found in a few cases a left bronchial artery related to a right intercostobronchial artery, mostly in a common trunk with a right bronchial artery. We found the presence of a separate subcarinal artery described by Nakamura in 7 of the 30 autopsy cases. In all cases, this artery has a very small orifice close to the aortic arch. In summary, we found consistency in the left bronchial arteries in that at least one left bronchial arose from the anterior wall of the descending thoracic aorta in over 90% of the cases and consistency in the right bronchial arteries in that a first right intercostobronchial artery was present in over 80% of the cases.

IV. Embryology of Pulmonary Circulation with Reference to Interconnections Between the Pulmonary and Bronchial Circulations

In lung transplantation, survival of the extrapulmonary airway may imply connections of the bronchial circulation and the pulmonary circulation. Experimentally, we could demonstrate neovascularization between the omental systemic blood supply and systemic bronchial vessels as early as 4 days after a lung transplant. In the meantime, the intrapulmonary airway is probably totally dependent on the pulmonary circulation for its nutrition. The existence of precapillary, capillary, and postcapillary connections between the pulmonary circulation and the bronchial circulation is assumed.

Human fetal bronchial arteries appear between the ninth and twelfth week as outgrowths of the aorta itself or its intercostal rami, constituting a secondary system implanted relatively late upon the peripheral coats of the airway and pulmonary vessels (Boyden, 1970). With later development of the pulmonary artery and veins, these vessels connect with a plexus around the developing lungs and establish anastomoses between the systemic and pulmonary circulations. Controversy still exists concerning the exact location and physiological function of the anastomosis between the pulmonary circulation and the bronchial circulation. Capillary anastomoses between the pulmonary circulation and the bronchial circulation have been demonstrated throughout the entire human airway (Miller, 1925). Verloop (1948) demonstrated two kinds of precapillary anastomoses between the pulmonary artery and the bronchial artery. Around the small bronchi, which have a few pieces of cartilage in the wall, there are arterial anastomoses between the two arterial systems of the lung. The bronchial arteries give off lateral branches to open into small branches of the pulmonary artery. In the visceral pleura, the bronchial arteries also communicate with the pulmonary artery, ending in intralobar branches of the pulmonary artery. Verloop was not able to demonstrate arteriovenous anastomoses. Marchand et al. (1950) also demonstrated pecapillary connections between the two arterial systems in nonemphysematous normal lungs. The physiological functions of these types of arterial connections between the pulmonary and bronchial arterial circulation is still unclear.

V. Experimental and Clinical Observations of Bronchial Circulation Following Lung Transplantation

The first single left lung allotransplantation in the canine model was reported by Metras (1950). He reestablished directly the bronchial circulation by attaching a button of aorta containing the orifice of the donor's bronchial artery to the recipient's subclavian artery. His lead in directly restoring bronchial circulation was not generally followed. In 1971, Derom and colleagues reported a 10 month survival following a human lung transplant (Derom et al., 1971). The recipient developed a 50% stenosis of the right bronchial anastomosis. Rejection, infection, ventilation-perfusion imbalance, improper donor and recipient selection, and bronchial complications due to ischemia made human lung transplantation unsuccessful until 1983.

Demikhov, in 1947 (Demikhov, 1960), experienced bronchial disruption in right lower lobe allotransplantation in the canine model. To avoid this he had to ligate or exteriorize the distal end of the bronchus, thereby impairing ventilatory function. Staudacher et al. (1950) also experienced disruption and necrosis of the bronchial anastomosis following right lower lobe allotransplantation in the canine model. Duvoisin et al. (1964) reported a 61% complication rate of bronchial necrosis and stenosis in 82 canine left lung autotransplantations. This autotransplantation model excluded rejection problems concerning the transplanted lung and airway. They concluded that the necrosis and stenosis appeared to be the result of interruption of the bronchial circulation. Veith and Richards (1970) were able to significantly reduce bronchial complications in canine allotransplantation by using a telescoping anastomotic technique. Other approaches have included reinforcing the bronchial anastomosis by surrounding mediastinal tissues or minimizing the length of the donor bronchus. Pinsker and colleagues (1979) reported a canine model in which they could control the degree of ischemic damage at the anastomotic site by varying the length of the donor bronchus. They postulated that the adequacy of retrograde collateral blood flow between pulmonary and bronchial circulations would increase at the anastomotic site as the donor bronchus was shortened. Lengthening the donor bronchus as much as possible would therefore provide a standard model of ischemic damage at the anastomotic site. They demonstrated a significant decrease in bronchial complications using an anastomosis at the level of the lobar bronchus. In left lower lobe reimplantation studies in the canine model, Huggins (1959) demonstrated that dividing the bronchus within 1 cm of the lobe could prevent bronchial necrosis.

VI. Spontaneous Restoration of the Bronchial Circulation After Division of Bronchus

Verloop demonstrated bronchial artery circulation to the tracheal bifurcation, the bronchial walls, the adventitia of the pulmonary artery and veins, the visceral pleura, and the lymph nodes, nerve fibers, and ganglia located in the bronchial wall (1948). Several studies were carried out to examine the fate of the bronchial circulation after its interruption in dogs (Table 3). Stone et al. studied bronchial circulation regeneration after radical right hilar stripping, simulating a lung reimplantation (1966). In 20 experiments, bronchoscopy showed evidence of impaired circulation in the bronchial mucosa distal to the line of reanastomosis, characterized by edema, cyanosis, and secretion retention. These changes disappeared within 6 weeks in 17 of the 20 animals; 1 dog developed severe bronchial stenosis, and 2 dogs developed bronchopleural fistulas. Ellis et al. demonstrated ischemia and necrosis in the bronchi of canine lungs in which the bronchial artery was filled with a dye cast to prevent pulmonary-to-bronchial collateral flow (1951). Experiments have demonstrated that regeneration of the bronchial circulation in a canine lung reimplantation

Table 3 Spontaneous Bronchial Vascular Regeneration After Complete Interruption of the Bronchial Circulation

Operation	Reference	Time required for bronchial artery regeneration (weeks)
Right hilar stripping	Stone et al. (1966)	4
Left autotransplant	Pearson et al. (1970)	4
Left allotransplant	Siegelman et al. (1977)	4
Left lobe autotransplant	Rabinovich (1970)	3–4

model occurs between 1 month and 1 year (Blank et al., 1966; Neveux et al., 1968).

Pearson et al. studied the bronchial artery regeneration in a left lung reimplantation model. All dogs had evidence of gross impairment of the circulation to the bronchial mucosa characterized by edema, cyanosis, and retained secretions distal to the anastomosis of the left main bronchus. In all the survivors, these abnormalities had completely resolved within 6 weeks of operation (1970). He was able to demonstrate by selective bronchial arteriography that fine regenerating vessels achieve communication with the bronchial arterial channels distal to the anastomosis after 4 weeks. The bronchial circulation is then reestablished through the original arterial channels on the distal side of the bronchial anastomosis. Siegelman et al. also demonstrated the same period to be necessary for reestablishment of the bronchial circulation in canine left lung allotransplantation. At 4–5 weeks postoperatively, they demonstrated a varying degree of filling of vessels beyond the bronchial anastomosis (1977).

The reestablishment of the bronchial circulation has also been studied in experimental left lower lobe autotransplantation (Rabinovich, 1972). Rabinovich demonstrated a diminishing of the hemorrhage and edema in the zone of the bronchial anastomosis 6–8 days after the operation with beginning of cicatrix formation. As early as the first 10 days, he found lymphatics and blood vessels growing across the bronchial anastomosis. In several animals, he could demonstrate reestablishment of the bronchial circulation as early as 3 weeks postoperatively. Routinely, the reestablishment of the bronchial circulation was quite distinct by 4 weeks. He further demonstrated that the reestablishment of the bronchial arterial network develops on the basis of the preexisting bronchial circulation of the transplanted lung.

In addition to reestablishment of the bronchial circulation after lung transplantation, spontaneous reestablishment of the lymphatic vessels has been demonstrated as early as 7–12 days postoperatively (Eraslan et al., 1964).

Injury to the nervous connections also results from hilar division. In a canine autotransplantation model, Esipova et al. (1967) demonstrated postoperative degeneration of medullated nerve fibers in the wall of the donor bronchus between the third and fifth day, whereas the majority of the nonmedullated fibers remained intact, as did the nerve cells in the nerve plexus of the bronchial wall. After 7 days, there was evidence of the ingrowth of regenerating nerve fibers and the gradual restoration of connections with the central nervous system, which was completed between 4 and 17 months postoperatively (Esipova et al., 1967). Transplantation of the lung thus does not disturb the integrity of the nerve cells and their connections within the lung, only those nerve pathways connecting the lung to the central nervous system. Histologically, Esipova et al. observed mucus to be absent from the lumen of bronchial glands as early as 2–8 days postoperatively, with dilated cells showing necrobiosis, differentiating within the first month to flattened regenerating structures.

Brody et al. studied canine mucociliary function after left lung radical hilar stripping with transection and reanastomosis of the left main bronchus (1972). Despite a 50% reduction in bronchial glands and despite histological and physiological evidence of diminished gland function, the submucosal glands continued to secrete mucus, which appeared to be sufficient in quantity to maintain normal particle clearance from the operated lung in the anesthetized dog. Physiological and histological studies showed that the submucosal glands of the operated lungs responded minimally to a dose of pilocarpine sufficient to stimulate excessive mucus production in the unoperated lung. Since pilocarpine acts at the postganglionic level and since ganglionic cells and their postganglionic fibers survive transplantation, the impaired response to pilocarpine is consistent with diminished gland size. Edmunds et al. demonstrated after reimplantation of the canine lung that vagal bronchoconstrictor nerves regenerate rapidly within 3–6 months postoperatively, whereas afferent and sympathetic efferent nerves do not regenerate sufficiently to restore physiological activity (1971). A weakly positive Hering-Brauer reflex and adrenergic reinnervation were demonstrated 45 months after canine lung reimplantation (Lall et al., 1973).

The mechanism by which the viability of the bronchial structures is maintained during the immediate postoperative period has not been conclusively demonstrated. It is assumed that the bronchus is supplied by collaterals between the pulmonary and bronchial circulations.

Injection studies with a radiopaque silicone compound (Microfil) in the pulmonary artery of six dogs and two human cadavers demonstrated by gross inspection and xeroradiography the presence of vessels along the side of the airways, from the hilum of the lung to the second tracheal cartilage (Ladowski et al., 1984).

VII. Experience with Indirect Revascularization

Lima and coworkers demonstrated early revascularization of the donor bronchus when an omental pedicle was wrapped around the bronchial anastomosis following left lung autotransplantation (1982). By the fourth postoperative day, multiple vessels were regenerated, originating from omental vessels communicating with the distal bronchial artery circulation (Figs. 1 and 2). Injection studies were performed postoperatively with silicone rubber (Microfil). Control animals underwent left lung autotransplantation without omentopexy. Aortic injection studies in these animals did not show any reestablishment of the bronchial circulation by the fourth day.

The ability of the omentum to impart new blood supply to ischemic tissue has long been known (Morrison, 1906). In the thorax, the omentum has

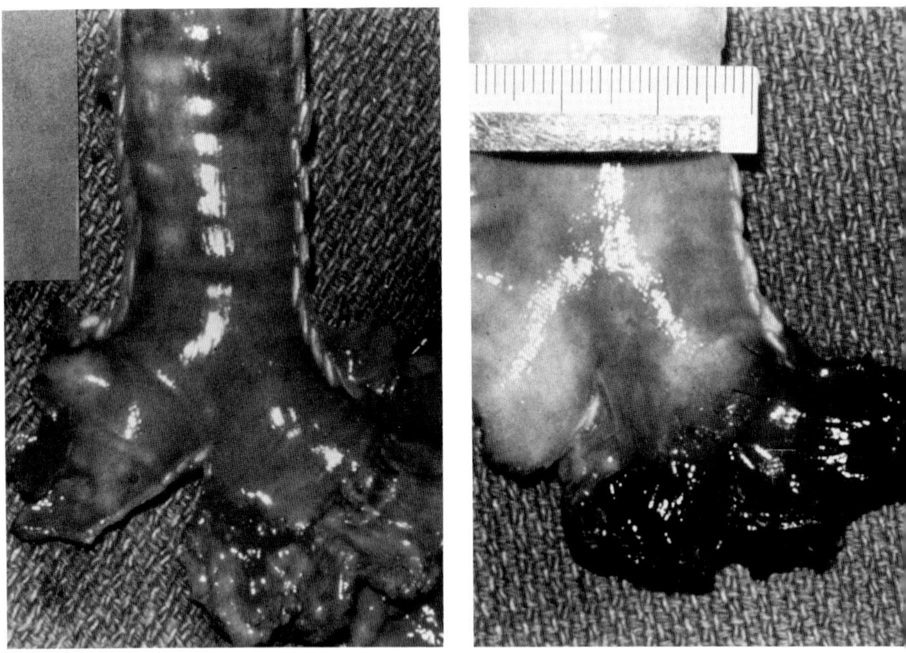

(a) (b)

Figure 3 (a) Bronchial stump reimplantation protected by omentopexy shown 23 days following procedure. The bronchial stump was viable with intact mucosa. (b) Necrosis and gangrene were the consequence in all animals with ischemic bronchial stump reimplanted without protection of the omentum. (From Morgan et al., 1982; used by permission.)

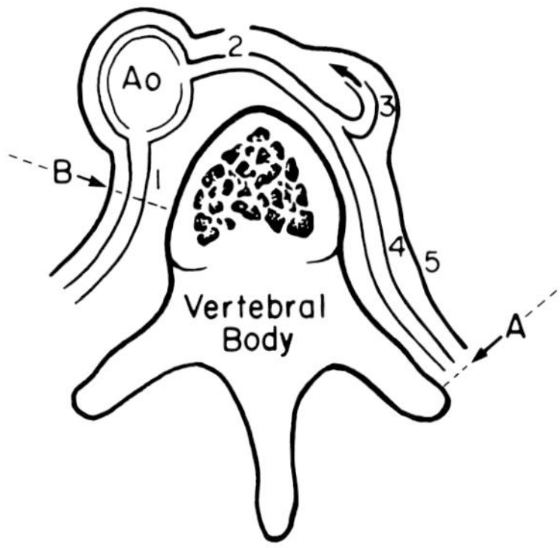

Figure 4 Transverse view showing relationship between intercostal arteries, aorta, vertabral bodies, and pleura. 1 = left intercostal artery; 2 = right intercostal bronchial artery; 3 = right bronchial artery; 4 = right intercostal artery; 5 = pleura; A_O = descending thoracic aorta at the level of T5–6. When the lungs are excised, together with the aorta and esophagus, the parietal pleural incisions are made at points A and B down to the vertebral bodies, and all tissue between these points, anterior to the vertebral bodies is taken with the specimen to avoid injury to the intercostal bronchial artery.

been used to repair bronchopleural fistulas and esophageal perforations or to cover bronchial stumps and to repair chest wall defects (Samson and Pasternach, 1979). Even lymphatic continuity has been established with relief of chronic lymphedema (Goldsmith et al., 1967). Furthermore, the presence of the omentum surrounding the bronchial anstomosis may well prevent major disruption or a bronchovascular fistula from occurring in the event that anastomotic healing is compromised. Morgan et al. evaluated the ability of the omentum to revascularize a totally ischemic bronchial autograft (1982). In five dogs without revascularization, 100% mortality occurred within a week as a result of bronchial necrosis. On the other hand, if a pedicled omental flap was wraped around the totally ischemic bronchial autograft, all animals demonstrated a well-healed graft when put to death at 23 days postoperatively (Fig. 3). Histological examination in animals without the omental pedicle demonstrated graft necrosis, whereas the animals in which the bronchial autograft was wrapped with omentum showed normal architecture at 23 days postoperatively. The beneficial effect of an omental pedicle wrap on bronchial anastomotic healing was also demonstrated following canine autotransplantation (Morgan et al., 1983). All dogs studied were put to death at 23 days. Four of six animals showed a normal bronchial mucosa, one a granular mucosal pattern, and one cyanosis of the bronchial mucosa due to compression of omental vessels by an incisional diaphragmatic hernia (technical failure).

In contrast, 8 of 10 animals in the control group, without an omentopexy, showed varying degrees of mucosal ulceration, necrosis, granulation tissue, or separation at the bronchial anastomosis. The cross-sectional area at the level of the bronchial anastomosis averaged 47% of normal in the control group and 81% of normal in the omentopexy group. The light microscopic findings paralleled the macroscopic findings in all animals.

The benefits of bronchial omentopexy for transplanted lungs was subsequently demonstrated (Dubois et al., 1984). Following left lung allotransplantation, the bronchial anastomosis had a cross-sectional area averaging 74% of normal. Al! animals in this study group received immunosuppressive agents (20 mg/kg/day of cyclosporine, and 1.5 mg/kg/day of imuran, discontinued after 14 days and replaced by 5 mg/day of oral prednisone). The immunosuppressive agents did not appear to interfere with the reestablishment of a collateral bronchial circulation from the omentum. The omentopexy provided an effective and simple method of improving local blood supply to the transplanted donor bronchus.

Immunosuppressive agents may play an important role in wound healing, however, Lima et al. evaluated the effect of immunosuppressive therapy upon the healing of the bronchial anastomosis following canine left lung autotransplantation (1981). The bronchial anastomosis was done just proximal to the bifurcation of the upper and lower lobes. A bolus injection of 125 mg methylprednisolone sodium succinate was given just before surgery. Each animal then received, orally, 2 mg/kg/day of methylprednisolone and 1.5 mg/kg/day of azathioprine until put to death. After sacrifice, the cross-sectional area (CSA) of the bronchial anastomosis was calculated ($CSA = a/2 \times b/2 \times \pi$, where a = sagittal diameter and b = coronal diameter) and expressed as a percentage of the CSA of the normal left bronchus just proximal to the anastomosis. The bronchial anastomosis was divided into strips 1 cm wide, perpendicular to the anastomosis, and the breaking strength of the wound was measured. The combination of methylprednisolone and azathioprine was shown to significantly affect the breaking strength of the bronchial anastomosis. At 23 days, the breaking strengths of the bronchial anastomosis in control animals was nearly twice that in immunosuppressed dogs. Both groups showed a similar incidence of moderate bronchostenosis. No correlation was found between bronchus breaking strength and cross-sectional area among groups. Using the same model to evaluate the effects of cyclosporine, it was demonstrated that immunosuppression with cyclosporine had no adverse effect on bronchial healing (Goldberg et al., 1983). The breaking strength of the anastomotic site in animals treated with cyclosporine was the same as in untreated animals. In subsequent studies, azathioprine and prednisone were evaluated separately and prednisone was found to be solely responsible for the inhibition of healing of the anastomotic wound. As a follow-up study, long-term bronchial anastomotic healing was evaluated in a canine left lung allotransplant model with cyclosporine as the primary immunosuppressive drug (Saunders et al., 1984). Early bronchial revascularization was achieved by wrapping an omental pedicle around the bronchial anastomosis. In these experiments, no significant bronchial complications occurred and late bronchostenosis was not seen in any of the six dogs surviving over 100 days. Documented rejection did not prejudice bronchial healing or result in bronchostenosis. Cyclosporine has little effect on tissue healing and, unlike steroids, does not alter the ultrastructural pattern of collagen at healing sites.

A review of the world experience with human lung transplantation revealed that until 1983 approximately 46 lung or lobe transplantations were attempted, with no long-term success and with only 1 patient discharged alive from the hospital. Of these 46 patients, only 13 lived more than 2 weeks, the majority dying in the third week of disruption of bronchial anastomosis. Only one recipient in this series underwent direct revascularization. This involved a left lung transplant with a subsequent right lung transplantation without revascularization in the same patient. This recipient died of right-sided bronchial disruption.

Since 1983, we have utilized an omental pedicle to protect and revascularize the donor bronchus in human single-lung transplantation. In the initial 21 single-lung transplants no fatality was caused by airway complications, although 2 patients developed late complications due to donor airway ischemia. We attribute our success to three factors: the use of omentopexy to provide early revascularization to the donor airway; the availability of cyclosporine as an immunosuppressive agent; and better recipient selection, with exclusion of steroid-dependent patients. Our first successful double-lung transplant was successfully performed in 1986, with a technique that utilized a tracheal anastomosis to attach the two lungs en bloc. Despite the use of an omental pedicle wrapped around the tracheal anastomosis, a significant number of airway complications have occurred with the use of this procedure (Patterson et al., 1990). We have recently modified the procedure, utilizing separate right and left lung implantation and bilateral bronchial anastomoses to eliminate the complications associated with the tracheal anastomosis.

VIII. Experience with Direct Revascularization of the Bronchial Circulation in Experimental Animals

Metras (1950) was the first to perform canine lung allotransplantation. He chose the left lung because of the more convenient bronchial artery connections that arise from one of the first four right intercostal arteries in dogs. The bronchial artery with a button of aorta containing its origin was excised with the donor lung and anastomosed to the subclavian artery (Metras, 1950). Nettleblad subsequently utilized direct bronchial artery revascularization in a pilot study in left lower lobe canine allotransplantation using a segment of aorta containing the bronchial artery. The segment of donor aorta was closed at either end and opened ventrally to anastomose side-to-side to the recipient's descending thoracic aorta (Nettleblad et al., 1964). This technique was also utilized successfully in canine whole-lung transplantation. In left lower lobe lung transplantation with direct revascularization of the bronchial artery, the patency of the vessels was documented by postmortem injection studies. This technique was abandoned in further experiments for several reasons: the role of the bronchial artery systemic supply in the maintenance of nutrition of lung parenchyma following lung transplantation was considered uncertain; the technique of using a donor segment of aorta increased the operative time; and the aortic-aortic anastomosis may introduce the hazard of bleeding in the recipient. Huggins demonstrated in left lower lobe canine autotransplantation that if the bronchus was divided within 1 cm of the parenchyma, no necrosis occurred, but that if the bronchus was divided at a distance of 1.5–2 cm from the parenchyma, many animals died from bronchial necrosis (1959).

Mills et al. undertook a controlled study of the effects of reconstitution of the bronchial arterial supply to the allotransplanted left lung in a canine model (1970). The bronchial artery supply to the donor left mainstem bronchus was followed proximally to its origin from an intercostal artery or from the aorta. Unrelated branches from the intercostal artery were ligated, and a button of aorta containing its origin was preserved. The left mainstem bronchus was transected 1 cm proximal to the origin of the upper lobe bronchus of the donor lung. After pulmonary circulation and ventilation were reestablished in the allograft, the bronchial circulation was restored by anastomosis of the button of donor aorta to the recipient's descending aorta. A control group underwent an identical lung allotransplantation without reconstitution of the bronchial circulation. Immunosuppression in both groups consisted of 10 mg/kg of daily Imuran, tapered to 4 mg/kg/day over the first 5 days. No anti-lymphocyte globulin or steroids were used. There was an 82–20% reduction in bronchial complication (Table 4). The bronchial complications observed were ulceration, disruption, and stenosis. Mills observed that no pneumonia occurred in transplanted animals without bronchial ulceration and that those animals with bronchial ulceration developed pneumonia in 50% of cases, probably due to desquamation of bronchial epithelium and impaired mucus clearance. This suggested that immediate reestablishment of bronchial circulation may decrease the incidence of pneumonia in the transplanted lung as well as the incidence of bronchial complications. Morales-Zuniga (1972) studied the effect of immediate reestablishment of the bronchial circulation in a

Table 4 Controlled Studies of the Incidence of Bronchial Complications After Canine Lung Transplantation With and Without Preservation of Bronchial Arteries

Reference	Operation	Number	Bronchial complications (%)
Mills et al. (1970)	Left lung allotransplantation		
	Control group	11	82
	Bronchial artery revascularization	10	20
Morales-Zuniga (1972)	Left lung autotransplantation		
	Control group	19	84
	Bronchial artery revascularization	11	9

Source: After Bartter et al. (1988).

canine left lung reimplantation model (Table 4). The left main bronchus was divided as proximal as possible to the takeoff of the left upper lobe. In preserving the bronchial arteries, a segment of aorta containing the orifice of the intercostal artery giving rise to the left bronchial artery was preserved. After reimplantation of the left lung and the reestablishment of the pulmonary circulation and of ventilation, the donor aortic segment was reanastomosed to the recipient aorta. Several studies of the anatomy of the bronchial arteries in dogs demonstrated the consistent finding that canine bronchial arteries arise from one of the first four right intercostal arteries (Notkovich, 1957). Both Mills et al. (1970) and Morales-Zuniga (1972) point to the fact that preparing a donor lung for left canine transplantation can incorporate an aortic button or segment that contains the bronchial arteries without great technical difficulty. Reestablishment of bronchial circulation after lung transplantation resulted in a significantly lower bronchial complication rate.

The left lung of a dog was transplanted into the right hemithorax in a canine model to facilitate immediate reconstruction of bronchial artery flow (Veith et al., 1978). In this canine model, the donor left lung was placed in the recipient's right hemithorax in an inverted position with the apex of the lung directed caudally. The aortic button containing the origin of the intercostal artery giving rise to the bronchial arteries was reanastomosed to the lateral wall of the recipient's right brachycephalic artery. In vivo and postmortem angiograms demonstrated the patency of the bronchial arterial system of the allotransplanted lung with effective perfusion from the recipient's brachycephalic artery. The experiments were performed with the assumption that preservation of a right bronchial artery in humans would be very difficult or impossible. In fact, in the dog model, the left bronchial artery arises from the right intercostal arteries, whereas in humans the left bronchial arteries only sporadically arise from the right intercostal arteries: specifically, the right bronchial artery in humans arises from the first right intercostobronchial artery in over 80% of cases, as discussed before (pp. 726–730).

Pinsker et al. demonstrated excellent bronchial healing in six dogs in which bronchial transection and reanastomosis at the level of the carina was performed while preserving the bronchial artery intact (1980). In contrast, animals who underwent the same procedure without saving the bronchial artery demonstrated poor healing with mucosal ulceration and exposed necrotic cartilage. In an additional group, a microsurgical technique was used to reanastomose the donor bronchial artery to a recipient's intercostal artery with similar excellent bronchial anastomotic healing. The feasibility of immediate revascularization of the bronchial circulation in left lower lobe transplantation has also been demonstrated by Rabinovich (1972), who proved the patency of the bronchial arteries with postmortem contrast x-ray studies. Thus, when evaluating bronchial ischemia as an isolated factor in the healing of a bronchial anastomosis, there seems no doubt that preservation or restoration of bronchial artery circulation results in excellent bronchial healing.

Based upon a number of laboratory studies, the time required for spontaneous reestablishment of the bronchial circulation is 2–4 weeks from the time of transplantation, whereas the time required for indirect reestablishment of the bronchial circulation with an omental pedicled flap wrapped around the bronchial anastomosis is about 4 days. In the case of the immediate reestablishment of the bronchial circulation by reanastomosing the bronchial arteries at the time of transplantation, the early bronchial ischemia is practically eliminated and the bronchial healing is not compromised by the ischemia factor.

IX. Clinical Experience with Direct Revascularization of the Bronchial Arteries

Despite consistent reports of success with immediate restoration of the bronchial circulation in experimental lung transplantation, only a few attempts have been made in human lung transplantation to restore the bronchial circulation at the time of transplantation. The apparent reasons for ignoring the systemic blood supply to the lung in lung transplantation may be laboratory reports regarding spontaneous restoration of the bronchial circulation, the extent of the assumed pulmonary circulation to bronchial artery collaterals, the presumed surgical difficulty and time delay required, concern about consistency in bronchial artery anatomic patterns, and uncertainty regarding the real function and importance of the bronchial arteries. Many of these concerns still apply to human lung transplantation. The first and only report of direct revascularization was of that performed in a left lung allograft using a donor aortic button containing the orifice of the bronchial artery and attaching it to the recipient's descending thoracic aorta (Haglin et al., 1973). During the same procedure a right pneumonectomy was performed. After 4 h, the patient's lung function deteriorated and a right lung transplant was performed using the right lung from the same donor without revascularization of the bronchial circulation. At the time of death, 10 days postoperatively, a well-healed left bronchus was found, whereas the right bronchial anastomotic site showed necrosis and disruption. It may be, however, that the prolonged ischemic time of the right lung influenced the bronchial healing on the right side. Nevertheless, it was significant that this recipient showed normal healing of the left bronchial anastomotic site.

X. Summary

In recent years, the field of lung transplantation has rapidly developed. Indications have broadened, techniques have been refined, and improvements made in the diagnosis and treatment of rejection, in lung preservation, and in postoperative care. Concomitant with these advances, the success rate of lung transplantation has significantly improved, and airway complications following transplantation have been reduced. In a recent review of 53 patients undergoing single or bilateral lung transplants, we observed a 14% incidence of bronchial complications. The mortality rate due to bronchial complications was 2%.

Despite improved results, however, the bronchial anastomosis continues to be a matter of real concern. There is no doubt that a safe, simple method for direct restoration of bronchial circulation at the time of transplantation would be an important advance. Such an approach may assume greater significance as the period of pulmonary preservation is extended. Two methods of direct bronchial revascularization have recently been employed with success. One involves preservation of a segment of aorta containing the origin of the bronchial arteries, with attachment of this aortic segment to the recipient aorta or subclavian artery. The second approach is an extension of the one originally demonstrated by Metras and involves preservation of the bronchial artery and an aortic button at its origin, with use of a vein graft between the recipient aorta and the origin of the donor bronchial artery. While awaiting a clinically applicable method for direct restoration of bronchial circulation, a better understanding of factors that effect collateral circulation between the bronchial and pulmonary arterial systems may further reduce posttransplant complications associated with airway ischemia.

References

Blank, N., Lower, R., and Adams, D. F. (1966). Bronchial dynamics and the reconstitution of bronchial artery supply in the autotransplanted lung. *Invest. Radiol.* **1**:363–370.

Botenga, A. S. J. (1970). Selective bronchial and intercostal arteriography. Baltimore, Williams & Wilkins, pp. 9–22.

Boyden, E. A. (1970). The developing bronchial arteries in a fetus of the twelfth week. *Am. J. Anat.* **129**:357–368.

Brody, J. S., Klempfner, G., Staum, M. M., Vidyasagar, D., Kuhl, D. E., and Waldhausen, J. A. (1972). Mucociliary clearance after lung denervation and bronchial transection. *J. Appl. Physiol.* **32**:160–164.

Cauldwell, E. W., Siekert, R. G., Lininger, R. E., and Anson, B. J. (1948). The bronchial arteries. An anatomic study of 150 human cadavers. *Surg. Gynecol. Obstet.* **86**:395–412.

Cooper, J. D. and the Toronto Lung Transplant Group. (1986). Unilateral lung transplantation for pulmonary fibrosis. *N. Engl. J. Med.* **314**:1140–1145.

Cudkowicz, L., and Armstrong, J. B. (1951). Observations on the normal anatomy of the bronchial arteries. *Thorax* **6**:343–358.

Deffebach, M. E., Charan, N. B., Lakshminarayan, S., and Butler, J. (1987). The bronchial circulation. Small, but a vital attribute of the lung. *Am. Rev. Respir. Dis.* **135**:463–481.

Demikhov, M. V. (1960). Experimental transplantation of vital organs. Moscow, Medgiz, pp. 129–135.

Derom, F., Barbier, F., Ringoir, S., Rolly, G., Berzenyi, G., Vermeire, P., and Vrints, L. (1971). Ten-month survival after lung homotransplantation in man. *J. Thorac. Cardiovasc. Surg.* **61**:835–846.

Dubois, P., Choiniere, L., and Cooper, J. D. (1984). Bronchial omentopexy in canine lung allotransplantation. *Ann. Thorac. Surg.* **38**:211–214.

Duvoisin, G. E., Fowler, W. S., Payne, W. S., and Ellis, F. H., Jr. (1964). Reimplantation of the dog lung with survival after contralateral pneumonectomy. *Surg. Forum* **15**:173–175.

Edmunds, L. H., Jr., Graf, P. D., and Nadel, J. A. (1971). Reinnervation of the reimplanted canine lung. *J. Appl. Physiol.* **31**:722–727.

Ellis, F. H., Grindlay, J. H., and Edwards, J. E. (1951). The bronchial arteries. I. Experimental occlusion. *Surgery* **30**:810–816.

Eraslan, S., Turner, M. D., and Hardy, J. D. (1964). Lymphatic regeneration following lung reimplantation in dogs. *Surgery* **56**:970–973.

Esipova, I. K., Denisov-Nikol'skii, Y. I., Kaufman, O. Y., and Rabinovich, Y. Y. (1967). Histological investigation of the experimentally autotransplanted lung. *Bull. Exp. Biol. Med.* **3**:320–323.

Goldberg, M., Lima, O., Morgan, E., Ayabe, H. A., Luk, S., Ferdman, A., Peters, W. J., and Cooper, J. D. (1983). A comparison between cyclosporin A and methylprednisolone plus azathioprine on bronchial healing following canine lung autotransplantation. *J. Thorac. Cardiovasc. Surg.* **85**:821–826.

Goldsmith, H. S., Santos de Los, R., and Beattie, E. J. (1967). Relief of chronic lymphedema by omental transposition. *Ann. Surg.* **166**:573–585.

Griffith, B. P., Hardesty, R. L., Trents, A., Paradis, I. L., Duqueznoy, R. J., Zeevi, A., Dauber, J. H., Dummer, J. S., Thompson, M. A., Gryzan, S., and Bahnson, H. T. (1987). Heart lung transplantation: Lessons learned and future hopes. *Ann. Thorac. Surg.* **43**:6–16.

Haglin, J. J., Ruiz, E., Baker, R. C., and Anderson, W. R. (1973). Histologic studies of human lung allotransplantation. In *Morphology in Lung Transplantation.* Edited by C. R. H. Wildervuur. Basel, S. Karger, pp. 13–22.

Hardy, J. D., Webb, W. R., Dalton, M. L., Jr., and Walker, G. R., Jr. (1963). Lung homotransplantation. in man: Report of the initial case. *JAMA* **186**:1065–1074.

Huggins, C. E. (1959). Reimplantation of lobes of the lung. An experimental technique. *Lancet* **2**:1059–1062.

Kasai, T., and Chiba, S. (1979). Macroscopic anatomy of the bronchial arteries. *Anat. Anz.* **145**:166–181.

Ladowski, J. S., Hardesty, R. L., and Griffith, B. P. (1984). The pulmonary artery blood supply to the supracarinal trachea. *Heart Transplant.* **4**:40–42.

Lall, A., Graf, P. D., Nadel, J. A., and Edmunds, L. H., Jr. (1973). Adrenergic reinnervation of the reimplanted dog lung. *J. Appl. Physiol.* **35**:439–442.

Liebow, A. A. (1965). Patterns of origin and distribution of the major bronchial arteries in man. *Am. J. Anat.* **117**:19–32.

Lima, O., Cooper, J. D., Peters, W. J., Ayabe, H., Townsend, E., Luk, S. C., and Goldberg, M. (1981). Effects of methylprednisolone and azathioprine on bronchial healing following lung autotransplantation. *J. Thorac. Cardiovasc. Surg.* **82**:211–215.

Lima, O., Goldberg, M., Peters, W. J., Ayabe, H., Townsend, E., and Cooper, J. D. (1982). Bronchial omentopexy in canine lung transplantation. *J. Thorac. Cardiovasc. Surg.* **83**:418–421.

Marchand, P., Gilroy, J. C., and Wilson, V. H. (1950). An anatomical study of the bronchial vascular system and its variations in disease. *Thorax* **5**:207–221.

Metras, M. H. (1950). Note preliminaire sur la greffe totale du poumon chez le Chien. C. R. Acad. Sci. III **231**:1176–1177.

Miller, W. S. (1925). The vascular supply of the bronchial tree. *Am. Rev. Tuberc.* **12**:87–93.

Mills, N. L., Boyd, A. D., and Gheranpong, C. (1970). The significance of bronchial circulation in lung transplantation. *J. Thorac. Cardiovasc. Surg.* **60**:866–874.

Morales-Zuniga, A. (1972). The importance of bronchial artery circulation in lung transplantation. Ph.D. Thesis, University of Minnesota.

Morgan, E., Lima, O., Goldberg, M., Ferdman, A., Luk, S. K., and Cooper, J. D. (1982). Successful revascularization of totally ischemic bronchial autografts with omental pedicle flaps in dogs. *J. Thorac. Cardiovasc. Surg.* **84**:204–210.

Morgan, E., Lima, O., Goldberg, M., Ayabe, H., Ferdman, A., and Cooper, J. D. (1983). Improved bronchial healing in canine left lung reimplantation using omental pedicle wrap. *J. Thorac. Cardiovasc. Surg.* **85**:134–139.

Morrison, R. (1906). Remarks on sonic functions of the omentum. *Br. Med. J.* **1**:76.

Nakamura, N. (1924). Zur anatomie der bronchial arterien. *Anat. Anz.* **58**:508–517.

Nathan, H., Orda, R., and Barkay, M. (1970). The right bronchial artery. *Thorax* **25**:328–333.

Nettleblad, S. C., Soroff, H. S., Sachs, B. F., Sharma, A. N., Bellas, A. E., Sherman, J., Harrison, H. N., and Deterling, R. A., Jr. (1964). Experimental studies of the response to homotransplantation of pulmonary tissues. *Ann. N. Y. Acad. Sci.* 689–709.

Neveux, J. Y., Bignon, J., Oancea, T., Rioux, C., and Mathey, J. (1968). Devenir de la circulation arterielle bronchique apres autotransplantation pulmonaire. *Ann. Chir. Thor. Car.* **7**:559–562.

Notkovich, H. (1957). The anatomy of the bronchial arteries of the dog. *J. Thorac. Surg.* **33**:243–253.

Patterson, G. A., Cooper, J. D., Goldman, B., Weisel, R. D., Pearson, F. G., Waters, P. F., Todd, T. R., Scully, H., Goldberg, M., Ginsberg, R. J., and Department of Surgery, University of Toronto. (1988). Technique of successful clinical double-lung transplantation. *Ann. Thorac. Surg.* **45**(6):626–633.

Patterson, G. A., Todd, T. R. J., Cooper, J. D., Pearson, F. G., Winton, T. L., Maurer, J., and Toronto Lung Transplant Group. (1990). Airway complications following double lung transplantation. *J. Thorac. Cardiovasc. Surg.* **99**(1):14–21.

Pearson, F. G., Goldberg, M., Stone, R. M., and Colapinto, R. F. (1970). Bronchial arterial circulation restored after reimplantation of canine lung. *Can. J. Surg.* **13**:243–250.

Pinsker, K. L., Koerner, S. K., Kamholz, S. L., Hagstrom, J. W. C., and Veith, F. J. (1979). Effect of donor bronchial length on healing. *J. Thorac. Cardiovasc. Surg.* **77**:669–673.

Pinsker, K. L., Montefusco, C., Kamholz, S. L., Hagstrom, J. W. C., Gliedman, M. L., and Veith, F. J. (1980). Improved bronchial anastomotic healing secondary to maintenance of restoration of bronchial arterial circulation by microsurgical techniques. *Surg. Forum* **31**:230–232.

Pump, K. K. (1963). The bronchial arteries and their anastomoses in the human lung. *Dis. Chest* **43**:245–255.

Pump, K. K. (1972). Distribution of bronchial arteries in the human lung. *Chest* **62**:447–451.

Rabinovich, J. J. (1972). Reestablishment of bronchial arteries after experimental lung lobe autotransplantation. *J. Thorac. Cardiovasc. Surg.* **64**:119–126.

Samson, R., and Pasternach, B. M. (1979). Current status of surgery of the omentum. *Surg. Gynecol. Obstet.* **149**:437.

Saunders, N. R., Egan, T. M., Chamberlain, D., and Cooper, J. D. (1984). Cyclosporine and bronchial healing in canine lung transplantation. *J. Thorac. Cardiovasc. Surg.* **88**:993–999.

Schreinemakers, J. H. J., Weder, W., Miyoshi, S., Harper, B. D., Shimokawa, S., Egan, T. M., McKnight, R., and Cooper, J. D. (1990). Direct revascularization of bronchial arteries for lung transplantation: An anatomic study. *Ann. Thorac. Surg.* **49**:44–54.

Siegelman, S. S., Hagstrom, J. W. C., Koerner, S. K., and Veith, F. J. (1977). Restauration of bronchial artery circulation after canine lung allotransplantation. *J. Thorac. Cardiovasc. Surg.* **73**:792–795.

Staudacher, V. E., Bellinazzo, P., and Pulin, A. (1950). Primary results in attempts at autoplastic reimplants and homoplastic transplants of pulmonary lobes. *Chir. Ital.* **5**:223.

Stone, R. M., Ginsberg, R. J., Colapinto, R. F., and Pearson, F. G. (1966). Bronchial artery regeneration after radical hilar stripping. *Surg. Forum* **17**:109–110.

Veith, F. J., and Richards, K. (1970). Improved technic for canine lung transplantation. *Ann. Surg.* **171**:553–558.

Veith, F. J., Torres, M., Colon, I., Pinsker, K., Koerner, S. K., Crane, R., and Paulson, D. (1978). Transplantation of the left lung into the right hemithorax to facilitate immediate reconstruction of bronchial artery flow. *J. Thorac. Cardiovasc. Surg.* **75**:141–146.

Verloop, M. C. (1948). The arteriae bronchiales and their anastomoses with the arteria pulmonalis in the human lung; a micro-anatomical study. *Acta. Anat. (Basel)* **5**:171–205.

Viamonte, M., Parks, R. E., and Smock, W. M., III. (1965). Guided catheterization of the bronchial arteries. I. Technical considerations. *Radiology* **85**:205–230.

AUTHOR INDEX

Italic numbers give the page on which the complete reference is listed.

C

H

K

L

N

O

Q

R

S

T

W

SUBJECT INDEX

A

B

C

F

G

N

O

P

U

V

W

X